Clinical Education: An Anthology Vol 2

American Physical Therapy Association
1111 North Fairfax Street
Alexandria, Virginia 22314-1488

ISBN # 1-887759-08-5

For more information about this and other APTA publications, contact the American Physical Therapy Association, 1111 North Fairfax Street, Alexandria, VA 22314-1488. [Publication No. E-30]

FOREWORD

An Era of Change in Clinical Education

We are pleased to present the second volume in our anthology series on clinical education. This volume is a collection of 81 articles representing the current state of knowledge about clinical education. Half of these articles were selected from the physical therapy literature since 1992, augmenting the first volume of the series. The remaining literature was obtained from other professional disciplines to further support the body of literature found in physical therapy clinical education and to affirm some of the critical questions being posed by other professional disciplines related to clinical education.

This second volume is organized similarly to the first volume in that it refers to the five dimensions addressed by the American Physical Therapy Association's Plans for Clinical Education (1989 to 1991, 1992 to 1994) with the addition of a new content area entitled "Student Issues in Clinical Education." As an added feature, this volume has an alphabetical listing of all articles by author, separated by content area. Volumes 1 and 2 together provide an excellent, comprehensive resource for all individuals involved with clinical education, whether academically or clinically based. This resource can be used to enhance clinical faculty training, clinical site development, clinical education research, professional curricular organization and design, students' knowledge about clinical education and clinical teaching, and our understanding of how students make career decisions.

In the past 3 years, the physical therapy literature has continued to grow significantly in these six dimensions, especially as related to issues of quality, productivity, outcomes, and measuring student competence in clinical education. Most remarkable since the first volume, however, is the advancement of knowledge in the area of design of clinical education using collaborative and cooperative learning approaches in response to a changing practice and health care environment. It would appear that the physical therapy profession, along with other professional disciplines, has acknowledged through investigative studies, the need to better understand diverse aspects of clinical education and its relationship to developing competent practitioners.

As the profession has sought answers to simple and complex questions in clinical education and to develop theories about student learning in the practice environment, alternative methods for exploring these issues have emerged. In the past 3 years, we have continued to make tremendous strides in physical therapy clinical education research in the United States and abroad, as reflected by this anthology. Likewise, this collection clearly indicates that many other disciplines, such as medicine, nursing, dentistry, occupational therapy, and speech therapy, are exploring similar issues and questions within their respective disciplines. Perhaps it is time to consider interdisciplinary and multidisciplinary collaborative studies to investigative some of the most challenging questions in clinical education that confront all health disciplines in this era of pervasive environmental changes in both health care and higher education. Given the complexity of some questions, it may require the knowledge and expertise of individuals from many disciplines to begin to arrive at answers that will benefit us all.

We hope that this second volume will serve as an inspiration and a source of pride for everyone involved with clinical education. Through critical and scholarly inquiry, exciting new opportunities for discovery await us only if we are open and willing to accept and respond to these challenges and to learn from our past failures and successes.

Jody Shapiro Gandy, PhD, PT
Director of Clinical Education
American Physical Therapy Association

Table of Contents

Clinical Environment and Resources

Design of Clinical Education

Evaluation and Research

Academic Resources

Student Issues in Clinical Education

CLINICAL
FACULTY

Academic Coordinator of Clinical Education

The Academic Coordinator of Clinical Education: Career Issues

Norene Clouten, EdD, PT

ABSTRACT: This study researched the career of the academic coordinator of clinical education (ACCE). Two investigator-developed questionnaires were mailed to current ACCEs and former ACCEs who had held the position within the previous 10 years. One hundred seven (91%) of the ACCE questionnaires and 63 (73%) of the former ACCE questionnaires were returned. The majority of ACCEs first considered the position when it was vacant or when desiring a job change. They came without formal preparation for the position and without an accurate perception of the role and responsibilities of the ACCE. One half of the ACCEs were very new or were planning to leave the position. Issues to be addressed in academic institutions include the socialization of physical therapy faculty to academia, clarification of the position and responsibilities of the ACCE, preparation of candidates for the ACCE position, and recognition of the ACCE as a full member of the academic community.

INTRODUCTION

In physical therapy education, the faculty member primarily responsible for the clinical education portion of the curriculum is the academic coordinator of clinical education (ACCE). Several authors have described the multiple roles and responsibilities of the ACCE.

Moore and Perry[1] described clinical education in physical therapy in 1976. They found that physical therapists were assuming the position and responsibility of ACCEs with little knowledge of the job. Their report included recommendations for the preparation and function of ACCEs. Booth[2] surveyed current and former ACCEs and reported that ACCEs were appointed with little background preparation and stayed a median of 3 years in the position. Myers[3] and Strickler[4] provided updates on the characteristics, status, and activities of ACCEs and of clinical education.

Dr Clouten is Associate Professor and Academic Coordinator of Clinical Education, Department of Physical Therapy, Andrews University, Berrien Springs, MI 49104.

Philips. McPhail. and Roemer[5] described the roles and functions of ACCEs. and Harris. Fogel, and Blacconiere[6] investigated job satisfaction among ACCEs. These authors included demographic characteristics of the ACCE. A focused study on the counseling function of ACCEs was reported by Kondela-Cebulski.[7]

The predicament of the ACCE as a misfit in academe was described by Deusinger and Rose[8] and by Strickler.[4,9] A recent compilation by Gandy[10] provided a model position description for the ACCE.

Related literature discusses career issues of college faculty and of physical therapy faculty. A national survey of college faculty conducted by the Carnegie Foundation for the Advancement of Teaching[11,12] found one fourth of the faculty dissatisfied with their profession. One half said they would seriously consider another academic job if one were offered.

Foegelle[13] compared the career planning of faculty members from different programs in schools of allied health. One third of the allied health faculty were planning a change in employment, primarily because of salary and work duties and responsibilities. The majority expected to remain in higher education, and many expected to become administrators. Radtka[14] examined voluntary job turnover of physical therapy faculty. The faculty turnover ranged from 8% to 11%. The majority of the faculty who left academia accepted clinical jobs and cited low salary as their reason for leaving.

Beyond these references, little has been published on the functions, career, or job satisfaction of the ACCE. This descriptive study focused on the career of the ACCE, the factors that attract individuals to the career of ACCE, and factors that influence them to either leave or remain in the position of ACCE. The specific questions addressed were as follows:

1. What are the personal characteristics and occupational status of current ACCEs and of former ACCEs?
2. In what ways are the ACCEs prepared for a career as an ACCE?

3. What are the major attractions for these individuals to become ACCEs?
4. What are the most and least attractive features of the ACCE position?
5. What are the future career plans of ACCEs?
6. What influenced former ACCEs to leave the position, and what has been their occupation after leaving?

METHOD

Subjects

The study population consisted of the 118 current (1990–1991) ACCEs from all American Physical Therapy Association accredited programs offering entry-level education for physical therapists, and former ACCEs who had held the ACCE position within the previous 10 years. Former ACCEs were identified from the responses of current ACCEs and from networking among physical therapists.

Procedure

Data were collected through two investigator-developed questionnaires, one for current ACCEs and another for former ACCEs. Both questionnaires contained sections dealing with biodemographic data and occupational status, preparation for a career as an ACCE, major attractions to the ACCE position, most and least attractive features of the ACCE position, and future career plans.

The ACCE Questionnaire and the Former ACCE Questionnaire were similar except for the last section, where current ACCEs were asked whether they were considering a job change and former ACCEs were asked about the circumstances surrounding their decision to leave. Items required a short factual answer, selection of a choice from a series of options or Likert-type statements, or written answers to open-ended questions. Each questionnaire also provided space for narrative comments. The questionnaires passed through many iterations, were pretested, and were reviewed by a panel of experts before the final printing.

A questionnaire packet was sent to the ACCE at each of the 118 entry-level programs. The packet contained a cover letter addressed to each ACCE by name, the ACCE Questionnaire booklet, a self-addressed and stamped return envelope, and a pen as an incentive. A follow-up letter was mailed to nonrespondents after 2 to 3 weeks, when replies had dwindled.

A similar packet containing the Former ACCE Questionnaire was mailed to each of the 86 former ACCEs identified..This mailing was completed 6 weeks after the distribution of the ACCE Questionnaire.

Interviews were held with current and former ACCEs, academic administrators, and other faculty members to complement or triangulate the data from the questionnaires. Some interviews were held in person at professional meetings, and others were telephone conversations. Interviews continued until the information received was repetitive.

Quantitative and narrative responses were classified, coded, and entered into the computer for analysis. The SPSS/PC+ program* was used for data analyses. Ranges, means, standard deviations, and percentages were calculated where appropriate.

RESULTS

One hundred seven (91%) of the ACCE Questionnaires and 63 (73%) of the Former ACCE Questionnaires were returned. More than three fourths of the respondents included additional narrative comments written on, or attached to, the questionnaires. The results are presented below in sections according to the specific questions, with numerical results preceding narrative results. Large differences between current and former ACCEs were not evident on most of the descriptive items. Current ACCE data are reported, and differences in responses from former ACCEs are noted.

Personal Characteristics and Occupational Status

Personal characteristics. Biodemographic information is presented in Table 1. Most of the ACCEs were female and between 30 and 44 years of age. The current ACCEs were older than the former ACCEs when they were in the same position. Slightly more than one half of the ACCEs reported that they were married.

The opinion that ACCEs were junior members of the faculty (both young and at the beginning of an academic career) occurred frequently in comments written on the questionnaires and interviews. Another theme that persisted in narrative data was that the ACCE is more free to fulfill the responsibilities of the position if single. Married ACCEs described

*SPSS Inc, 444 N Michigan Ave, Chicago, IL 60611.

Table 1

Personal Characteristics: Current and Former Academic Coordinators of Clinical Education (ACCEs) (N=170)

Characteristic	Current ACCE (%)	Former ACCE (%)
Age (yr)		
<30	7	18
30-34	24	33
35-39	27	27
40-44	20	13
45-59	6	6
60+	15	4
Women	81	87
Married	52	57

Table 2

Occupational Status of Current and Former Academic Coordinators of Clinical Education (ACCEs) (N=170)

Variable	Current ACCE	Former ACCE
Time as ACCE (yr) (mean ± SD)	4.6 ± 5.4	5.2 ± 3.3
Academic rank (%)		
Lecturer	5	2
Instructor	34	30
Assistant professor	38	46
Associate professor	12	10
Professor	3	3
Other	8	9
Tenure status (%)		
Tenure available at institution	90	86
Tenured	15	18
Not tenured, on tenure track	19	30
Not tenured, not on tenure track	56	47
No response	10	5
Appointment (%)		
Faculty	79	69
Administrative	8	8
Combined	13	23
Share ACCE position (%)	24	16
ACCE position full-time (%)	73	73
Program degree award (%)		
Certificate	0	5
Baccalaureate	57	84
Master's	30	3
Transition	13	8

adjustments that they and their spouse were able (or unable) to make.

Occupational status. Table 2 presents occupational status information. Current ACCEs had held the position for a mean of 4.6 years, with a range from 1 month to 27 years. Twenty-four current ACCEs had held the job for less than 1 year, most of these for less than 6 months.

While ACCEs worked in a variety of academic environments, the majority were untenured instructors or assistant professors with faculty appointments. There were some administrative appointments, and others described combinations of academic, administrative, and professional appointments.

Of the current ACCEs, 15% had earned tenure, and another 19% were on a tenure track. The ACCEs who had tenure status had been in the ACCE position for a mean of 11 years, while the ACCEs who were on a tenure track had been in the position for a mean of 3.7 years. Thirty percent of the former ACCEs had been on a tenure track but had failed to receive tenure or had left the position prior to a tenure decision.

There was considerable variation in appreciation for the nontenure track position. Some ACCEs claimed that it was a distinct advantage, often because they were relieved of the pressure for doctoral education and the traditional requirements for tenure, while others believed that the nontenure track put them in the position of second-class faculty without the respect, privileges, security, and responsibilities of tenured faculty.

More current than former ACCEs shared the position with another ACCE, either by one acting as an assistant ACCE or by sharing the position as co-ACCEs. Most of the former ACCEs had been associated with baccalaureate-degree programs. Current ACCEs were more likely to be associated with master's-degree or transitioning programs.

The results reported in Table 3 indicate that the majority of ACCEs are away from home overnight several times a year for work-related causes. Most ACCEs visit distant clinical sites and students, but others place students within commuting distance of the academic institution and do not visit more distant sites.

The ACCEs perceive that tenure is more difficult for them to achieve than for other physical therapy faculty. They also perceive that they work longer hours, enjoy their work more, experience more stress in their work, and have more freedom than other physical therapy faculty.

Career Preparation

Few ACCEs received formal preparation for the position, but they came with relevant work, educational, and life experiences.

Work experience. All respondents reported clinical experience as a physical therapist prior to accepting the position. Current ACCEs had a mean of 9½ years and former ACCEs of 7½ years in clinical practice. One half (53%) reported some previous teaching experience, and one half (52%) had at some time been a center coordinator of clinical education (CCCE). Twelve percent reported previous experience as an ACCE.

Of the current ACCEs, almost two thirds (62%) listed their previous occupation as a physical therapist in the clinical setting. One third (33%) listed physical therapy faculty, including some who were an ACCE at another institution. Others were graduate students or administrators in settings other than physical therapy. By comparison, more of the former ACCEs were clinicians (79%) and less (18%) were faculty.

The previous occupational level varied from that of staff to director and from instructor to professor. Immediately before accepting the ACCE position, almost one third (31%) of current ACCEs were at the director or assistant-director level, primarily in clinical departments.

Formal education. Of the 107 current ACCEs responding to this questionnaire,

15% held a baccalaureate degree, 76% held a master's degree, and 9% held a doctorate. Of current ACCEs at the baccalaureate level, one half were continuing their education in a master's-degree program. Nine ACCEs currently holding a master's degree were involved in a doctoral program.

At the master's degree level, areas of study varied widely, but at the doctoral level two thirds of the ACCEs majored in education or administration.

Previous association with physical therapy education. Three fourths of the ACCEs reported having been a clinical instructor and one half had been a CCCE, but 17% of the ACCEs reported neither clinical instructor nor CCCE experience. More than one third of the ACCEs had participated in occasional lecture or laboratory sessions for educational programs.

Career planning. Among the ACCEs, the most popular career goal at the time of physical therapy graduation was director of physical therapy in a hospital setting. The point at which the ACCEs first considered an academic position varied widely. The range included after working with students as a clinical instructor (21%), when wanting a job change (15%), when the position was vacant or offered (14%), after being a CCCE (14%), during graduate school (14%), around the time of graduation as a physical therapist

(13%), and after part-time or occasional teaching involvement. (9%).

The ACCE position itself was not recognized as a career goal at graduation. Sixty-two percent of the respondents first considered the ACCE position when it was vacant or when desiring a job change. Some of these respondents were looking for a faculty position, and others were encouraged to fill a vacancy. Six percent of ACCEs claimed that they were not attracted to accept the position but were forced to do so by circumstances.

Prior knowledge of the ACCE position. The ACCEs were asked to reflect on the moment when they decided to accept their current (or former) position as ACCE and to rate how much they really knew about the position at that time. Of the current ACCEs, 21% considered that they were very well informed, and 11% considered themselves uninformed. Twenty percent of the current ACCEs felt very well prepared for the position of ACCE, and 11% felt unprepared. Only 20% of the ACCEs rated their perception of the ACCE position before they accepted it as accurate. The former ACCEs considered themselves better informed and more prepared than did the current ACCEs, and the former ACCEs were equally accurate in their perception of the position.

Recommendations for ACCE preparation. The ACCEs ranked a list of courses or experiences according to their perceived value in preparation for the ACCE position (Tab. 4).

Table 3

Number of Nights per Year That Work Causes the Academic Coordinator of Clinical Education (ACCE) to Be Away From Home: Current and Former ACCEs (N=170)

Number of Nights	Current ACCE (%)	Former ACCE (%)
0-10	34	32
11-20	44	30
21-30	13	24
Over 30	6	14
No response	3	0

Table 4

Value of Courses or Experience as Preparation for Position of Academic Coordinator of Clinical Education (ACCE) (N=170)[a]

Course or Experience	Current ACCE		Former ACCE	
	Mean	Range	Mean	Range
Communication	3.8	2-4	3.9	2-4
Counseling	3.4	2-4	3.6	2-4
Clinical instructor	3.4	2-4	3.4	1-4
Center coordinator of clinical education	3.2	1-4	3.2	1-4
Teaching	2.9	1-4	3.0	2-4
Clinical expertise	2.8	1-4	2.9	2-4
Administration	2.8	1-4	2.9	1-4
Research	1.9	1-4	1.9	1-3

[a]1=no value, 2=some value, 3=more valuable, 4=most valuable.

The highest recommendations were given to courses or experiences in communication and counseling, as well as to work experience as a clinical instructor and CCCE.

Major Attractions to the Position

From a list (adapted from Foegelle[13]) of possible reasons for selecting an employment opportunity, ACCEs checked as many as they considered appropriate. The most frequently checked reasons were "duties and responsibilities of the job" and "ready for a change" (Tab. 5).

Another item on the questionnaires sought responses to the question, "How actively did you seek the position of ACCE?" On a 5-point scale, a response of 1 signified that the ACCE actively sought the position, and a response of 5 indicated that the ACCE was persuaded to accept. Twenty-nine percent of the ACCEs actively sought the position, and 18% were persuaded to accept.

In response to an opportunity to list four major attractions that becoming an ACCE held for them, one half (52%) of the ACCEs mentioned some aspect of the job. The flexible schedule, opportunity to travel, and variety of responsibilities were attractive, particularly in contrast to a more rigid schedule in clinical practice.

One half (51%) of the ACCEs mentioned an attraction to working in the university setting or to becoming part of a faculty. Many of these responses mentioned academia in a way that implied status or prestige. There was esteem for colleagues who were faculty and a desire to join this select group. In particular, knowing and admiring the program chair or previous ACCE made the position attractive. Several noted that the ACCE position was an opportunity to evaluate academia as a member of the academic faculty. A specific academic institution was mentioned as an attraction by 21% of the ACCEs. The convenience of the geographic location, the institution as the alma mater, commencement of a new program, and respect for a program's faculty were cited.

Many ACCEs (38%) were attracted because they had enjoyed working with students in another capacity, for example as a clinical instructor or as a part-time lecturer or laboratory assistant. Others wanted to work more closely with students as individuals or sought the opportunity to make an impact on the profession through students.

Continued contact with many physical therapy clinicians and a variety of clinical sites was mentioned by more than one third (35%) of the ACCEs. They anticipated that they would have reason to visit a broad array of clinics to keep up with changing physical therapy practice.

Personal and professional advancement was an attraction (25%) in the form of advanced education, contact with faculty, and keeping abreast of the latest developments at the university and clinics. The ACCEs welcomed the opportunity to be part of a strong physical therapy program and to gain from the strengths of that program. Almost one fourth (21%) mentioned their personal need to change jobs or get out of a particular job or readiness to develop a new career. Some ACCEs (21%) felt prepared and able to hold the position following preparation in graduate school or experience as a clinical instructor, CCCE, or teaching faculty.

Seventeen percent were attracted to a challenge to change clinical education. They wanted to improve the quality or increase the program emphasis on clinical education. This was often in response to their unsatisfactory experiences as a student.

Most and Least Attractive Features

Each ACCE was asked to list the four most attractive and the four least attractive features of the ACCE position. Other items on the questionnaires asked about aspects of the ACCE position that were unexpected, providing a rating of the enjoyment of a variety of ACCE experiences. The many additional comments written by ACCEs and the interviews provided further insight into this area.

Most attractive features. The most attractive features of the ACCE position were associated with students and clinics. Working with clinical instructors in the various clinics and contact with a variety of clinics through site visits were mentioned as a most attractive feature of the position by 66% of the ACCEs. Working with students, seeing student growth, and the challenge of student problems were attractive to 65% of the respondents. One half (56%) of the ACCEs noted that the job included a variety of activities and that there was flexibility in the work schedule and autonomy in decision making. A form of the word "flexible" was used in 34% of the responses.

Least attractive features. Unattractive features of the job concerning paperwork, scheduling, contract negotiation, phone time, and salary were mentioned by a majority of the ACCEs. The paperwork was described as "massive," "overwhelming," "constant," "voluminous," and "requiring infinite attention to detail." Many mentioned the routine nature of some time-consuming tasks that "could be delegated if you had a good secretary," or "could be done by a well-organized administrative assistant." Many ACCEs (44%) mentioned the "long hours" and "hectic pace" required of the ACCE position.

Some ACCEs (21%) enjoyed "limited" travel, but for 24% of current ACCEs and 32% of former ACCEs, it had lost its appeal and had become a burden. Travel was mentioned as an attraction to the ACCE position, as a most attractive feature of the position, and as a least attractive feature of the position.

In response to the structured question of the enjoyment of a variety of ACCE experiences, both current and former ACCEs gave the highest score to visiting students and the lowest score to paperwork (Tab. 6).

Surprises. The most frequently mentioned unexpected aspects of the ACCE position related to the work load ("the work is never

Table 5

Reasons for Selecting Position of Academic Coordinator of Clinical Education (ACCE) (N=170)

Reason	Current ACCE (%)	Former ACCE (%)
Duties and responsibilities of job	80	91
Ready for a change	58	64
Educational opportunities for self	43	29
Congeniality of colleagues	40	40
Geographic location	38	44
Competence of colleagues	29	29
Mission and philosophy of institution or unit	29	25
Status and prestige	22	27
Potential for advancement	21	24
Fringe benefits	13	10
Salary	11	5
Policies and practices of administration	9	10
Educational opportunities for family	8	2
Physical facilities	3	3
Employment opportunities for spouse	2	0

Table 6

Academic Coordinators of Clinical Education (ACCEs) Score Their Enjoyment of Various ACCE Experiences (N=170)[a]

Experience	Current ACCE		Former ACCE	
	Mean	Range	Mean	Range
Visiting students	3.3	2-4	3.6	2-4
Classroom teaching	3.2	2-4	3.2	2-4
Laboratory teaching	3.2	1-4	2.8	1-4
Counseling	3.2	1-4	3.4	1-4
Clinical instructor	3.1	1-4	3.1	1-4
Public relations	3.1	1-4	3.3	1-4
Clinical practice	2.8	1-4	2.7	1-4
Challenging students	2.8	1-4	2.9	1-4
Travel	2.7	1-4	2.9	1-4
Evaluation of sites	2.7	1-4	3.1	2-4
Evaluation of students	2.6	1-4	2.7	1-4
Research	2.3	1-4	1.8	1-4
Scheduling	1.9	1-4	1.9	1-4
Telephone time	1.7	1-4	1.8	1-3
Paperwork	1.4	1-3	1.7	1-4

[a]1=not enjoyable, 2=okay, 3=enjoyable, 4=most enjoyable.

Table 7

Reasons Current Academic Coordinators of Clinical Education (ACCEs) Seek to Leave Position, and Reasons Former ACCEs Left Position (N=170)

Reason	Current ACCE (%)	Former ACCE (%)
Duties and responsibilities of job	48	37
Potential for advancement	48	27
Salary	38	24
Ready for a change	31	55
Geographic location	28	11
Policies and practices of administration	24	24
Mission and philosophy of institution or unit	17	23
Status and prestige	14	17
Educational opportunities for self	10	31
Congeniality of colleagues	10	11
Competence of colleagues	7	8
Physical facilities	7	2
Educational opportunities for family	3	2
Employment opportunities for spouse	0	8

done"), various ACCE responsibilities including legal aspects and paperwork, academia and job problems ("the politics of academia," "tenure requirements"), problems with affiliating clinics, and student problems.

Future Career Plans

What would cause you to leave? In response to an open-ended question, the ACCEs described the situations that would cause them to leave their current ACCE position. Several ACCEs gave more than one response, providing a list of frustrations. Forty-five percent of the ACCEs wrote that they would leave seeking a change in environment. They were attracted to the clinic, teaching, a doctoral program, administration, or retirement.

Frustrations with the physical therapy program could cause 36% to leave, one half of these because of lack of support for the position and the other half if they were given any added responsibilities. An additional 21% of the ACCEs mentioned the work load, including burnout, as the factor that could cause them to leave. A lack of financial reward was mentioned along with frustration because of an inability to receive tenure.

Reasons for job change. Current ACCEs were asked whether they were seriously considering or actively pursuing a job change. Of the 107 respondents, 29 (27%) checked a positive response. A list of possible reasons for selecting a new employment opportunity

was provided, and the ACCEs who were planning to leave checked as many as appropriate to indicate their reasons for leaving (Tab. 7). The reasons most often given were the duties and responsibilities of the job (48%), potential for advancement (48%), salary (38%), and readiness for a change (31%).

Prediction of next job. All ACCEs, including the 29 who were pursuing a job change, were asked for a realistic prediction of their next job. Of the current ACCEs, 37% expected to choose a faculty position, 32% expected to return to clinical practice, 11% expected to retire, 10% expected to stay where they were or were unwilling to make a prediction, and 4% expected to choose an administrative position possibly outside physical therapy.

Factors Influencing Former ACCEs

Former ACCEs left the ACCE position for a variety of reasons, and many gave more than one reason. One half of the former ACCEs left when they were ready to change to another area such as doctoral study, administration, classroom teaching, or clinical practice. One third of the former ACCEs mentioned frustration with the ACCE position (academics and politics), one third mentioned family responsibilities (relocation, marriage, or children), and one third listed overwork, high stress, burnout, or lack of vacations as an ACCE. Seventy percent of the former ACCEs had actively sought to leave the position, and 11% were recruited away.

Occupation. Forty percent of the former ACCEs listed physical therapy faculty as their next position, 35% listed physical therapist, 11% administrator, 7% retirement, and 7% graduate student. The faculty category included academic administrators, teaching faculty, and ACCEs. The physical therapist category included department directors, senior physical therapists, and staff physical therapists. Several former ACCEs made notations that they were involved in multiple roles (eg, graduate study while practicing as a clinician).

Since leaving the ACCE position, one half of the former ACCEs had held administrative positions. Most of these remained in academia, but others were based in a variety of clinical facilities and in other settings. The ACCE has many administrative duties, and several current ACCEs were also acting academic administrators of an education program.

Involvement with physical therapy education. All but two of the 63 former ACCEs have been involved with physical therapy education at the same or a different institution since they left the ACCE position. This involvement has been as full-time and part-time academic faculty, as clinical faculty, or as a graduate student.

DISCUSSION

Previous studies described several demographic characteristics of ACCEs, and the findings of this study are comparable to those reported.[3-9] The data also were compared to those available for physical therapists, physical therapy faculty, and college faculty in general. In comparison with other physical therapy faculty, ACCEs were more likely to be female, less likely to be tenured, and more likely to consider themselves in a trial or entry-level faculty position. Over 80% of the ACCE respondents were female, a slightly higher percentage than for physical therapists as a group (75% female[15]). The ACCEs were much more likely to be female than were the physical therapy full-time teaching faculty as a whole (62% female[16,17]) and college faculty in general (30% female[18]).

Most of the former ACCEs were associated with baccalaureate-degree programs, while the current ACCEs were from baccalaureate-degree, postbaccalaureate-degree, and transitioning programs. This probably reflects the change to postbaccalaureate-degree education rather than an exodus from baccalaureate-degree programs.

Tenure is the traditional key to job security and status as a full member of academe. Others have drawn attention to difficulties experienced by ACCEs in obtaining tenure and to the need to restructure the role of the ACCE to comply with the demands of higher education.[4,8,9] At the time of this study, only 15% of the ACCEs were tenured. The ACCEs were less likely to be tenured than the physical therapy full-time teaching faculty (31% tenured[16,17]) or than the college faculty in general (64% tenured[18]). Most ACCEs can become part of the academic community through involvement in scholarly activities and through contribution of service to the university. Innovative methods for analyzing the work of the ACCE and scholarship in clinical education should be explored in efforts toward attaining tenure.

The ACCE position has been used as an entry-level or trial faculty position. Almost two thirds of the ACCEs were physical therapy clinicians before accepting the position, and most were recruited without deliberate preparation for the position. The majority of ACCEs held a master's degree and were untenured instructors or assistant professors. In the view of the academic institution, they were junior faculty. The professional education and socialization of physical therapists

provide limited preparation for academe. Instead of clinical skills, the university values scholarly activities, classroom teaching, and service activities for promotion and tenure.

The physical therapy faculty struggle with the transition from the clinic, but ACCEs with their various roles and responsibilities often find a fit in academia to be even more complex. Any faculty position may be used as an entry-level position, and all faculty—including the ACCE—may be involved in continuing education and research. The results of this study show that research was not valued in preparation for the ACCE position and that few ACCEs enjoyed research activities. This is attributed to a variety of factors, including inadequate preparation and understanding of research and a demanding schedule.

The Carnegie Foundation study[11,12] found one fourth of the faculty dissatisfied with their position, but most of these faculty were not actually leaving. Physical therapists, both clinicians and faculty, are in demand and frequently receive offers of other positions. There are those who enjoy clinical education and the position of ACCE and plan to continue, but others seeking advancement are attracted away from academia by higher salaries in clinical practice or seek advancement in academia through other faculty or administrative positions. One half of the ACCEs were new or were planning to leave the ACCE position.

The ACCE is the liaison between the clinical and academic settings, and a lack of stability in this vital role can lead to instability of the education program. One third of the ACCEs expected that their next move would be to another faculty position, but the academic institution's special relationship with multiple clinical sites is interrupted even when the former ACCE moves within a faculty.

No ACCE had a career goal of becoming an ACCE at the time of graduation as a physical therapist, and only one fourth actively sought the position. Physical therapy educators have recognized the need to educate students as well as clinicians to be clinical instructors. There also is a need to prepare those who demonstrate interest and ability to become ACCEs. Various consortia have developed programs to meet the needs of clinical instructors and CCCEs, and those who show good potential to assume the ACCE role would benefit from similar encouragement.

To prepare for the position, the ACCEs highly recommended experience or course work in communication and counseling, as well as work experience as a clinical instruc-

tor and CCCE. Moore and Perry[1] made similar recommendations in 1976. Kondela-Cebulski[7] reported that, while most of the ACCEs found counseling to be a part of their role, only half of them believed that they were prepared for this role.

The professional preparation of the physical therapist candidate for the position of ACCE alone will not suffice. Individuals and committees responsible for recruiting and/or selecting ACCEs must better understand the roles and function of the position. Too many ACCEs accepted the position when someone who really did not know what it involved told them that they could do it.

The position of the ACCE must be clarified. Physical therapy faculty members are at a premium, and many tasks performed by ACCEs could be accomplished by qualified support staff, allowing the ACCE to invest more effort in traditional faculty activities. The amount of secretarial support and the expectations for student visitation, classroom teaching, clinical practice, graduate study, research, and service activities vary in different institutions and departments. An ACCE Position Description compiled by Gandy[10] after these data were collected provides a useful guide to the role responsibilities and expectations for the position.

The ACCE's schedule often intrudes into personal lives. Duties and responsibilities of the job was the most-cited reason for selecting the ACCE position and also the most common reason for leaving. Once-attractive features of the job—such as travel opportunities and a flexible schedule—became problems when travel became a burden, and the flexible schedule was evidenced by long hours of work and late-night phone calls.

There is potential for redesigning some of the expectations. The amount of travel expected of the ACCE varies widely and may be decreasing. Fewer current ACCEs than former ACCEs had been away from home for more than 20 nights per year. Some programs require travel to each clinical site whenever a student is affiliating, but alternatives such as visits by other faculty and alumni, telephone contacts, and clustering of clinical sites may reduce travel by the ACCE.

It is important to educate the faculty and the administration as to the role and responsibilities of the position. Academic faculty, including the ACCEs, are expected to think, investigate, reflect, and explore. The ACCEs are role models for both students and clinicians, and it is important that they have the time to model these behaviors.

CONCLUSION

Although considerable variation exists among ACCEs, the majority were untenured instructors or assistant professors with a master's degree. They were female and had held the position for a mean of 4.6 years. Almost two thirds of the ACCEs came from the clinical setting, and one third came from a faculty position.

No ACCE recognized the position as a career goal at the time of graduation as a physical therapist, and the majority first considered the position when it was vacant or when desiring a job change. They came without formal preparation for the position and without an accurate perception of the role and responsibilities of the ACCE. The ACCEs gave the highest recommendation for courses or experience in communication as preparation for the position.

Attractions to the position included the duties and responsibilities of the job itself, working at the university setting with students and faculty, and continuing contact with clinicians. The most attractive features of the ACCE position were associated with students and clinics. The least attractive features were the routine, time-consuming tasks such as paperwork, scheduling, and "telephone tag." Difficulties with recognition and tenure and excessive time spent in travel also were unattractive. Factors that were originally attractions to the position were mentioned as least attractive features of the position and as reasons for leaving.

More than one fourth of the ACCEs were seriously considering or actively pursuing a job change. The primary reasons for leaving were the duties and responsibilities of the job and a lack of potential for advancement. One third of the ACCEs expected to leave the position for another faculty position and one third to return to the clinic.

Of the former ACCEs, over one third listed physical therapy faculty as their next position, and one third listed physical therapist. Since leaving the ACCE position, one half of the former ACCEs had held administrative positions.

Issues for further discussion in academic institutions include the problems of tenure, travel, and routine tasks. There should be identification and preparation of potential ACCEs, clarification of the position and responsibilities of the ACCE, and the potential for the ACCE to become a full member of the academic community through teaching, involvement in scholarly activities, and contribution of service to the university.

REFERENCES

1. Moore ML, Perry JF. *Clinical Education in Physical Therapy: Present Status/Future Needs.* Washington, DC: Section for Education, American Physical Therapy Association; 1976:2:17–19.

2. Booth JA. *Factors Influencing the Mobility of Academic Coordinators of Clinical Education in Curricula for the First Professional Degree in Physical Therapy.* Richmond, Va: Virginia Commonwealth University; 1979. Thesis.

3. Myers RS. *Current Patterns for Providing Clinical Education in Physical Therapy Education.* Alexandria, Va: Department of Education, American Physical Therapy Association; 1985.

4. Strickler EM. The academic coordinator of clinical education: current status, questions, and challenges for the 1990s and beyond. *Journal of Physical Therapy Education.* 1991;5:3–9.

5. Philips BL Jr, McPhail S, Roemer S. Role and functions of the academic coordinator of clinical education in physical therapy education: a survey. *Phys Ther.* 1966:66:981–985.

6. Harris MJ, Fogel M, Blacconiere M. Job satisfaction among academic coordinators of clinical education in physical therapy. *Phys Ther.* 1987;67:958–963.

7. Kondela-Cebulski PM. Counseling function of academic coordinators of clinical education from select entry-level physical therapy educational programs. *Phys Ther.* 1982;62:470–476.

8. Deusinger SS, Rose SJ. Opinions and comments: the dinosaur of academic physical therapy. *Phys Ther.* 1988;68:412.414.

9. Strickler EM. The role of the academic coordinator of clinical education: a dilemma in academe. *Journal of Allied Health.* 1990:19:95–101.

10. Gandy J. *Position Description—Physical Therapist Program.* Alexandria, Va: Department of Education, American Physical Therapy Association; 1993.

11. Carnegie Foundation for the Advancement of Teaching. Change: the faculty: deeply troubled. *Change.* 1985;17(5):31–34.

12. Carnegie Foundation for the Advancement of Teaching. Change: trendlines. The satisfied faculty. *Change.* 1986;18(2):31–34.

13. Foegelle WE. *Characteristics of Allied Health Faculty in Academic Health Centers.* Indianapolis, Ind: Indiana University; 1984. Dissertation.

14. Radtka S. Predictors of physical therapy faculty job turnover. *Phys Ther.* 1992;73:243–253.

15. *Physical Therapy Practice: General Information.* Alexandria, Va: Department of Practice, American Physical Therapy Association; 1988.

16. *Physical Therapy Education: Physical Therapist Entry-level Programs.* Alexandria, Va: Department of Education, American Physical Therapy Association; 1990.

17. *Physical Therapy Education: Physical Therapist Entry-level Programs.* Alexandria, Va: Department of Education, American Physical Therapy Association; 1991.

18. National Center for Education Statistics. *Digest of Education Statistics.* Washington, DC: Office of Education Research and Improvement; 1991.

SCHOLARLY PAPER

Managing Clinical Education: The Programme

Joy Higgs

Key Words

Clinical education, management, programme development.

Summary

A management framework for the design, implementation and evaluation of clinical education programmes in physiotherapy is presented. The framework has its basis in systems theory, management theory and adult learning theory. In using the CIPP (context, input, process, product) evaluation model as a starting point, the framework proposes that the evaluation of a programme's context and input should be conducted during the planning stages of the curriculum, and evaluation of the programme's process and products should be conducted both during implementation as part of programme development and after the programme for judgement and accreditation of the programme. This framework provides a relevant and comprehensive guide to clinical education programme management.

This paper is a sequel to 'Managing clinical education: The educator-manager and the self-directed learner' (Higgs, 1992), which discussed the application to the clinical education context of management principles and theories and research related to adult and self-directed learning.

Introduction

Clinical education is an essential element of physiotherapy education programmes. Effective management of clinical education is therefore important in the education of future physiotherapists. This paper presents a framework for managing clinical education programmes, which is based on systems theory and the CIPP (context, input, process, product) model of programme evaluation. In this framework the clinical teacher* is presented as a manager of the clinical education programme and the student as a self-directed learner who also participates in programme management. The framework provides the basis for the effective management of clinical education programmes including their design, implementation and evaluation.

Across the health professions the term 'clinical education' has many forms and connotations. The wide variety of approaches to clinical education includes the apprenticeship system, competency-based learning, problem-based learning, clinical simulation in laboratories, the use of simulated patients, contractual learning, on-campus clinics and supervised clinical practice in real health care settings (Henley et al, 1981; Holzman, 1982; Fox and West, 1983; Oppelaar et al, 1983; Sasmor, 1984; Day, 1985). The central element of these approaches, and the core of clinical education, is the experience by students of their clinical/professional role

*The term (clinical) 'teacher' in this paper refers to physiotherapists who are engaged in teaching students in the clinical context, and includes both educators from educational institutions and clinicians.

in real or simulated settings. In this paper the framework for clinical education management focuses on clinical education in the form of supervised clinical practice in real health care settings. The framework is directed primarily at situations which involve the treatment of patients.

Systems Theory

Clinical education programmes function like systems. This is evident from examining the following definitions. 'A system is essentially a set or assemblage of things that are interconnected, or interdependent, so as to form a complex whole' (Koontz et al, 1982). An open system occurs when inputs received from the environment are processed and new products are returned to the environment (Von Bertalanffy, 1969). This is illustrated in the figure below.

The concept and image of an open system is an appropriate representation of a learning programme (Romiszowski, 1970). Inputs such as the programme design and learners with their existing characteristics, enter the system or learning programme. During the programme the inputs undergo transformation (eg learning occurs). The changed products/people then return to the environment. The connection between clinical education and systems is very evident on examination of the concept of 'soft systems' which was introduced by Checkland (1981) to refer to those systems in which goals may be unrecognisable and outcomes ambiguous.

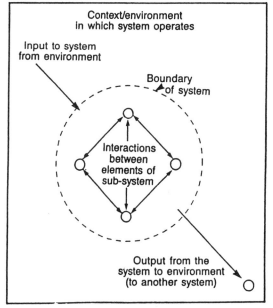

An open system (based on Romiszowski, 1970, p 13)

In clinical education settings, for instance, participants frequently face ill-defined problems, goals that are complex and outcomes that are difficult to predict clearly.

There are three main advantages of using a systems approach to examining and managing clinical education programmes. The first of these is that the study of human behaviour as a purposeful system makes it possible to investigate behavioural or living phenomena as a whole (Ackoff and Emery, 1972). According to Emery (1969) it is only by using an open systems approach to studying living phenomena that we can reveal the 'gestalten' properties which characterise living systems. (A system is seen as being 'gestalten' when the effects of the whole system are greater than the aggregate of the effects of the parts of the system.)

Secondly, systems theory provides us with the concept of the individual as a purposeful subsystem operating within a larger system such as a learning programme. Purposeful subsystems or participants engage in goal-directed behaviour as part of the socio-cultural system, in accordance with their perceptions of environmental conditions. In professional clinical education programmes, learners and clinical teachers can be viewed as purposeful subsystems. Both parties have responsibilities and are accountable for their actions. This is compatible with the principles of adult learning which emphasise the need for learners to be active, responsible, decision-making participants in the learning process. It is also consistent with the concept of the teacher in a learning programme being the overall 'manager' and the learner becoming increasingly more competent and autonomous (Higgs, 1992).

Another important characteristic of successful systems or learning programmes is the congruence of their elements. In educational programmes congruence between such elements as leadership, goals and programme organisation is highly desirable (Torbert, 1978). Similarly, congruence between the system's goals, roles, procedures and interpersonal factors, promotes effective system operation (Rubin, 1980). The greater the degree of congruence, the greater the likelihood of achieving the programme's goals (Nadler and Tusham, 1979).

Creating congruence between elements in a clinical education programme is therefore very important. The messages that students receive, for instance via teacher behaviour, learning goals and assessment instructions, should be consistent in order to promote effective achievement of clinical education goals.

In summary, there are several characteristics of 'open system' learning programmes which are very applicable to clinical education in physiotherapy curricula. These include: the goal of promoting individual purposefulness or self-direction in learning, the integrated yet multidimensional nature of such programmes, the value of open learning environments which promote and support change, the recognition of learners' individual perceptions of and responses to their environment, the dynamic nature of learning programmes/systems and the importance of congruence between key elements of systems. The clinical educator's role includes creating a learning programme which acts as an effective open system in order to facilitate learning.

The CIPP Model of Programme Evaluation and Development

Having established the value of taking a systems approach to the design, implementation and evaluation of clinical education, the next step is to develop a framework within which this approach can be operationalised. The CIPP model of programme evaluation, which follows a systems approach, can provide such a framework (Stufflebeam, 1983). This model can be used as a means of proactive and formative evaluation during programmes to improve rather than prove the value and nature of the programme, as a means of programme accreditation, and as a tool to assist in programme design. Using this model the programme's structure and nature can be defined by identifying the context (needs and goals) of a programme and the input (design) of a programme. In addition, the programme can be evaluated and developed by examining the actual process which is implemented and the products or outcomes which result. The parallel between this model and open systems as described above is apparent. The CIPP model enables the learning programme to be viewed as a whole, with both intended and actual process and outcomes.

The context of a programme can be viewed as a source of needs for that programme. Within physiotherapy education, needs may relate to the nature of the profession, the current expectations of the workforce (eg for a commitment to lifelong learning) and where appropriate, to the needs of individual learners. Evaluation of these needs can identify the 'intended ends/outcomes' (goals) of a programme.

The programme's input/design should be created to achieve these outcomes. That is, the input is the 'intended means' of accomplishing the stated goals. The programme participants may be selected, on the basis of appropriate entry characteristics, to enable programme goals to be accomplished. Alternatively, the programme could be designed around the specific needs of a target group. Input design and evaluation should also take into consideration the availability of resources and any limitations within the situation.

The 'actual means' or process of the programme refers to the way the designed programme is implemented. Evaluation of the process allows for programme modification during implementation. In addition, evaluation of process and outcome can occur after the programme as part of summative evaluation. The outcomes or products of a programme can be referred to as the 'actual ends' of the programme. They are the sum of the intended and unintended effects of the programme.

A Framework for Clinical Education Management

There are several steps in the application of systems theory and the CIPP model to the design, implementation and evaluation of clinical education programmes. These implementation stages along with the theoretical basis provided by systems theory and the CIPP model comprise a framework for clinical education management.

Stage 1: Understanding the theory

The first stage in using this framework is to understand the relevance of systems theory and the CIPP model to clinical education. This is explained above.

Stage 2: Defining the context of the clinical education programme

The 'context evaluation' aspect of the CIPP model can be used to plan a clinical education programme or to evaluate an existing programme. The context of a programme includes the needs that a programme addresses and the way these needs are reflected in the programme's goals and objectives. Context evaluation asks the question: 'What are, or should be, the intended outcomes of the programme?' A number of methods can be used to answer this question. Stufflebeam (1983) provides a discussion of the following list of methods: system analysis, survey, document review, hearings, interviews, diagnostic tests and the Delphi technique (Madaus et al, 1983).

The context of physiotherapy education can be described as follows. Entry-level physiotherapy curricula are vocational programmes which have several key purposes. They aim to prepare students to become physiotherapists with responsibilities to their professions and to the community they serve, to be applied scientists in a context which values scientific evidence and justification, and to develop as skilled lifelong learners and innovators in a rapidly changing world. During this process it is hoped that the traditional role and values associated with physiotherapists as care-givers are fostered and indeed enhanced. This is particularly important within today's age of consciousness of the humanitarian and environmental concerns of the 'world-community'.

The literature provides many insights into the nature and goals of physiotherapy education. The need to prepare health science students for a professional role is emphasised by Guilbert (1981). He argues that key elements in educational programmes for the health sciences are a focus on the code of ethics and the knowledge base or principles which underpin the profession in question. Similarly, Anderson (1990) asserts that 'most professions require a high standard of specialised technical knowledge before the recruit (student) will be licensed to practise.'

A number of common goals for clinical education can be identified. Of particular importance is the development of clinical competencies relevant to physiotherapy (Marcoux and Pinkston, 1984). Clinical competence includes assessment skills, record-keeping skills, patient education skills and skills in managing oneself and others (Heath, 1978; Colwell and Smith, 1985).

The development of self-knowledge and interpersonal skills is another key goal of clinical education. It relates to interactions with patients, clients, families and other health-care team members. These skills are discussed widely in the literature under the headings: communication skills, self-awareness, interpersonal skills and the ability to cope with one's own feelings and act professionally (Pratt and Seddon, 1979; Kahn et al, 1981; Gartland, 1984; Levin and Riley, 1984; Dobbelaere and de Volder, 1987).

Within the current context of rapidly expanding knowledge there has been an increasing emphasis in physiotherapy in recent decades on the skills of clinical reasoning and self-directed learning. The following skills have therefore become very important goals in physiotherapy curricula: problem-solving, knowledge integration and decision-making skills (Day, 1985; Henry, 1985a; Hammond and Collins, 1991). Similarly, the acquisition of skills in self-evaluation, skills in self-directed learning and a commitment to personal and professional growth, are regarded as central curricular goals (Fox and West, 1983).

An associated goal is the development of the student's ability to be able to respond to changing health-care needs of the community (Foreman, 1986). Cox (1988), for instance, identifies the need to maintain the relevance of health science curricula to the needs of the community with its changing patterns of disease and illness and changing government policies and economic conditions. He also argues that health-care systems should meet society's expectations in terms of such factors as effectiveness and efficiency of intervention, utility to the patient, humanity, patient autonomy, responsibility for ongoing care and equity of access. The achievement of these outcomes begins within undergraduate physiotherapy education programmes.

Clinical education is a major element in physiotherapy curricula and has an important role to play in achieving the above goals. The importance of clinical education is strongly supported in the literature. Engel (1976) argues that clinical skills 'provide the medium for the human interaction that is the heart of patient care'. The acquisition and development of such skills is a central goal of clinical education. Wells and Lessard (1986) describe clinical education as 'an intricate, but essential, process in the physical therapy education programme'. Holmes (1975) contends that clinical education is vital to help students gain confidence in handling patients, develop their clinical/technical skills and acquire skill in clinical decision-making.

A recent exploratory study by the author and colleagues (Higgs et al, 1991) led to the development of a list of goals of clinical education programmes which have relevance to physiotherapy and a list of components of clinical education programmes which can assist in the achievement of these goals. (The components will be discussed in stage 3). The aim of the study was to develop guide lines to facilitate the achievement of educational and management effectiveness within clinical education programmes.

In this study 90 clinical teachers from the Faculty of Health Sciences at Sydney University were surveyed. The clinical education experience of the respondents ranged from one to ten years. They represented the following disciplines: physiotherapy, occupational therapy, nursing, health information management, medical radiation technology, orthoptics and diversional therapy. In a semi-structured questionnaire respondents were asked to indicate their perception of the importance of a set of goals and components to clinical education in their profession. These initial goals and components of clinical education had been developed by four academics who each had considerable experience (five to 15 years) as

Table 1: Goals of clinical education

To contribute to the development of students'

Understanding of health, illness and the health care system.
Awareness of own attitudes, values and responses to health and illness.
Ability to cope effectively with the demands of the professional role.
Understanding of the interrelated roles of health care team.
Clinical competencies relevant to the student's discipline, including clinical reasoning skills, psychomotor competencies, and interpersonal and communication skills.
Ability to provide a sound rationale for intervention/actions.
Skills in the education of relevant people, eg patients, clients, the community, staff.
Self-management skills, eg time and workload management.
Ability to process, record and use data effectively.
Abilty to evaluate critically and develop own performance.
Ability to review and investigate the quality of clinical practice.
Professional accountability commitment to clients/self/employers.
Commitment to maintain and develop professional competence.
Skills necessary for lifelong professional learning.
Ability to respond to changing community health care needs.

Table 2: Components of clinical education or factors contributing to the effectiveness of clinical education

The students

The students and their abilities, needs and interests.
Preparation of students prior to clinical placements (including learning theory and practical skills, orientation to clinical education).

Links between clinical and academic programmes

Integration of clinical/academic aspects of the curriculum (during curriculum design, implementation and evaluation).
Opportunities for clinical educators to participate in staff development activities.

The clinical education programme

Organisation of the clinical education programme.
The design of clinical education programme (ie sequencing, proportioning and linking of all aspects of the programme).
Clear programme goals.
Time allocated to clinical education.
The quality of clinical education (ie effectiveness of the use of time allocated to clinical education).

Resource people, and resources in the clinical education setting

Teachers (academic and clinical), and other clinical resource people who participate in clinical education.
The venue (ie setting within which clinical education occurs).
Material resources and facilities (ie the materials and space that exist at the clinical education venue).

Learning activities, supervision and learning climate

Learning activities and opportunities (ie the activities and events that are either designed or utilised by teachers and students in clinical education to facilitate student learning).
The learning climate (ie nature or atmosphere of the clinical learning environment and the extent to which it is conducive to student learning).
Supervision (ie monitoring and guiding student behaviour).

Assessment and feedback

The establishment of expected standards of performance.
The summative assessment process (ie the process of evaluating and accrediting students' performance).
Feedback to students (ie the process of providing constructive feedback based on evaluation of students' performance).
Encouragement of students to evaluate their own performance and discuss this with their clinical teachers.

Evaluation of the clinical education programme

Evaluation of the programme (ie determining the programme's effectiveness, including teaching effectiveness).

clinical teachers and/or clinical education administrators. The preliminary lists were based on a comprehensive review of the literature and the experience of this group. Respondents were also invited to review the lists and propose changes if necessary.

The results of this study supported the original lists of goals and components with minor modifications. Tables 1 and 2 provide the revised lists of goals and components. They are presented here not as a definitive description of clinical education goals and programme elements but as a starting point for designing and managing clinical education programmes.

The goals (as listed in table 1) can be used as a guide to planning the 'intended ends' of clinical education programmes and evaluating the 'actual ends' (outcomes or products) of these programmes. They represent the scope of aims of clinical education which have relevance to the current context of physiotherapy education. Clinical education programme managers and clinical teachers planning specific programmes for their own situation would need to examine the precise relevance of these goals to their given situation. The goals would need to be expressed in terms which are situation-specific. Where desired, a complementary set of objectives could also be formulated which are highly specific to the physiotherapy curriculum in question. Finally, within specific programmes it would also be desirable to introduce goals which meet the needs of individual students in identifying their own learning goals. Watts (1990) provides useful exercises to help clinical teachers identify what students want and need to learn.

Stage 3: Designing the clinical education programme

Input evaluation addresses the question: 'What plan or programme design is best suited to address the needs and achieve the goals identified by the context evaluation?' To answer this question clinical programme managers need to consider the relative merits, for their situation, of alternative programme designs. This review should consider the nature of any existing programme as well as programmes conducted or described elsewhere. Also, it is necessary to identify clearly the capabilities of the situation/system in which the programme will operate in terms of the opportunities, resources and limitations it provides to achieve the programme's goals. For instance, the following factors could be identified: the range of patient groups available to participate in the clinical education programme, the level of access to quality clinical education sites, financial or resource constraints, the number of actual or potential clinical teachers available and the nature of their clinical and teaching abilities.

Methods to evaluate or plan for a programme's input include: conducting an inventory and analysing the relevance, feasibility and economy of utilising available human and material resources, solution strategies and procedural designs (Stufflebeam, 1983). Furthermore, alternative designs could be reviewed by searching and reading relevant literature, visiting exemplary programmes, conducting pilot trials and examining alternatives via advocate teams. Students have a valuable role to play in designing clinical learning programmes, particularly within progammes which aim to foster the development of self-directed learning skills and behaviour.

Many factors which contribute to the design and implementation of effective clinical education programmes have been examined in the literature. In particular, clinical teachers play a major role in ensuring the entry-level competence (Wells and Lessard, 1986) and lifelong learning ability of graduates from these programmes. Therefore, the effectiveness of clinical teachers as clinicians and teachers is very important to the success of clinical education programmes. The need for clinical teachers to be well prepared for their roles as teachers and managers has received extensive support (Greenberg et al, 1984; Morgan, 1986; Griffiths, 1987).

A number of studies have examined aspects of the competence of clinical teachers. Irby (1978), for instance, identified seven factors which influenced the effectiveness of clinical supervision. These are organisation/clarity, group teaching skills, enthusiasm, knowledge, clinical supervision, clinical competence and modelling of professional characteristics. A study of medical students by Stritter et al (1975) identified six effective clinical teaching behaviour areas: the promotion of active student participation, a preceptor attitude towards teaching, an emphasis on applied problem-solving, the use of student-centred instructional strategies, a humanistic orientation and an emphasis on references and research. Conahan et al (1981) identified 41 attributes of effective clinical teachers. Four of these were regarded as being most important to clinical teachers and learners: clinical judgement, accuracy of information, emphasis on clinical reasoning and supervisor availability.

Among the many roles assigned to clinical supervisors several receive particular attention in the literature. These include the importance of the clinical teacher as a role model (Jacobson, 1978) and the value to students of opportunities to assume responsibility for their own learning (Farquhar and Holdman, 1982).

The nature and importance of assessment also receives particular attention in the literature. The integral part played by feedback and evaluation in promoting learning (Henry, 1985b) is stressed along with the role and methods of assessing student performance in relation to learning and summative assessment (May, 1978; Harper et al, 1983; Palmer et al, 1985; McCoy, 1991; Davis, 1991). In addition, assessment can strongly influence the way students perceive the value and credibility of what they are learning and their ability to transfer learning between classroom and clinical contexts. These outcomes are fostered by links between the clinical and academic programmes, particularly links which deal with the assessment of student performance (Coates, 1991).

During the design phase it is important to plan opportunities for programme evaluation and for feedback to clinical teachers as well as to students. Feedback to teachers is regarded as an important influence on the effectiveness of clinical education (Cimorell-Strong and Ensley, 1982) as is self-evaluation (Watts, 1990). Planned programme evaluation should also address evaluation of the content and teaching methods contained in clinical education programmes (Kern and Mickelson, 1971; Irby, 1983).

Previous work by the author and a colleague (Romanini and Higgs, 1989) led to the development of a 'teacher-manager model' which had its origin in experience and research related to health science education. The principal argument underlying this model is that teachers can achieve the goals of health science education, such as promoting learners' self-directed learning, and promote effective learning, by acting as facilitative managers and co-managers (with the learners) of learning programmes. In this model the teacher is seen as being a proactive facilitator of the overall learning programme. This involves a number of management roles including management of the learning environment, learner participation in the learning task, group process and individual learner development. Learners are encouraged to act independently as well as interactively (with other learners and the teacher) and to take an increasing level of responsibility for their own learning. Each of these roles are employed in the various stages of the learning programme, ie planning, implementation and evaluation.

In the exploratory study on clinical education discussed above (Higgs et al, 1991) a set of components of clinical education programmes was developed (table 2). These programme components identify the various aspects of clinical education programmes which the co-ordinator of such programmes is responsible for managing. They can be used to plan and evaluate the 'means' of achieving a programme's goals.

The programme components need to be operationalised to serve the unique situational needs of a given programme. As part of this process managers and teachers involved in the programme would need to identify which educational and management principles they wished to adhere to, and build these elements into the programme. It is recommended that adult learning and a management approach which focuses on empowerment and situational relevance are used as the basis for clinical education management, since these are highly consistent with the goals and context of physiotherapy education. In addition, it is desirable that the programme should be designed around the characteristics of effective open systems — in particular, congruence between goals and programme design, and opportunities for learners to behave purposefully.

Stage Four — Conducting and evaluating the process of the clinical education programme

The implementation of a clinical education programme can be described as the 'actual means' or process of achieving the programme's goals. Process evaluation serves three purposes. The programme as designed can be examined prior to implementation, to predict and avert potential problems and to avoid programme design defects. During programme implementation, process evaluation can be performed to provide information which can be used to improve the programme during operation. After implementation, process evaluation is part of programme accreditation. The basic questions to be addressed are: 'Are there potential defects in the procedural design of the programme?' 'If so, how can these be. addressed?' 'How was the programme implemented and to what extent was the programme implemented as planned?' 'If changes were made to the original design what were they and why were they made?' 'Was the programme design well received by participants?'

Methods for conducting process evaluation (Stufflebeam, 1983) include monitoring the programme's potential and actual procedural barriers, remaining alert to unanticipated barriers, describing the actual process to obtain specified information to make decisions relating to ongoing implementation and accreditation, and constant interaction with and observation of programme participants in action. Rotem and Bandaranayake (1983) emphasise the role of collecting information about a programme and evaluating this information as part of making decisions about the programme. In a variation of the CIPP model they propose that programme evaluators identify specific questions to be asked about the programme, for instance: 'Do students understand what is expected of them in the assessment of their learning during field experience?' These authors recommend that evaluators identify and collect information, including indicators and criteria for judging the worth of the programme, in order to provide the answers to these questions. This process could readily be applied to clinical education programme evaluation and management.

Stage 5: Evaluating products and outcomes of the clinical education programme

Product evaluation of the clinical education programme asks the questions: 'What were the positive and negative, intended and unintended results of the programme?' 'How do people involved with the programme (ie the programme's stakeholders) judge the worth and merit of the programme's outcomes?' 'To what extent did the programme meet the needs that the programme sought to address?' 'What changes to the programme are indicated by the observed outcomes?' Stages 4 and 5 can occur simultaneously.

The goal list provided in table 1 and the specific goals of the programme in question can be used to assess the extent to which the programme is achieving its intended outcomes, producing desirable or undesirable outcomes, and meeting the needs of the stakeholders and target population it serves. Methods of product evaluation (Stufflebeam, 1983) include describing programme outcomes, defining outcome criteria operationally and measuring these, collecting judgements of outcomes from stakeholders, and performing qualitative and quantitative analysis of information collected. A discussion of the merits of different forms of data collection and evaluation is provided by Rotem and Bandaranayake (1983).

Discussion of the Framework

This framework was created to provide management guide lines for clinical education. As stated at the beginning of the paper the framework has most relevance to clinical education situations which could be described as 'supervised clinical practice' but could be adapted to most learning programmes. It is a tool for facilitating the effective design, implementation and evaluation of clinical education programmes. When applying the framework it is advisable to employ adult learning and management principles to create a 'facilitative manager' role for clinical teachers and a self-directed learning role for students.

The model is based on an open system approach and is derived from the CIPP model of programme evaluation. In using the CIPP evaluation model as a starting point, the framework proposes that the evaluation of a programme's context and input be conducted during the planning stages of the curriculum and evaluation of the programme's process and products be conducted both during implementation as part of programme development and after implementation for judgement and accreditation of the programme.

This framework has value in terms of its relevance and comprehensiveness. The systems approach is directly applicable to physiotherapy education and emphasises the wholeness and congruence of educational programmes. The list of goals is relevant to physiotherapy education in general and to clinical education in particular. The components list covers the major elements within clinical education programmes and provides a mechanism for applying management and educational principles to suit the specific goals and situational variables of programmes to which it is applied.

It is not the intention of the framework to provide definitive answers. Rather, it presents directions for clinical education, management guide lines for conducting clinical education programmes and the flexibility to adapt to many different clinical education situations. It becomes the task of clinical teachers to use this framework to design and implement clinical education programmes which are relevant to their needs. By using this framework such programmes should be characterised by relevance, congruence in structure and function, effective operation as an open human activity system (being responsive to and interactive with their environments) and a sound basis in educational and management principles.

Conclusion

Clincial education has moved a long way from being simply the means of practising in clinical settings, those skills already learned in the classroom. Neither is clinical education now seen as the process of apprentices seeking to acquire the expertise of their masters. Instead, clinical education has become an integral part of physiotherapy curricula, which both extends prior learning and provides opportunities for creating new knowledge.

Managing clinical education programmes to achieve these goals is a complex task. The framework in this paper is presented as a means of facilitating effective learning programmes. Clinical teachers are encouraged to be creative teachers, efficient managers and co-operative participants in dynamic clinical education systems. Learners are also challenged to be purposeful participants in clinical education, playing an active and responsible role in creating and implementing effective clinical learning programmes.

Acknowledgements

The author wishes to thank colleagues (Mary Glendinning, Fran Dunsford and Judy Panter) who were co-researchers in the exploratory study referred to in this paper.

Author and Address for Correspondence

Joy Higgs PhD GradDipPhty MPHEd is Head, School of Physiotherapy, Faculty of Health Sciences, University of Sydney, PO Box 170, Lidcombe, 2141, Australia.

References

Ackoff, R L and Emery, F E (1972). *On Purposeful Systems*, Tavistock, London.

Anderson, D S (1990). 'The undergraduate curriculum: Educating recruits to the professions' in: Moses, I (ed) *Higher Education in the Late Twentieth Century: Reflections on a changing system*, Higher Education Research and Development Society of Australasia, Sydney, pages 168–187.

Checkland, P B (1981). *Systems Thinking: Systems practice*, John Wiley and Sons, New York.

Cimorell-Strong, J and Ensley, K G (1982). 'Effects of student clinician feedback on the supervisory conference', *Australian Speech and Hearing Association*, January 24, pages 23–29.

Coates, H M (1991). 'The integration of clinical education with academic assessment', *Proceedings of the World Confederation for Physical Therapy 11th International Congress*, WCPT, London, page 311.

Colwell, C B and Smith, J (1985). 'Determining the use of physical assessment skills in the clinical setting', *Journal of Nursing Education*, 24, 333–339.

Conahan, T J, Rubeck, R F and Anderson, D O (1981). 'Rating the importance of clinical teacher attributes', *The Arizona Medical Educator*, 11, 1–3.

Cox, K (1988). 'Professional and educational context of medical education', in: Cox, K R and Ewan, C E (eds), *The Medical Teacher* (2nd edn) Churchill Livingstone, Edinburgh, pages 4–8.

Davis, C M (1991). 'Evaluating student clinical performance in the affective domain', *Proceedings of the World Confederation for Physical Therapy 11th International Congress*, WCPT, London, pages 315–317.

Day, J A (1985). 'Beyond lecture and laboratory in the physical therapy classroom', *Physical Therapy*, 65, 1214–16.

Dobbelaere, R I M C and de Volder, M L (1987). 'Affective objectives and their assessment in physiotherapy education', *Physiotherapy*, 73, 12, 623–625.

Emery, F E (1969). *Systems Thinking*, Penguin Books, Middlesex.

Engel, G L (1976). 'Are medical schools neglecting clinical skills?' (editorial) *Journal of the American Medical Association*, 236, 861–863.

Farquhar, L J and Holdman, H (1982). 'Preferred styles of clinical teaching: Measuring physician control over students in patient care encounters', *Medical Teacher*, 4, 104–109.

Foreman, S (1986). 'The changing medical care system: Some implications for medical education', *Journal of Medical Education*, 61, 11–21.

Fox, R D and West, R F (1983). 'Developing medical student competence in lifelong learning: The contract learning approach', *Medical Education*, 17, 247–253.

Gartland, G J (1984). 'Teaching the therapeutic relationship', *Physiotherapy Canada*, 36, 24–28.

Greenberg, L W, Goldberg, R M and Jewett, L S (1984). 'Teaching in the clinical setting: Factors influencing residents' perceptions, confidence and behaviour', *Medical Education*, 18, 360–365.

Griffiths, P (1987). 'Creating a learning environment', *Physiotherapy*, 73, 328–331.

Guilbert, J J (1981). *Educational Handbook for Health Personnel* (2nd edn) World Health Organisation, Geneva.

Hammond, M and Collins, R (1991). *Self-directed Learning: Critical practice*, Kogan Page, London.

Harper, A C, Roy, W B, Norman, G R, Rand, C A and Feightner, J W (1983). 'Difficulties in clinical skills evaluation', *Medical Education*, 17, 24–27.

Heath, J R (1978). 'Problem oriented medical systems', *Physiotherapy*, 64, 269–270.

Henley, E C, Hodges, M A and Brooks, B (1981). 'A working model for allied health clinical practice', *Journal of Allied Health*, February, pages 23–27.

Henry, J N (1985a). 'Identifying problems in clinical problem solving: Perceptions and interventions with non-problem-solving clinical behaviours', *Physical Therapy*, 65, 1071–74.

Henry, J N (1985b). 'Using feedback and evaluation effectively in clinical supervision', *Physical Therapy*, 65, 354–357.

Higgs, J (1992). 'Managing clinical education: The educator-manager and the self-directed learner', *Physiotherapy*, 78, 11, 822–828.

Higgs J, Glendinning M, Dunsford F, Panter J (1991). 'Goals and components of clinical education in the allied health professions', *Proceedings of the World Confederation for Physical Therapy 11th International Congress*, WCPT, London, pages 305–307.

Holmes, B (1975). 'The compleat physiotherapist', *Physiotherapy Canada*, 27, 90–91.

Holzman, G B (1982). 'Clinical simulation', in: Cox, K R and Ewan, C E, *The Medical Teacher*, Churchill Livingstone, Edinburgh, chapter 27.

Irby, D M (1978). 'Clinical teacher effectiveness in medicine', *Journal of Medical Education*, 53, 808–815.

Irby, D M (1983). 'Evaluating instruction in medical education', *Journal of Medical Education*, 58, 844–849.

Jacobson, B F (1978). 'Characteristics of physical therapy role models', *Physical Therapy*, 58, 560–566.

Kahn, E, Lass, S L, Hartley, R and Kornreich, H K (1981). 'Affective learning in medical education', *Journal of Medical Education*, 56, 646–652.

Kern, B P and Mickelson, J M (1971). 'The development and use of an evaluation instrument for clinical education', *Physical Therapy*, 51, 540–546.

Koontz, H, O'Donnell, C and Weihrich, H (1982). *Essentials of Management* (3rd edn) McGraw-Hill, New York, page 9.

Levin, M F and Riley, E J (1984). 'Effectiveness of teaching interviewing and communication skills to physiotherapy students', *Physiotherapy Canada*, 36, 190–194.

Madaus, G F, Scriven, M S and Stufflebeam, D L (1983). *Evaluation Models*, Kluwer-Nijoff, Boston.

Marcoux, B and Pinkston, D (1984). 'Clinical experience and cognition of a physical therapy procedure', *Physical Therapy*, 64, 1545–48.

May, B J (1978). 'Competency-based evaluation of student performance', *Journal of Allied Health*, summer, 232–237.

McCoy, M P (1991). 'Assessment of clinical competence of physiotherapy students', *Proceedings of the World Confederation for Physical Therapy 11th International Congress*, WCPT, London, pages 312–314.

Morgan, W L (1986). 'The environment for general education', *Journal of Medical Education*, 61, 47–59.

Nadler, D A and Tusham, M (1979). 'A congruence model for diagnosing organizational behaviour', in: Kolb, D A, Rubin, IM and McIntyre, J M (eds) *Organizational Psychology: An experiential approach* (3rd edn) Prentice-Hall, New Jersey, pages 443–458.

Oppelaar, L, Bleys, F C and Gerritsma, J G M (1983). 'Use of stimulation techniques in an intermediate course linking up preclinical and clinical students', *Medical Teacher*, 5, 96–102.

Palmer, P B, Henry, J N and Rohe, D A (1985). 'Effect of vidoetape replay on the quality and accuracy of student self evaluation', *Physical Therapy*, 65, 497–501.

Pratt, J W and Seddon, V (1979). 'Sensitivity training with pre-clinical students', *Physiotherapy*, 65, 10, 310–311.

Romanini, J and Higgs, J (1989). 'The teacher as manager in continuing and professional education', *Studies in Continuing Education*, 13, 41–52.

Romiszowski, A J (1970). *A Systems Approach to Education and Training*, Kogan Page, London.

Rotem, A and Bandaranayake, R (1983). 'How to plan and conduct programme evaluation', *Medical Teacher*, 5, 127–131.

Rubin, I (1980). 'Team development', in: Schenke, R (ed) *The Physician in Management*, The American Academy of Medical Directors, Virginia, chapter 19.

Sasmor, J L (1984). 'Contracting for clinical', *Journal of Nursing Education*, **23**, 171–173.

Stritter, F T, Hain, J D and Grimes, D A (1975). 'Clinical teaching re-examined', *Journal of Medical Education*, **50**, 876–881.

Stufflebeam, D L (1983). 'The CIPP model for program evaluation', in: Madaus, G F, Scriven, M S and Stufflebeam, D L (eds) *Evaluation Models*, Kluwer-Nijoff, Boston, pages 117–142.

Torbert, W R (1978). 'Educating toward shared purpose, self-direction and quality work — the theory and practice of liberating structure', *Journal of Higher Education*, **49**, 109–135.

Von Bertalanffy, L (1969). 'The theory of open systems in physics and biology' in: Emery, F E (ed) *Systems Thinking*, Penguin Books, Middlesex, chapter 4.

Watts, N T (1990). *Handbook of Clinical Teaching*, Churchill Livingstone, Edinburgh.

Wells, P A and Lessard, E (1986). 'Survey of student clinical practice', *Physical Therapy*, **66**, 551–554.

Role Modeling Behaviors and the Effective Clinical Teacher

Rewards of Teaching Physical Therapy Students: Clinical Instructor's Perspective

Jan Gwyer, PhD, PT

ABSTRACT: *Physical therapy clinical instructors were surveyed to determine the most important factors influencing their decision to continue to participate in clinical teaching. Three hundred forty-nine clinical instructors from five types of clinical settings rated 34 items in terms of their importance as rewards for clinical teaching. Six categories of rewards for clinical teaching were identified: intellectual stimulation, professional rewards, adjunct university amenities, status, altruistic motivations, and enhanced self-image. Intangible rewards associated with altruistic motivations and intellectual stimulation were rated substantially higher than were tangible rewards associated with use of university facilities or financial compensation for teaching.*

INTRODUCTION

In physical therapy education, the clinical education portion of the professional curriculum comprises, on average, 30% of the total number of weeks in the curriculum.[1] Students spend these hours under the direct supervision of clinical instructors (CIs) who are physical therapists in various health care settings. The complex administrative and educational relationships between the academic institutions and these approved clinical education centers have been described in the literature.[2-6]

A more detailed understanding of the CI's motivation to teach students in the clinic has yet to be described. This is of interest to the profession as we experience changes in health care reimbursement and as the ability to support professional educational costs decreases.[7] Information on the reward structure associated with clinical teaching will assist in planning for clinical education in the future and may lend insight into the job satisfaction of physical therapists.

Physical therapy clinical education in the United States includes a system of exchanges of costs and benefits between academic edu-

cation programs and clinical education centers.[8-11] The costs of clinical education are borne by the clinical center, the educational institution, and the student. The benefits accrue to the institutions involved, the students, and the CIs.

The benefits of clinical education to CIs can be categorized as either tangible or intangible; the former consists of direct benefits and resource exchanges, and the latter consists of professional or social exchanges that result in increased satisfaction.

Educational institutions have developed numerous methods to compensate either the clinical center or the CI directly for their participation in the clinical education program. The tangible benefits range from continuing education tuition vouchers for CIs or continuing education provided by university faculty, to discounts on purchases from university stores. The purpose of these benefits is to provide a desired and tangible reward to the CIs within the resources of the institution. As financial resources of educational institutions decrease and the number of clinical education centers grows, the range and quantity of these tangible benefits may decrease.

Intangible motivators for CIs include fulfilling a sense of responsibility and commitment to the profession, continuing learning by teaching students, and improving the quality of care to patients.[12] Clinical instructors find preparing for and implementing a clinical education program to be an excellent mechanism to remain current.[9]

A better understanding of which types of rewards and benefits are most meaningful to CIs is important as the educational institution's ability to provide tangible rewards

decreases. Clinical education programs rely on the personal commitment of each CI. An understanding of how best to foster that commitment is important to physical therapy educators. This descriptive study examined the relative importance of various benefits and rewards of teaching physical therapy students in the clinic.

METHOD

Subjects

A sample of CIs for this study was constructed in a two-stage sampling design. The academic coordinators for clinical education (ACCEs) at all entry-level physical therapy education programs accredited in January 1990 were contacted by mail in the first stage (n=122). Each ACCE was asked to identify, in a random fashion, one affiliating clinical education center in each of five practice settings: hospital (larger than 500 beds), hospital (smaller than 500 beds), inpatient rehabilitation, outpatient clinic (specialized or general practice), long-term care (skilled nursing), and home health.

The subjects were stratified by practice setting to allow for the varied influence of practice setting on attitudes of clinical instructors toward the benefits of clinical teaching. The five categories of practice setting represented the most frequently used clinical education practice settings in the United States.[6]

The names and addresses of the center coordinators for clinical education (CCCEs) at these five centers were returned to the investigator. Seventy percent of the ACCEs responded, submitting an unduplicated total

Dr Gwyer is Assistant Professor and Director of Graduate Studies, Graduate Program in Physical Therapy, Duke University Medical Center, Box 3965, Durham, NC 27710.

Table 1

Frequency of Respondents by Practice Setting

Practice Setting	Percentage of Respondents
Hospital (>500 beds)	19
Hospital (<500 beds)	24
Inpatient rehabilitation	22
Outpatient clinic, specialized or general practice	22
Long-term care (skilled nursing) or home health	13

Table 2

Frequency of Rating of Importance of Items to Respondents' Decision to Participate in Clinical Education

Item	Rating (%)[a]			
	0	1	2	3
To teach students, I must keep my knowledge and skills up to date; it's good motivation to stay current.	0	1	15	84
Interaction with the student causes me to constantly analyze the care I'm giving my patients.	0	2	18	80
The students stimulate me to learn more.	0	1	19	79
I enjoy one-on-one teaching.	0	2	20	78
Students are appreciative of my teaching efforts.	0	1	24	75
I want to give something back to the profession, and I can do this by teaching students, as someone taught me when I was a student.	0	3	24	73
I have a responsibility to ensure the competence of new professionals entering the field.	0	3	24	72
Students need to see physical therapists working in this practice setting.	0	4	23	72
Teaching students makes my work more interesting and less routine in nature.	0	3	31	65
I feel a professional obligation to teach students.	0	5	30	65
I learn best by teaching others.	0	3	42	54
Student feedback results in an improved level of care for our patients.	2	9	40	49
Students teach me new skills and techniques.	2	8	44	47
I get recognition of my clinical skills from the students.	1	24	53	21
I can call on the academic faculty as resource persons for clinical problems or research projects.	30	17	36	17
I value the prestige of being associated with the university.	21	38	31	10
I appreciate the in-service educational programs the academic faculty provides at my center.	58	13	19	10
I enjoy feeling like an expert in the student's eyes.	0	49	41	9
I am able to use the university library.	42	25	25	8
I receive discounted registration to continuing education sponsored by the university.	66	12	15	6
I can receive financial support from the university for attendance at a continuing education meeting of my choice.	80	9	6	6
I value the books and audiovisual materials given to the center by the university.	72	12	11	4
I can have an academic appointment as a member of the clinical faculty of the university.	57	21	18	4
Students help carry the load when we have staff shortages or staff out sick.	14	60	21	4
I can have free tuition for university courses.	82	9	6	4
When I have a student, I actually have more free time to do other things I enjoy at work.	28	53	16	3
I enjoy having the academic faculty members in our clinic occasionally, treating patients and providing coverage during staff vacations.	83	8	7	3
I receive professional resource material from the academic faculty (articles, research abstracts).	72	10	14	3
I am eligible for university and association awards for outstanding clinical teacher.	62	26	10	2
I have access to the university's recreational facilities (pools, athletic fields, etc.)	69	22	7	2
I have access to university sports events.	80	15	3	2
I receive financial support from the university for teaching their students in the clinic.	89	7	3	1
I appreciate the equipment the university has given us or loaned us to use with students.	89	7	3	1
I receive discounts at the university's bookstore.	88	9	2	1

[a] 0=not applicable to me, because to my knowledge, this benefit is not available to me in my center; 1=not at all important to me; or I do not consider this to be a reward for clinical teaching; 2=somewhat important to me; or I do consider this to be a reward, but of limited value to me; 3=very important to me; or I consider this to be one of the most valued rewards I receive from clinical teaching.

of 400 CIs as subjects for the study. This mechanism of sampling, while subject to bias, was the most appropriate manner of selecting a nationwide sample of CIs, as no national sampling frame of clinical education sites or CIs existed.

Instrument

A self-administered mail questionnaire was developed for this study, comprised of 34 statements of potential benefits or rewards for CIs identified in the literature. The questionnaire was pretested with five CIs (nonsample participants) in each practice setting and was revised based on their feedback. The respondents were asked to rate how important each item was to their personal decision to continue to participate in clinical teaching.

A 3-point scale was developed with the following ratings: 1=not at all important, or I do not consider this to be a reward; 2=somewhat important, or I do consider this to be a reward but of limited value to me; and 3=very important, or I consider this to be one of the most valued rewards I receive from clinical teaching. Because some benefits are not offered at all centers, a "not applicable" rating (0) was provided. In addition, data describing the respondent's age, gender, entry-level physical therapy education, highest earned degree, work status, CI experience, and practice setting were collected.

Data Collection

The mail questionnaire was sent to the 400 CCCEs, with the instructions that they should complete the questionnaire only if they had personally served as a CI for a student within the past year. If they were not qualified, they were asked to randomly select an active CI in their center to complete the questionnaire. One follow-up mailing was performed three weeks after the initial mailing.

Data Analysis

Data were analyzed using the Statistical Analysis System.* Descriptive statistics were calculated for all scale items and for the demographic data. Significant relationships between practice setting and ratings of each scale item were examined using the Kruskal-Wallis nonparametric analysis of variance test. A conservative level of significance for these inferential tests was set at .01. Factor analysis of the 34 scale items was performed to determine whether common themes existed in the data.

---

*SAS Institute, Inc. Box 8000 SAS Circle, Cary, NC 27512.

RESULTS

Three hundred forty-nine usable responses were received (87%). Eighty-two percent of the responding CIs were women. The mean age of the respondents was 33.2 years (SD=6.9), and the mean number of years of experience as a CI was 6.8 (SD=5.1). Almost all of the CIs worked full time (97%).

Eighty-two percent of the CIs were educated at the baccalaureate-degree level in physical therapy, with 9% each at the certificate and master's-degree level. Twenty-six percent of the CIs held a master's degree as their highest earned degree, and one held a doctorate. The stratification of the sample based on work setting functioned to achieve a well-distributed group of respondents (Tab. 1).

The respondents' rating of the 34 scale items is reported in Table 2. The number of respondents for each item ranged from 344 to 349, with very few missing data. More than 75% of the respondents rated the following factors as very important, or some of the most valued rewards they receive from clinical teaching: to teach students, I must keep my knowledge and skills up to date (84%), interaction with the student causes me to constantly analyze the care I'm giving my patients (80%), the students stimulate me to learn more (79%), and I enjoy teaching one on one (78%).

Seven tangible rewards were rated by more than 75% of the respondents as not available to them: financial support for teaching students (89%), equipment loaned from the university (89%), bookstore discounts (88%), having academic faculty in the clinic to treat patients (83%), free tuition for university courses (82%), access to university sports events (80%), and financial support from the university for attendance at continuing education meetings (80%).

Responses to the scale items were analyzed for differences in ratings based on practice setting. In only 2 of the 34 scale items were statistically significant differences found. Clinical instructors in long-term care or home health settings were more likely than CIs in other settings to rate giving something back to the profession ($P=.001$) and teaching students makes my work more interesting ($P=.01$) as somewhat or not at all important in their decision to teach.

The scale items were submitted to a principal components factor analysis with varimax rotation, and six identifiable factors emerged with eigenvalues higher than 1. The factor names and scale item factor loadings are presented in Table 3. Scale items with factor loadings greater than .40 were retained to define the factors.

Table 3
Factor Analysis of 34 Scale Items

Factor	Eigenvalue	Scale Item	Factor Loading
Intellectual stimulation	2.886	Stimulate to learn more	.75
		Stay current	.71
		Analyze patient care	.68
		Work is more interesting	.55
		Improved patient care	.51
		Learn by teaching others	.49
		Students teach me new skills	.44
Professional rewards	2.754	Discount on books	.64
		Financial support for any continuing education	.63
		Free tuition	.59
		Financial support to teach students	.52
		Loan of equipment	.52
		Financial support for university-sponsored continuing education	.46
Adjunct university amenities	1.745	Use of recreational facilities	.57
		Use of library	.55
		Books and audiovisuals given to center	.52
		Access to sports events	.42
		In-service in center by faculty	.40
Status	1.742	Faculty can be resources	.61
		Receive a faculty appointment	.52
		Enjoy prestige	.50
Altruistic motivations	1.398	Give back to the profession	.63
		Professional obligation	.53
		Students need to see practice in this setting	.44
		Responsible to ensure competence	.43
Enhanced self-image	1.241	Feel like an expert in student's eyes	.61
		Gain recognition of skills from student	.47

The first factor represents the rewards associated with the *intellectual stimulation* of teaching students in the clinic. The second factor represents the tangible, *professional rewards* rated by the respondents. Factor three consists of the rewards that accompany association with a university and is termed *adjunct university amenities*. The fourth factor reflects the rewards of increased *status* enjoyed by the CIs. Factor five represents the *altruistic motivations* for clinical teaching held by CIs. The last factor represents the perception of enhanced self-image reported by the CIs.

To assess the relative importance of the factors, the average frequencies with which each item comprising the factors was rated as a very important reward are summarized in Table 4. The items comprising the factors "altruistic motivations" and "intellectual stimulation" were rated as very important with the highest frequency.

DISCUSSION

The CI respondents in this study were similar in demographic characteristics to previous studies of CIs in physical therapy.[13] The typical CI is a 33-year-old woman, is educated in physical therapy at the baccalaureate-degree level, and works full time.

The respondents' rating of the importance or perceived reward of these items provides a current assessment of the existence and value of previously cited benefits of participation in clinical education activities. Although an exchange of tangible benefits is cited in the literature,[7,11] over 80% of these respondents stated that free university tuition, discounts on books, financial support for continuing education, financial support for teaching students, loan of equipment, and access to university sports events were not available to them. Fourteen of the 18 tangible benefits were rated as not available by over 50% of the respondents.

The lack of availability of many of the tangible rewards of clinical teaching may reflect the geographic proximity of the clinical site to the school. Individual CIs also may be unaware of the tangible benefits available to them. The study respondents were not

Table 4

Average Frequency With Which Items in Each Factor Were Rated as "Very Important"

Factor	Frequency
Altruistic motivations	70
Intellectual stimulation	65
Enhanced self-image	15
Status	10
Adjunct university amenities	5
Professional rewards	3

asked to identify themselves as either CCCEs/CIs or CIs, so it is not possible to determine whether their role had an influence on their awareness of the benefits available to them.

Several of the tangible rewards that were available to CIs, however, received consistently low ratings of importance. Library facilities were rated, as available to 58% of the respondents; however, only 8% rated this item as very important. Similarly, academic appointments and eligibility for awards were available to 43% and 38% of the respondents, respectively, but these were rated as important by only 4% and 2%, respectively.

The intangible benefits were uniformly rated higher than the tangible benefits. All but two intangible benefits were rated as very important by over 45% of the respondents: I enjoy feeling like an expert in the student's eyes (9%), and I get recognition of my clinical skills from the students (21%). These two items comprised the "enhanced self-image" factor and had a mean very important frequency rating of 15%.

The factor analysis provided a categorization of rewards that simplifies the discussion of variables important to a physical therapist's decision to continue to participate in clinical teaching. Three of the factors represent intangible rewards: intellectual stimulation, altruistic motivations, and enhanced self-image. Two of the factors represent tangible rewards: professional rewards and adjunct university amenities. The fourth factor, status, is a combination of two tangible rewards (receiving a faculty appointment and having faculty available as resources) and one intangible reward (valuing the prestige of being associated with a university).

In comparing the relative importance of the six factors in determining a clinician's continuing participation in clinical teaching, the three intangible factors were rated higher than the tangible or mixed factors. Of the intangible rewards, altruistic motivations and intellectual stimulation were routinely rated much higher than was enhanced self-image. This latter factor does not appear to describe identified needs of CIs or needs that are met through clinical teaching.

These data support the conclusion that CIs continue to participate as clinical teachers largely because of a sense of responsibility and obligation to the profession and to the student, and because of the intellectual stimulation that surrounds the clinical teaching experience. These findings support the future of our current model of clinical education, which depends heavily on the CI as an important resource in determining the quality of the learning experience. Academic educators can reinforce the perceived benefits of clinical teaching during the entry-level curriculum by helping students develop teaching skills and by acknowledging clinical teaching as a valuable professional development activity that can promote continued competency and learning for physical therapists.

Clinical administrators may use this information to justify their center's participation in clinical education, as CIs appear to be practitioners who are motivated to remain current and who seek intellectual stimulation. ACCEs may emphasize these intangible benefits more strongly with new CIs and increase their use of methods acknowledging and reinforcing the personal commitment made by experienced CIs.

CONCLUSION

Clinical instructors in physical therapy rated the importance of various items to their decision to participate in clinical education. Six factors were identified that included tangible and intangible rewards for clinical teaching. Intangible rewards, including altruistic motivations and a sense of intellectual stimulation, were rated frequently as very important rewards. Tangible rewards were not rated as important to the CIs' participation in clinical education. Academic and clinical educators may use these data to discuss appropriate resources to share in creating the needed reward structure for clinical teachers.

REFERENCES

1. *Physical Therapy Education*. Alexandria, VA: American Physical Therapy Association Department of Education; 1991.
2. Windom PA. Developing a clinical education program from the clinician's perspective. *Phys. Ther.* 1982;62:1604–1609.
3. Kondella PM, Darnell RE. Trends in compensation and benefits provided to physical therapy students during clinical education. *Phys. Ther.* 1979;59:1234–1237.
4. Perry JF. Model for designing clinical education. *Phys. Ther.* 1981;61:1427–1432.
5. Gandy JS. Fiscal implications for clinical education. In: *Pivotal Issues in Clinical Education: Present Status/Future Needs*. Alexandria, VA: American Physical Therapy Association; 1988.
6. Myers RS. *Current Patterns for Providing Clinical Education in Physical Therapy Education*. Alexandria, VA: American Physical Therapy Association; 1985.
7. Holder L. Paying for clinical education: fact or fiction? *J Allied Health*. 1988;17:221–229.
8. Moore, ML, Perry JF. *Clinical Education in Physical Therapy: Present Status/Future Needs*. Washington, DC: American Physical Therapy Association; 1976.
9. Baker MA. Rewards and benefits for clinical faculty. In: *Pivotal Issues in Clinical Education: Present Status/Future Needs*. Alexandria, VA: American Physical Therapy Association; 1988.
10. Hawken PL, Hillestad EA. Weighing the costs and the benefits of student education to service agencies; parts 1 and 2. *Nursing and Health Care*. April 1988; 223–227; May 1988; 277–281.
11. Gandy JS, Sanders B. Costs and benefits of clinical education. *Journal of Physical Therapy Education*. 1990;4(2):70–75.
12. Scully RM, Shepard KF. Clinical teaching in physical therapy education: an ethnographic study. *Phys. Ther.* 1983;63:349–358.
13. *Report on the Clinical Education Faculty in Physical Therapy Education: 1985*. Alexandria, VA: American Physical Therapy Association; 1986.

Clinical Educators

"INSIGHTS YOU Can't FIND IN A TEXTBOOK"

t could be said that all physical therapy practitioners are teachers. They teach patients good health behaviors, they teach family caregivers how to assist patients, and they teach each other as clinicians.

Clinical educators will tell you that working with students is a challenge in and of itself. They like to say that working with students keeps you on your toes; that it requires patience and an ability to verbalize the "hows" and "whys" of clinical practice; that successful clinical affiliations take time, practice, and an ability to relinquish full control of patient care. Whether it's a love of teaching or practice that drives them, clinical educators seem to genuinely enjoy having a hand in crafting a student's practical and clinical skills.

Explains Susan Serbinski, PT, a Center Coordinator of Clinical Education (CCCE) at Cook County Hospital in Chicago, "Working with students brings you back to basics." Serbinski, who was a clinical instructor (CI) at the hospital until assuming the role of CCCE last March, finds that her background as a physical education instructor helped make the transition to clinical educator easier once she became a physical therapist. "Teaching keeps my

As part of this month's focus on education, PT looks at the clinical educator, the person who takes a student's classroom experiences and applies them to the "real world" of patient care.

skills fresh. It motivates me and keeps my enthusiasm going," she says.

As part of her responsibilities as CCCE, Serbinski coordinates the CIs on staff, maintains contracts with 7 to 10 schools of physical therapy, arranges continuing education and inservice programs for staff, selects instructors who will best fit students'

by Beth Monahan

needs, fills in as an instructor in the general acute care department, and treats patients in her specialty area, foot care. "I have to be a generalist in my position," she says. "But I have the best of both worlds; I get to work with students and also treat patients."

At Ranchos Los Amigos Medical Center in Downey, Calif, physical therapist Debbie Diaz claims her position is "the best job we have here." As a Physical Therapy Instructor who supervises 22 CIs in the spinal injury service, Diaz is responsible for orienting all new staff to the service and supervising 33 of the 100 students who walk through Ranchos' doors each year. (Three other Physical Therapy Instructors teach the remaining students in other diagnostic-related treatment areas.) Diaz also teaches observational gait analysis at inservice programs and outside workshops.

With four new students starting clinical affiliations with her every 6 weeks, Diaz works to find them "experience that is realistically close to what they will face in practice." Her goal by the end of each affiliation is to have students working with six to eight patients, roughly a full caseload. "The most rewarding part of my job is seeing students leave our facility as professionals,"

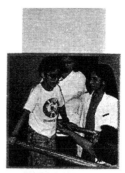

Clinical instructor
Carmen Abril (kneeling)

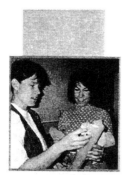

Clinical instructor Debbie Diaz (right)
with USC intern Karen Gosling

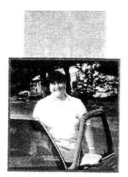

Home health PT and clinical instructor
Marla Tonseth

she says. "I especially enjoy working with students who are having difficulty mastering their clinical skills, working first to identify what the problem is and then to help the students apply what they've learned in school. For many students, success in the clinic is often a matter of building confidence, not competence, in their hands-on abilities."

As the sole proprietor of a subcontract-based private practice in Warminster, Pa, Marla Tonseth, MBA, PT, is both a CI for students at Temple University and a CCCE for her one-person practice. Most of her contracts are for people in home health and nursing homes, but she also has a contract with Bucks County, which includes treating patients at a maximum-security prison. "I have very fond memories of my own affiliations and the challenges they presented, and I wanted to give some of that back," she says. "Certainly, going to a prison as part of your first clinical affiliation is unique, but every clinical affiliation presents new challenges."

Tonseth says that in her role as a home health CI, her main objective is to teach students adaptation skills and to supervise range-of-motion testing, goniometric measurement, and gait training. "The setup in a patient's home is never as ideal as it is in a hospital, so I have to teach students adaptation, creative thinking, and safety—how to make the home safe for patients and also accomplish goals as a clinician despite the limitations."

Part of the reason Tonseth likes taking students on their first affiliation is that "my practice doesn't offer enough autonomy for senior students, and I wouldn't want to stifle anyone as a clinician. I can offer students a learning experience that provides constant

feedback and consistency, which is great for students in their early learning experiences." Although she acknowledges that working with students involves more preparation time, she says it's also a lot of fun. "As a clinical instructor, you are being challenged, so you're getting back what you're giving."

Carmen Abril, a private practitioner in San Juan, Puerto Rico, feels she is doing her part to help ease the shortage of physical therapists in her homeland. "Puerto Rico is losing many therapists to the United States because the salaries here are two to three times less, which makes it hard to retain new therapists and recruit new clinical instructors." Abril was a faculty member at the University of Puerto Rico before starting her own practice 10 years ago; she now works with two students per semester at her facility.

A specialist for children with brain injury, Abril works to provide students with a broad overview of her area of practice. From evaluation in the home to training family members to shopping for adaptive equipment for the client, she says the rewards of being a CI are twofold: Having a student in her clinic helps her organize both her thoughts and her paperwork. "In the end, it makes me much more organized and efficient," she says. "Plus, I always feel the need to review the literature more when I'm working with a student, so it's a great educational motivator."

Abril says she chose to bring students to her pediatric practice "out of a responsibility to my profession. I also wanted to share the insights I've gained from working with patients over the years, insights that you can't find in a textbook."

As one of the Academic Coordinators of

Clinical Education (ACCE) for Boston University (BU), physical therapist Nancy Peatman's job is to ensure that BU students are placed in clinical experiences that will 1) give them well-rounded exposure to physical therapy, 2) help them develop clinical decision-making skills, and 3) foster socialization into the profession. She also acts as BU's representative to clinical sites across the US and keeps the sites informed of where the students are academically. With 100 students in each graduating class, Peatman's schedule gets "a little crazed" juggling the tasks of visiting sites, interviewing students about their clinical "wish lists," coordinating affiliation arrangements, and checking up on students who are already onsite. She also co-teaches a professional issues course at the University and develops clinical education policies and procedures for the physical therapy department.

As both matchmaker and troubleshooter for BU, Peatman is the one who students and CCCEs contact when there is difficulty on a clinical affiliation. "We choose sites that have an interest in educating students, not sites that want students simply because they're short-staffed. Sometimes students or CIs find that they need assistance during the affiliation; then it's my job to go in and problem-solve with the student, the CI, and the CCCE." On the academic side, Peatman also brings site feedback to the University on areas for improving student curriculum.

Peatman, who also developed the clinical education program as the ACCE for the University of Massachusetts in Lowell, finds it a pleasure to work for academic institutions "that place a high value on clinical education."

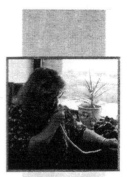

Nancy Peatman, an ACCE at Boston University

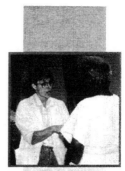

Cook County Hospital's CCCE Susan Serbinski

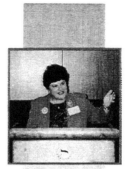

Former clinical educator Meredith Drench

Collaborative Learning

With only 5,500 clinical sites in the US and more than 12,000 students of physical therapy (who will each have three to four affiliations), a recent trend in large institutions is toward a 2:1 or 3:1 ratio of students to CIs. With these models, the CI typically gives up his or her caseload to 2 or more students and then supervises the treatment plan. Despite some early reservations from both clinicians and students, these alternative models appear to be working successfully.

"We were responding to a double-edged sword," says Serbinski. "We would cry to the schools that we needed bigger classes, but then we didn't have enough sites to send students to for their clinicals." Although the 2:1 model was a logical solution, "trying to sell the CIs here on the 2:1 model took some time because many felt that they could not teach as effectively when they had responsibility for more than one student." She adds that the 2:1 model has worked well in her main department and has been tried in the intensive care unit on a limited basis.

At Boston University, students are being sent to an increasing number of clinical sites in which the new model is being utilized, notes Peatman. "Students are telling us they like the collaboration with one another and with the CI. The CIs are reporting that the model is time-intensive at the beginning of the affiliation, but evens out in the end as students learn to problem-solve for themselves. The model is effective because collaboration reinforces adult learning patterns."

Now in its first year of the 2:1 model, the spinal injury service at Ranchos Los Amigos has made the transition fairly smoothly, says Diaz. "Initially I had some hesitations about it, but now we've all adjusted well. We've found that it's much more true-to-life because PTs rarely have only one supervisor at a facility; we're always working collaboratively."

Other Rewards

One of the added benefits of being a clinical educator is the potential to see future practitioners in action on a trial basis. Tonseth, Abril, and Serbinski all were recruited for their first job by one of their clinical affiliations. Says Tonseth, "It gives the person in charge of hiring you a chance to look you over for 4 to 8 weeks to see how your clinical skills improve, if you mesh with the other staff, if your paperwork is acceptable, and if the patients like you. Clinical affiliations are one of the best ways to know exactly what you're getting as a future employer."

Clinical educators also have the satisfaction of seeing some of their former students pass on the tradition by becoming clinical educators themselves. "It's rewarding to think that, as a clinical instructor, you may have had a hand in recruiting another teacher into the profession," says Abril.

The Future

What will it take to attract more clinical educators into the profession? According to Meredith Drench, PhD, PT, who over the years has been a CI, a CCCE, and an ACCE and who now runs her own consulting practice, "It's going to take more nurturing of good teachers, more clinicians who are given the opportunity to work with students." (For more on Drench, see "Clinical Education: The Academic-Clinical Faculty Exchange Model," page 74.)

"Clinical educators need to know how to assess a student's needs, much like they would assess a patient's needs. They must be able to establish learning objectives, plan learning experiences based on a student's educational needs and level of learning, and evaluate student performance outcomes. Too many people in our profession underestimate their ability to transfer patient assessment skills to teaching students.

"To those who say that they can't become a clinical educator because their focus is on pediatrics, sports medicine, manual therapy, or any other specialty field, I say, 'There's room for students in all of those areas.' Students travel from clinic to clinic much like ambassadors. They bring something new to our patients and to us."
—*Beth Monahan is Associate Editor—News/Photo Editor*

For More Information
Collaborative efforts in clinical education have resulted in the formation of clinicial education consortia. To date, 30 such groups exist for ACCEs, CIs, and CCCEs at the statewide or regional level. For information on the consortium nearest you, call APTA's Department of Education at 800/999-2782, ext 3203.

Research Being Gathered on Why PTs Become Clinical Educators

Kelli Koga, PT, currently is writing her master's thesis on factors that influence whether clinicians participate in clinical education. Koga chose the project after an extensive literature review turned up a great deal of data on the medical profession, but none on physical therapy. Koga's thesis for the University of Health Sciences at the Chicago Medical School will be completed this spring.

Role Modeling for Clinical Educators

Ellen Richter Ettinger, O.D., M.S.

Abstract:

Role modeling is a basic component of the educational process. In order to become better role models, clinical educators should be conscious of the behaviors they demonstrate, and the broad range of activities and attitudes that students observe and emulate.

Key Words: Role model, teaching by example, professional demeanor.

Introduction

Students learn from what they see. Do clinical educators serve as positive role models?

Research has shown the significance of role modeling in the development of professionals in many areas. In medicine,[1-3] nursing,[4] administration,[5] and education,[6-8] for example, the impact of role modeling has been recognized. A program at the Indiana University School of Medicine[1] presented faculty members, staff, students, and administrators with an opportunity to discuss and share thoughts, attitudes and techniques of role modeling. It was hoped that following the program, "the participants would be more cognizant of their influence as role models and would be motivated to become better role models."

Role modeling is a basic component of the learning process. As students observe clinical educators, they learn more about how a health professional

Dr. Ettinger is associate professor at the State University of New York—State College of Optometry. This paper was presented at the American Academy of Optometry meeting in December 1990.

works and behaves, and as they observe, they begin to emulate what they see. The basic definition of role modeling (Table 1) is a function of teaching by example. The clinical educator teaches, in part, by *demonstrating* polished clinical skills, sharp analytical reasoning, effective decision-making, comprehensive record-keeping, and caring doctor-patient interactions. The student looks to the educator, in a position of authority, and learns how one functions as a clinician.

Educators are not always aware of the influence that they have, by their example, in developing their students' skills, competence and professionalism. Although faculty members may be *most* conscious of demonstrating good clinical care, the student may be observing many other aspects of the clinican's behavior and performance, as well. By virtue of their authorized and respected position as educators, they may be looked upon as examples and models of how the clinician should act; their behaviors, attitudes and actions are looked upon as standards.

It should be noted that role models can be positive or negative. The educator who approaches patient care hurriedly, who writes incomplete records, or who acts insensitively to patients is as much an example to students as the one who demonstrates patience, competence, and sensitivity. Even if they are carried out inadvertently, the former behaviors can be seen by students and mistakenly interpreted as appropriate, usual, acceptable professional responses.

To students, interns, and residents, the manner in which educators carry themselves is a reflection of the profession; as students learn more about the clinical discipline they are entering, doctors with whom they come into contact are likely to be used in the formation of the image they develop of their profession.

By becoming more aware of their influence as role models, clinical educators can be more conscious of (1) the behaviors they demonstrate, (2) the broad range of activities that students observe in authority figures, and (3) improvements they can make to become better role models.

Role Modeling vs. Mentoring

The terms role modeling and mentoring are often used synonymously, although there are some important differences (Table 1). The role model is a person who is observed by others, as an example. In theory, a learner may watch someone's actions and performance intently, without ever speaking to that person individually. (Athletes and prominent leaders, for example, are often thought of as role models for children, although they may never meet in

---

TABLE 1
Terms Associated With Modeling

Role Model — a person in a position to set an example for others (usually someone in a position of authority).

Mentor — an expert in a particular field (or fields) who works to develop the skills and abilities of another person.

Mentee — the person who works, under the guidance of a mentor, to develop his or her skills.

---

person). In addition, the person functioning as the role model may not always be aware that he or she is being observed, and may not be conscious of all the behaviors that are being monitored. Thus, whether or not the role model is aware of it, his or her function as model continues because the observer is watching.

The mentor[9,10] is an expert who spends designated time with a learner, the mentee. He or she is usually very observant in identifying the mentee's strengths and weaknesses, and helpful in providing direction and support. The mentor must be accessible to meet with the mentee, and provides guidance and feedback.

One may serve as both a mentor and a role model, if both functions are carried out; the two terms, however, are not equal and there are important characteristics that differentiate them. Mentoring is more of an *active* process, in which the mentor deliberately takes the time to meet with the mentee to work on specific skills or projects. Role modeling, on the other hand, frequently is more of a *passive* process on the side of the professional. By virtue of his or her position, the role model is observed by the student, who learns from the model's example, *whether or not the model is conscious of this.*

Within institutions of clinical education, there are many faculty members who take on the active responsibility as trusted mentors. *All* faculty members, however, have a significant—though not always obvious—function as role models. Students are attentive onlookers, carefully analyzing, and often "shadowing," emulating, echoing, imitating and following the actions, attitudes, and behaviors they observe.

Components of Role Modeling for the Clinical Educator

1. *Clinical Competence* — The clinical educator must emit a strong sense of competence, confidence and proficiency in the clinic. There is no substitute for competence. The educator must consistently demonstrate mastery and facility in carrying out clinical tests, analyzing test results, and advising patients.

The educator should demonstrate the act of being a "life-long" learner. By bringing recent articles and journals into the clinic, applying relevant findings from the current literature to patient care, discussing continuing education lectures they have attended, and describing other post-graduate learning experiences, the educator can show, by example, that the most capable clinician is one who continues to learn throughout the years of one's professional career.

2. *Professional Demeanor* — Everything the educator says or does in the clinic can be interpreted by students as a model of how one *ought* to act. From the way he or she dresses, to the attitudes displayed towards patients, the educator reflects an image of appropriate conduct and behavior for the clinician. Areas of professional demeanor that students observe include:

- Appearance and dress
- Attitudes towards patients and students
- Punctuality
- Attendance Record
- Organization of equipment, records and physical space
- Clinical habits

What sense of professional conduct does the clinical teacher display? By watching the instructors in their clinics, students build on their developing image of how one should practice as a health professional. Does the educator arrive on time for clinical care and proceed in a timely manner? Does he or she introduce him- or herself to the patient personally, and appear open and receptive to patient concerns? Does he or she maintain an organized examination room, with a neat working space and clean equipment? Does he or she always display good clinical habits, such as washing hands between patients?

The educator must demonstrate a sense of professionalism.

One of the best ways students have of learning about "professionalism" is by watching doctors in the clinic. It would be difficult to start a course in the didactic curriculum of our schools and colleges of optometry called "Professionalism 101: A Guide to Professional Conduct." Such a course would probably only be able to touch the surface of certain clinical practices which may seem logical and obvious, but which are not always carried out, in the ideal form, in reality. Discussing these areas may be beneficial, but what students discuss in theory is not always applied, in practice. By observing appropriate professional behavior in the clinic, students gain a sense of *how* these behaviors fit in with the delivery of clinical care.

The education of professionalism is probably taught very effectively where it can be observed and applied most readily and directly - in the clinic.

3. *Doctor-Patient Interactions* — It has been said that "patients don't care how much you know, until they know how much you care."

Experienced clinicians know that the effectiveness of the doctor-patient relationship can actually elevate the quality of the care provided by making the patient more relaxed, cooperative, responsive and confident in the doctor. The level of patient compliance also may be enhanced.

When they first start working in the clinics, students are often more concerned with the mechanical aspects of clinical care than with their communication skills and interpersonal interactions; their ability to reach patients, however, relies so heavily upon their ability to form a successful doctor-patient rapport. In addition to mastering the technical and analytical components of clinical care, students also must recognize how important it is to provide a supportive, sensitive environment for their patients, and to exhibit caring, compassionate attitudes.

All patients deserve sensitive, humane, compassionate health care. By demonstrating these qualities *in our own actions,* clinical educators can help our students learn more about the art of caring for patients.

4. *Ethical Values* — One of the difficulties of teaching medical ethics is that it would be difficult to present every situation and decision that students will ever encounter in their careers; even if one could do so, it would be inappropriate to establish "correct responses" or "standard answers" because the area of ethics involves deeply personal decisions. One cannot dictate the decisions of others; however, one can *demonstrate* the *processes* of ethical decision-making and clinical performance as students train in the health care environment.

Educators must be respectable (worthy of the respect of others) and respectful (showing respect to other people). They must display a sense of integrity, honesty, decency and trustworthiness. By demonstrating ethical values in the decisions and recommendations made, instructors can facilitate the development of ethical and moral attitudes in their students.

Areas of medical and biomedical ethics have been examined,[11-15] and there is strong support for educating students about ethics during their clinical training programs.[16-19] As discussed, one way students learn about ethics is by watching their instructors. Educators should be conscious of the messages they convey to students with respect to the following questions.

Do I:

- always act in the best interests of the patient?
- see that my patient has access to all necessary services, and that *only* those services that are necessary for the patient are provided?
- make appropriate referrals, when necessary, and choose competent and qualified referral sources?
- provide the patient with truthful, adequate information about the status of his or her health?
- maintain the confidentiality of my patient's medical status and clinical data?
- stay up-to-date with new clinical and scientific findings so I can provide my patients with modern, high quality clinical care?

5. *Social Consciousness* — Health professionals should care about other individuals, and should possess an interest in the social issues within our society. The economic, social, political, environmental, and medical dilemmas within our communities require involvement and action by those trained in the health professions.

The major focus of clinical education is on the patient-doctor encounter, and the development of good clinical skills. Such attention and rigorous training is appropriate, but often little (or no) attention is given to the social concerns of the community. Students graduate, often in significant debt as a result of the high costs of clinical education, with substantial financial pressures and obligations. Often, though, no notice is paid to the problems of the world. The resulting disposition is frequently referred to as the "me first" generation, or the sentiment of "looking out for number one."

Although new graduates and practicing clinicians must respond to the realistic personal pressures and responsibilities that exist, a sense of concern for humanity, and for the problems of others, must also exist. In the community, the nation, and the world, problems abound. The plight of the homeless, the poor, and the abused continues to grow, and patients with AIDS and other debilitating illnesses look for answers to their daily hurdles. Such challenges within communities warrant the attention of involved individuals.

The development of social consciousness should be part of the education of clinical students. The significance of

faculty role models in demonstrating responsible, committed actions must be recognized. A new "Faculty Committee on Social Concerns and Community Relations" has been established at the State University of New York—State College of Optometry, under the leadership of Dr. Martin Birnbaum, to recognize this facet of clinical education. Faculty on the committee meet to discuss and identify the problems that exist in our area, and they consider how members of our college community can contribute to the needs of our local community. Through special projects (e.g. food and clothing drives, with collection baskets in our lobby; lecture programs on social issues and concerns; volunteer vision screenings and eye care for underserved and needy populations in our vicinity), faculty members demonstrate *through their actions* that aside from being good doctors and educators, they are also concerned citizens.

Summary

Patterning one's behavior after a respected individual is a common behavior. Clinical instructors should be aware of the five important areas, discussed here, in which they serve as role models for their students:

- Clinical Competence
- Professional Demeanor
- Doctor-Patient Interactions
- Ethical Values
- Social Consciousness

Educators should be aware that part of their role, as teachers, is to teach by example.

References

1. Ficklin FL, Browne VL, Powell RC, and Carter JE. "Faculty and House Staff Members as Role Models." *J. Med Educ.* 1988; 63:392-396.
2. Levinson W, Tolle SW, and Lewis C. "Women in Academic Medicine." *N. Engl. J. of Med.* 1989; 321(22):1511-1517.
3. Roeske, NA and Lake K. "Role Models for Women Medical Students." *J. Med. Educ.* 1977; 52:459-66.
4. Erickson HC, Tomlin EM, and Swain MA. *Modeling and Role-Modeling - A Theory and Paradigm for Nursing.* Englewood Cliffs, N.J: Prentice Hall, 1983.
5. Josefowitz N. *Paths to Power.* Reading, MA: Addison-Wesley Publishing, 1980.
6. Eble KE. *The Craft of Teaching.* San Francisco: Jossey-Bass Publishers, 1988.
7. Wilkinson J. "Varieties of Teaching," In: Gullette MM, ed. *The Art and Craft of Teaching.* Cambridge, MA: Harvard University Press, 1984; 19.
8. Wilson RC, Gaff JC, Dienst ER, Wood L, and Bavry JL. *College Professors and Their Impact on Students.* New York: John Wiley and Sons, 1975.
9. Phillips-Jones L. *Mentors and Protegees.* New York: Arbor, 1982.
10. Ettinger, ER. "Reaching for Excellence: Mentoring and Networking." *J. of Amer. Opt. Assoc.* (In press).
11. Warner, R. *Morality in Medicine: An Introduction to Medical Ethics.* Sherman Oaks, California: Alfred Publishing, 1980.
12. Center for Vision Care Policy of the State University of New York - Policy Insight. "Ethical Challenges in the New Optometry." New York: Spring/Summer, 1986.
13. Bulger EB. "The Need for an Ethical Code for Teachers of the Basic Biomedical Sciences." *J. Med. Educ.* 1988; 63:131-133.
14. Dunstan GR, and Shinebourne EA. *Doctor's Decisions - Ethical Conflicts in Medical Practice.* New York: Oxford University Press, 1989.
15. Phillips M and Dawson J. *Doctor's Dilemmas - Medical Ethics and Contemporary Science.* New York: Methuen Inc., 1985.
16. Puckett AC, Doyle GG, Pounds LA and Hash FT. "The Duke University Program for Integrating Ethics and Human Values Into Medical Education." *Acad. Med.* 1989; 64:231-235.
17. Miles SH, Lane LW, Bickel J, Walker RM, and Cassel CK. "Medical Ethics Education: Coming of Age." *Acad. Med.* 1989; 64:705-714.
18. Walker RM, Lane LW, and Siegler M. "Development of a Teaching Program in Clinical Medical Ethics at the University of Chicago." *Acad. Med.* 1989; 64:723-729.
19. Barnard D and Clouser KD. "Teaching Medical Ethics in Its Contexts: Penn State College of Medicine." *Acad. Med.* 1989; 64:743-746.

SCHOLARLY PAPER

Managing Clinical Education:
The Educator-manager and the Self-directed Learner

Joy Higgs

Key Words

Clinical education, self-directed learning, management.

Summary

Clinical educators and learners have important roles in managing clinical education programmes. This paper discusses the roles of clinical educators as facilitators and managers of student learning and the role of students as self-directed learners and co-managers of learning programmes in achieving effective learning in the clinical setting.

Introduction

Clinical education plays a very important part in physiotherapy education. It is in clinical settings that learners can truly appreciate their roles and responsibilities as health care providers and evaluate their readiness for autonomous professional practice after graduation. The clinical environment provides the situational, task and human complexities of the real world as a context for new learning and for the practice and evaluation of previous learning. Both clinical educators as teachers, programme managers and role models, and students as self-directed learners, play critical roles in promoting learning.

Clinical education programmes contribute to the achievement of overall curricular goals. Common goals in physiotherapy education include the development of technical competence, clinical reasoning competence, interpersonal skills, knowledge and self-directed learning skills for lifelong learning. Self-directed learning skills and the ability to perform as adult learners are particularly important attributes of physiotherapy students in this age of rapid technological advancements. They provide learners with the ability to generate

knowledge and skills in order to deal both proactively and responsively with their own learning needs and with changes in society's health care needs.

This paper will examine the role of clinical educators as managers of clinical education programmes and the role of physiotherapy students as self-directed learners in the clinical setting. Several areas of literature will be examined: adult learning and self-directed learning theory, research into student learning, management theory in relation to teaching, and literature dealing with knowledge generation. Proposed roles and responsibilities of teachers and learners will be discussed.

Clinical Teachers as Facilitators and Managers of Student Learning

Facilitating Adult Learning and Self-directed Learning

Clinical educators need to be effective teachers as well as skilled clinicians. This entails becoming facilitators of adult learning since adult learning is highly relevant to achieving the goals of professional education. In addition, the adoption of adult learning and self-directed learning as an educational framework for clinical education creates the need for clinical educators to be viewed as managers of learning. That is, by acting as learning programme managers, educators can create adult learning environments, facilitate adult and self-directed learning, and promote the achievement of learning programme goals. To promote students' self-directed learning, clinical educators need to encourage students to act as co-managers of their learning programmes.

Numerous authors have reported their experiences and hypotheses concerning conditions which facilitate adult learning (Knox, 1977; Bagnall, 1978; Knowles, 1980;

Table 1: Conditions which promote adult learning

Environmental conditions	Decision making/management factors
Motivation	Shared goals
Acceptance of the learner as a person	Mutual decision-making/planning
Freedom/autonomy	Shared management
Individuality	Shared resource acquisition
Emphasis on abilities and experience	Learner involvement in diagnosing learning needs and
Learning via experiences relevant to the learner	evaluating learning
Student-centred learning	Effective communication
Resource rich environment	Choice in participation
Security/support	Collaborative facilitation
Mutual respect/trust	Learner direction in posing questions/seeking answers
Teacher support/facilitation	Ongoing review by teacher and learner
Praxis — integrating theory, practice, experience and	Learner identification of community goals and needs as part of the
reflection in action	context of their own learning
Integrated learning in real-life situations.	Learner acceptance of responsibility
Effective interaction between learners	

Mezirow, 1985; Brookfield, 1986; Engel, 1991; Hammond and Collins, 1991). The work of these authors supports the following contentions. First, it can be argued that a number of (theoretically) 'accepted' conditions which promote adult learning can be identified. These can be subdivided into two groups: environmental conditions and conditions related to the decision-making and management strategies employed in the programme. Table 1 presents these conditions as derived from the work of the authors identified above.

Second, the role of teachers in adult learning programmes is to create these conditions by means of programme management. Learners also have a role in creating these conditions. According to the above authors these conditions result in adult learning behaviours as listed in table 2. These behaviours are highly compatible with the goal of developing effective learning skills and lifelong learning behaviours.

Table 2: Adult learning behaviours

Problem-solving
Experiential learning
Empowered self-direction
Self-correction
Progressive mastery
Active seeking of meaning
Critical reflection
Individual pacing
Active involvement in learning
Interaction with teachers and other learners
Reciprocal learning (with teachers and other learners)
Identifying own learning goals within the context of
    community goals and needs

Long (1990, p 29) argues that 'what lifelong learning seeks to do is to provide a framework within which an individual can reflect on the past and prepare for the future in terms of learning experiences'. As part of this process learners need the ability to cope effectively with change and indeed to initiate change (Tough, 1983). Candy emphasises the strong need for self-directed learning in our education systems as a means of coping with change. He argues:

'Rapid social change and technological changes have become so commonplace that their ability to shock has diminished. . . . However, one thing has remained more or less constant; the limitations to people's ability to cope with change. The effect has been not only to throw into sharp relief our human frailty, but even more to highlight the apparent inadequacy of educational systems to cope with people's hunger for new skills and information' (Candy, 1991, p xiii).

The teacher's role in effective adult learning programmes includes the roles of facilitator (Rogers, 1969) and change agent (Havelock, 1973). The concept of the teacher as a facilitator rather than an information giver is fundamental to adult learning (Candy, 1988a; Heron, 1989). Schon argues that students can be *helped* in their learning. They cannot be *taught* what they need to know to deal with 'the complex, unstable, uncertain, and conflictual worlds of practice' (Schon, 1987, p 12).

Clinial educators are ideally situated to enable students to learn to cope with change, to deal with the complexities of real-world clinical practice, and to develop and satisfy their hunger for new learning. Teachers can use the opportunities provided by a clinical setting (such as real cases) and its realities and constraints (including time pressures). Within this stimulating learning environment clinical teachers can also foster students' inquiry behaviour and help them learn from experience.

The concept of teachers as facilitators includes the ideas of sharing of management, power, control and responsibility for learning with students, and the creation of a learning environment which allows these behaviours to occur. Learning programmes which involve high levels of unilateral decision-making and responsibility by teachers promote learner passivity and dependence. By comparison, programmes which emphasise adult learning facilitate students taking responsibility for their own progress.

In sharing decision-making about programmes with learners, teachers become managers who delegate some power and responsibilities to students by promoting learner self-direction and involving learners in negotiating and managing learning experiences. The success of such endeavour (such as negotiated learning contracts) in the promotion of independent behaviour, cognitive achievement and autonomous learning has been reported in the literature (Tompkins and McGraw, 1988).

Negotiation of learning goals and activities is well suited to clinical settings, for several reason. For instance, in clinical education there are likely to be smaller numbers of students which allows for more individualised programme planning and management. Also the context of a clinic is dynamic and often unpredictable, making it necessary for clinical teachers to work within the limitations of available learning resources and to take advantage of opportunistic learning situations.

Promoting Effective Learning Behaviour

Clinical as well as academic teachers have a major role in creating learning environments which promote effective learning behaviour and meaningful learning. A large body of educational research has been conducted in recent years on the nature of effective student learning and the effects of learning contexts on student approaches to learning (Pask, 1976; Entwistle, 1981; Biggs, 1982). An important focus of this research has been on the differences between deep or meaningful approaches to learning and superficial or rote approaches, and on factors within the learning environment which promote these. According to Ramsden (1988, p 20) 'only through using [deep] approaches can students gain mastery of concepts and a firm hold on detailed factual knowledge in a given subject area' and develop 'imaginative and adaptive skills and the wide sphere of interests that are increasingly demanded in the world of work'.

Entwistle and Ramsden (1983) examined associations between learning environments and student learning. Tertiary students' approaches to learning were found to be influenced by the context in which they were studying. These authors identified that deep approaches occur most often in contexts characterised by freedom in learning, less formality, good teaching input, a good social climate and clear goals. By comparison, surface or rote learning approaches are more likely to be adopted where there are heavy workloads. Clinical environments by their very nature, therefore, provide excellent opportunities to promote deep learning, so long as excessive workloads and a lack of time to process learning experiences are avoided.

As part of their role in creating learning environments which promote meaningful learning, clinical teachers are responsible for managing students' learning experiences. Experiential learning (Kolb, 1984) is at the heart of clinical education. However, clinical experience alone does not guarantee learning. Boud (1988) identifies reflection as being a critical element of experience-based learning. Reflection should occur firstly as a behaviour of learners throughout learning experiences. Second, reflection should be a planned element of experiential learning programmes. This could be accomplished by debriefing sessions, for instance.

Similarly, Schon (1987) contends that we need to be educating 'reflective practitioners'. He argues that it is not enough to teach students how to withdraw from the real world to examine well-structured problems using established research practices. The professional person dealing with and immersed in the 'messiness' of reality (such as occurs in the clinic) needs to develop the ability to cope with the uniqueness, uncertainty and conflict inherent in real problems. Schon contends that professional educational programmes should focus on enhancing students' facility for 'reflection-in-action', that is, reflection during activity. Such reflection helps learners to examine aspects of behaviour and context, and thereby reshape actions as required by the context. Reflection, then, should be an important element of clinical education.

Managing Student Learning in Clinical Education Programmes

Clinical educators have a clear role in programme management and in the management of student learning. The value of applying management principles to education programmes as a means of enhancing the effectiveness of education practice is evident in the literature (Magill *et al*, 1986; Long, 1990). Davies (1971) used the term 'teacher-manager' to describe a teacher's role in terms of managing learning resources. By comparison in this paper the concept of the teacher as manager is used in a broader sense. It focuses on the management of people, on enabling learners to participate in the management of their own learning and on promoting the growth and development of individuals. Particularly in clinical education, clinical educators are ideally situated to empower learners, because of the flexibility of the learning environment, and the close association between students and teachers. This association provides teachers with the opportunity to know in detail the learning needs and strengths of learners and to spend time in providing feedback and encouragement.

The study of leadership and management forms a key part of the exploration of social systems and the management of human resources in organisations and programmes (Gordon, 1977; Hunt, 1979). Leadership or management involves several factors. Managers require the ability to influence people to achieve goals (Robbins, 1979). Leadership involves the art of promoting willing and enthusiastic participation in goal achievement (Koontz *et al*, 1982). In addition, effective managers are able to work both with and through individuals to achieve the goals of the programme or organisation (Hersey and Blanchard, 1982). Thus, there is a clear similarity between managers and teachers of adult learners. The latter seek to facilitate learning by encouraging learners to engage enthusiastically in their learning task, by empowering learners to participate in the management of their own learning and by promoting the learners' growth and development (Romanini and Higgs, 1989).

The first step in learning from leadership/management theory is understanding what it means to be an effective leader/manager. Since the 1960s the dominant leadership theory has been contingency leadership. These theorists aimed to identify situational variables that allowed leader behaviour to be effective in given situations (Evans, 1970; Fiedler, 1971; House and Mitchell, 1974).

Situational leadership is a concept that has particular relevance to education since it seeks to relate leader (or teacher) behaviour to 'follower' (or learner) readiness. The term 'learner task maturity' was developed by the author as part of research into self-directed learning (Higgs, 1991). It refers to a learner's readiness for the specific task in hand. Such task maturity varies with the experience of students as independent learners, with their ability to employ effective approaches to learning, and with their previous experience and success with similar learning tasks.

Where the learners' task maturity is low, teachers need to provide a structure or framework for the learning programme which will 'liberate' the learners' self-directed learning behaviour. For instance, in the clinical setting teachers could begin with close supervision of students' clinical practice, accompanied by positive and constructive feedback, and gradually increase the level of student autonomy as the students gain in competence and confidence.

Where learners' task maturity is high, there is greater scope and need for them to participate in the management of their learning programmes. That is, they are capable of being, and should be encouraged to be, co-managers of the learning programmes. In the clinical setting, once clinical teachers have identified a high level of student competence the next step is to negotiate with the students about which learning goals and activities could best enhance the students' development and experience. The teachers would then allow a higher level of student freedom and risk-taking in learning, while at the same time maintaining supervisory responsibility for the health and well-being of students and patients.

Thus, encouraging development of self-directed learning skills and promoting lifelong learning attitudes and ability does not mean allowing students excessive independence which results in isolation. The clinical setting in particular is one in which it is valuable to promote interdependence in learning and the sharing of knowledge gained from previous experience.

Interdependent learners need to work effectively in groups. This is common in clinical education. The literature provides a rich resource of theory, research and experience-based material which can help educators to promote effective learner interaction or effective group dynamics (McLeish *et al*, 1973; Shaw, 1981). A useful set of characteristics of effective groups was developed by

Likert (1984). These are listed in table 3. Part of a clinical teacher's role is to foster effective group dynamics so that learning can result from effective interactions between participants in the learning programme. In clinical education programmes such players would include teachers, clinicians, learners, patients and their families.

Table 3: Properties and performance characteristics of the ideal highly effective group (Likert, 1984, page 156)

1. The members are skilled in all the various leadership and membership roles and functions required for interaction between leaders and members and between members and other members.

2. The group has been in existence sufficiently long to have developed a well-established, relaxed working relationship among all its members.

3. The members of the group are attracted to it and are loyal to its members, including the leader.

4. The members and leaders have a high degree of confidence and trust in each other.

5. The values and goals of the group are a satisfactory integration and expression of the relevant values and needs of its members. They have helped shape these values and goals and are satisfied with them.

6. In so far as members of the group are performing linking functions, they endeavour to have the values and goals of the groups which they link in harmony, one with the other.

7. The more important a value seems to the group, the greater the likelihood that the individual members will accept it.

8. The members of the group are highly motivated to abide by the major values and to achieve the important goals of the group.

9. All the interaction, problem-solving, decision-making activities of the group occur in a supportive atmosphere.

The Learner's Role in Self-directed Learning and Knowledge Generation in Clinical Education

The ideas of learners' responsibility for their own learning and learner autonomy have been slower in coming to clinical than to academic education. In the same way that clinicians who participate in clinical education have needed to acquire the title and role of educator, the role of physiotherapy students in clinical education has had to change from practising or apprentice clinician to student.

What is expected of physiotherapy students in clinical settings today? Within clinical learning environments which both allow and expect self-directed learning behaviour and learner responsibility, learners need to come to terms with several factors if they are to receive greatest benefit from this opportunity. In preparing for adult learning programmes clinical teachers need to develop an understanding of the nature of self-directed learning and to assess and if necessary redress their readiness for this type of teaching. Their programme planning needs to incorporate adult learning principles and strategies. During programme implementation clinical teachers should participate actively in programme management as well as in learning activities, facilitate student involvement in programme management, and act as effective agents for change.

Understanding Self-directed Learning

Physiotherapy students will be familiar with the idea of professional autonomy as a central concept of professional practice. This term connotes independence in decision-making and action, acceptance of responsibility for actions taken and the demand for accountability towards those who receive the services of the professional.

Self-directed learning by its very nature encourages each of these factors. It can be defined (Higgs, 1988) as an approach to learning in which the behaviour of the learner is characterised by:

● Responsibility for and critical awareness of, his or her own learning process and outcome, and for developing his or her learning abilities.
● Self-direction in performing learning activities and solving problems which are associated with the learning task.
● Active input to decision-making regarding the learning task.
● Learning with and through others (eg teachers and other learners).

Two other aspects of the nature of self-directed learning programmes are especially important from the learner's perspective. The first of these is that learner self-direction does not mean learning in isolation. Rather it is based on internal motivation. While learners may elect to learn by themselves, effective learning usually involves interaction with others. This view is discussed by Griffith (1987) who examined the concept of independence versus interdependence in learning programmes. She stresses the importance of learners valuing the contributions each can make to the other's learning. Similarly, Heron (1989) argues that learners can be self-directing only in reciprocal relations with other self-directed persons.

Learners and teachers also need to realise that self-directed learning does not represent a single mode or pattern of behaviour. Rather, self-directed learning occurs through a number of phases and involves a variety of learner behaviour. Through an investigation of a group of undergraduates, Taylor (1987) identified four phases and phase transitions which occurred during self-directed learning programmes. The phases identified were disorientation, exploration, reorientation and equilibrium. The phase transitions were disconfirmation, naming the problem, reflection and sharing the discovery. Taylor found, for instance, that self-directed learners encountered periods of confusion as well as times when they found their direction again. Similarly, the students needed to learn how to identify problem areas and limitations in knowledge, and to share what was learned with other learners.

When learners are allowed or seek autonomy in learning they become even more accountable for their learning process and outcomes. In the clinical setting students can relate this to taking responsibility for their professional decisions and actions. As part of self-directed learning, students in clinical settings can take responsibility for their learning through actions such as monitoring what they have learned in relation to programme objectives and their own goals, evaluating their clinical performance, identifying their learning needs and seeking assistance from teachers and clinicians to address these needs.

A difficulty can arise in this area if teachers are also assessors. That is, students may be reluctant to seek help in relation to their weaker areas for fear of being 'marked down' by their teachers. This problem needs to be addressed and as far as possible avoided. This can be achieved through appropriate teacher behaviour such as encouraging students to identify learning needs and clearly differentiating between formative and summative assessment sessions. Similarly learners can help in dealing with this problem by negotiating a change to the way the clinical programme is conducted. For instance, a different examiner or a co-examiner could be requested.

Readiness for Self-directed Learning

Another important factor in independent learning contexts is the extent to which learners are ready for the demands and benefits of self-directed learning in the current situation. This readiness is influenced by past and current educational experiences. Learners and clinical teachers have a responsibility to assess and ensure an appropriate level of 'learner task maturity' (Higgs, 1991).

To gain greatest benefit from their clinical education programme learners need to be able to evaluate their level of readiness for the current learning programme. This involves identifying whether they have the required learning skills and experience of related clinical tasks. For instance, have they learned in the classroom or in previous clinical education sessions, the technical skills needed to manage effectively the patients they will encounter in the current session?

A realistic assessment of their own 'task maturity' will enable learners to redress gaps in their learning, to set appropriate learning goals, and to seek assistance from others, especially their clinical teachers. Learners also need to identify what level of autonomy they desire in learning and in clinical practice. It is important to discuss this with clinical teachers to avoid an over-confident approach which may be hazardous to patients or an under-confident, cautious approach which could limit the scope for learning. Students need to develop confidence and a base of experience which will help them know how far to experiment and take risks in their learning without compromising their patients' well-being. They also need to be able to trust their clinical teachers to guide and facilitate them in this endeavour.

Sharing in Learning and in Learning Programme Management

In self-directed learning programmes learners need to take responsibility for their learning by contributing to programme design and content. Griffith's (1987) experience and research in the area of sharing power and creating interdependence in learning situations has led her to the conclusion that both dependent and independent learning situations are limited. Dependent learners are guided by external criteria while independent learners are more inner-directed. She argues that in interdependent learning situations, power becomes a more positive factor through the empowerment of oneself and others. By comparison, dependency situations involve being under the control of another and independence involves striving for control by self.

The question of learners taking control of their learning is not without difficulties. Candy (1987) investigated this question in a review of self-directed learning research (Parlett, 1970; Witkin et al, 1977; Entwistle et al, 1979). He reported that learners have been found to have a limited desire or ability for self-direction and a tendency to seek or rely on direction or external control.

This finding was identified despite other research which found that the majority of adults engage in independent learning activities outside educational institutions (Tough, 1978, 1979; Brookfield, 1982). Candy (1987) concluded that the willingness of learners 'to accept increased control will depend on whether or not, in any particular case, they judge it to be a valid strategy and a situation from which they can learn' (page 174).

In seeking to be effective self-directed learners in the clinical context, therefore, physiotherapy students should address two goals. These are to understand the relevance and effectiveness of self-directed learning approaches and to recognise the value of promoting effective interdependent learning. In practice, this means that learners in clinical education programmes need to assess their learning situations and to determine the value to themselves of learning in an interdependent mode with other learners, the clinical teacher and other clinicians. In addition they need to be able to appreciate the benefits of participating in programme management, including such activities as goal setting and planning of learning activities. Clinical educators play an important part in enabling learners' activities and goals related to self-direction and co-management to succeed. In particular, clinical educators need to adopt a facilitating and empowerment approach to teaching in which the learners are encouraged to share in programme management and to overcome any previous conditioning which encouraged them to act dependently in teacher-controlled situations.

Effecting Change

In becoming a competent clinician and an effective self-directed learner the physiotherapy student becomes an agent of change. Tough (1978) argues that self-planned learning involves people trying to learn and trying to change. Learning then, becomes a means to change oneself, to adapt to external changes or to create external changes. Havelock (1973, page 5) describes a change agent as 'a person who facilitates planned change or planned innovation' by acting as a catalyst, a solution giver, a process helper and a resource linker. In a world of constant change, physiotherapy students need to prepare themselves for each of these change agent roles.

A similar concept to that of the change agent is put forward by Hammond and Collins (1991, page 13) who describe 'critical self-directed learning' as being within the tradition of emancipatory adult education. This approach to learning involves learners who are engaged in meeting their individual needs, being 'informed and guided by a critical analysis of prevailing social needs'. Physiotherapy students need to view their professional development within the context of the society they serve and within the time-frame of lifelong learning. In developing the desire and skills to manage their own learning, students become more able to make sense of their world, to change themselves, and to change the world around them (Candy, 1991).

Seeking and Generating Knowledge

Without adequate knowledge, learning skills and problem-solving skills have limited value. To become effective clinicians, physiotherapy students need to develop a sound knowledge base which is relevant to physiotherapy and is organised into meaningful patterns (Norman, 1990; Grant, 1991).

Knowledge is not something that we discover but is a construction of the human mind (Novak and Gowin, 1984) seeking to make sense of the world. The term knowledge has several meanings. These include objective knowledge or knowledge of the discipline, and subjective knowledge or experiential knowledge which represent the meaning the learner derives from his/her experiences. Polanyi (1958) also identified tacit knowledge which refers to knowledge which is understood, where we know far more than we can put into words and where our understanding is based on an interpretative framework. Each of these types of knowledge is valid and requires testing against other forms of knowledge, against changes in our understanding arising from further learning and against the knowledge of others.

The clinical setting provides an important opportunity for physiotherapy students to generate and test their knowledge and to develop a knowledge base which is sound and well-organised. This can be done by students seeking to discover their own meaning through self-directed learning, and by endeavouring to make sense of their clinical learning experiences. Achieving these goals entails students questioning what they are learning or have learned, reflecting on their thoughts and actions, exploring the validity and effects of different ways of achieving their clinical goals, experimenting with new ideas and discussing thoughts and experiences with others. Reflection on what has been learned is especially valuable. Boud *et al* (1985), for instance, argue that reflection allows learners to bring their ideas to consciousness which enables the evaluation of these ideas. Such evaluation is a necessary part of forming and refining knowledge and determining actions. The importance of reflection in self-directed learning is also stressed by Harris (1989) and Brookfield (1986) who regard reflection as an integral part of the self-directed learner's pursuit of meaning.

The goal of knowledge generation is to attain subject matter autonomy. This term was developed by Candy (1988b) to refer to the ability to make judgements, to determine viewpoints and to be able to defend a position in a given knowledge area. Such subject matter autonomy is vital to today's health professionals. Seeking knowledge in the learning environment is the first step towards achieving the ability to generate knowledge (and skills) throughout one's professional career.

Conclusion

To move from being a clinician to becoming an effective clinical educator requires the development of skills in the facilitation and management of learning. Clinical educators can learn a great deal to assist them in implementing these roles from the literature dealing with adult and self-directed learning, effective student learning in higher education and management theory. In essence the primary roles of clinical educators are to provide competent clinical role models, to facilitate and manage students' learning and to empower students to learn and to take control of and responsibility for their learning.

The combination of an appropriate learning environment and the desire and ability of learners to act as self-directed learners provides the optimal context for effective clinical education. Physiotherapy students may have limited ability to act as self-directed and interdependent learners due to previous conditioning to act passively in teacher-directed situations, or due to their perceptions of potential rewards or punishments for independent learning behaviour. For successful self-directed learning to occur students need to develop an understanding of self-directed learning and of their own readiness for this type of learning, to participate in programme management and to seek knowledge. In this way they will become effective agents for change within their own lives as lifelong learners and within the lives of others as health care professionals.

Author

Joy Higgs PhD GradDipPhty MPHEd is head, School of Physiotherapy, Faculty of Health Sciences, University of Sydney.

Address for Correspondence

Dr J Higgs, Head, School of Physiotherapy, Faculty of Health Sciences, University of Sydney, PO Box 170, Lidcombe, 2141, Australia.

References

Bagnall, R G (1978). 'Principles of adult education in the design and management of instruction', *Australian Journal of Adult Education*, **28**, 19–27.

Biggs, J B (1982). 'Student motivation and study strategies in university and college of advanced education populations', *Higher Education Research and Development*, **1**, 33–55.

Boud, D (1988). 'How to help students learn from experience' in: Cox, K and Ewan, C E (eds) *The Medical Teacher* (2nd edn) Churchill Livingstone, Edinburgh, pages 68–73.

Boud, D, Keogh, R and Walker, D (1985). *Reflection: Turning experience into learning*, Kogan Page, London.

Brookfield, S D (1982). *Independent Adult Learning*, Adults: Psychological and Educational Perspectives No 7, Department of Adult Education, University of Nottingham.

Brookfield, S D (1986). *Understanding and Facilitating Adult Learning*, Jossey-Bass, San Francisco.

Candy, P (1987). 'Evolution, revolution or devolution: Increasing learner-control in the instructional setting' in: Boud, D and Griffin, V (eds) *Appreciating Adults Learning: From the learners' perspective*, Kogan Page, London, pages 159–178.

Candy, P C (1988a). 'Key issues for research in self-directed learning', *Studies in Continuing Education*, **10**, 104–124.

Candy, P (1988b). 'On the attainment of subject-matter autonomy' in: Boud, D (ed) *Developing Student Autonomy in Learning* (2nd edn) Kogan Page, London, pages 59–76.

Candy, P C (1991). *Self-direction for Lifelong Learning: A comprehensive guide to theory and practice*, Jossey-Bass, San Francisco.

Davies, I K (1971). *The Management of Learning*, McGraw-Hill, London.

Engel, C E (1991). 'Not just a method but a way of learning' in: Boud, D and Feletti, G (eds) *The Challenge of Problem-based Learning*, Kogan Page, London, pages 23–33.

Entwistle, N J (1981). *Styles of Learning and Teaching*, John Wiley & Sons, London.

Entwistle, N J, Hanley, M and Hounsell, D J (1979). 'Identifying distinctive approaches to studying', *Higher Education*, **8**, 365–380.

Entwistle, N J and Ramsden, P (1983). *Understanding Student Learning*, Croom Helm, London.

Evans, M G (1970). 'Leadership and motivation: A core concept', *Academy of Management Journal*, **13**, 91–102.

Fiedler, F E (1971). 'Validation and extension of the contingency model of leadership effectiveness', *Psychology Bulletin*, **76**, 128–148.

Gordon, T (1977). *Leader Effectiveness Training*, G P Putnam's Sons, New York.

Grant, E R (1991). 'Obsolescence or lifelong education: Choices and challenges', *Proceedings of the 11th International Congress of the World Confederation for Physical Therapy*, London, pages 145–159.

Griffith, G (1987). 'Images of interdependence: Authority and power in teaching/learning' in: Boud, D and Griffin, V (eds) *Appreciating Adults Learning: From the learners' perspective*, Kogan Page, London, pages 51–63.

Hammond, M and Collins, R (1991). *Self-directed Learning: Critical practice*, Kogan Page, London.

Harris, R (1989). 'Reflections on self-directed adult learning: Some implications for educators of adults', *Studies in Continuing Education*, **11**, 102–116.

Havelock, R G (1973). *The Change Agent's Guide to Innovation in Education*, Educational Technology Publications, New Jersey.

Heron, J (1989). *The Facilitators' Handbook*, Kogan Page, London.

Hersey, P and Blanchard, K (1982). *Management of Organizational Behavior: Utilising human resources* (4th edn) Prentice-Hall, New Jersey.

Higgs, J (1988). 'Planning learning experiences to promote autonomous learning' in: Boud, D (ed) *Developing Student Autonomy* (2nd edn) Kogan Page, London, chapter 2.

Higgs, J (1991). 'The role of the teacher and learner in fostering self-direction in indepedent learning programmes', *Proceedings of the 11th International Congress of the World Confederation for Physical Therapy*, London, pages 177–179.

House, R J and Mitchell T R (1974). 'Path-goal theory of leadership', *Journal of Contemporary Business*, **3**, 81–97.

Hunt, J W (1979). *Managing People at Work: A manager's guide to behaviour in organisations*, McGraw-Hill, London.

Knowles, M S (1980). *The Modern Practice of Adult Education — From pedagogy to andragogy*, Cambridge — The Adult Education Company, New York.

Knox, A B (1977). *Adult Development and Learning*, Jossey-Bass, San Francisco.

Kolb, D A (1984). *Experiential Learning — Experience as the source of learning and development*, Prentice-Hall, New Jersey.

Koontz, H, O'Donnell, C and Weihrich, H (1982). *Essentials of Management* (3rd edn) McGraw-Hill, New York.

Likert, R (1984). 'The nature of highly effective groups' in: Kolb, D A, Rubin, I M and McIntyre, J M (eds) *Organizational Psychology: Readings on human behavior in organizations*, Prentice-Hall, New Jersey.

Long, D G (1990); *Learner Managed Learning: The key to lifelong learning and development*, Kogan Page, London.

Magill, M K, France, R D and Munning, K A (1986). 'Educational relationships', *Medical Teacher*, **8**, 149–153.

McLeish, J, Matheson, W and Park, J (1973). *The Psychology of the Learning Group*, Hutchinson University Library, London.

Mezirow, J (1985). 'Concept and action in adult education', *Adult Education Quarterly*, **35**, 142–151.

Norman, G R (1990). 'Problem-solving skills and problem-based learning', *Physiotherapy Theory and Practice*, **6**, 53–54.

Novak, J D and Gowin, D B (1984). *Learning How to Learn*, Cambridge University Press.

Parlett, M R (1970). 'The syllabus-bound student' in: Hudson, L (ed) *The Ecology of Human Intelligence*, Penguin Books, Harmondsworth, Middlesex, pages 272–283.

Pask, G (1976). 'Styles and strategies of learning', *British Journal of Educational Psychology*, **46**, 128–148.

Polanyi, M (1958). *Personal Knowledge*, Routledge Kegan Paul, London.

Ramsden, P (1988). 'Studying Learning: Improving teaching' in: Ramsden, P (ed) *Improving Learning: New perspectives*, Kogan Page, London, pages 13–31.

Robbins, S P (1979). *Organizational Behavior: Concepts and controversies*, Prentice-Hall, New Jersey.

Rogers, C R (1969). *Freedom to Learn: A view of what education might become*, Charles E Merrill, Ohio.

Romanini, J and Higgs, J (1989). 'The teacher as manager in continuing and professional education', *Studies in Continuing Education*, **13**, 41–52.

Schon, D A (1987). *Educating the Reflective Practitioner*, Jossey-Bass, San Francisco.

Shaw, M E (1981). *Group Dynamics: The psychology of small group behavior* (3rd edn) McGraw-Hill, New York.

Taylor, M (1987). 'Self-directed learning: More than meets the observer's eye' in: Boud, D and Griffin, V (eds) *Appreciating Adults Learning: From the learners' perspective*, Kogan Page, London, pages 179–196.

Tompkins, C and McGraw, M (1988). 'The negotiated learning contract' in: Boud, D J (ed) *Developing Student Autonomy in Learning* (2nd edn) Kogan Page, London, pages 17–39.

Tough, A M (1978). 'Major learning efforts: Recent research and future directions', *Adult Education*, **28**, 250–263.

Tough, A M (1979). *The Adult's Learning Projects: A fresh approach to theory and practice in adult learning*, Ontario Institute for Studies in Education, Toronto.

Tough, A (1983). 'Self-planned learning and major personal change' in: Tight, M (ed) *Adult Learning and Education*, Croom Helm, London, pages 141–152.

Witkin, H A, Moore, C A, Goodenough, D R and Cox, P W (1977). 'Field-dependent and field-independent cognitive styles and their educational implications', *Review of Education Research*, **47**, 1–64.

REVIEW PAPER

From Clinical Supervisor to Clinical Educator:
Too Much to Ask?

Vinette Cross

Key Words

Clinical education, professional development, educational relationships.

Summary

Clinicians involved in clinical education have been required to adopt a variety of roles in relation to physiotherapy students. These roles are defined and some of the reasons for the changes which have taken place are considered. The paper goes on to question the feasibility of further developments in the face of current pressures within the health service.

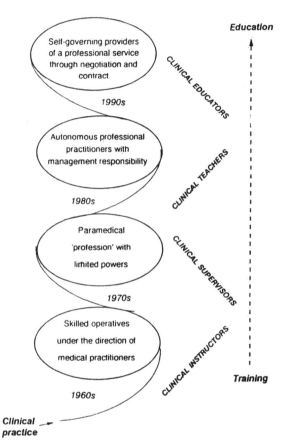

The development of physiotherapy practice and clinicians' roles in clinical education

Introduction

Much has been written about the changes which have taken place in physiotherapy practice and education during the past three decades (Kaiser, 1968; CSP, 1979; Pagliarulo, 1986; Jensen, 1988; Walker, 1991; Richardson, 1992; Thornton, 1994). These changes have been necessary and important developments in the growth of the profession. The word 'development' is appropriate, implying not only change but *direction*. Human development has been described as occurring not in a gradual linear manner, but in a series of spiralling plateaux, each a qualitative improvement on its predecessor (Daloz, 1986). The left side of the figure shows this concept applied to physiotherapy practice, from the dependency of the 1960s to the autonomy of the 1980s. There is a purpose and direction to this movement which may or may not continue into the uncertainties of the 1990s, uncertainties which are explored in more detail below.

Set alongside the developmental spiral of practice in the figure are the roles which clinical practitioners have been required to adopt in relation to students' learning in the clinical setting. The word 'required' is deliberately chosen. While the world of clinical practice has apparently developed in the sense of qualitative improvements building one on another, the world of the clinician involved in student learning seems to have stumbled through a variety of roles each teetering only precariously on the one before. Why should this be so? In 1979 the CSP Education Committee expressed the

view that the profession had developed an autonomy which had gone ahead of professional training. There was a need for 'professional training to be . . . liberalised and deepened to catch up with the tasks expected of the physiotherapist'. One might postulate that this asynchrony in development fostered an occasional lack of empathy between practitioners and educationists in relation to their needs and expectations of each other.

Some Effects of Professional Development on Clinical Education

The instructor of the 1960s was quite adequate in drilling learners to reproduce traditional procedures and enough of the ethos of the 'enthusiastic amateur' (Wagstaff, 1988) still remained to make this no great burden to the clinicians involved. The 1970s saw increasing numbers of students and a broadening curriculum. This demanded

Reprinted with permission from *Physiotherapy*. 1994; Vol 80; No 9; pp 609-611; UK ISSN 0034 9106.

more in the way of organisational skills from clinicians who might be required to supervise the activities of several students. Important in this supervision, from the clinicians' viewpoint, was minimising disruption to the normal running of departments in which greater clinical responsibilities and increasing external pressures were becoming the norm.

As the notion of professional autonomy took firm hold throughout the 1980s, the need to improve status and credibility drove educational establishments towards degree-based programmes grounded in a core curriculum; 'training' was transformed into 'education'. Clinicians were expected to take on the role of teachers of students in the field. Drilling and role-modelling — the established way of doing things — were no longer appropriate. Active teaching in a widening variety of clinical locations, giving and receiving feedback, encouraging initiative and a greater focus on individuals were now the way to foster professional practitioners of the future. Unfortunately, increasing student numbers, coupled with the need for clinicians to acquire more secure teaching skills to meet the challenge of changed student expectations, did not always sit comfortably with a concomitant increase in clinical workloads (Nosworthy, 1990).

What of the 1990s? Some would argue that the notion of development through qualitative improvement fails to stand up against an avalanche of NHS management upheaval, a market-place mentality and a private sector onslaught. Perhaps 'survival' is the word of choice here? Richardson (1992) suggests that physiotherapy as a profession has reached a watershed in its development; that it will be exposed to searching scrutiny from other disciplines. It will be called upon to respond to conflicting ideologies while trying to maintain a clear sense of its own. Certainly a situation has been created in which clinical expertise alone may not be enough to justify survival. In order to 'fight the corner' for a physiotherapy service in which practitioners can take honest pride, staff must develop expertise in a range of interpersonal communication and management skills. In the future it is the exercise of these skills in fora well beyond the professional reference group of physiotherapy which could determine the profile and credibility of clinical expertise. While many existing physiotherapy managers have been forced by circumstance to acquire management skills under fire, training opportunities in stress management, time management, communication skills, facilitation and evaluation of learning, collaborative skills, etc, are now de rigeur for even the most junior staff.

Physiotherapy educators within the schools have a responsibility to equip students fully to take up the cause of quality physiotherapy in the future. Making them aware of the need to develop basic management expertise is an increasingly important part of this responsibility. That being so, educational strategies and resources must be devised and evaluated which will enable students to explore the nature of the skills involved and practise them in protected circumstances, in precisely the same way as they do in relation to clinical skills. Such a change of emphasis, involving as it does experimentation with new educational models, creates a yet more challenging role for clinicians involved in student learning.

Role Definitions

As much as anything else, the prevailing vocabulary embodies the changes taking place. 'Conflict', 'collaboration', 'facilitation', 'ideology', negotiation, etc, are a long way from the formal classwork and traditional therapeutic measures of yesterday. 'Clinical educator' is the term now being used to describe those clinicians responsible for leading students towards this new millenium (CSP, 1991). It is these clinical educators who are 'ideally situated to enable students to learn to cope with change, to deal with the complexities of real-world clinical practice' (Higgs, 1992). The change from 'supervisor' to 'educator' defines the greater complexity of this new role. Education is very different from supervision; 'Learning is very different from being taught' (Thomas, 1985). Daloz's (1986) view that 'Education is something we neither "give" nor "do" to our students. It is a way we stand in relation to them', prompts speculation on the way in which terminology might define role in clinical education.

Reference to dictionary definitions can often lead to oversimplification of complex situations, but by the same token they can be of help in clarifying apparently overlapping concepts. 'Supervision' is defined as 'directing or inspecting; exercising control' (Onions, 1973), and as such could be seen as something 'done to' students. Thus control over what is done lies in the hands of the supervisor. The extent to which individual student needs or demands are allowed to disrupt the established pattern of what is done can be fairly easily controlled within the role definition. 'Teaching', on the other hand, is defined as 'imparting or conveying knowledge or skill' (Onions, 1973). Thus clinical teachers have a more 'giving' role in so far as they impart their own knowledge and skill to students, using a variety of techniques designed to help their transmission. Both supervision and teaching in these definitions appear confined in terms of the clinicians' input and passive in terms of the students' response (interestingly, 'teachable' is defined as docile). Their relationship seems limited and one-sided.

In contrast, among the definitions of 'education' is found 'the process of nourishing or rearing; development of powers; formation of character' (Onions, 1973). The clinical 'educator' enters into a relationship which embodies these definitions; an active one based on the provision of care as well as the transmission of knowledge or skill. More significantly, it involves a different balance of power.

Power Sharing in a Clinical Education Relationship

Brown (1993) focuses on three key elements in a power sharing educational relationship: approachability, self-disclosure and respect. Approachability involves clinical educators in negotiating, acting as mentors and supporting students in their own efforts to achieve educational outcomes. In this relationship it is implicit that on-going mutual respect cannot be taken for granted, it must be earned. The reciprocity of the relationship makes it legitimate and desirable for clinical educators to share their own concerns, weaknesses and limitations with students, through appropriate self-disclosure. The linkage between these three elements holds the potential to empower the clinician/student relationship in a way which supports students in their early attempts to develop basic management skills. As qualified practitioners they will be required to use these skills in facilitating power sharing relationships with patients, negotiating with and on behalf of patients, as well as in determining the quality of the physiotherapy service which is ultimately available to those patients. Logical and desirable though this change of emphasis seems to be, it nonetheless involves a return to uncertainty for clinicians who may only just be coming to terms with the role of 'clinical teacher'.

Conclusions

In this Centenary year Brook (1994) warns that emerging issues in physiotherapy education could give rise to 'a sharp intake of breath!'

'New policies in health care will inevitably influence both the syllabus and the educational process so as to attempt continually to meet the demands of newly qualified physiotherapists' (Brook, 1994).

These demands will always include the highest standards of clinical expertise grounded in a sound and credible theoretical base. However, new policies are creating additional demands, as those currently practising are being made relentlessly aware. Justifiable concern has been voiced that the need to introduce students to management skills through their clinical education could be at the expense of hands-on experience. Nevertheless, graduates emerging without such skills are more likely to see themselves as 'threatened . . . misrepresented . . . and hamstrung by fate' (Lane, 1992) than as self-governing practitioners with the power to orchestrate a quality future for the students who follow in their footsteps.

It is ironic that the very political and economic situation which provides such a convincing rationale for the advances in clinical education strategies discussed above, is also a major factor in obstructing their implementation. Lack of time, lack of staff, business plans which make only reluctant provision for clinical education, all conspire to hold back the liberalisation of physiotherapy education urged by the CSP a decade ago. The question: 'Is it too much to ask clinicians to accept and fulfil the role of clinical educator at this time?' is one which should be at the top of the agenda in any discussions between practitioners and educational institutions. The answer could determine the future direction of the profession.

Author and Address for Correspondence
Vinette Cross MMedEd MCSP DipTP is a senior teacher with responsibility for course evaluation at the School of Physiotherapy, Queen Elizabeth Medical Centre, Edgbaston, Birmingham B15 2TH.

References

Brook, N (1994). 'A sharp intake of breath: Inspiration in education — Some of the issues', *Physiotherapy*, **80** A, 20A–23A.

Brown, G D (1993). 'Accounting for power: Nurse teachers' and students' perceptions of power in their relationship', *Nurse Education Today*, **13**, 111–120.

Chartered Society of Physiotherapy (1979). 'The CSP's policy on degree courses', *Physiotherapy*, **65**, 11, 353–354.

Chartered Society of Physiotherapy (1991). *Standards for Clinical Education Placements*, CSP, London.

Daloz, L A (1986). *Effective Teaching and Mentoring*, Jossey-Bass, London.

Higgs, J (1992). 'Managing clinical education: The educator-manager and the self-directed learner', *Physiotherapy*, **78**, 11, 822–828.

Jensen, G M (1988). The work of accreditation on-site evaluators. Enhancing the development of a profession', *Physical Therapy*, **68**, 10, 1517–25.

Kaiser, H L (1968). 'Today's tomorrow', Fifth Mary McMillan Lecture presented at 45th Annual Conference of American Physical Therapy Association, *Physical Therapy*, **71**, 5, May 1991, 407–414.

Lane, R (1992). 'Management — The enabling function'. *Physiotherapy*, **78**, 12, 885–890.

Nosworthy, J (1990). 'Physiotherapy education: The fight for the future', *Australian Journal of Physiotherapy*, **36**, 1, 4.

Onions, C T (ed) (1973). *Shorter Oxford English Dictionary, On Historical Principles*, Oxford University Press.

Pagliarulo, M A (1986). 'Accreditation. Its nature, process and effective implementation', *Physical Therapy*, **66**, 7, 1114–18.

Richardson, B (1992). 'Professional education and professional practice today — Do they match? *Physiotherapy*, **78**, 1, 23–26.

Thomas, L F (1985). 'Nothing more theoretical than good practice: Teaching for self-organised learning' in: Bannister, D (ed) *Issues and Approaches in Personal Construct Theory*, Academic Press, London, chapter 13.

Thornton, E (1994). '100 years of physiotherapy education', *Physiotherapy*, **80**, A, 11A–19A.

Wagstaff, P (1988). 'The great debate', *Proceedings of Association of Teachers of Chartered Society of Physiotherapy*, Spring Conference, pages 16–18.

Walker, A (1991). 'Clinical education — Funding and standards', *Physiotherapy*, **77**, 11, 742–743.

SCHOLARLY PAPER

Clinicians' Needs in Clinical Education:
A report on a needs analysis workshop

Vinette Cross

Key Words

Institutional model, needs analysis, adult learning, clinical education.

Summary

The move towards an undergraduate honours degree programme prompted the Queen Elizabeth School of Physiotherapy to reappraise its approach to the provision of learning experiences for clinicians involved in the clinical education of its students. The framework of Knowles' assumptions regarding the nature of the adult learning process allowed parallels to be drawn between the changes in thinking and strategy generated by the new undergraduate course and those required by a revised clinical education development programme.

A needs analysis workshop provided a means by which an inventory of clinicians' learning needs, in relation to the demands of the degree course, could be compiled. At the same time it created a climate in which consideration of the clinicians' perceived needs alongside the educational priorities of the institution could become an illuminative and genuinely collaborative process.

Introduction

The start of an undergraduate honours degree course marked a turning point in physiotherapy education at the Queen Elizabeth School of Physiotherapy. It necessitated a change in direction in the way academic staff thought about and organised course content, teaching strategies, the students and themselves as educators. For parallel changes in the clinical education component of the course to be successful, there was a need for collaboration at all stages between academic staff based in the school and practitioners dealing with students in clinical locations.

While involvement of clinicians in the development of clinical education had obviously occurred in the past, a review of the school's attempts to facilitate this process through short courses and study days indicated only limited success. In a study of teaching outcomes of a typical clinical supervisors' course run by the school, Cross (1991) looked at the nurturant and instructional effects of the course on both clinical and academic staff. In relation to the clinical staff, nurturant effects were considered to be those which served to revitalise enthusiasm for involvement in the clinical education process from the point of view of the clinician as a learner and a provider. Equally important was the need for such interest and motivation to be sustained over time, in order that the clinical education objectives of the course could be achieved. For the academic staff, nurturant effects were those which sustained motivation to continue to facilitate clinical education on a regular basis and to be involved in planning learning experiences for clinicians. Instructional effects were concerned with consolidating practitioners' previous learning while exposing them to different ideas, particularly in relation to educational methods and assessment. The provision of useful insights into the contextual variables related to different clinical locations and an opportunity to develop strategies to deal with these were viewed as desirable instructional effects for the academic staff.

The results of the study painted a disappointing picture with the course showing most poorly in relation to long-term effects, both nurturant and instructional. Thus, while there was some evidence of a brief kindling of enthusiasm on the basis of the immediate post-course evaluation, just over a year later the flame appeared to have flickered and almost died. The effect of this was concern on all sides that the clinical objectives of the course were not being consistently achieved.

The reasons underlying this failure were thought to lie in the disjunction between the institutional model of programme development being used by the school and the contextual variables of professional practice over which the school had little control. Brookfield (1986) describes four main procedural features inherent in the institutional model of programme development:

1. Institutional definition of needs.

2. Institutional choice of programme content and format.

3. Placement and management of the programme within previously designated, institutionally convenient time periods.

4. Institutional choice of evaluation criteria.

A review of the outcomes of the existing programme, described above, led to an acknowledgment by the school (the institution) of a tendency to define clinicians' learning needs in relation to *its* perception of the objectives of clinical education and choose content and format accordingly. The choice of institutionally convenient time periods contributed to generally poor uptake of a limited programme and the choice of evaluation criteria provided only information regarding immediate impact, which usually demonstrated a brief upsurge of enthusiasm which failed to be sustained. Among the wide variety of contextual variables of professional practice which might account for this failure to endure, changes of personnel and different levels of appropriate experience were particularly relevant along with political and administrative issues. Inequities in available resources and managerial support, increasing administrative burdens, and greater or lesser degrees

Reprinted with permission from *Physiotherapy*. 1992; Vol 78; pp 758-761; UK ISSN 0034 9106.

of motivation and learning readiness were among the influencing factors.

During the negotiations leading up to the validation of the new course, a small number of practitioners provided valuable clinical representation on the course planning team. In the full-scale development of the clinical education component of the course it was seen as essential that as many clinicians as possible should be able to express their views and take an active part in achieving the highest possible standards of clinical education for physiotherapy students in the 1990s. To this end a needs assessment workshop was held with the objective of involving all clinicians in compiling an inventory of staff development from *their* perspective, in relation to the demands of clinical education to degree level.

The Workshop

In order to accommodate the numbers involved, the workshop was repeated on four separate occasions. A total of 71 clinicians from 37 locations attended. Their areas of expertise covered the full range of students' clinical practice experience. The duration of experience in clinical education ranged from one to 25 years, the average length of time being 4.5 years.

The two-hour workshop began with an introduction by the workshop leader, outlining the philosophy of the degree course and a description of the teaching strategies being employed. This incorporated a discussion of the participants' own learning experiences since qualification. Two small-group activities followed, the outcomes of which would be used in planning the development of the clinical education programme. At the end of the workshop the participants completed an evaluation form.

In the introduction, some of the assumptions made about the 'adult learning' process, as represented by the work of Malcolm Knowles on the theory and practice of adult education (table 1), were presented and their applicability

Table 1: Some assumptions about the adult learning process (Knowles, 1980)

Adults are aware of specific learning needs generated by real-life tasks or problems.

Adults' learning is affected by their past experience which provides a rich resource for learning.

Adults are generally self-directing and the learning encounter should reflect this tendency.

Adults are competency-based learners, wishing to apply newly-acquired skills/knowledge to their immediate situation.

to undergraduate physiotherapy education considered. Reflecting upon their own experiences of learning since qualification, participants noted the variety of motives, past experiences and styles of learning involved and their effects on learning outcomes. Attention was drawn to the increasing numbers of mature students entering undergraduate physiotherapy courses, whose expectations and learning needs demanded greater flexibility in course structure and teaching strategies than had previously been the case. The need for systems to assess experiential learning, guidance in

self- and peer-assessment, student-centred approaches and the development of self-directed learning skills were all highlighted (Young, 1990). Discussing the view that the rather confusing term 'adult learning' applied more to an *approach* to learning rather than chronology, it was acknowledged that such strategies were as relevant to school leavers as to 'mature' students, and that because optimal learning experiences could not be provided for all learners simultaneously, it was important to provide them with the intellectual skills which would enable them to learn in ways which suited their personal style (Collins and Hammond, 1987).

The foregoing discussion gave rise to some misgivings among clinicians attending the workshop, as to the relevance of 'idealised models' of learning to the reality of their day-to-day contact with students. However, it was acknowledged that, for their relationship to be one of equal partnership in professional education, just as academic staff must be conversant with the realities and contextual variables of contemporary practice, while not necessarily being fully involved in them, so must clinical staff have a measure of awareness of the thinking underlying educational change, while not allowing undue concern for educational theory to impede their ability to deal with practical teaching problems in the clinic (Barnett *et al*, 1987). Indeed, by experiencing and reflecting upon such problems, practitioners might be encouraged to generate their own educational theories out of the realities of their everyday practice with students (Fish, 1988). This element of the discussion strongly reinforced the view that any attempt to initiate a new clinical education development programme must take account not only of the prescribed needs of the institution (the 'professional educators' within the school) but must be rooted in the perceived needs of practising clinicians who, for the most part, are not professional educators in the same sense, and for whom 'patient-primacy' and student education must always make uneasy bedfellows (Shepard and Jensen, 1990). This view makes even more worthy of attention Thomas-Edding's (1985) assertion that, although the survival and growth of the physiotherapy profession depends on a variety of people, 'no more significant role will be taken than that of the clinician who teaches. In the final analysis, it is in the clinic that learning really takes place'.

The Needs Analysis Process

Implicit in making a needs workshop the starting point for the development of clinical education to degree level, was the recognition that both academic and clinical staff must allow themselves to be cast in the role of 'adult learner' at various points in the ensuing programme, while at other times acting as facilitators of each other's learning. This way lay the path to true collaboration. Hence, the workshop activities set out to identify needs and strengths among the participants, which sprang out of Knowles' assumptions about the adult learning process.

Participants took part in two activities designed to reveal their strengths and needs in relation to the educational demands of the course, as they perceived them, in the light of the information and discussion in the first part of the workshop. In other words, in order to sustain their clinical teaching role in the changed educational climate, what were the specific areas related to students' education, which they would like to see addressed in any ensuing development programme?

The first activity — identification of 'key incidents' — focused on the first of Knowles' assumptions, the aim being for each individual to identify a learning need generated by a real-life problem. Participants were asked to reflect individually and anonymously on their experience in clinical education, identifying one or more incidents or situations related to student learning which they remembered as causing them discomfiture, anxiety or difficulty, and to list questions raised by the incidents. The clinicians were asked to think not only in terms of crises or serious confrontations. What was required was a wide spectrum of experiences including those seen as serious and also those which, although only mildly disconcerting, nonetheless raised interesting issues.

Seventy-two incidents were documented raising such questions as those shown in table 2. The key incidents fell into five major categories of concern (table 3).

Table 2: Questions raised by student learning experiences

Should clinicians receive prior warning of students' difficulties?

How can clinicians cope with guilt feelings about students?

Do all clinicians fail students when they think they should?

How can we help students to grasp the concept of constructive criticism and involve them in the process more?

What are students' expectations before they start clinical work?

Are clinicians able to spend enough time to meet the needs of students?

How do you convert 'theorists' into clinicians?

Table 3: Concerns raised by key incidents

Category of concern	No of incidents documented
Counselling students in distress	21
Assessment of students' performance	20
Need for specific teaching skills	17
Adequacy of pre-clinical preparation	8
Coping with the rival demands of clinical workload and student education	6

The second workshop activity focused on the assumption that adults' past experience should provide a rich resource for learning and hence brought attention to more positive aspects of the clinician's role. In small groups participants considered what particular qualities or strengths each one possessed which could contribute to effective student learning in the clinical situation. They were urged to view themselves holistically, taking into account not only 'professional' expertise or knowledge, but such personal qualities as empathy, kindness, being a good listener, as well as their life experience. Each small group produced a combined list of strengths which was displayed for the larger group to discuss. Individuals then ticked those items on each list which were of interest to them and which reflected a personal need. The results of this activity (table 4) clustered into categories which echoed those produced by the key incidents.

Table 4: Number of participants expressing interest in strength categories

Perceived strengths	No of ticks
Ability to facilitate learning in some way (including research skills)	66
Skills of performance assessment and evaluation	26
Counselling/mentorship skills	23
Stress management skills	20
Time management skills	16
Experience of other cultures	9
Good standards of record-keeping	7
Ability to liaise well with the school	5

Participants' Evaluation of the Workshop

The participants were asked for their immediate reaction to the workshop by indicating the extent to which they agreed or disagreed with each statement on a pro-forma (table 5); 68 out of the 71 clinicians who attended completed the evaluation form. The results are shown in the figure opposite.

Table 5: Possible effects of the workshop: Participants' evaluation form

1. It gave a clear picture of the educational philosophy and teaching strategies underlying the degree course.
2. It provided a useful opportunity for me to express my own needs in relation to my role as a clinical supervisor.
3. It did not affect the way I think about my role as a clinical supervisor.
4. It provided a useful insight into other people's needs as clinical supervisors.
5. It caused me to feel anxious/threatened by proposed changes which could affect my role as a clinical supervisor.
6. It enabled me to identify particular strengths which I am able to bring to the learning situation.
7. It kindled my enthusiasm for involvement in the forthcoming development programme.

The use of the term 'clinical supervisor' in the evaluation points up the need for changes in the approach to clinical education to keep pace with academic development. The evolution of clinical supervisors into the wider role of 'clinical educators' is a definitive objective of future learning programmes.

Most of the participants found the workshop effective in providing information and a forum in which to express and exchange views. While a number of people were stimulated to reconsider the way they thought about their role as a clinical supervisor, only a very few indicated that they felt in any way anxious about their role in the future. More opportunity to discuss the key incidents in small groups might have enabled participants to gain wider insights into other people's needs. Despite widespread diffidence at being asked to identify personal strengths during the workshop, this activity appeared to be particularly worth while, revealing a reservoir of abilities and experience which could provide the 'rich resource for learning', of which Knowles (1980) speaks.

In general the results of the evaluation indicated satisfactory short-term nurturant and instructional effects on the participants, who ended the workshop with positive attitudes and new information. Short-term

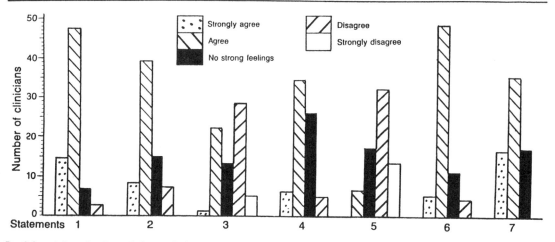

Participants' evaluation of the workshop by responses to statements

effects on the academic staff involved were considered to be similarly favourable. Staff felt they had gained new insights into both the needs, interests and abilities of their clinical partners and the contextual variables which influenced their work with students (instructional effects). They also came away with positive attitudes to the prospect of future involvement in similar activities (nurturant effects).

The workshop was brought to its conclusion with the suggestion that the change in direction of physiotherapy education at the Queen Elizabeth School meant that all those involved — academic staff, clinical staff *and* students — found themselves in a position in which each could learn from the other in real collaboration. The next step would be to generate a learning programme from the agenda provided by the clinicians themselves, which reflected the needs and utilised the strengths identified in the workshop. Three major principles were emphasised: first, that the clinical education development programme should be continuous in nature; second, for the programme to be sensitive to and responsive to contextual variables it should foster negotiation and creativity, with the focus of interaction in developing clinical education skills shifting from the physiotherapy school into the clinical workplace; the third principle — that evaluation of the programme's relevance and effectiveness should be collaborative and integral to the process — was seen as the most effective way to foster long-term nurturant and instructional effects in both clinical and academic staff.

Conclusion

The workshop was successful in generating an agenda for development which sprang directly from the clinicians' interpretations of their experiences and the academic staff were able to share in this interpretation, gaining insights from it. The application of the first two elements of Knowles' theory of adult learning (table 1) facilitated this illuminative process. It is now hoped that by creating a clinical education development programme alongside clinicians, in their specific workplaces rather than *en masse* in the school, they will be enabled to direct their own learning more effectively, further facilitating

institutional insights. Moreover, they will be able to apply the acquired skills to their immediate situation in keeping with Knowles' last two assumptions.

Such an approach clearly echoes that advocated for the undergraduate programme discussed above. It supports the view of physiotherapy education as a three-way learning partnership in which both academic staff, clinical staff *and* students may be cast at different times in the role of adult learner or facilitator according to need and circumstance.

Author

Vinette Cross MCSP DipTP DipMedEd is a teacher at the Queen Elizabeth School of Physiotherapy, Birmingham.

Address for Correspondence

Mrs V Cross MCSP DipTP DipMedEd, The School of Physiotherapy, Queen Elizabeth Medical Centre, Edgbaston, Birmingham B15 2TH.

References

Barnett, R A, Becher, R A and Cork, N M (1987). 'Models of professional preparation: Pharmacy, nursing and teacher education', *Studies in Higher Education*, **12**, 1, 51–63.

Brookfield, S D (1986). *Understanding and Facilitating Adult Learning*, Open University Press, Milton Keynes, chapter 5.

Collins, R and Hammond, M (1987). 'Self-directed learning to educate medical educators. Part 2: Why do we use self-directed learning?' *Medical Teacher*, **9**, 4, 425–431.

Cross, V (1991). 'Teaching outcomes of a clinical supervisors' course for physiotherapists'. Unpublished paper for Diploma in Medical Education.

Fish, D (1988). *Turning Teaching into Learning: TRIST and the development of professional practice*, West London Press, London.

Knowles, M S (1980). *The Modern Practice of Adult Education: From pedagogy to androgogy*, Cambridge Books, New York, cited in Brookfield, S D, *op cit*.

Shepard, K F and Jensen, G M (1990). 'Physical therapist curricula for the 1990s: Educating the reflective practitioner', *Physical Therapy*, **70**, 9, 44–55.

Thomas-Edding, D (1985). 'Educating the professional educator', *Physiotherapy Canada*, **37**, 5, 295–300.

Young, J N (1990). 'Mature students in physiotherapy undergraduate education', *Physiotherapy*, **76**, 3, 127–131.

Characteristics of Effective Clinical Teachers of Ambulatory Care Medicine

DAVID M. IRBY, Ph.D., PAUL G. RAMSEY, M.D., GERALD M. GILLMORE, Ph.D., and DOUG SCHAAD, Ph.D.

Abstract—This study identified characteristics of clinical teachers in ambulatory care settings that influenced ratings of overall teaching effectiveness and examined the impacts of selected variables of the clinic environment on teaching effectiveness ratings. A survey instrument derived from prior research and observations of ambulatory care teaching was sent to 165 senior medical students and 60 medicine residents at the University of Washington School of Medicine in 1988. A total of 122 (74%) of the seniors and 60 (71%) of the residents responded. Results indicate that the most important characteristics of the ambulatory care teachers were that they actively involved the learners, promoted learner autonomy, and demonstrated patient care skills. Environmental variables did not have a substantial influence on these ratings. *Acad. Med.* 66(1991):54–55.

As faculty spend more time teaching and providing patient care in outpatient settings,[1-3] research on clinical teaching of ambulatory care medicine is needed in order to create valid and reliable forms for rating teaching in the ambulatory care environment. Research on clinical teaching previously has been conducted predominantly in inpatient settings.[4-7] The objectives of the present study were (1) to identify characteristics of clinical teachers in ambulatory care settings that have the most influence on ratings of overall teaching effectiveness, and (2) to determine the impacts of selected clinic environment variables on ratings of overall teaching effectiveness.

Method

A panel of experts, consisting of a team of five clinicians who were rated as excellent teachers in ambulatory care settings and four medical educators, identified behaviors characteristic of effective teaching performed by attending physicians in ambulatory care settings. The educators (in teams of two) conducted six half-day observations of ambulatory care teaching and interviewed medical students and residents about the best attending physicians they had encountered in an ambulatory care setting.

The results of these inquiries were combined to create a 44-item survey instrument that clustered teachers' behaviors under seven factors of teaching effectiveness: knowledge, organization and clarity, enthusiasm, group instructional skills, clinical supervision skills, clinical competence, and modelling professional characteristics. Five variables of the clinic environment that might influence teaching were also included: case mix of clinic, work load (pace), structured time for teaching, space for teaching, and organization of clinic. One open-ended question was used to identify the one to three most significant characteristics that made an effective teacher stand out in the respondent's mind.

The questionnaire was designed for medical students and residents. It requested them to think of the most recent clinic teacher they had encountered in an ambulatory care setting and to assess the teaching effectiveness of that person by rating how fully that person exhibited each of a variety of teaching behaviors listed on the questionnaire, using a scale of 1 (not at all descriptive) to 7 (very descriptive), or to indicate that a particular listed behavior was not observed. The respondent was then asked to rate the influence of each of several variables of the clinic environment on the overall performance of their teacher, using a rating of 1 (not at all influential) to 7 (highly influential), or to indicate that he or she could not assess this.

The survey was mailed in 1988 to all graduating medical students at the University of Washington School of Medicine, in Seattle. Of the 165 senior students, 122 (74%) responded. Sixty medicine residents (71%) also completed the inventory.

Results

The first research objective was to identify the characteristics of clinical teachers in ambulatory care settings that have the most influence on ratings made by medical students and residents of overall teaching effectiveness. Using stepwise regression analysis, the following four characteristics of ambulatory care teachers best predicted overall teaching effectiveness: involved me in the learning process ($R^2 = .779$), communicated expectations for my performance ($R^2 = .846$), stimulated my interest ($R^2 = .864$), and interacted skillfully with patients ($R^2 = .876$). All subsequent items explained less then 1% of the variance in the data. The top four items reflect instructional skills (active involvement, clarity of expectations, and stimulation of interest) and role modeling of clinical competence.

The most important characteristics of teachers in ambulatory care settings identified in open-ended comments were as follows: possessed broad knowledge of medicine, seemed to enjoy teaching and patient care, demonstrated caring concern for pa-

Dr. Irby is professor, Department of Medical Education; Dr. Ramsey is associate professor and acting chairman, Department of Medicine, and a Henry J. Kaiser Family Foundation Faculty Scholar in general internal medicine; Dr. Gillmore is associate professor, Department of Psychology, and Director, Office of Educational Assessment; and Dr. Schaad is research assistant professor, Department of Medical Education. All are at the University of Washington in Seattle.

Reprinted with permission from *Academic Medicine*. Irby DM, Ramsey PG, Gillmore GM, Schaad D. 1991;66(1):54–55.

tients, was personable and approachable, showed respect for others, and was enthusiastic. The students and residents responded similarly, with the exception of breadth of knowledge in medicine, which was mentioned more frequently by residents.

Using factor analysis, the underlying structure of the survey items (minus the clinic environment variables) was investigated. Two factors were identified using a varimax rotation following a principal-component solution on the teacher's behaviors items. Factor 1 relates to learner-centered instruction and accounts for 33% of the variance. These behavior items reflect the attending physician's instructional skills of establishing rapport with the learner, actively involving the learner in the learning process, and encouraging the learner's autonomy and responsibility. Factor 2 is associated with the attending physician's patient care skills and accounts for 25% of the variance. These items relate to the attending physician's clinical skills in the context of teaching and patient care. For each of these two factors, item loadings of .60 or greater are reported in the footnote.*

The second research objective was to determine the impacts of selected variables of the clinic environment on ratings of overall teaching effectiveness. This was examined by correlating the environment items with the overall ratings of teaching effectiveness. None of the environment items was strongly correlated with the overall rating of teaching effectiveness. R values ranged from −.07 for structured time for teaching to .12 for space for teaching, to .19 for clinic case mix, to .20 for organization of clinic, to .27 for workload. All environmental variables were combined

to predict overall teaching effectiveness using multiple regression. The resulting multiple correlations were found not to be statistically significant.

Discussion

One of the most notable findings in the present study is the clustering of items associated with learner autonomy in factor 1. Respecting the autonomy of the learner and nurturing self-directed learning appear to be key elements of teaching effectiveness in the ambulatory care setting. In addition, factor 1, associated with learner-centered instruction, represents a composite of three factors found in prior research: supervisory skills, knowledge and clarity, and interpersonal relations.[6] Factor 2, associated with attending patient care skills, relates to a fourth factor in the

---

*For factor 1, the loadings are, in descending order, .84 (involved me in learning process), .82 (showed a personal interest in me), .82 (overall teaching effectiveness), .80 (provided constructive feedback), .80 (communicated expectations), .79 (asked me for my plans before making recommendations), .78 (allowed me to find answers for myself), .76 (used questions effectively), .73 (allowed me to maintain responsibility), .70 (helped me to analyze complicated cases), .70 (allowed teaching to flow naturally from patient interactions), .68 (was enthusiastic about teaching), .65 (provided underlying reasons for recommendations), .64 (directed me to useful literature), .63 (stimulated my interest), .63 (listened attentively to my questions), and .62 (treated me with respect).

For factor 2, the loadings are .85 (showed respect for patients), .80 (demonstrated concern for patients), .78 (demonstrated respect for others), .77 (interacted skillfully with patients), .76 (provided information on outpatient care), .73 (seemed to enjoy patient care), .64 (showed how to involve patients in decision making), and .60 (provided insight into psychosocial aspects of care).

previous research: demonstrating clinical competence.

The relatively slight impact of various characteristics of the clinic environment on students' ratings of teaching is congruent with findings on ratings of classroom teaching.[8]

In conclusion, the characteristics of clinical teachers in ambulatory care settings were similar to those found in prior studies of ward teaching. Generic rating forms for clinical teaching may be used in many kinds of ambulatory care settings, although specific rating forms for each setting will provide more targeted feedback on critical teaching behaviors in each environment.

The authors acknowledge the contributions of the following persons to this research: Wylie Burke, M.D., Tom Inui, M.D., Tom Greer, M.D., Jan Carline, Ph.D, and Mark Guthrie.

References

1. Perkoff, G. T. Teaching Clinical Medicine in the Ambulatory Setting: An Idea Whose Time May Have Finally Come. *N. Engl. J. Med.* **314**(1986):27–31.
2. Schroeder, S. A., Showstack, J. A., and Gerbert, B. Residency Training in Internal Medicine: Time for a Change? *Ann. Intern. Med.* **104**(1986):554–561.
3. Wooliscroft, J. O., and Schwenk, T. L. Teaching and Learning in the Ambulatory Setting. *Acad. Med.* **64**(1989):644–648.
4. Irby, D. Clinical Teacher Effectiveness in Medicine. *J. Med. Educ.* **37**(1978):258–261.
5. Irby, D. Evaluating Teaching Skills. *Diabetes Educator* **11**(1986):37–46.
6. Irby, D., and Rakestraw, P. Evaluating Clinical Teaching in Medicine. *J. Med. Educ.* **56**(1981):181–185.
7. Irby, D., Gilmore, G., and Ramsey, P. Factors Affecting Ratings of Clinical Teachers by Medical Students and Residents. *J. Med. Educ.* **62**(1987):1–7.
8. Feldman, D. A. Consistency and Variability among College Students in Rating Their Teachers and Courses: A Review and Analysis. *Res. Higher Educ.* **6**(1977):223–274.

Clinical Education:
Students' and Clinical Tutors' Views

SUSAN NEVILLE BA MCSP DipTP

Principal Lecturer, Division of Physiotherapy, Polytechnic of East London

SALLY FRENCH

BSc MSc(Psych) MSc(Soc) DipGradPhys DipTP

Lecturer, Department of Health and Social Welfare, Open University

Key words: Education, clinical experience.

Summary: Various studies have shown that clinical education is a rewarding yet problematic area of education for both physiotherapy students and clinical tutors. In this study 40 third-year BSc(Hons) physiotherapy students and 64 clinical tutors were asked for their views regarding what constitutes a 'good' and a 'poor' clinical experience. The main factors highlighted by the students were the attitude and behaviour of the tutors, the environment and social atmosphere and the quality of the learning experience. The main factors highlighted by the clinical tutors were the attitude and ability of the students, student development, and personal and professional growth. It was concluded that there is far more to the role of clinical tutor than excellence in clinical practice and that a more structured education for clinical tutors, to help them in this role, needs to be developed.

Biography: Susan Neville qualified as a physiotherapist at the Royal Victoria Infirmary, Newcastle on Tyne, and after working at home and abroad joined the staff of The London Hospital School of Physiotherapy in 1972. When the school became part of the Polytechnic of East London (formerly NELP) in 1981, she became clinical education tutor and is presently researching into the teaching and learning of students in the clinical environment.

Sally French qualified as a physiotherapist from the Royal National Institute for the Blind School of Physiotherapy in 1972 and completed her physiotherapy teacher training in 1978. While working as a teacher she gained degrees in psychology and sociology and has a particular interest in the application of the behavioural sciences to illness and disability. She is now a lecturer in the Department of Health and Social Welfare at the Open University.

> "The 'clinicians' are the members of the profession who are spending the majority of their time treating patients, achieving the mastery level of their clinical skills and becoming familiar with modern equipment. It is these members of our profession who have so much to offer the students and who should be at the forefront of the clinical education process."
> — Coates (1986)

Introduction

CLINICAL work is usually viewed as the most enjoyable and rewarding aspect of physiotherapy students' education, and it is likely that the attitudes, skills and behaviour patterns acquired clinically are more profound and lasting than those acquired in the college setting. This puts considerable responsibility on to physiotherapists engaged in clinical teaching, yet they tend to receive little if any instruction regarding teaching and learning, and may be uncertain of what students and academic staff expect of them.

There is little information on the perceptions and views of physiotherapy clinical tutors regarding clinical education and their role within it, and a similar dearth of information on the attitudes and perceptions of physiotherapy students to their clinical education. Emery (1984) asked physical therapy students, who had completed their clinical education, to rate the importance and frequency of 43 previously identified clinical tutor behaviours. These behaviours were classified as relating to communication,

interpersonal relationships, professional skills and teaching skills. The students considered all the skills valuable but the tutors' interpersonal skills and their ability to communicate were considered more important than their teaching capabilities. Clinical skills were considered least important even though they were demonstrated most frequently. In a similar study Orton (1984) found that student nurses rated highly considerate and understanding sisters who treated them as learners rather than workers and who generated a team spirit. Best (1988) argues that concentrating entirely on clinical skills can be destructive. She states:

> 'Some supervisors are exacting task-masters and in their determination to produce competent clinicians often destroy the students' developing confidence so that they are unable to perform.'

Scully and Shepard (1983) conducted an observational study of physical therapists in the USA which included semi-structured interviews. With regard to their role as clinical tutors the respondents mentioned negative and positive aspects. They commented on lack of privacy, reduced contact with patients and difficulty managing time, but also mentioned the enriching effects students had on them and the whole department. Sotosky (1984) found that clinical tutors had very positive attitudes towards tutoring though they were dissatisfied with the training they received.

The aim of this small study was to investigate the views of physiotherapy students and clinical tutors on what they regard as a 'good' and a 'poor' clinical experience. Throughout this paper the term 'clinical tutor' will be used in preference to 'clinical supervisor' as it is felt that it describes the role of these senior physiotherapists more accurately.

Method and Procedure

This investigation was carried out in two parts, which will be referred to as 'study 1' and 'study 2'. The data collected in study 1 were originally intended simply to provide physiotherapy lecturers, in one institution, with an insight into the views of students undergoing clinical education. They were also used later as material on a course for clinical tutors. The data used in study 2 were gathered during a teaching session of a one-day workshop for clinical tutors which was repeated two weeks later. It was only later that the authors considered that the information from these two sources might be of interest to other physiotherapists and physiotherapy lecturers. For this reason the research methodology is less rigorous than it would ideally be.

Study 1

On their first day back in college after completing an eight-week clinical placement, a third-year cohort of 40 students following a BSc(Hons) physiotherapy course were asked to take part in this study. They had all completed 12 weeks of clinical practice in the preceding year. They were presented with the following question:

> 'Consider your last clinical placement. If it was a "good" clinical placement can you identify why it was good? If it was a "poor" clinical placement can you identify why it was poor?'

Reprinted with permission from *Physiotherapy*. 1991; Vol 77; No 5; pp 351-354; UK ISSN 0034 9106.

The question was presented to the students in a written form and they were asked to write their answers in the style of an essay. They were given no preparation time and were allowed 20 minutes to complete the task. Some students asked if they could include information from previous clinical placements and this was allowed. The essays were collected and analysed by means of content analysis by one of the authors who is experienced in clinical education.

Study 2

The subjects comprised 64 clinical physiotherapists who attended a one-day workshop on clinical education. They were all involved in the clinical teaching of physiotherapy students. As part of a small group exercise they were asked to consider what they regarded as a 'positive' and a 'negative' tutoring experience. The small group discussions lasted for about 15 minutes and the ideas were then shared and discussed with the other participants in a large group. The information was recorded by one of the course tutors.

Results

Study 1

Students valued their clinical tutors if they were friendly, encouraging, helpful, forthcoming with information and approachable. Many students liked to be regarded as 'another therapist' and as members of the team. They valued a positive, pleasant and relaxed approach with good rapport with their clinical tutors and other members of staff. Their satisfaction was greatly enhanced if they were well integrated in the department and allowed to use the staffroom.

Regarding their learning experiences, students appreciated and enjoyed student-centred teaching and learning methods as well as regular teaching sessions. They rated highly frequent, constructive feedback from their clinical tutors and time with them for observation, questioning and the sharing of ideas. They liked tutors to be encouraging and to use a variety of learning materials such as books and hand-outs. They also considered their placement to be 'good' if they were given opportunities to see surgery, visit clinics and interact with other professional people. A personal interest in the clinical area and a varied and carefully planned case load also led to satisfaction. The students liked to be given responsibility, space, freedom and independence, along with guidance and availability of help if required.

Factors constituting a 'poor' clinical placement included being 'talked down to', being treated as an inconvenience and a burden, and enduring constant criticism. This type of behaviour often led to feelings of intimidation and insecurity. They were dissatisfied if they were treated like outsiders in the department, for example, not being allowed to use the staffroom. The learning experience was seen to be less than adequate if the clinical tutor 'took over the treatment' or if they were not challenged to justify their choice of treatment. A lack of teaching sessions and feedback, and either too much or too little responsibility, were also mentioned as producing a 'poor' clinical placement. Many students could appreciate that staff shortages and lack of time often lay at the root of these problems.

Other factors giving rise to a 'poor' clinical placement included long travel times, inadequate college preparation, too few patients, an unvaried case load and the subjective nature of the assessment at the end of the placement, which many students regarded as unfair. They expressed dislike of unplanned visits by college staff and conflict between academic and clinical tutors.

Study 2

Tutors felt positive if the students were enthusiastic, interested, questioning and receptive. They preferred conscientious students and those who used their initiative. They found the experience 'good' if students were responsible, respectful, knowledgeable, challenging and evaluative. Seeing the students develop professionally was also viewed as a positive experience. The clinical tutors enjoyed watching students putting theory into practice and developing good interaction skills and rapport with their patients.

Another area of positive satisfaction for the clinical tutors was their own personal and professional development. They believed that work in this field improved their skills in personal communication, teaching, time management, organisation, and assessment. They also felt they had become more self-aware and flexible. Positive interaction with the students was viewed as important in order for this development to occur. They needed to be motivated and stimulated by students, to exchange ideas and perspectives with them and to receive positive feedback.

The characteristics which gave rise to a negative clinical experience included lack of enthusiasm and interest on the part of the students, over-confidence, inability to take criticism, lack of commitment and an orientation to theory. Other negative features related to reduced patient contact, lack of college back-up and lack of time. Clinical tutors regretted the loss of patient contact which having students entailed and some were concerned that patients might be disadvantaged by receiving treatment from students rather than experienced physiotherapists. Other negative factors were lack of support and information from academic staff and conflict between recent clinical developments and the material taught in college. They also complained of considerable stress brought about by lack of time to spend with students.

Discussion

The views and opinions of the clinical tutors and physiotherapy students in this study broadly mirror those of the research mentioned above. Although the students want tutors who can teach well and are knowledgeable and skilful clinically, of equal or more concern is that they should be friendly, approachable and communicative. Although the reliability and validity of student ratings can be questioned, in this case their validity is strengthened by the fact that many of the points raised by the students are covered extensively in the literature on learning environments, where it is recognised that a relaxed and supportive atmosphere, where students feel secure to ask questions and are supported if they make mistakes, is essential to effective learning.

Students must constantly adjust to new tutors and new clinical situations where they will encounter differing work practices, rules and expectations. They must strike a delicate balance between acting like students and acting like therapists, between being independent and being over-demanding, and between caution and over-confidence. This is no easy task as expectations differ from one department and one clinical tutor to another, an issue which clinical tutors should keep in mind.

Clinical tutors have an important, exacting and multi-faceted task and frequently work in less than ideal conditions where time is short, support is lacking and little opportunity is given to study the theory and practice of teaching and learning. They must strike a delicate balance between providing sufficient help and being over-controlling, of giving students too much or too little to do and of providing a relaxed atmosphere which is free from anxiety yet simultaneously full of challenge.

Best (1988) maintains that clinical tutors must strike a balance between concern for students and concern for physiotherapy tasks. She believes that high concern for physiotherapy tasks coupled with low concern for students gives rise to anxiety-provoking and thoroughly dissatisfying learning experiences. High concern for students with low concern for physiotherapy tasks, on the other hand, gives rise to clinical placements which are relaxed but not particularly challenging. Best suggests that high concern for both students and physiotherapy tasks provides highly interesting and valuable experiences which benefit both parties.

However the tutor role is demanding, for tutors must adapt and adjust to each new student and at the same time cope with clinical and administrative responsibilities. It is fortunate that clinical physiotherapy contains many of the skills required of a good teacher which can, to some extent, be transferred to the tutoring role.

It should be noted that some dissatisfaction voiced by both students and clinical tutors concerned relationships and interactions with academic tutors. In fact, academic tutors were only mentioned in relation to conflict. More recent investigations by one of the authors, however, have shown that both students and clinical tutors feel strongly that there is a need for academic tutors to visit clinical areas. This dual input, known in management as a matrix structure (Arnold and Feldman, 1986) can be beneficial to students in terms of reinforcing and broadening their experience, but at the same time it can generate power conflicts causing stress and confusion and impeding decision making. Clearly more research needs to be done to identify the optimum characteristics of this double process. Despite the practical difficulties posed by students working in geographically distant departments and the time constraints imposed on both clinical and academic staff, it is vital that contact and channels of communication are not only maintained but strengthened.

The complex yet rewarding relationship between clinical tutors and students might be enhanced if they communicated their needs, difficulties and expectations more clearly to each other. It is, for example, unlikely that many students would realise the importance of giving positive feedback to clinical tutors or the stimulation and motivation they can provide by sharing their ideas. Likewise the experienced clinical tutor may have forgotten the anxiety of treating patients with a given condition for the first time, or of the practice required to learn new skills. The evaluation of learning should also involve students. Heron (1988) suggested that negotiations between students and clinical tutors could go some way to reducing the unfairness felt by students with regard to assessment procedures. This is yet another area worthy of investigation.

It was noted above that one of the causes of dissatisfaction among the clinical tutors was the inability on the part of students to link theoretical with practical knowledge. This is by no means an easy task, however, and is one with which the clinical tutor must assist. Mason (1984) believes that understanding the subject matter is a major dimension of successful teaching and studies which have looked at the process of learning in a clinical setting (Gardiner, 1989) have emphasised the importance of realising that the theory/practice link constantly changes. Theory is developed from practice as well as practice being guided by theory. This awareness of the need to reflect on practice actively involves

students in the learning process, which should be as much their responsibility as that of the clinical tutors (Ilot, 1990).

Environmental factors play an important part in the facilitation of students' learning. Beard and Hartley (1984) pointed out that under-achievement is caused by many factors unrelated to intellect such as debilitating anxiety and lack of security. In the view of the students in this study there is clearly far more to being competent clinical tutors than being good and knowledgeable clinicians, though these skills are highly valued by them.

For a further discussion of learning environments and how to create them the reader is referred to Orton (1984), Mathews (1987), Whiteley (1988), Griffiths (1989) and Marsen (1990).

It is evident from this small study that clinical tutoring can be a rewarding occupation and one which provides physiotherapists with the opportunity for considerable personal and professional development. Most of the negative factors highlighted by the clinical tutors were in terms of their working conditions, for example, lack of time and lack of support. Many of the students were well aware that these problems lay at the root of most of their dissatisfactions, for example, the quality of teaching they received. It is clear that the working conditions of clinical tutors are less than ideal and need to be improved.

Teaching is a skill which can be learned and although many clinical tutors have a natural flair for teaching, a more structured education is almost certainly overdue and needs to be developed. May (1983) found that most of the physical therapists he surveyed had learned to teach through 'trial and error' with few believing teaching to be a natural skill. The enhancement of teaching skills and the ability to create an environment conducive to learning, will not only benefit students but also junior staff and patients, in fact anyone in the department who is keen to learn. In addition many of the qualities clinical tutors need are those of effective managers, thus the skills are not specific to teaching but can be generalised to other aspects of physiotherapists' work.

Conclusion

Many of the students and clinical tutors express views compatible with the literature on adult learning. There should preferably be a climate which is collaborative and mutually respectful as opposed to one which is autocratic and formal. Planning the learning experience should involve negotiation between the parties, rather than being controlled by the clinical and academic tutors, and methods should involve experiential learning and inquiry as opposed to transmittal techniques of teaching (Warren-Piper, 1984). This is not easy to achieve when one considers the circumstances in which many clinical tutors work and the limited education in teaching they receive. It is important that academic staff do their utmost to ensure that both clinical tutors and students are adequately supported and informed. Students should be treated like the intelligent adults they are and, with guidance, be granted greater responsibility for their own learning in the clinical situation.

REFERENCES

Arnold, H J and Feldman, D C (1986). *Organisational Behaviour*, McGraw-Hill International Editions, New York.

Beard, R and Hartley, J (1984). *Teaching and Learning in Higher Education* (4th edn) Paul Chapman Publishing Ltd, London.

Best, D (1988). 'Physiotherapy clinical supervision: Effectiveness and the use of models', *Australian Journal of Physiotherapy*, 34, 4, 209–214.

Coates, F (1986). 'Clinical supervision — No! Clinical teaching — Yes!' *Bulletin of the Association of Teachers of the Chartered Society of Physiotherapy*, **5**, Spring, 5.

Emery, M J (1984). 'Effectiveness of the clinical instructor: Students' perspective', *Physical Therapy*, **64**, 1079–83.

Gardiner, M J (1989). *The Anatomy of Supervision — Developing learning and professional competence for social work students*, Society for Research into Higher Education/Open University, Milton Keynes.

Griffiths, P (1989). 'Creating a learning environment', *Physiotherapy*, **73**, 335–336.

Heron, J (1988). 'Assessment revisited'. in: Boud, D (ed) *Developing Student Autonomy in Learning* (3rd edn) Kogan Page, London.

Ilott, I (1990). 'Facing up to the fear of failure', *Therapy Weekly*, **17**, 10, 6.

Marsen, S (1990). 'Creating a climate for learning', *Nursing Times*, **66**, 17, 53–55.

Mason, S N (1984). 'Developing the teaching role of the ward sister', *Nurse Education Today*, **4**, 1, 13–16.

Mathews, A (1987). *In Charge of the Ward*, Blackwell Scientific Publications, Oxford.

May, B J (1983). 'Teaching a skill in clinical practice', *Physical Therapy*, **63**, 10, 1627–33.

Orton, H D (1984). 'Learning on the ward — How important is the climate?' in: Skevington, S (ed) *Understanding Nurses*, John Wiley and Sons, Chichester.

Scully, R M and Shepard, K F (1983). 'Clinical teaching in physical therapy education', *Physical Therapy*, **63**, 3, 349–358.

Sotosky, J R (1984). 'Physical therapists' attitudes towards teaching', *Physical Therapy*, **64**, 3, 347–349.

Warren-Piper, D (1984). 'Sources and types of reform' in: Goodlad, S (ed) *Education for the Professions*, Society for Research into Higher Education and NFER-Nelson, Guildford.

Whiteley, A J (1988). 'Using the ward as a classroom', *Nursing Standard*, **41**, 2, 31.

Perceived Differences in the Importance and Frequency of Practice of Clinical Teaching Behaviors

Crystal L. Dunlevy
Kay N. Wolf

ABSTRACT: The purpose of this study was to identify whether or not discrepancies existed between the importance of clinical teaching behaviors and the frequency with which those behaviors were practiced in the clinical setting. Surveys listing clinical teaching behaviors were distributed to preceptors and their students. Both groups completed the survey twice, ranking their perception of the importance of each behavior, as well as the frequency with which it was practiced in the clinical setting. Four different allied health disciplines from four, four-year undergraduate institutions in Ohio participated in the study. Means and standard deviations were calculated for each item. Two-tailed t-tests were applied to each set of responses, with $p<0.05$ considered statistically significant. Results revealed that while both students and preceptors agreed on the importance of the items, they differed significantly ($p<0.05$) with regard to the frequency with which effective clinical teaching behaviors were practiced.

Clinical teaching is a major component in the majority of allied health/medical educational programs, and it involves numerous clinicians in its implementation. At The Ohio State University alone, the School of Allied Medical Professions (SAMP) utilizes the services of approximately 200 nonsalaried adjunct instructors at various academic ranks to provide clinical education. Further, the programs that rely heavily on clinical education collectively require approximately 5200 clinical practice hours annually. Many of the clinical faculty involved in providing these experiences have little or no training in educational methods, and often are chosen as clinical preceptors on the basis of their will-

Reprinted with permission from the *Journal of Allied Health.* Dunlevy CL, Wolf KN. 1992;21:175-183.

ingness to participate or their clinical expertise.[1] However, these two conditions may not consistently translate into effective clinical teaching behavior.

A review of the literature revealed limited resources available on the evaluation of clinical teaching in allied health. The majority of articles dealing with clinical teaching concentrate on eliciting perceptions of effective teaching behaviors.[2-6] However, few of these utilized valid, reliable instruments in order to identify those behaviors. Further, these studies have not moved beyond the identification of effective clinical teaching behaviors, to offering practical suggestions for implementation of the effective behaviors. An earlier study by the authors identified 34 desirable clinical teaching behaviors, and 8 commonly cited students problems, through open-ended questionnaires sent to clinical preceptors.[7] The questionnaire used in the previous study also solicited suggestions for implementing the effective teaching behaviors in the clinical setting. These suggestions were outlined previously by the authors.[7]

The literature generally recognizes the use of scales or forms that list effective clinical teaching behaviors as an acceptable means of evaluation for clinical educators.[8-10] Such scales are generally completed by both peers and students, and are subsequently used to evaluate clinical educator effectiveness. Although the articles are helpful in pointing out effective behaviors, they generally make no attempt to offer practical suggestions for the implementation of those behaviors. One institution, however, has recently developed an entry-level course specifically designed to instruct clinical educators on the roles and responsibilities associated with clinical instruction.[11] Zimmerman and Westfall identified 43 "effective clinical teaching behaviors" (ECTB), and assessed the factors for content and construct validity through factor analysis, internal consistency, and test-retest reliability. The ECTB scale was found to possess both content and construct validity as well as test-retest reliability.[12]

The purpose of the study described in this paper was to determine clinical teaching behaviors deemed effective and the frequency with which they were actually implemented in daily clinical instruction. By identifying clinical teaching behaviors that were ranked as important but infrequently practiced, awareness of important clinical teaching behaviors can be increased among clinical faculty and preceptors. Improved awareness of effective teaching behavior has great potential to affect student learning in the cognitive, affective, and psychomotor domains.

MATERIALS AND METHODS

With the authors' permission, the 43-item ECTB survey instrument developed by Zimmerman and Westfall was sent to 102 senior students enrolled in four-year programs of physical therapy, respiratory therapy, coordinated dietetics, and medical technology, and 125 of the senior students' preceptors at four different undergraduate institutions throughout Ohio. The importance and frequency of implementation of these behaviors were rated on a Likert-type scale.

The students and preceptors completed the survey twice. The first time, respondents were asked to indicate the importance of each of the 43 behaviors listed, responding with 1 (not at all important), 2 (of little importance), 3 (somewhat important), 4 (important), and 5 (very important). Respondents were then asked to rate the frequency with which these behaviors were actually practiced in the clinical setting, relative to their own experience, on the following scale: 1 (never), 2 (seldom), 3 (occasionally), 4 (often), and 5 (always).

The response rate was 72% (n=90) for clinical preceptors, and 100% (n=102) for students. Means and standard deviations were calculated for each of the 43 items listed on the ECTB instrument. Two-tailed t-tests were performed within and between student and preceptor responses, with $p<0.05$ considered to be statistically significant.

RESULTS AND DISCUSSION

Means and standard deviations for the frequency and importance of each ECTB are listed in Table 1. Students and preceptors agreed on the importance of items 96% of the time ($p>0.05$). For example, both students and preceptors agreed that honesty, patience, strong knowledge base, and dedication to patient care were important; they also agreed that research to improve the quality of patient care, skill in leading large group discussions, and encouragement of critical thinking were of lesser importance. However, the two groups differed significantly ($p<0.05$) in their perceptions of the frequency with which these behaviors were implemented on 65% (n=28) of the items. In each of these cases, preceptors reported that they actually practiced the behaviors more often than students reported observing the practices in the clinical setting.

Differences between students' and preceptors' perceptions of the ECTBs can be found in Table 2. There was no statistically significant difference between student or preceptor responses among the four disciplines surveyed. Items that revealed the largest statistically significant difference ($p<0.001$) between students' and preceptors' perceptions regarding frequency of practice included communication skills, tolerance, and availability.

Differences among students' and preceptors' perceptions of ECTBs are reported in Table 3. Although preceptors believed most of the items listed were important, they reported that they were able to practice only 30% of the 43 items more than "occasionally" (n=13). Items that preceptors ranked as important or very important, but occasionally or never practiced, included the following: acts as a resource person; identifies principles basic to practice; uses skill in group discussion; is objective in evaluation; assists students in understanding their professional responsibilities; is honest with students; corrects students tactfully; conducts clinical conferences in a productive manner; shows concerned understanding for students; tells students when they have done well; keeps self available when students are in stressful situations; helps students to identify their needs; demonstrates enthusiasm; encourages students to feel free

TABLE 1

Effective Clinical Teaching Behaviors

	STUDENT MEAN (SD) IMPORTANCE	STUDENT MEAN (SD) FREQUENCY	PRECEPTOR MEAN (SD) IMPORTANCE	PRECEPTOR MEAN (SD) FREQUENCY
1. Acts as a resource person during clinical.	4.49 (.667)	3.97 (.74)	4.65 (.54)	4.36 (.69)
2. Identifies principles basic to practice.	4.43 (.70)	3.93 (.71)	4.51 (.59)	4.25 (.72)
3. Uses skill in group discussion process.	3.94 (.72)	3.44 (.76)	3.85 (.76)	3.56 (.98)
4. Is honest with students.	4.72 (.56)	4.13 (.76)	4.78 (.44)	4.59 (.64)
5. Is objective in evaluation.	4.66 (.53)	4.11 (.71)	4.75 (.48)	4.41 (.70)
6. Assists students in understanding their professional responsibility.	4.36 (.65)	3.84 (.83)	4.4 (.64)	4.14 (.76)
7. Corrects students tactfully.	4.62 (.54)	4.20 (.68)	4.59 (.57)	4.24 (.66)
8. Conducts clinical conferences in a manner that is productive.	4.26 (.74)	3.76 (.87)	4.26 (.69)	3.86 (.93)
9. Shows concerned understanding for student.	4.31 (.70)	3.86 (.86)	4.28 (.7)	4.45 (.64)
10. Tells student when he/she has done well.	4.42 (.68)	3.9 (.96)	4.59 (.55)	4.37 (.71)
11. Keeps self available when students are in stressful situations.	4.32 (.69)	3.75 (.90)	4.58 (.59)	4.33 (.71)
12. Communicates knowledge to student.	4.55 (.55)	4.14 (.77)	4.3 (.63)	4.23 (.67)
13. Permits freedom of discussion.	4.53 (.62)	4.06 (.86)	4.54 (.58)	4.37 (.83)

TABLE 1 (continued)

Effective Clinical Teaching Behaviors

	STUDENT MEAN (SD) IMPORTANCE	STUDENT MEAN (SD) FREQUENCY	PRECEPTOR MEAN (SD) IMPORTANCE	PRECEPTOR MEAN (SD) FREQUENCY
14. Helps students to identify own learning needs/objectives.	4.24 (.76)	3.59 (.9)	4.26 (.65)	3.95 (.91)
15. Demonstrates enthusiasm that is "catching", making student interested.	4.13 (.73)	3.59 (.90)	4.31 (.63)	4.16 (.75)
16. Is a good role model for students.	4.38 (.72)	3.97 (.72)	4.59 (.54)	4.31 (.65)
17. Encourages students to feel free to ask for help.	4.66 (.50)	4.12 (.87)	4.63 (.52)	4.51 (.68)
18. Clearly defines expectations.	4.51 (.65)	3.55 (.81)	4.62 (.55)	4.08 (.84)
19. Stimulates students to think about using research to improve quality of care.	3.78 (.95)	2.86 (1.1)	3.61 (.84)	3.03 (1.0)
20. Encourages students to think critically.	4.39 (.66)	3.79 (.86)	4.25 (.77)	3.91 (.9)
21. Assists students to apply theoretical content to clinical.	4.24 (.77)	3.55 (.95)	4.17 (.72)	3.98 (.82)
22. Is realistic in expectations.	4.55 (.55)	3.91 (.73)	4.49 (.63)	4.21 (.66)
23. Encourages students to achieve to their highest level.	4.4 (.7)	3.86 (.76)	4.28 (.66)	4.12 (.75)
24. Provides helpful feedback on documentation.	4.44 (.74)	3.85 (.87)	4.35 (.58)	4.21 (.73)

TABLE 1 (continued)

Effective Clinical Teaching Behaviors

	STUDENT MEAN (SD) IMPORTANCE	STUDENT MEAN (SD) FREQUENCY	PRECEPTOR MEAN (SD) IMPORTANCE	PRECEPTOR MEAN (SD) FREQUENCY
25. Interacts well with students on a one-to-one basis.	4.41 (.66)	4.04 (.81)	4.33 (.59)	4.38 (.63)
26. Supervises in new experiences for students.	4.37 (.72)	4.01 (.87)	4.3 (.69)	4.31 (.78)
27. Is flexible.	4.34 (.71)	3.95 (.78)	4.29 (.66)	4.22 (.66)
28. Provides timely feedback on clinical performance process.	4.4 (.57)	3.87 (.72)	4.42 (.57)	4.22 (.80)
29. Interacts well with students in a group situation.	4.0 (.81)	3.77 (.77)	4.04 (.65)	3.85 (.91)
30. Demonstrates activities/procedures when appropriate.	4.5 (.58)	4.10 (.80)	4.27 (.62)	4.25 (.79)
31. Provides timely feedback on documentation.	4.43 (.70)	3.95 (.82)	4.33 (.66)	4.15 (.83)
32. Interacts well with patients.	4.36 (.67)	4.24 (.66)	4.50 (.60)	4.41 (.74)
33. Gives guidance in new and/or difficult situations.	4.54 (.61)	4.01 (.8)	4.51 (.54)	4.40 (.74)
34. Is receptive to students' input.	4.55 (.58)	3.86 (.91)	4.45 (.56)	4.31 (.75)
35. Facilitates students' own self-evaluation.	4.24 (.76)	3.74 (.94)	4.12 (.82)	3.73 (.88)
36. Interacts well with staff.	4.22 (.69)	4.07 (.65)	4.24 (.62)	4.27 (.65)
37. Assists students to see alternatives.	4.39 (.74)	3.69 (.81)	4.24 (.67)	3.87 (.74)

TABLE 1 (continued)

Effective Clinical Teaching Behaviors

	STUDENT MEAN (SD) IMPORTANCE	STUDENT MEAN (SD) FREQUENCY	PRECEPTOR MEAN (SD) IMPORTANCE	PRECEPTOR MEAN (SD) FREQUENCY
38. Asks stimulating questions of students.	4.29 (.70)	3.7 (.87)	4.29 (.73)	3.89 (.76)
39. Is organized with clinical instruction.	4.46 (.67)	3.79 (.81)	4.28 (.67)	4.01 (.79)
40. Is patient with students.	4.58 (.6)	4.15 (.68)	4.4 (.62)	4.3 (.66)
41. Helps students to recognize his/her own errors.	4.49 (.69)	3.91 (.77)	4.3 (.61)	4.05 (.63)
42. Shows genuine interest in patients and their care.	4.49 (.76)	4.14 (.73)	4.67 (.50)	4.59 (.61)
43. Attempts to ensure the selection of appropriate experiences to meet objectives.	4.36 (.73)	3.77 (.80)	4.36 (.59)	4.26 (.75)

to ask for help; clearly defines expectations; stimulates students to use research to improve patient care; encourages students to think critically; assists students in applying theory to practice; is realistic in expectations; encourages students to achieve to their highest level; provides helpful and timely feedback; interacts well with students in a group setting; facilitates students' self-evaluation; assists students to see alternatives; asks stimulating questions; is organized with regard to clinical instruction; and helps students to recognize their own mistakes. Many preceptors reported that time was the major barrier to implementation of these behaviors.

SUMMARY AND CONCLUSION

Survey results revealed numerous inconsistencies between the importance of clinical teaching behaviors and the frequency with which they were actually practiced, as well as inconsistencies between those behaviors which preceptors reported that they routinely practiced in the clinical setting, and those behaviors that students reportedly observed in their preceptors. Due to the limited

TABLE 2

Differences Between Students' and Preceptors' Perceptions of Effective
Clinical Teaching Behaviors

	STUDENT MEAN (SD) (All items combined) n = 102	PRECEPTOR MEAN (SD) (All items combined) n = 90	t-test	P
IMPORTANCE	4.39 (0.19)	4.37 (0.22)	1.11	0.28
FREQUENCY	3.86 (0.25)	4.15 (0.3)	11.55	0.00

TABLE 3

Differences Among Students' and Preceptors' Perceptions of Effective
Clinical Teaching Behaviors

	t-test	P
STUDENTS: IMPORTANCE VS FREQUENCY n = 102	20.58	0.00
PRECEPTORS: IMPORTANCE VS FREQUENCY n = 90	8.83	0.00

geographic area surveyed, the results here may not be true for areas, or disciplines, other than those surveyed. Implications for further research include the development of curricula and/or materials designed to assist clinical preceptors in implementing clinical behaviors identified as effective, and offering practical suggestions that may be easily incorporated into everyday practice.

Because many graduates of allied health programs assume the role of clinical preceptor within one year after graduation, the development of an undergraduate course segment designed to instruct students on effective clinical education is indicated. Through the identification of teaching behaviors deemed most effective, individuals who possess those attributes should be encouraged to enter clinical instruction. The opportunity also exists for the development of instructional opportunities to assist clinical preceptors in improving the quality of their instruction. By working to improve the teaching skills of clinical faculty and preceptors, there is great potential to affect student learning in the cognitive, affective, and psychomotor domains, ultimately producing more competent practitioners who may one day serve their disciplines as clinical preceptors.

REFERENCES

1. Yonke AM. The art and science of clinical teaching. *J Med Educ.* 1979;13(2):86-90.
2. Wooley AS, Costello SE. Innovations in clinical teaching. *National League of Nursing Publication.* 1988;15:89-105.
3. Pugh EJ. Soliciting student input to improve clinical teaching. *Nurs Educ.* 1988; 13(5):28-33.
4. Wong J, Wong S. Towards effective clinical teaching in nursing. *J Adv Nurs.* 1987;12(4):505-513.
5. Irby DM. Clinical teaching and the clinical teacher. *J Med Educ.* 1986;61(9):35-45.
6. Jarski RW, Kulig K, Olson RE. Allied health perceptions of effective clinical instruction. *J Allied Health.* 1989;18(5):469-478.
7. Dunlevy C, Wolf K. Perspectives on teaching practices in clinical/field settings. *American Association For Respiratory Care Distinguished Papers Monograph.* 1992;1(1):39-44.
8. Castleden WM. An audit of clinical teaching: an approach to one performance indicator of educational competence. *J Med Educ.* 1988;22(5):433-437.
9. Fallon SM, Croen LG, Shelov SP. Teachers' and students' ratings of clinical teaching and teachers' opinions on use of student evaluations. *J Med Educ.* 1987;62(5):435-438.
10. Bergman K, Gaitskill T. Faculty and student perceptions of effective clinical teachers: an extension study. *J Prof Nurs.* 1990;6(1):33-44.
11. Halcarz PA, Marzouk DK, Avila E, Bowser MS, Hurm L. Preparation of entry-level students for future roles as clinical instructors. *J Phys Ther Educ.* 1991;5(2):78-80.
12. Zimmerman L, Westfall J. The development and validation of a scale measuring effective clinical teaching behaviors. *J Nurs Educ.* 1988;27(6):274-277.

Crystal L. Dunlevy, EdD, is assistant professor, Respiratory Therapy Division; and Kay N. Wolf, MS, is instructor, Medical Dietetics Division, both at the School of Allied Medical Professions, The Ohio State University, 1583 Perry Street, Columbus, Ohio 43210-1234.

Education Feature

Congruence of student, faculty and graduate perceptions of positive and negative learning experiences

GLEN C. RAMSBORG, CRNA, MA
Park Ridge, Illinois
RICHARD HOLLOWAY, PhD
Houston, Texas

A total of 163 nurse anesthesia clinical instructors, student/graduates* and students were surveyed regarding characteristics of specific positive and negative learning experiences. Results suggested there was an extraordinary degree of congruence among students, student/graduate, and clinical instructor perceptions of positive and negative teaching/learning experiences. Results suggest that instructors may assume that students will respond to their efforts to improve clinical instruction by setting goals and expectations, motivating, stimulating memory, gaining attention, communicating effectively, providing opportunities for practice, and evaluating performance.

Do students and teachers agree on what makes for positive and negative learning experiences? The answer to such a question could have significant implications for the structure of nurse anesthesia education. There is significant evidence that congruence in the learning situation may lead to improved learning outcomes.[1] Therefore, it might be reasonably expected that congruence in perception of positive and negative learning experiences by students and instructors would also lead to improved performance on the part of both students and instructors. The study reported here begins by asking if students and instructors agree on characteristics of positive and negative learning experiences, and also examines what characteristics cause agreement or disagreement.

Nurse anesthesia education is an intensive 24-month postgraduate didactic and clinical curriculum for the registered nurse. The Council on Accreditation of Nurse Anesthesia Educational Programs/Schools requires a nurse anesthesia student to have either a baccalaureate degree in nursing, an associate degree in nursing or a diploma in nursing plus 30 semester hours (45 quarter hours) of additional college work.** In addition, one year of nursing experience in an acute patient care setting is required. Nurse anesthesia education has developed a significant commitment to faculty development and improved educational experiences by requiring continuing education for clinical instructors in the areas of curriculum, instruction and evaluation. The study reported here has implications for professional education in general and nurse anesthesia education specifically, because the clinical instructor might be able to plan for meeting student needs with greater precision.

---

*Student/graduates refers to a group of people who were surveyed once while they were students and immediately after they had graduated.

**By July, 1987, the individual must possess a bachelor's degree in nursing or other appropriate science.

Theoretical background

Professional education has become a significant component of higher education. Specifically, this type of education includes both cognitive and noncognitive indoctrination into the traditions of the profession.[2]

Blauch identified stages in the evolution of professional education. Initially, the philosophy of education was predominantly professional training, based on the apprenticeship approach. Gradually, there was a separation of formal training from practical application. As professional education has progressed, there has been integration of theory-based programs incorporating traditional subject-matter and apprenticeship experiences into the educational system.[3]

Dependence upon theory has become the distinguishing characteristic of the professions. The profession develops the theories that later become the standards by which the profession is practiced. Thus, theory has become the basis of the profession's educational programs, and knowledge of theory characterizes the professional.[2]

Mayhew described three educational experiences that are common to most professional educational programs. These experiences generally include the basic arts and sciences, typical problems and activities of the profession, and practical application—the link between theory and practice.[4]

Many professions with a limited educational research data base have devoted a significant amount of time and energy to research experiences and anecdotes. Currently, attention is being focused more on the instructional process which begins with observation of the learner. This observation is perceptive and thoughtful but seldom empirical. It has usually evolved out of a concern by the professionals about the direction of the profession and the education of its future members.[2]

Research activities in professional education initally focused *retrospectively* on prerequisite coursework, academic records, admission criteria, curriculum differences, records and/or student personal experiences. Now, professions are attempting to *predict* success in professional schools based on these topics.

In 1961, McGlothlin observed that instructors varied widely in their use of past clinical experiences to present concepts of professional practice. During the apprenticeship approach, the aspiring professional learns the many aspects of professional practice. Exposure to complex learning situations results in the acquisition of knowledge, development of attitudes and perfection of acquired skills.

The success of this approach to professional education is due in part to the prerequisite student attributes, preparatory educational experiences, variety of clinical sites, characteristics and instructional behaviors of clinical instructors, supplementary teaching strategies, evaluation of student performance and instructional evaluation.[5]

Yonke[6] and Daggett, Cassie and Collins[7] identified sources of information for determining effective instructional characteristics and behaviors. First, the experienced and successful clinical instructor describes what has worked best in the past or seemed most appropriate for the situation at hand. Second, students identify instructor characteristics and behaviors that most often facilitated their clinical learning. Third, educational researchers who are knowledgeable about instructional psychology currently are investigating clinical instruction through observation in the clinical environment. However, analysis of instructional outcomes, a complicated process which correlates cause and effect, is difficult in this type of learning environment.

The success of the instructor in professional education's clinical component is dependent upon his skill in both the *art* of teaching and the *science* of teaching. Both elements must be present in order for a therapeutic learning environment to exist.

The *art* of teaching has been described as the instructor's attitude toward teaching and interest shown in the student. Additionally, learners often emulate clinical instructors who are excellent role models and who have had a significant impact on the student. Professional competence is the role model's most important characteristic, coupled with the ability to observe and analyze the student's practice. Interaction with the student to find out what he or she knows and believes about anesthesia practice is as important as examining how the student practices. Proficiency in the art of clinical teaching enhances the instructor/student relationship.[2]

The *science* of teaching—organization, practice and evaluation—can be consciously learned and/or modified. The organized clinical instructor assists the student in establishing goals and expectations for learning, motivates the student toward problem-solving with dynamism and energy, and directs the student's attention through the correlation of previously taught concepts and practical experiences.[2]

Open, two-way communication between instructor and student allows each individual to discuss practical applications, strengths and weaknesses, and personal feelings and values which ultimately influence important decisions in regard to patient care. This type of interactive process greatly improves the learning situation, and the practice in communication helps the student to solidify the knowledge, attitudes and/or skills to be learned in each clinical situation.[8]

The instructor must guide the student's practical experiences toward a set of predetermined concepts—the theory supporting the learning experience. As the student moves along the learning continuum, the instructor is less involved in directing instruction and more involved in the supervision and evaluation of the student's performance.[9]

The final and probably most important part of the process is evaluation of student performance. Giving the student prompt and systematic feedback is paramount. A student's difficulties in learning should always be privately discussed with him and a mutually agreed upon plan for corrective action should be developed. In addition to evaluating student performance, the instructor should introspectively evaluate his own teaching strategies, obtain verbal and/or written feedback from the student and make modifications in his approach to the teaching/learning process. This ultimately will enhance the responsibility and independence of the student and will result in a safe, competent practitioner.[8]

In most clinical environments, a one-to-one relationship exists between the instructor and student which can become a "mentor-protege" model for instruction. The staff anesthetist or clinical instructor is the mentor. The mentor must focus on the care of the patient, but must ensure that the needs of the protege are met as well. In this situation, the mentor must demonstrate a dual advocacy for the patient and the protege. It is important to understand that the mentor-protege model is congruent with the daily practice of the staff anesthetist. While some may find themselves unable or unwilling to adopt this model, they must be able to recognize, extract, and use the principles of the model, which often requires sensitivity and practice.[10]

Method

The study was conducted with students and teachers from 22 schools of nurse anesthesia which were randomly chosen from the "List of Recognized Educational Programs," as published by the Council on Accreditation of Nurse Anesthesia Educational Programs/Schools in July, 1982. A total of 272 questionnaires were used of which 163 were usable, for a response rate of 59.92%. Included in the sample were 27 clinical instructors, 13 student nurse anesthesia graduates of the Minneapolis School of Anesthesia, and 123 current students in schools across the country.

Respondents were asked to recall a specific instance of a negative or positive learning experience and then respond to 26 items culled from a questionnaire by Stritter and Flair[8] which encompassed areas of (1) establishing goals and expectations, (2) motivation, (3) memory stimulation, (4) attention, (5) communication, (6) practice and (7) evaluation. Each item was scored on a four-point scale, assessing whether a behavior was extremely well done, fairly well done or not done at all.

The authors hypothesized that for all areas of clinical teaching, positive experiences would be rated significantly higher than negative ones. These differences were expected to be greatest in the areas of "establishing goals and expectations" and evaluating and reinforcing the student. Discrepancies were also expected to be greater for graduates than students.

Results

Of the 163 questionnaires returned, 85 related a positive teaching/learning experience and 78 related a negative teaching/learning experience. There was a 31-year span in graduation dates of the clinical instructors and student/graduates. Graduations occurred from 1951 to 1982, with a mean of 1977, a median of 1979 and mode of 1981.

The Council on Accreditation of Nurse Anesthesia Educational Programs/Schools requires that clinical instructors have preparation in the areas of curriculum, instruction and evaluation.[11] Clinical instructor respondents reported that 52% (14) had completed the curriculum component, while 70% (109) had completed the instruction and evaluation component. Student respondents indicated 15% (19) had completed the curriculum component while 17% (21) had completed the instruction and evaluation components. The student/graduate population revealed that 38% (5) had completed the curriculum component and 62% (8) had completed both the instruction and evaluation components.***

The information obtained about the highest academic achievement for all three groups was

***This research was completed in 1984; presently there is near 100% compliance of the curriculum, instruction and evaluation requirements.

compiled together. The results were as follows: associate degree in nursing - 31; diploma - 39; baccalaureate - 87; master's - 2; doctorate - 0; and, no degree in this category - 4. The breakdown of respondents according to highest academic achievement earned in anesthesia was as follows: certificate - 86; baccalaureate - 8; master's - 29; doctorate - 0 and, no degree in this category - 40. The breakdown of the highest academic achievement in an academic field related to nursing or anesthesia was: baccalaureate - 53; master's - 4; doctorate - 1; and, no degree in this category - 105.

The number of months each student was in a nurse anesthesia program ranged from 5-30 months. The mean and mode were 14.2 months and the median was 18 months.

Survey analysis

Table I contains obtained reliability estimates (Cronbach's alpha) for the seven scales for each of the three populations and for the total. As is evident, the reliabilities were uniformly excellent in those scales for which estimates could be made (two scales were not calculated for reliability because they contained one and two items, respectively). The authors have concluded that the scales had achieved an acceptable level of reliability to allow continuation with further analyses.

Analysis of variance was performed using a 2x3 factorial design (2 levels of learning experience: positive or negative x 3 levels of respondent type: clinical instructor, student or student/graduate) to determine if differences in perceptions existed between the instructors and students on positive and negative experiences. Each of the subscales (goals and expectations, motivations, and the like) was treated as a separate dependent measure.

Table I
Reliabilities (Cronbach's Alpha)

Scale	Clinical Instructor	Student/ Graduate	Student	All
Goals	.83	.94	.86	.87
Motivation	.83	.97	.89	.90
Memory stimulation	*	*	*	*
Attention	*	*	*	*
Communication	.83	.93	.89	.88
Practice	.83	.93	.89	.88
Evaluation	.94	.97	.94	.94
Total	.96	.99	.97	.97

*Number of items were too low for accurate reliability estimates.

Scale 1 (Establishes goals and expectations). Significant differences were found between positive and negative experiences (F=31.211, df 1, 67, p< .001), but not between types of respondents.

Scale 2 (Motivates the student). Again significant differences were found between positive and negative experiences (F=5.3, df 1, 105, p< .05), but not between types of respondents.

Scale 3 (Stimulates the student's memory). As before, significant differences were found only for the positive vs. negative learning experience difference (F=7.084, df 1, 58, p<.01)

Scale 4 (Directs student's attention). Positive-negative dimension was significant (F=19.806, df 1 38, p<.001).

Scale 5 (Communicates with student). Positive-negative dimension was significant (F=9.996, df 1 92, p<.002).

Scale 6 (Providing practice for the student). Positive-negative was significant (F=12.749, df 1, 73, p<.001).

Scale 7 (Evaluating and reinforcing the student). Positive-negative was significant (F=7.429 df 1, 103, p<.01).

Discussion

Each clinical instructor and student was asked to give a brief description of his or her most positive or most negative teaching/learning experience. Responses were to relate to one specific situation, and generalizations were to be avoided. Each response was analyzed and categorized first as a positive or negative teaching/learning experience and then as clinical or instructional in nature.

Content analysis of the clinical situations written on each questionnaire suggest that positive and negative learning experiences may be due to clinical problems (such as responsibility for procedures or patient difficulty) or instructional problems (such as instructor or student attitudes or guidance). Specific feedback to students and instructors regarding these experiences may well prove useful to enhance the acquisition of skills in the clinical setting.

Clinical instructors most often noted that positive teaching experiences resulted when the student was motivated and exhibited an enthusiasm for learning, and possessed the ability to correlate and apply didactic material in the clinical environment. Students and student/graduates most often noted that mastering a new skill or technique, having an instructor who projected confidence into the situation and winning a degree of independence in practice made for positive clinical learning experiences.

Clinical instructors stated that conflict between members of the anesthesia care team and dislike for instructing students created negative clinical teaching experiences. Students and student/graduates repeatedly expressed frustration at not being able to use techniques or anesthetic plans they suggested. This was further compounded by the instructor's insistence on personal preferences over concrete principles of practice. Additionally, several students noted that instructors who did not offer support when a problem occurred and berated a student's judgment created negative learning experiences.

Negative instructional experiences identified by clinical instructors were most often caused by students with a "know-it-all" attitude, argumentative students and students who were unable to meet expectations.

Negative instructional experiences from a student and student/graduate perspective included condescending comments by instructors in the presence of others, frustration with the instructional technique utilized by the clinical instructor, lack of positive feedback and insensitivity to the student's personal needs.

Clinical instructors noted that their most positive instructional experiences came from watching students mature and grow, as they moved through the program, changing from beginning students requiring extremely close supervision to safe, competent graduate practitioners.

Students and student/graduates indicated that managing a case with minimal supervision using problem-solving skills resulted in positive learning experiences from an instructional perspective. Students responded positively to open communication and dialogue regarding case management, constructive feedback and reinforcement.

These results suggest that there is nearly complete congruence among faculty, students, and graduates regarding positive and negative learning experiences. Furthermore, results suggest that this instrument is extremely capable of differentiating between positive and negative learning experiences.

Future research

The three groups surveyed reported that they highly value the items identified in each scale. The authors suggest that future research investigate the actual utilization of the skills valued by clinical instructors.

Additional investigations currently being performed attempt to determine if students actually learn best through the characteristics they claim to value highest.

REFERENCES

(1) Boshier R. 1973. Educational participation and dropout: A theoretical model. *Adult Education*, 23 (4) : 255-282.
(2) Dinham SM, Stritter FT. 1984. *Third Handbook of Research on Teaching*. New York: MacMillan Publishing Company.
(3) Blauch LE. 1962. A centruy of the professional school. In W. W. Brickman & S. Lehrer (Eds.), *A Century of Higher Education*. New York: Society for the Advancement of Education.
(4) Mayhew LB. 1971. *Changing Practice in Education for the Professions*. Atlanta: Southern Regional Educational Board.
(5) McGlothlin WJ. 1961. Insights from one profession which may be applied to other professions. In G. K. Smith (Ed.), *Current Issues in Higher Education*. Washington, D.C.: Association for Higher Education.
(6) Yonke AM. 1979. The art and science of clinical teaching. *Medical Education*, 13, 86-90.
(7) Daggett CJ, Cassie JM, and Collins GF. 1979. Research on clinical teaching. *Review of Educational Research*, 49: 151-169.
(8) Stritter FT and Flair MD. 1980. *Effective Clinical Teaching*. Bethesda: National Medical Audiovisual.
(9) Gunn IP. 1977. Unpublished paper. Presented at the AANA Assembly of School Faculty meeting, February, 1977.
(10) Tobias R. 1981. Learning anesthesiology made less stressful by increasing teacher effectiveness. *Journal of the American Association of Nurse Anesthetists*, 386-388.
(11) Council on Accreditation of Nurse Anesthesia Educational Programs/Schools. 1980. *Standards and Guidelines for the Accreditation of Nurse Anesthesia Educational Programs/Schools*, p. 32.

SUGGESTED READING

(1) Knowles MS. 1978. *The Adult Learners A Neglected Species*. 2nd edition. Houston: Gulf.
(2) Cross KP. 1981. *Adults as Learners*. San Francisco: Jossey-Bass, Inc.

AUTHORS

Glen C. Ramsborg, CRNA, MA, received his anesthesia education at Northwestern Hospital School of Anesthesia in Minneapolis, Minnesota, and his BS in nurse anesthesia and MA from the University of Minnesota. Currently, he is a PhD candidate in educational administration at the College of Education at the University of Minnesota. He is a lieutenant colonel in the United States Air Force Reserve, and serves as military consultant for the U.S. Air Force to the Surgeon General. Mr. Ramsborg is deputy executive director of the AANA.

Richard L. Holloway, PhD, received his MS and PhD from Syracuse University, Syracuse, New York. He has been widely published and has presented papers to a variety of professional groups. He is a member of the Research Committee of the Society of Teachers of Family Medicine, and a member of the Committee on Research and New Techniques of the Minnesota Academy of Family Physicians. He is the recipient of several research grants. Currently, he is research coordinator and associate professor, Department of Family Medicine, Baylor College of Medicine, Houston, Texas.

Ratings of Clinical Clerkship Feedback by Allied Health Faculty and Students

Patricia A. Hageman

ABSTRACT: The purpose of this survey study was to investigate allied health faculty members' and students' ratings of the clinical educational feedback process. Faculty members and students from seven allied health programs at the University of Nebraska Medical Center, who were currently involved with clinical education, were asked to indicate their feelings on a seven-point scale for each of 22 feedback characteristics. An ANOVA and a Scheffe's test for post hoc analysis were used for data analyses. The results indicated that while both faculty members and students perceived eight feedback characteristics as equally important, they differed significantly (p < .01) in their ratings of actual feedback provided in the characteristics of specific, timely, encouraging, and recommending improvement. Other significant faculty/student discrepancies were found in the area of student reception of feedback provided. The results are useful to guide and direct improvements in the clinical education of allied health students.

Clinical education of allied health students incorporates learning by doing in the presence of a clinical model. Feedback and evaluation, though they differ, are integral components of the daily communication that clinical faculty members use to help students learn. True feedback is characterized as being direct, descriptive, accepting and respecting an individual's freedom, and immediate. Henry[1] states that it is difficult to give true feedback because it is

Patricia A. Hageman is assistant professor of physical therapy education at the University of Nebraska Medical Center, Omaha, Nebraska 68105.

Manuscript received April 28, 1987; accepted October 27, 1987.

often confused with judgements made during evaluation.

The literature defines feedback as useful as an instructional technique if it is explicit and done without delay.[2] Feedback must be relevant, verifiable, impactive, and focused in order to be effective.[3] Feedback is essential, especially in handling the problem student, because it gives the student the opportunity to recognize deficits and then change.[4] In addition, the faculty learn about the professional attitudes of students by observing their responses to the feedback provided.

Despite its instructional importance, few studies are found in medical or allied health education that focus on feedback processes,[5-7] or that separate the feedback process from the evaluation process in clinical teaching.[1] For this study, feedback is defined as information conveyed from faculty members to students about their past performance in the clinics which serves to enhance or modify future actions of the learners.[7] The purpose of this study was to investigate allied health faculty members' and students' perceptions of the feedback process within the clinical educational setting.

METHOD

In February 1987, a feedback questionnaire was sent to all faculty members (n = 140) and all students (n = 115) from seven professional programs within the School of Allied Health Professions (SAHP) at the University of Nebraska Medical Center, who were currently involved with clinical education. The SAHP programs of Medical Nutrition (MN), Medical Technology (MT), Nuclear Medicine (NM), Physical Therapy (PT), Physician Assistant (PA), Radiation Therapy Technology (RTT), and Radiologic Technology (RT) were represented.

The questionnaire sent to both the faculty and students was identical in form and content except that the faculty were asked to respond regarding feedback they provided to students, and the students were asked to respond regarding feedback they received from faculty. Faculty members and students were asked to rate their perceptions of 22 feedback characteristics representing four categories: importance of feedback, feedback provided or received, faculty feedback procedures, and student reception of feedback. The respondents were asked to indicate their feelings on a seven-point scale in which 7 = very important or always, and 1 = not important or never.

The first three categories of this questionnaire were formatted in a similar fashion to a 1984 study of clinical clerkship feedback by Gil et al[7] of medical students and medical faculty. In this study, an extensive review of the literature revealed a repeated emphasis on certain criteria for effective feedback. These criteria were used to establish feedback areas in their questionnaire, and subsequently in the questionnaire used in the present study.

The first category of the survey asked the respondents to indicate the importance they felt each of eight feedback characteristics had in the clinical education of allied health students. The eight characteristics describing the feedback were: sufficient, specific, timely, regular, relevant, encouragement, recommendations for improvement, and reciprocity; each of these was followed by a statement clarifying its meaning. Clarifying statements for each of the characteristics are included in Table 2.

The second category of the questionnaire requested the respondents to rate the feedback provided or received during the clinical clerkships within the past two months on the same eight feedback characteristics.

Within the third category, the respondents were asked about their feelings on whether faculty took enough time to provide feedback, based their feedback on direct observations of clinical performance, and took feelings of students into account when providing feedback.

The fourth category was incorporated into this study to identify the role of students in the reception and interaction to feedback provided by the faculty. In this section of the survey, the respondents were asked whether students acknowledged the feedback provided by faculty, whether a student advised an instructor of feedback needs, and whether the feedback received by the student modified behavior.

A one-way analysis of variance was conducted on the faculty members' and students' ratings for each of the 22 feedback characteristics to determine the significance of the main effects. The main effects were type (student or faculty) and program (MN, MT, NM, PT, PA, RTT, or RT). Post hoc analyses were completed using a Scheffe's test. The significance level was 0.05 for all analyses.

RESULTS

Sixty-nine faculty members (49.3%) and fifty students (43.5%) responded to the questionnaire. All programs were represented in the returns for both faculty and students except for medical nutrition education which had no responses from their student group (see Table 1).

Descriptive statistics for faculty members' and students' ratings for all of the 22 feedback characteristics are included in Table 2. No significant differences were observed between the faculty members' and students' ratings of importance for any of the first eight feedback characteristics. The highest rated area was reciprocating feedback and the lowest rated area was regular feedback.

Significant differences (df = 1; p < .01) were observed between faculty members' and students' ratings on the amount of feedback provided or received for these characteristics of feedback: specific, timely, encouraging, and recommended improvement. Sufficient feedback and regular feedback were also significantly different (df = 1; p < .05) between faculty and students.

Significant differences were observed between faculty and students responses on the questions that asked whether the students advised their instructors of feedback needs (df = 1; p < .01), and whether the faculty feedback modified or reinforced behavior (df = 1; p < .05).

Program was found to be a significant effect (df = 6; p < .05) for 14 feedback

TABLE 1
Breakdown of Survey Responses by Program

SAHP Program	Faculty			Student		
	Number of Surveys Mailed	Number of Surveys Returned	% return	Number of Surveys Mailed	Number of Surveys Returned	% return
Medical Nutrition	4	4	100.0%	4	0	0.0%
Medical Technology	36	14	38.8%	30	5	16.6%
Nuclear Medicine	24	9	37.5%	7	1	14.3%
Physical Therapy	36	22	61.0%	40	31	77.5%
Physician Assistant	20	13	65.0%	20	8	40.0%
Radiation Therapy Technology	7	2	28.6%	4	4	100.0%
Radiologic Technology	13	5	38.5%	10	1	10.0%
	140	69		115	50	

characteristics: characteristics 1, 2, 3, 6, 7, and 8 in the category of importance of feedback; characteristics 9, 11, 13, 15, and 16 in the category of feedback provided or received; characteristic 19 in the category of faculty feedback procedure; and characteristics 20 and 22 in the category of student reception to feedback.

A post hoc analysis revealed significance ($p < .05$) between specific programs in only 5 of these 14 feedback characteristics: between physical therapy and physician assistant programs in feedback characteristics 1, 3, and 8; between medical technology and radiation therapy technology programs in feedback characteristic 13; and between physical therapy and radiation therapy technology programs in characteristics 6 and 13.

DISCUSSION

The results indicated that while both faculty members and students perceived the eight feedback characteristics as equally important, they differed significantly in their ratings of the actual feedback provided or received. Students perceived significantly less feedback provided in the characteristics of sufficient, specific, timely, regular, encouraging, and recommended improvement than did faculty; yet all the ratings for these descriptions were above the median score of 4. These faculty/student discrepancies are similar to responses observed in a 1984 study by Gil et al[7] of medical faculty and students.

There are several possible reasons for these faculty/student discrepancies.

TABLE 2
Ratings by SAHP Faculty and Students of Feedback Categories.

Feedback Category	Student Ratings Mean	Faculty Ratings Mean	F Value Type (df = 1)	p	F Value Program (df = 6)	p
RATINGS OF IMPORTANCE						
1. Sufficient (enough to meet the needs of the situation)	6.14 (n = 50)	5.94 (n = 69)	1.07	NS	2.95	.05
2. Specific (adapted to a particular instance or purpose)	6.08 (n = 49)	6.16 (n = 69)	0.17	NS	2.55	.05
3. Timely (occurs at appropriate or within reasonable time)	6.24 (n = 49)	6.30 (n = 69)	0.13	NS	3.63	.05
4. Regular (evenly distributed during an interval)	5.49 (n = 49)	5.59 (n = 69)	0.21	NS	0.96	NS
5. Relevant (bearing upon the matter at hand)	6.22 (n = 49)	6.14 (n = 69)	0.19	NS	1.74	NS
6. Encouragement (stimulating, inspiring)	6.16 (n = 50)	6.26 (n = 69)	0.38	NS	5.98	.05
7. Recommended Improvement	6.34 (n = 50)	6.24 (n = 69)	0.00	NS	3.73	.05
8. Reciprocating (encourages 2-way communication between faculty and students)	6.38 (n = 50)	6.26 (n = 69)	0.53	NS	6.04	.05
RATINGS OF FEEDBACK PROVIDED AND RECEIVED						
9. Sufficient	4.73 (n = 49)	5.15 (n = 69)	4.42	.05	3.68	.05
10. Specific	4.90 (n = 50)	5.65 (n = 69)	13.39	.01	1.89	NS
11. Timely	4.78 (n = 50)	5.45 (n = 69)	10.30	.01	2.64	.05
12. Regular	4.40 (n = 50)	4.98 (n = 69)	4.69	.05	0.55	NS
13. Relevant	5.34 (n = 50)	5.72 (n = 69)	3.66	NS	2.83	.05
14. Encouragement	4.84 (n = 50)	5.84 (n = 69)	20.40	.01	1.80	NS
15. Recommended Improvement	4.78 (n = 50)	5.56 (n = 69)	16.19	.01	2.94	.05
16. Reciprocating	4.90 (n = 50)	5.07 (n = 69)	0.50	NS	2.75	.05
FACULTY FEEDBACK PROCEDURES						
17. Faculty spent enough time	4.70 (n = 49)	4.73 (n = 64)	0.02	NS	0.81	NS
18. Faculty based feedback on direct observations	4.96 (n = 49)	5.28 (n = 64)	1.67	NS	0.42	NS
19. Faculty took feelings of students into account	5.00 (n = 48)	5.31 (n = 64)	1.93	NS	2.31	.05
STUDENT RECEPTION OF FEEDBACK						
20. Student acknowledged feedback	5.50 (n = 50)	5.37 (n = 69)	0.41	NS	4.57	.05
21. Student advised instructor of feedback needs	4.77 (n = 49)	3.98 (n = 69)	7.72	.01	0.41	NS
22. Feedback modified or reinforced student behavior	5.08 (n = 49)	5.55 (n = 69)	5.40	.05	2.33	.05

The structure of medical care and tight patient scheduling in the clinical setting often do not allow faculty the opportunity to provide timely and regular feedback to students. In addition, many allied health clinical faculty do not have any formal training in the provision of feedback to students.[3,8] Departments rarely have clear policies about providing feedback, and this process may be neglected.[8]

Frequently, clinicians, regardless of their personal interest in teaching, are required to participate in clinical faculty roles because they are employed by teaching medical facilities. Even clinicians who are interested in teaching and who recognize the importance of clinical education are not automatically prepared to assume the role of a clinical instructor.[8] Finally, clinicians may expect students in professional training to be more mature and independent, thus requiring less feedback.[7]

The students' ratings may be influenced by their expectations of faculty members to be extremely supportive. Gil et al[7] suggested that students may expect formal feedback sessions and may not recognize feedback experiences when they are not announced. The sensitivity of the faculty to student feelings was an issue in medical education;[7] however, in this study, no faculty/student discrepancies concerning the faculty feedback procedures were observed.

The low faculty score of 3.98 for the feedback characteristic 21 implies that the faculty did not receive or did not recognize communication from students of their feedback needs. A significant difference between student and faculty ratings for this feedback characteristic suggests that barriers occur in the educational communication process. An open communication process is important because a student's provision of feedback to faculty members significantly improves the instruction and the educational experience.[9]

Variance in the ratings from all programs accounted for the significance of program as a main effect in 14 feedback characteristics. Specific programs were identified as being significantly different by a post hoc analysis in only 5 of the 14 feedback characteristics. Possible reasons for the observed significance of program as a main effect include the variety in the scope of clinical education and differences in the nature of clinical education between the seven allied health programs represented.

Caution is advised when extrapolating the results of this study to other populations. The potential for response bias exists in this study because fewer than 100% of the subjects repsonded. The results imply that feedback is an important process in clinical education and that mismatched perceptions occur between faculty members and students, although variability in the responses from different programs diminishes these generalizations to allied health as a whole.

Sheffield[10] suggested that effective teaching is a question of finding a correct match between the style of the teacher and the preferred style or needs of the student. An active feedback process between faculty members and students assists the matching of each group's needs. The results of this study are useful for highlighting specific feedback characteristics which should be acted upon for improvement of the feedback process.

Other allied health programs may find this method of investigation useful for reviewing their faculty/student feedback process. Future research should focus on what constitutes an adequate feedback process for the clinical instruction of the allied health student.

CONCLUSIONS

Seven allied health programs were represented in this investigation of allied health faculty members' and students' ratings of the feedback process in the clinical educational setting. The results indicated that while both faculty members and students perceived eight feedback characteristics as equally important, they differed significantly in their ratings of actual feedback provided or received in the following feedback characteristics: sufficient, specific, timely, regular, encouraging, and recommending improvement. A significant faculty/student discrepancy was also observed in the perception of communication by students to their instructors of their feedback needs.

Educators of allied health may find these results useful when developing methods to strengthen the clinical education process.

REFERENCES

1. Henry JN: Using feedback and evaluation effectively in clinical supervision: Model for interaction characteristics and strategies. *Phys Ther* 1985 65:354–357.
2. Wessels IR: What in the senior student's view makes a good and what makes a bad teacher at a medical faculty? *S Afr Med J* 1973 47:2085–2086.
3. Irvy D, Evans J, Larson L: Trends in clinical evaluation, in Morgan MK, Irby DM (eds): *Evaluating Clinical Competence in the Health Professions.* St. Louis, Mosby, 1978 pp 20–29.
4. Moeller P: Clinical supervision: Guidelines for managing the problem student. *J Allied Health* 1984 13:205–211.
5. Stritter F: Clinical teaching re-examined. *J Med Educ* 1975 50:876–882.
6. Irby D: Clinical teacher effectiveness in medicine. *J Med Educ* 1978 53:808–815.
7. Gil DH, Heins M, Jones P: Perceptions of medical school faculty members and students on clinical clerkship feedback. *J Med Educ* 1984 59:856–864.
8. Emery MJ: Effectiveness of the clinical educator: Students' perspective. *Phy Ther* 1984 64:1079–1083.
9. Cohen PA: Effectiveness of student-rating feedback for improving college instruction: A meta-analysis of findings. *Res High Educ* 1980 13:321–341.
10. Sheffield EF (ed): *Teaching in Universities: No One Way.* Montreal, Canada, McGill-Queen's University Press, 1974.

Allied Health Perceptions of Effective Clinical Instruction

Robert W. Jarski
Kornelia Kulig
Ronald E. Olson

ABSTRACT: Clinical instruction is a critical component of allied health education. The purposes of this study were to identify those behaviors of clinical instructors perceived as both most effective and most hindering in facilitating learning, to identify and compare the behaviors of clinical instructors as perceived by two different allied health groups, and to categorize into meaningful domains the behaviors identified. A published 58-item questionnaire was completed by 311 clinical students and instructors from eight physical therapy and ten physician assistant programs. Results were analyzed by multivariate analysis of variance. Instructor behaviors rated as most helpful in learning included answering questions clearly, taking time for discussion and questions, and providing opportunities for practicing skills. Behaviors most hindering to learning were asking questions in an intimidating manner and correcting student errors in front of patients. Ratings were significantly different ($P \leq .001$) between the physical therapy and physician assistant groups on 13 items, and posed important considerations for allied health educators.

Clinical teaching constitutes a major portion of most allied health educational programs, and many clinicians are involved in this phase of student education. The clinical phases of physical therapy (PT) and physician assistant (PA) education are where the theoretical and practical components of the educational process are integrated into real life situations. Clinical instructors are role models for students and should exemplify excellent humanitarian and interpersonal skills.

A number of common characteristics are shared by PTs and PAs.[1-3] Both evaluate and treat patients in a variety of outpatient and inpatient settings, and have educational programs that typically require patient contact experience prior to application for study. During the formal program, the clinical practi-

Reprinted with permission from the *Journal of Allied Health*. Jarski RW, Kulig K, Olson RE. 1989;19:469-478.

cums of each follow an intense course of theoretical instruction. The two professions attract students with an aptitude in the biological sciences and a desire to devote themselves to a career in the helping professions.

There are also some notable differences between these health care professions.[1,2] Physical therapy education typically emphasizes assessment and treatment of the musculoskeletal, neurological, and cardiopulmonary systems, while PA education covers the broad field of primary care medicine.

However, more similarities than differences exist between these two professional groups. Physical therapy and PA programs are frequently located in the same institutions and sometimes share faculty. In addition, some allied health "core curricula" have been implemented. However, it is not known if, or to what degree, individuals in these professions differ in their perceptions of effective clinical teaching.

Clinical teaching requires a unique subset of teaching skills,[4-8] and although many clinical instructors lack formal preparation in education, many academic programs place significant emphasis on the quality of clinical instruction. Because clinical teaching skills have not been completely defined in behavioral terms,[7] they are often difficult to assess. In addition, without accurate information about their own clinical teaching behaviors, clinical instructors may lack direction in planning their professional enrichment activities.

The purposes of this study were: 1) to identify those behaviors of clinical instructors perceived as most effective and most hindering in facilitating learning; 2) to identify the behaviors of clinical instructors perceived differently by those in PT and PA programs; and 3) to categorize into meaningful domains the behaviors identified. These domains were then used to analyze the characteristics of effective clinical instruction.

METHODS

Survey Instrument

A list of 58 effective or ineffective teaching behaviors were identified by Gjerde and Coble[4] based on the theoretical work of Stritter, et al.[6] With permission, the Gjerde and Coble questionnaire, originally developed for use in family medicine or family practice medicine, was adapted for use in allied health education by changing some of the terminology. For example, the word "resident" was changed to "student," and the scale range was expanded from 1-5 to 1-7. One item was not used because of a printing error. Questions regarding professional degrees and student or faculty status in the program were added to the beginning of the instrument. An additional item was added at the end of the instrument concerning active and regular involvement in clinical practice.

The ratings for each item were weighted as follows: 1=very helpful, 2=moderately helpful, 3=slightly helpful, 4=neither helpful nor hindering, 5=slightly hindering, 6=moderately hindering, and 7=very hindering. Multivariate analysis of variance was calculated to determine if there were overall significant differences in subjects' ratings. Wherever a significant F-statistic was found, a follow-up t-test was calculated to identify individual items that differed significantly. A conservative alpha level of 0.001 was selected to minimize the probability of detecting chance differences between the groups compared.

Sampling Method

To increase the accuracy and general applicability of the findings, eight PT programs representing eight different states in various US geographic regions, and ten PA programs from ten different states in various regions, were sampled (Table 1). Instruments with instructions and postage-paid return envelopes were mailed to the 18 program directors. A cover letter attached to each questionnaire explained the general purpose of the study and indicated that participation was voluntary. Program directors received letters asking them to distribute an instrument to each of their students involved in clinical learning and to their clinical instructors.

Subjects. One hundred thirty-nine PT students, 33 PT instructors, 107 PA students, and 32 PA instructors returned completed instruments. The subjects'

TABLE 1

Description of Subjects

		P.A.	P.T.
Number of Programs Represented		10	8
Number of States Represented		10	8
Number of Student Respondents		107*	139
Regions			
Northwest		25	28
Northeast		35	58
Southwest		21	37
Southeast		26	16
Months of Clinical Instruction	Range:	1 to 36	1 to 24
	Mode:	(N=22) 9	(N=30) 2
Number of Instructor Respondents		32	33
Physician Assistants		20 (63%)	0
Physical Therapists		0	31 (94%)
Physicians		7 (22%)	0
Other (B.S., M.S. or Ph.D.)		5 (16%)	2 (6%)
Years as a Clinical Teacher	Range:	1 to 28	1 to 20
	Mode(s):	(N=6) 1	(N=4,4) 1,8
	Next Highest Frequency:	(N=5) 9	—
Percent Time as a Clinical Teacher	Range:	2 to 100	5 to 50
	Mode:	(N=7) 20	(N=9) 10
	Next Highest Frequency:	—	(N=8) 20

*Three student questionnaires were not included in this number because zero months of clinical instruction were recorded.

characteristics are outlined in Table 1. The percentage of questionnaires returned from each program varied from approximately 14% to 100%. It was not possible to determine the exact percentage returned from most programs because questionnaire distribution was handled by program directors. In addition, the majority of students and instructors were at distant clinical sites, and it was not known how many actually received the questionnaires.

Checks on Sampling Methods. Varying return rates could have affected the results of the study. To test for possible rating differences between programs with high and low return rates, instrument ratings by PA students from the programs known to have the two highest response rates (94% and 60%; n=38) were compared to responses from the five programs having the lowest return rates (28% to 33%; n=34). In comparing the mean ratings by *t*-tests, there was no significant difference found for any of the 58 questionnaire items ($P \leq 0.05$). Thus, it was concluded that the different return rates did not significantly affect the results.

Table 1 shows that a significant number of the 32 PA instructor respondents were not PAs. Seven (22%) identified themselves as physicians, and five (16%) reported having BS, MS, or PhD degrees. Rating differences attributable to the professional backgrounds of the respondents were identified using *t*-tests. Physician assistant and non-PA ratings differed significantly ($P \leq 0.05$) on three items: 1) "creates practice opportunities for students," 2) "discusses practical applications of knowledge and skills," and 3) "demonstrates sensitivity to patient needs." In all three cases, PAs considered these behaviors more helpful than non-PA clinical instructors. It was concluded that the remaining items were not rated differently by respondents due to their backgrounds. Physical therapy instructor respondents were not compared in a similar way because only two of 33 did not identify themselves as PTs.

Behavior Classification

A simple and well-defined system was devised for classifying teaching behaviors into meaningful domains. It was determined a priori that criteria for such a system should include not only the optimum conditions for conveying knowledge and skills, but should also take into account the various relationships among all those involved in clinical education (the student, the patient, and the clinical instructor). Emery's 1984 report[7] closely delineated the essential categories. The present study used a precise definition for each term to help differentiate each teaching behavior into a clearly defined domain.

The following classification system was synthesized from various literature sources to encompass the essential conditions unique to clinical education:

1) *Interpersonal skills* include the four characteristics described by Barrett-Lennard[9] (empathy, level of regard, congruence, and conditionality). Empathy is the intellectual apprehension of another person's condition or state of mind; level of regard is the degree of one person's affective response to another; congruence is the extent to which a person appears self-

consistent; and conditionality refers to one's interest in a relationship. The Barrett-Lennard Relationship Inventory uses these four characteristics, and it has been validated on a variety of populations and used in over 100 studies, including several on health care personnel. It is probably the most suitable instrument of its kind for use in the health sciences.[10]

2) *Professional skills* are defined as the practitioner's possession and use of those qualities and traits necessary in caring for patients, and in executing any other tasks associated with the professional role. This includes scientific knowledge and technical skills gained through continuing education, scientific writing, and research.

3) *Communication skills* incorporate the methods for exchanging information by way of mutually understood messages and behaviors.[11] The instructor must be capable of expressing himself/herself in alternative ways to assure that the learner perceived the information accurately. Information refers to content as well as processes, such as clinical decision making.

4) *Andragogic or adult instructional skills* are defined as the use of appropriate educational strategies in teaching adults,[12] (ie, pedagogy) using known theories of adult education. Clinical students should be considered adults because high levels of maturity and responsibility are required of clinical students. Effective use of objectives, instructional aids, adult-to-adult discussion, and constructive feedback are examples of appropriate strategies in the adult educational process.

Without knowledge of the survey results, a group of three experienced allied health professors classified each of the teaching behaviors contained in the instrument. Each item was ascribed to one of the four skill domains: interpersonal, professional, communication, or andragogic. Consensus on item classification was achieved through group discussion.

RESULTS

The 20 items identified as most helpful by the combined PT and PA program groups are rank-ordered and listed in Table 2. The two highest-rated items were in the communication skills domain. Of the 20 behaviors, 40% were andragogic skills, 30% were communication skills, 20% were interpersonal skills, and only 10% were professional skills.

The most hindering behavior ("questions students in an intimidating manner") was in the interpersonal domain, and had a mean rating of 5.91. The overwhelming majority (60%) of the most hindering behaviors were in the interpersonal domain. The remaining domains together constituted only 40% of the behaviors perceived as most hindering. The other most hindering clinical teaching behaviors are listed in Table 3.

Thirteen items were rated very differently ($P \leq 0.001$) by the PT and PA groups (Table 4). Fifty-four percent were in the andragogic skills domain, 23% in interpersonal, 15% in communication, and 8% in professional. The greatest difference was found in the mean ratings for the item, "sets expectations which

TABLE 2

Twenty Teaching Behaviors Identified as Most Helpful

Behavior	Rank	Mean Rating*	S.D.	Domain**
Answers questions clearly	1	1.31	0.59	C
Takes time for discussion and questions	2	1.32	0.66	C
Provides students with opportunities to practice both technical and problem-solving skills	3	1.42	0.76	A
Provides constructive feedback	4	1.43	0.89	A
Discusses practical applications of knowledge and skills	5	1.46	0.77	A
Is willingly accessible to students	6	1.46	0.81	I
Shares his/her knowledge and experience	7	1.53	0.78	C
Creates practice opportunities for students	8	1.54	0.83	A
Asks questions that stimulate problem solving	9	1.55	0.81	A
Demonstrates skills for students	10	1.56	0.85	P
Demonstrates a genuine interest in the student	11	1.57	0.85	I
Demonstrates enthusiasm for teaching	12	1.59	0.83	I
Deals with students in a friendly, outgoing manner	13	1.59	0.87	I
Summarizes major points at the conclusion of the teaching session	14	1.61	0.86	A
Demonstrates sensitivity to patient needs	15	1.61	0.88	P
Is well prepared for teaching session	16	1.61	0.92	A
Actively promotes discussions	17	1.64	0.82	C
Explains clinical problems in a comprehensible manner	18	1.65	0.86	C
Emphasizes problem solving approaches rather than solutions per se	19	1.69	0.94	A
Encourages students to ask questions	20	1.72	0.90	C

*Based on the combined ratings by 311 clinical students and teachers from 10 physician assistant and 8 physical therapy programs. 1=very helpful, 2=moderately helpful, 3=slightly helpful, 4=neither helpful nor hindering, 5=slightly hindering, 6=moderately hindering, 7=very hindering.

**A=Andragogic Skills, C=Communication Skills, I=Interpersonal Skills, P=Professional Skills.

take the student's background into account." Physician assistant program respondents, with a mean rating of 2.64, did not consider this behavior as helpful as did PT respondents, with a mean rating of 2.02 (lower scores indicated that the behavior was more helpful in facilitating learning). Respondents from PT programs rated all 13 items with consistently more extreme and lower scores than did the respondents from PA programs.

DISCUSSION

The mean ratings indicated that the most helpful items were in the andragogic and communication skill domains. However, most of the behaviors perceived

TABLE 3

Ten Teaching Behaviors Identified as Most Hindering

Behavior	Rank	Mean Rating*	S.D.	Domain**
Questions students in an intimidating manner	58	5.91	1.48	I
Corrects student's errors in front of patients	57	5.62	1.48	I
Bases judgments of students on indirect evidence	56	5.33	1.51	I
Fails to adhere to teaching schedule	55	5.21	1.34	A
Fails to recognize extra effort	54	5.03	1.58	A
Is difficult to summon for consultation after hours	53	4.88	1.33	I
Discusses medical cases in front of patients	52	4.77	1.69	I
Appears to discourage student/faculty relationships outside of clinical areas	51	4.64	1.27	I
Gives general answers to specific questions	50	4.62	1.59	C
Fails to set time limits for teaching activities	49	4.49	1.51	A

*Based on the combined ratings by 311 clinical students and teachers from 10 physician assistant and 8 physical therapy programs. 1=very helpful, 2=moderately helpful, 3=slightly helpful, 4=neither helpful nor hindering, 5=slightly hindering, 6=moderately hindering, 7=very hindering.

**A=Andragogic Skills, C=Communication Skills, I=Interpersonal Skills, P=Professional Skills.

as hindering were in the interpersonal domain. These findings supported the conclusion that while good teaching and communication skills facilitate learning, good interpersonal skills alone may not.

It is possible that even if a clinical instructor has good andragogic and communication skills, poor interpersonal behaviors may hinder learning. All clinical instructors are not equally skilled in all four domains, and many appear to excel in one domain or another. According to Moore and Perry,[13] most teaching clinicians are not outstanding educators, but are excellent patient care providers. Many new clinicians serve as clinical instructors early in their careers and establish reputations as knowledgeable professionals; after a short period of service, many decline further requests to teach. Community clinical resources can add an important real world dimension to theoretical education. Because of this valuable contribution, further study is required in 1) adjunct faculty attrition patterns, and 2) motivators to increase the number of community clinical sites available to academic programs.

The present study showed that having excellent skills in one domain but seriously lacking skills in another may disrupt the teaching/learning process, resulting in a hindering rather than helping experience. For example, if an excellent clinician questions students in an intimidating manner, the clinician will be perceived as hindering learning. Future studies should investigate the degree to which one of the four domains might interfere with or compensate for

TABLE 4

Behaviors Ratings That Differed Significantly* Between
Respondents from Physician Assistant and Physical Therapy Programs

Behavior	Domain**	P.A. Mean	S.D.	P.T. Mean	S.D.	Difference in Means
Sets expectations which take the student's background into account	A	2.64	1.42	2.02	1.03	0.62
Emphasizes his/her personal research	P	3.87	1.28	3.27	1.25	0.60
Cites mistakes of students for teaching purposes	A	3.07	1.55	2.49	1.49	0.58
Compliments others for good performance	I	2.22	1.22	1.73	0.93	0.49
Demonstrates sensitivity to student needs (e.g., feelings of inadequacy, frustration)	I	2.06	1.22	1.57	0.72	0.49
Emphasizes conceptual comprehension rather than factual recall	A	2.22	1.32	1.74	0.87	0.48
Maintains atmosphere which encourages expression of differenct viewpoints	I	2.04	1.29	1.57	0.74	0.47
Emphasizes problem solving approaches rather than solutions per se	A	1.94	1.11	1.48	0.71	0.46
Compliments students for good performance	A	2.01	1.15	1.58	0.86	0.43
Provides constructive feedback	A	1.65	0.95	1.26	0.65	0.39
Shares his/her knowledge and experience	C	1.73	0.89	1.38	0.64	0.35
Asks questions that stimulate problem solving	A	1.73	0.97	1.41	0.62	0.33
Takes time for discussion and questions	C	1.47	0.80	1.20	0.50	0.28

*$P \leq 0.001$; N=311
**A=Andragogic Skills, C=Communication Skills, I=Interpersonal Skills,
.P=Professional Skills.

another. Clinical instructors lacking skills in a particular area could improve their teaching effectiveness by enhancing their skills in that area. Such factors should be considered when clinical instructors and institutions plan their continuing education offerings.

Although PTs and PAs shared a number of common characteristics, 13 of 58 (22%) teaching behaviors were perceived very differently. The PT respondents considered the research interests (professional skills domain) of clinical instructors more helpful than did the PA respondents. This was not surprising because all PT programs require a research course as part of their entry-level curriculum,[1] whereas such course work is not required in PA programs, and entry-level research courses are infrequent.[14] From this, it appeared that exposure to specific coursework in a discipline can result in positive attitudes toward that discipline.

Because physical therapists and physician assistants differed widely in their perceptions of some clinical teaching behaviors, educators should consider these differences in planning "core curricula," and in teaching important and frequently critical skills in the clinical setting.

SUMMARY

This study identified clinical teaching behaviors perceived as most effective and most hindering in facilitating learning. The behaviors were categorized and compared using well-defined, educational domains. Among the most helpful behaviors, 40% were in the andragogic skills domain and 30% were communication skills. Sixty percent of the most hindering behaviors were interpersonal skills. It was concluded that good teaching and communication skills facilitate learning, and good interpersonal skills alone do not. However, even if a clinical instructor possesses good andragogic and communication skills, poor interpersonal behaviors may hinder the learning process.

The behaviors that were perceived differently by subjects in PT and PA programs were compared. Thirteen items were rated very differently, and educators should take into account these differences when planning allied health "core curricula."

REFERENCES

1. Tammivaara J, Yarbrough P, Shepard KF: *Assessing the Quality of Physical Therapy Education Programs.* Alexandria, Va, American Physical Therapy Association, 1986.
2. Schafft GE, Cawley JF: *The Physician Assistant in a Changing Health Care Environment.* Rockville, Md, Aspen Publishers, Inc, 1987.
3. Hislop HJ: The not-so-impossible dream. *Phys Ther* 1975;55(10):1069-1080.
4. Gjerde CL, Coble RJ: Resident and faculty perceptions of effective clinical teaching in family practice. *J Med Educ* 1982;14(2):323-327.
5. Irby DM: Clinical teacher effectiveness in medicine. *J Med Educ* 1978;53:808-815.
6. Stritter FT, Hain JD, Grimes DA: Clinical teaching reexamined. *J Med Educ* 1975;50:876-882.
7. Emery MJ: Effectiveness of the clinical instructor: Students' perspective. *Phys Ther* 1984;64(7):1079-1083.
8. Scully RM, Shepard KF: Clinical teaching in physical therapy education: An ethnographic study. *Phys Ther* 1983;63(3):349-358.
9. Barrett-Lennard GT: Dimensions of therapist response as casual factors in therapeutic change. *Psychol Monographs* 1962;76(43):Hole No. 562.
10. Jarski RW, Gjerde Cl, Bratton BD, et al: A comparison of four empathy instruments in simulated patient-medical student interactions. *J Med Educ* 1985;60:545-551.
11. *Webster's Ninth New Collegiate Dictionary.* Springfield, Mass, Merriam-Webster, Inc, 1983.
12. Knowles MS: *Andragogy in Action: Applying Modern Principles of Adult Learning.* San Francisco, Jossey-Bass Publishers, 1985.

13. Moore ML, Perry JF: *Clinical Education in Physical Therapy: Present Status/Future Needs.* Washington, DC, American Physical Therapy Association, 1976.
14. Oliver DR: *Fourth Annual Report on Physician Assistant Educational Programs in the United States, 1987-88.* Alexandria, Va, Association of Physician Assistant Programs, 1987.

Robert W. Jarski, PA-C, PhD, is associate professor; Kornelia Kulig, PT, PhD, is assistant professor; and Ronald E. Olson, PhD, is professor and dean, all in the School of Health Sciences, Oakland University, Rochester, MI 48309-4401.

This project was funded in part by a grant from the Oakland University Educational Development Fund.

Manuscript received February 20, 1989; accepted August 7, 1989.

Comparing Students' Feedback about Clinical Instruction with Their Performances

DAVID C. ANDERSON, M.D., ILENE B. HARRIS, Ph.D.,
SHARON ALLEN, M.D., Ph.D., LEON SATRAN, M.D., CAROLE J. BLAND, Ph.D.,
JOAN A. DAVIS-FEICKERT, M.A., GREGORY A. POLAND, M.D., and
WESLEY J. MILLER, M.D.

Abstract—Validation of students' feedback as a measure of teaching effectiveness has been problematic for courses teaching clinical skills. This is true in part because establishing a valid and reliable method of assessing students' mastery of clinical skills has been a stumbling block. Reported here is the correlation of students' performances on an objective structured clinical examination (OSCE) with previously and independently collected feedback from students. In 1987–88, 190 second-year medical students at the University of Minnesota Medical School —Minneapolis spent one fourth of a second-year clinical skills course on neurology randomly assigned to one of four teaching sites — hospitals A, B, C, and D. Following their rotations, 180 of the students completed usable feedback forms. The students were consistently and significantly more positive about the teaching at hospital A. At the end of the year, all 190 students were tested using an OSCE having 20 stations, four of which presented neurologic problems. The students who had the neurology course at hospital A performed better on all four neurology problems, and differences were statistically significant for two of the problems. Feedback in this case accurately reflected a more effective teaching program. *Acad. Med.* 66(1991):29–34.

Teaching is an important mission of academic medicine, and "good" teaching, like "good" research, should be considered worthy of respect and reward. Teaching effectiveness, however, is generally viewed as more difficult to evaluate than the quality of research. This is particularly true of clinical teaching occurring at the bedside. The most readily available data for evaluating teaching is feedback collected from students. There is concern, however, that such assessments may be "popularity polls" that lack validity as measures of actual teaching effectiveness. Approaches for examining the validity of students' feedback as a measure of teaching and program effectiveness have not been readily available.

Theoretically, it seems most appropriate to evaluate teaching by its product or outcome, that is, by assessing students' mastery of the content and goals of the instruction. Measurement of clinical performance is typically undertaken by faculty instructors based on observation of students' examinations of assigned patients and evaluation of oral presentations and writeups. Such assessments are unstandardized and may therefore be subjective, inaccurate, and unreliable.[1] At times, moreover, faculty members do not directly observe students' clinical performances.[2] As a result, they tend to base evaluations of such skills as history taking and physical examination on the behaviors they do observe, such as students' interest in learning, aggressiveness in patient care, and verbal skills in presenting cases. Use of such product or outcome data to assess teaching effectiveness is obviously limited by potential inaccuracy and bias.[3]

The development of the objective structured clinical examination (OSCE) has provided an alternative to traditional assessment of learned clinical skills with potential for more valid and reliable performance evaluation.[4-5] In this station-to-station testing format, each student is evaluated in the same series of situations and problems. Assessment is based on observation by trained observers using standardized checklists. This test format maximizes the potential for validity and reliability and minimizes the potential for bias.

In 1988 we administered an OSCE at the conclusion of the second-year clinical skills course at the University of Minnesota Medical School—Minneapolis (UMMS). The examination results provided an opportunity to assess teaching and program effectiveness by what is generally viewed as the "gold standard" for such evaluations: valid, reliable outcome measures. In this paper, we report the relationship of feedback from students about the neurology component of the course to their subsequent performances on the neurology stations of the final OSCE.

The Course

The goal of the Introduction to Clinical Medicine course taken during year two at UMMS is for students to master clinical skills to prepare for their externships in year three. In the third segment, Clinical Medicine III (CMIII), students perfect their bed-

Dr. Anderson is associate professor of neurology, Hennepin County Medical Center, Minneapolis, Minnesota; Dr. Harris is associate professor of medical education; Dr. Allen is assistant professor of family practice and community health; Dr. Satran is assistant professor of pediatrics; Dr. Bland is professor of family practice and community health; Ms. Davis-Feickert is research assistant of laboratory medicine and pathology; and Dr. Miller is associate professor of medicine; all at the University of Minnesota Medical School—Minneapolis. Dr. Poland is assistant professor of medicine, Mayo Medical School, Rochester, Minnesota.

Correspondence and requests for reprints should be addressed to Dr. Anderson, Department of Neurology, Hennepin County Medical Center, 701 Park Avenue South, Minneapolis, MN 55415.

Another article about the validity of student feedback appears on page 26.

Reprinted with permission from *Academic Medicine*.
Anderson DC, Harris IB, Allen S, Satran L, Bland CJ, Davis-Feickert JA, Poland GA, Miller WJ. 1991;66(1):29–34.

side data-gathering skills by working with actual patients, then analyze the cases based on bedside and record data and present their findings and assessments orally and in writing. The segment is divided into four six-week periods sponsored by the family medicine, internal medicine, neurology, and pediatrics departments. The students in the year two class are grouped randomly into four quarters; each quarter rotates through the four departments in a different sequence. students spend two half-days weekly in CMIII activities.

Neurology Component

During the neurology component of CMIII, students are assigned randomly to one of the four public teaching hospitals. designated here as A, B, C, and D, in the UMMS system. The neurology goals, which are outlined in a course guidebook and communicated to students and faculty, are intended to apply across all four hospital sites. In brief, the goals are (1) mastery of neurologic examination techniques; (2) understanding of basic concepts of localization and pathophysiology in developing differential diagnoses; and (3) familiarity with clinical approaches to abnormal mental behavior, spells, coma, and motor deficits. The course is supervised at each hospital by a neurologist site coordinator.

By both design and natural evolution within scheduling limitations, considerable uniformity in the way the course is conducted exists across the four hospitals. The first week is devoted to review of the neurologic examination. During weeks two through six, the student divides one half-day weekly between attending one of the five core lectures of the course (principles of case formulation, mental status assessment, motor localization, spells, coma) and interviewing and examining assigned neurology patients. He or she prepares a written report to be turned in to the tutor, with whom the student meets the second half-day each week for supervised bedside presentations and discussions. From four to six students are assigned to each tutor, and the tutorial groups remain intact

throughout the rotation. Site coordinators are responsible for recruiting tutors from among the full-time faculty, clinical faculty, and fellows. Over the course of the year, each site uses five to ten different tutors.

Evaluation

At the conclusion of each period, tutors and site coordinators submit a performance evaluation and a pass/fail grade for each student, based on their observations of the students over the six weeks. Almost without exception, students pass all components of the CMIII course. Each student, in turn, completes a feedback form designed specifically for the neurology rotation. The form identifies the hospital site and the period during which the neurology component was taken. For all rating categories on the form, the student indicates his or her assessment of each aspect of the training using a five-point Likert-type scale, where 1 means "very strongly agree" and 5 means "very strongly disagree."

Using the form the students first give an overall assessment of the educational value of the rotation. Each student rates the effectiveness of the classroom component (initial orientation, lectures) and the degree to which his or her tutor manifested a number of characteristics considered important in stimulating learning. Second, the student is requested to judge how well the course prepared him or her to perform in various aspects of the bedside process of data collection and analysis. Third, the student provides data about the actual work requirements of the rotation, in the form of written case reports, hours spent in outside reading, and the like. Finally, the student is asked about several administrative issues, e.g., how often patients were discharged between the time of the student's workup and the opportunity for the student to present the patient to the staff two days later.

Method

The OSCE was administered to the entire UMMS year two medical

school class (190 students) at the conclusion of the complete CMIII sequence in the spring of 1988. The OSCE was administered as a 20-station examination. Four stations were devoted to neurology material: two were "skills stations" and two were "interpretive stations." In one of the skills stations (for which ten minutes rather than five were allowed), a simulated patient portrayed an acute confusional state. The student was required to perform a formal mental status examination, and his or her proficiency was evaluated by an observer using a point-based, standardized checklist. The subsequent station was an interpretive station, where the student answered five multiple-choice questions based on his or her findings. In the second neurology skills station, left upper extremity paresis was simulated by a normal individual. A limited motor and reflex examination was required of the student, whose skill was again appraised by an observer with a standardized checklist. In the subsequent interpretive station, the student answered five multiple-choice questions about his or her findings. Perfect scores for the four stations were 90, 50, 45, and 50 points, respectively.

For analysis, we averaged the feedback ratings the students had given about their neurology rotations; the students were those assigned to each of the four hospitals (A, B, C, and D). We also averaged the same students' scores on their performances at the four neurology stations in the final OSCE. We tested for between-hospital differences in (1) the averaged feedback of the students about the neurology rotations and (2) the averaged performance scores of the same students on the OSCE by using one-way analyses of variances (ANOVAs) with Scheffe-paired comparisons.

Results

In the following paragraphs, we have presented, first, the students' feedback about their educational experiences, averaged for each of the four hospitals, and second, the students' performances on the neurology items of the OSCE, averaged for each hospital.

Table 1
Students' Mean Ratings of 20 Aspects of Their Neurology Rotations at Four Hospitals, University of Minnesota Medical School—Minneapolis, 1988*

Aspect	Training Hospital (n = no. students trained who gave ratings)							
	A (n = 44)		B (n = 44)		C (n = 44)		D (n = 48)	
	Mean	SD	Mean	SD	Mean	SD	Mean	SD
Overall assessment								
Valuable learning experience	1.41	.58	1.84	.82	2.02†	.71	2.63†‡§	.82
Consistent with guidelines	1.49	.59	2.00†	.73	2.23†	.65	2.77†‡§	.84
Initial orientation/lectures								
Effective orientation	1.56	.69	2.09†	.80	2.28†	.73	3.02†‡§	.88
Lectures achieved goals	1.57	.72	1.91	.77	2.39†‡	.75	2.94†‡§	.75
Lectures delivered effectively	1.52	.73	1.75	.86	2.48†‡	.76	2.90†‡	.78
Tutor's characteristics								
Set clear goals/responsibilities	1.66	.71	2.11	.83	2.34†	.83	2.71†‡	.82
Was flexible to meet needs	1.67	.88	1.89	.85	2.18	.97	2.74†‡§	.93
Had reasonable expectations	1.52	.72	1.82	.88	2.18†	1.06	2.49†‡	.80
Was accessible for discussion	1.39	.69	1.89	.93	2.16†	.94	2.90†‡§	1.04
Supervised/observed adequately	1.89	.96	2.39	1.08	2.73†	1.04	3.02†‡	1.09
Gave regular feedback	1.84	.93	2.11	1.01	2.39	.87	2.98†‡	1.20
Made useful critiques of write-ups	1.81	.89	1.98	1.02	2.25	.94	2.72†‡	1.19
Asked challenging questions	1.50	.66	1.86	.86	2.05†	.75	2.48†‡	.87
Encouraged student's questions	1.64	.88	1.77	.84	1.98	.89	2.38†‡	.76
Gave clear, succinct explanations	1.57	.78	1.73	.76	2.05	.86	2.42†‡	1.03
Demonstrated concern for progress	1.66	.79	1.80	.91	2.20†	.88	2.77†‡§	.95
Inspired enthusiasm for neurology	1.68	.76	1.84	.87	2.43†‡	.89	2.85†‡	1.11
Was a positive role model	1.36	.65	1.82	.95	1.86	.80	2.43†‡§	1.13
Excelled as a teacher	1.60	.75	1.79	.92	2.19	.94	2.64†‡.	1.19

*The table gives 180 second-year students' feedback data about the training programs at the hospitals (A, B, C, or D) to which they had been assigned. The students provided feedback using a five-point Likert-type scale where 1 = very strongly agree and 5 = very strongly disagree. These data show that the hospital A students rated most aspects of their training more favorably than did the students at the other three hospitals. The authors correlated these data with the same students' performances on an objective structured clinical examination in order to validate the students' feedback as a measure of the effectiveness of the neurology training.

†Different from the corresponding mean rating of hospital A training at the .05 level.
‡Different from the corresponding mean rating of hospital C training at the .05 level.
§Different from the corresponding mean rating of hospital B training at the .05 level.

Feedback

Feedback forms were available for 180 of the 190 students, and return rates were similar for the four hospitals: hospital A—44/46 (number returning forms/number assigned to hospital); hospital B—44/47; hospital C—44/47; hospital D—48/50.

While the educational experiences were rated highly at all sites, the students at hospital A rated all aspects —overall assessment, initial orientation/lectures, tutor characteristics—more favorably than did the students who took their neurology rotations at hospitals B, C, and D (Table 1). Differences were statisti-

cally significant in all aspects compared with hospital D. Differences from the other two hospitals were also significant for the students' perceptions of the degree to which the rotation proved to be consistent with written course guidelines and the effectiveness of the initial orientation.

Differences by hospital assignment in the students' perceptions of their own growth in clinical skills as a result of their neurology rotations were also obtained for six of seven items (Table 2). It is noteworthy that the relative average rating of personal learning outcomes across hospitals paralleled the average ratings of the educational experiences shown in

Table 1.

Differences in the work requirements for the neurology rotation of CMIII by hospital assignment were not significant. Consistent differences in administrative matters were not detected.

Performance

Because of the large number of students, the 20-station (plus two rest stops) OSCE was administered simultaneously at three sites and repeated three times. (That is, approximately 22 students per site multiplied by three sites multiplied by three repetitions equals 198 students, which pro-

Table 2

Students' Mean Ratings of Their Growth in Clinical Skills at Four Hospitals, University of Minnesota Medical School—Minneapolis, 1988*

| | Training Hospital (n = no. students trained who gave ratings) | | | | | | | |
| | A (n = 44) | | B (n = 44) | | C (n = 44) | | D (n = 48) | |
Skill That Improved	Mean	SD	Mean	SD	Mean	SD	Mean	SD
Communicating with patients	2.14	.78	2.20	.77	2.25	.84	2.66†‡	.89
Obtaining medical histories	1.95	.71	2.13	.81	2.36	.72	2.73†‡	.89
Conducting physical examinations	1.70	.69	1.89	.84	2.02	.82	2.42†‡	.94
Applying basic science knowledge	1.86	.69	2.16	.85	2.23	.77	2.77†‡§	.79
Developing differential diagnosis	1.66	.71	2.39†	.95	2.32†	.83	2.92†‡§	.89
Organizing and communicating data	2.04	.71	2.09	.87	2.25	.65	2.91†‡§	.83
Learning independently	1.93	.75	2.16	.85	2.07	.79	2.27	.77

*The table gives 180 second-year students' feedback data about their skills improvements at the hospitals (A, B, C, or D) to which they had been assigned for neurology training. They provided feedback using a five-point Likert-type scale where 1 = very strongly agree and 5 = very strongly disagree. The table shows differences in their perceptions according to hospital assignment for six of the seven skill areas. The authors correlated these data with the same students' performances on an objective structured clinical examination in order to validate the students' feedback as a measure of the effectiveness of the neurology training.

†Different from the corresponding mean rating of hospital A training at the .05 level.

‡Different from the corresponding mean rating of hospital C training at the .05 level.

§Different from the corresponding mean rating of hospital A training at the .05 level.

vided sufficient spaces for the 190 students.) The students were assigned randomly to the OSCE sites and test session times, irrespective of their hospital assignments for CMIII rotations.

Test item reliability was assessed for the entire OSCE by using ANOVAs to compare the mean scores for each station across the three different test sites. There was no significant difference in the mean ratings across sites for the multiple-choice stations that assessed the students' interpretations of data they had acquired at the preceding skills stations with simulated patients. In several cases involving students' performances at skills stations, however, there were significant differences in the students' mean scores across sites. These differences could be attributable to variability in ratings among the examiners at the different sites—that is, imperfect interrater reliability. On the other hand, the use of ANOVAs showed that there was no significant difference in the mean ratings across sessions. This suggests high intrarater reliability, since the same raters served for all three sessions at the same site. Of the two neu-

rology skills stations, an intersite difference in scores was found for one, the mental status skills station.

The two neurology interpretive stations were each composed of five multiple-choice questions related to the previous neurology skills stations. Although one would not expect written examinations composed of five items to yield reliable total scores, it is noteworthy that each of the ten items was highly discriminating, with point biserial correlations ranging from .32 to .60.

Displayed in Table 3 are the average performances at the neurology stations of students who took the neurology rotations at the four hospitals. Students assigned to hospital A tended to perform better on all four stations. The difference was statistically significant compared with all three other hospitals for the motor/reflex skills station. One possible explanation for these differences might be that the students assigned to hospital A for neurology were simply superior. Arguing against this is the fact that the average scores on the entire OSCE were no different (by ANOVAs) for the students assigned to hospital A for neurology than for

the other students. Finally, the students were asked to rate the OSCE itself as a learning experience. Students assigned to hospital A did not rate it higher than did the others, suggesting further that as a group they were not more generous raters of teaching effectiveness.

Discussion

The students assigned to hospital A for their neurology rotation performed better on average on the neurology items of the final OSCE than did the students assigned to hospitals B, C, and D. These differences paralleled very distinct differences in the students' perceptions of the educational experience provided during the neurology rotation at hospital A compared with the other sites, especially hospital D. We would argue that the parallelism of the differences is more than coincidence, implying that the educational product offered at hospital A was superior and that the students recognized and reported this qualitative difference in their feedback. If so, these data represent a validation of students' feedback as a measure of teaching and program

Table 3

Students' Mean Scores on an Objective Structured Clinical Examination (OSCE) at Four Neurology Stations, by Students' Hospital Training Site, University of Minnesota Medical School—Minneapolis, 1988*

Skill Area Tested at Station	Highest Possible Score	Training Hospital (n = no. students trained at each hospital)							
		A (n = 46)		B (n = 47)		C (n = 47)		D (n = 50)	
		Mean	SD	Mean	SD	Mean	SD	Mean	SD
Mental status—performance	90	60.22	15.15	59.45	13.39	56.07	14.61	58.78	13.87
Mental status—interpretation	50	37.83	8.14	34.68	11.40	35.12	8.56	31.80†	10.04
Motor/Reflex—performance	45	30.12	4.01	26.28†	6.22	26.81†	5.36	27.00†	5.42
Motor/Reflex—interpretation	50	38.91	9.94	37.87	10.62	37.87	9.54	33.40	11.71

*The table gives 190 students' mean scores on the OSCE; the scores were combinations of ratings given by faculty members in the performance stations and of students' responses in the interpretation stations. The authors correlated these data with 180 of the same students' feedback about their neurology training in order to validate the students' feedback as a measure of the effectiveness of the neurology training, as measured by the OSCE.

†Different from the corresponding mean score for those trained at hospital A at the .05 level.

effectiveness.

Meaningful assessment of the quality of education endeavors of medical school faculty is important as a diagnostic process in faculty development as educators, as a means for providing information upon which to base administrative decisions about teaching programs, and as a source of data that may bear on the evaluation and promotion of individual faculty.[6] Assessment tools used for these important purposes should be valid—i.e., measure what they are supposed to measure, quality of education—and reliable—i.e., consistent and reproducible under the conditions in which they will be used.[7]

Considerable data support the reliability of student feedback about their clinical teachers.[7] Qualities of good clinical teaching have been derived by a process of extrapolation from other teaching situations and by consensus.[8,9] Nonetheless, they have demonstrated acceptable reliability.[9-11] More difficult has been validation of feedback about teaching and program effectiveness. Little has appeared in the literature regarding the relationship between students' feedback about their clinical education and actual learning outcomes.[9,12,13] In one report,[12] students' feedback about instructors failed to correlate with their subsequent performances on a final written clinical simulation. In another,[13] however, feedback about

instructors in an introductory clinical sequence predicted performance of the same students during the next sequence of a basic clinical skills course.

The difficulty of validating students' feedback against learning outcomes results from several conditions common to clinical courses: unclear concepts of the desired outcomes, multiplicity of instructors and other learning sources, and lack of valid and reliable measures of outcome. The circumstances reported here minimized the impact of some of these conditions. The neurology component of CMIII is an introduction to the neurologic clinical process; almost all students take six more weeks of neurology later. Hence, the focus of the course has remained clear and limited. Students are exposed to a standard curriculum of lectures and have one tutor throughout the rotation, thus minimizing the diversity of instructional sources. The outcome measure, the OSCE, has been shown to have high reliability and validity compared with other assessment tools.[14,15] An additional advantage in detecting a meaningful relationship between students' feedback and learning outcomes was the large number of students involved.

Despite these advantages, it is remarkable that these relationships were detected, given other potential sources of variance. Students spend only 10–20% of their time and ener-

gies in CMIII. Differences in interest, personal commitment, and clinical aptitude obviously influence the impact of the quality of the educational experience on outcome. Finally, the OSCE was administered at the conclusion of the six months of CMIII; quarters of the class had completed the neurology component 18, 12, and six weeks or immediately prior to taking the OSCE. The variation in recentness of exposure represents yet another potential influence on variation in average performance. That the site assignment influence remained apparent suggests quite different educational experiences in hospital A, attested to by the large differences in student feedback.

Although not the subject of this report, the virtues of the program at hospital A deserve comment. Among the most significant differences perceived by the students across the hospital sites were in the classroom area: initial orientation to the course and site, consistency with guidelines, and effectiveness of the lecture series. Moreover, at least five different tutors were involved at hospital A, suggesting that at the time of this study, programmatic quality and teaching climate were important aspects of the educational experience in CMIII and may have influenced the effectiveness of tutors.

In conclusion, the positive relationship between students' feedback and their performances on the OSCE stations reported here contributes to the literature on validation of students' feedback as an assessment of teaching and program effectiveness. Moreover, the positive relationship between students' feedback, averaged by hospital site, and their OSCE performances suggests the importance of instructional programs and milieu, as well as the importance of teaching, in providing effective clinical education.

References

1. Elliot, D. L., and Hickam, D. H. Evaluation of Physical Examination Skills: Reliability of Faculty Observers and Patient Instructors. *JAMA* 258(1987):3405–3408.
2. Payson, H. E., and Barchas, J. D. A Time Study of Medical Teaching Rounds. *N. Engl. J. Med.* 273(1965):1468–1471.
3. Borman, W. C. Evaluating Performance Effectiveness on the Job: How Can We Generate More Accurate Ratings? In *Evaluation of Noncognitive Skills and Clinical Performance*, J. S. Lloyd, ed., pp. 179–193. Chicago, Illinois: American Board of Medical Specialties, 1982.
4. Harden, R. M., Stevenson, M., Downie, W. W., and Wilson G. M. Assessment of Clinical Competence Using Objective Structured Examination. *Brit. Med. J.* 1(1975):447–451.
5. Newble, D. I., Elmslie, R. G., and Baxter, A. A Problem-Based Criterion-Referenced Examination of Clinical Competence. *J. Med. Educ.* 53(1978):720–726.
6. Irby, D. M. Evaluating Instruction in Medical Education. *J. Med. Educ.* 58(1983): 844–849.
7. Rippy, R. *The Evaluation of Teaching in Medical Schools.* New York: Springer, 1981, pp. 32–56.
8. Irby, D. M. Clinical Teacher Effectiveness in Medicine. *J. Med. Educ.* 53(1978): 808–815.
9. Skeff, K. M., Campbell, M., and Stratos, G. Process and Product in Clinical Teaching: A Correlational Study. In *Research in Medical Education: 1986, Proceedings of the Twenty-Fourth Annual Conference*, Stephanie Kerby, compiler, pp. 25–30. Washington, D.C.: Association of American Medical Colleges, 1985.
10. Irby, D. M., Gillmore, G. M., and Ramsey, P. G. Factors Affecting Ratings of Clinical Teachers by Medical Students and Residents. *J. Med. Educ.* 62(1987):1–7.
11. Donnelly, M. B., and Woolliscroft, J. O. Evaluation of Clinical Instructors by Third-Year Medical Students. *Acad. Med.* 64(1989):159–164.
12. Benbassat, J., and Bachar, E. Validity of Students' Ratings of Clinical Instructors. *Med. Educ.* 15(1981):373–376.
13. Petzel, R. A., Harris, I. B., and Masler, D. S. The Empirical Validation of Clinical Teaching Strategies. *Eval. and the Health Professions* 5(1982):499–508.
14. Newble, D. I., Hoare, J., and Elmslie, R. G. The Validity and Reliability of a New Examination of the Clinical Competence of Medical Students. *Med. Educ.* 15(1981): 46–52.
15. Petrusa, E. R., Blackwell, T. A., Rogers, L. P., Saydjari, C., Parcel, S., and Guckian, J. C. An Objective Measure of Clinical Performance. *Am. J. Med.* 83(1987):34–42.

Clinical Teaching and Leadership Development

The Journal of Continuing Education in the Health Professions, Volume 13, pp. 85-98. Printed in the U.S.A.
Copyright © 1993 The Alliance for Continuing Medical Education and the Society of Medical College Directors of Continuing Medical Education. All rights reserved.

Original Article

How Expert Clinical Educators Teach What They Know

SONIA CRANDALL, PH.D.
Assistant Professor
Department of Family Medicine
University of Oklahoma Health Sciences Center
Oklahoma City, Oklahoma 73104

Abstract: *Schön's Model of Reflective Practice is based on how physicians think, and it emphasizes learning from experience. In this study, 13 "above average" clinical teachers were interviewed, exploring the question "How do good teachers transmit to learners the knowing-in-action that is imbedded in experience?"*

The findings indicate that physicians think like the other professionals studied by Schön and that the stages of his model are apparent in the way good physician-teachers help residents learn from patient care experiences.

This paper discusses characteristics of the physician-teachers, examples of how their responses fit Schön's model, ways this teaching method can be incorporated into existing curricula, and implications of the model for other components of the medical education continuum.

Key Words: teaching reflective practice, characteristics of expert clinical teachers, continuing professional education, medical education

Background

Some exciting presentations and keynote addresses at recent national conferences such as Third Congress on CME and the Society of Teachers of Family Medicine could indicate a growing groundswell within academic medicine. Schön's Model of Reflective Practice[1] seems to be gaining support as a useful model for medical education because it emphasizes learning from experience. The model lends itself easily to medical education and is already being piloted in a number of residency programs. A project is underway at the University of Oklahoma that, through a charting system based on the five stages of Schön's model, tracks residents' progress in becoming reflective practitioners.

Sonia Crandall

Schön's model is highly theoretical and is open to interpretation in terms of how it is applied to professional practice. Further study is needed to determine how the process can be most effectively woven into the continuum of medical education, i.e., undergraduate (predoctoral), graduate (residency), and continuing medical education. A strong argument can be made that the model has merit for residency education and continuing medical education, because, as Schön asserts, it reflects how practitioners think. Those of us who are "believers" contend that we should go one step further and begin using the model earlier in the medical education process, i.e., with medical students.

This paper presents a study that explores how the reflective practice model pertains to medical education and how we can translate the process to apply it to the continuum of professional education.

In traditional medical education the master clinician-teacher imparts knowledge to the novice learner through what appears to the learner to be a mysterious, even mystical, process—the master at work. Many medical educators criticize this approach because it is inadequate in preparing future practitioners for the ever changing world of taking care of patients, and it is antithetical to accepted tenets of adult education. One can argue that what physicians do in practice is related to how they were taught in medical school, and certainly in residency. If we educators believe that change is needed in how physicians practice, then we need to help change the process by which they are trained.

Medical schools in several countries are embracing a new vision for training physicians, one based on the medical culture's acceptance of a new philosophy, problem-based learning (PBL). Although PBL is an improvement over traditional methods, it has shortcomings in that the tutoring so often takes place in a nonclinical vacuum. PBL prepares students to collect and to appraise information critically, a process that is fundamental to framing and solving clinical problems, but it does not necessarily prepare the learner to function in the real clinical world.

Interestingly, the training of residents is very different from medical school training. In residency education, clinical teaching—the process of transferring expert knowledge (the artistry of medicine) to learners by helping them to develop problem-solving strategies that reconstruct their knowledge around patient problems—is live. It more closely mimics the real world where real doctors see real patients in a practice setting. Arguably, this is the process by which all medical education should occur.

How do expert clinical teachers teach? How do they transmit to learners what they do as practitioners, no matter where the learners are situated on the

How Expert Clinical Educators Teach What They Know

learning curve? Schon's Model of Reflective Practice provides a conceptual framework for answering these questions. The reflective practice model combines the science of medicine (the zone of mastery) with the art of medicine (a zone characterized by uniqueness, conflict, and ambiguity.)[1] By using this model, clinical teachers can help learners : (1) organize their knowledge and skill around practice; (2) recognize and address the conflict, ambiguity, and uniqueness characteristic of each case; (3) construct and reconstruct knowledge and skill around the surprises they encounter in patient care and other aspects of the health care role; (4) experiment carefully, wisely, and effectively to address conflict, ambiguity and uniqueness; and (5) reflect on their professional performance and alter practices appropriately.[2]

Schön's model implies that professional practice is not routine and that expert clinicians frame problems well because they have practical knowledge that is fundamental to "wise action."[3] Professionals frame problems in ways that help solve them. According to Schön, as professionals solve problems they work through five stages: (1) knowing-in-action, (2) surprise; (3) reflection-in-action, (4) experimentation, and (5) reflection-on-action.

Knowing-in-action refers to the tacit knowledge that practitioners bring to the clinical encounter. Most clinical encounters contain some element of surprise: "A familiar routine produces an unexpected result; an error stubbornly resists correction; or, although the usual actions produce the usual outcomes, we find something odd about them because . . .we have begun to look at them in a new way."[1]

Professionals may react to surprise either by reflecting-in-action or reflecting-on-action, depending on the nature of the surprise. In reflection-in-action, the practitioner thinks about how to affect the situation without interrupting what he or she may be doing at the time. His or her thinking "leads to an on-the-spot experiment"[1] to resolve the surprise. He or she may alter a patient's medication, try a new procedure, or take a wait-and-see stance where time becomes a clinical trial. Reflection-on-action refers to practitioners "thinking back on what they have done in order to discover how their knowing-in-action may have contributed to an unexpected outcome,"[1] how their experiments altered the outcome, and whether to change practice because of the outcome.

For an in-depth analysis of the concepts of the reflective practitioner, refer to recent articles by Cervero,[3] Fox,[4] and Shapiro and Talbot.[5]

Some questions arise. How does Schön's framework translate to the real world of clinical teaching in undergraduate and graduate medical education? What implications does this model have for continuing medical education (CME)?

Sonia Crandall

Methods

The intent of the study was to explore the relevance of Schön's model to the education of physicians. A grounded theory approach[6] employing ethnographic interviewing was used to explore the above questions. Although this approach is ordinarily used to generate theory, it was used here in accordance with the suggestion of Glaser and Strauss[6] that it can be used simply to explore an area under study.

The predominant research question for this study was: "How do good clinical teachers translate and express to learners their *knowing-in-action* that is embedded in experience?" Purposive sampling was used to select physician-teachers for interview. Family medicine and surgery residents from two university-based programs, one in the Northeast and the other in the Southwest, were asked to identify their "above average" clinical teachers and to specify why they were thought to be above average. Faculty members who were selected by at least two residents were contacted, told they had been identified as good clinical teachers, and asked if they would agree to be interviewed about how they teach. Those who agreed to participate were sent the first four interview questions two weeks prior to the interview date in order to stimulate their thinking about clinical teaching encounters.

The author conducted all interviews during 1991 and 1992. The interviews were taped and transcribed. The interviews were fairly unstructured, allowing individuals to explore and to reflect on what they do to promote learning, what they do to help residents learn from their experiences, what they do to socialize them into the culture of medicine, and how they do all of this. The Critical Incident Technique (CIT)[7] was used to guide the interviews. The interviewer began by asking physicians to recall a teaching encounter that they believed had gone exceptionally well—in terms of the learner progressing in understanding and/or clinical expertise—and to describe everything they remembered about that encounter. They were then asked to describe in similar fashion an encounter they thought had gone exceptionally poorly.

Results

Of 14 physicians contacted for interviews, 13 agreed to participate in the study; one surgeon declined on the grounds that he did not consider himself an outstanding teacher and would thus have nothing to contribute to the study. Twelve males and one female were interviewed: four males were surgeons, the remaining nine were family practitioners. The physicians had had from two to 34 years of clinical teaching experience, with an average of about nine years. Eight of the physicians had private medical practices before entering academic

How Expert Clinical Educators Teach What They Know

medicine. The physician who had had 34 years of teaching experience has been in academia his entire career. To serve as pilot for the interview, two other physicians were interviewed first: a pathologist who has won several teaching awards and a family practitioner from another country.

The study interviews were conducted in the author's office, the physician's office, or over the telephone, and lasted from 45 minutes to two hours. Constant comparative method[6] was used to analyze the tape transcripts. Credibility (trustworthiness) of the findings was addressed primarily through peer debriefing and member checking:[8] (1) four educators, three in medical education and one from a college of education, reviewed the transcripts—peer debriefing; (2) all physicians received a copy of their interviews to give them an opportunity to provide the author with additional feedback on what they had said; and (3) all physicians were given a copy of this manuscript to assure that none of the information had been misrepresented or misconstrued—member checking.

The following sections discuss the characteristics of the physician-teachers; examples of how physician responses fit Schön's model; how this method of teaching can be incorporated into existing curricula, whether PBL or traditional; and implications of Schön's model for the continuum of professional education.

Characteristics of Physician-Teachers

Several themes emerge that reflect common characteristics of excellent clinical teachers; a few of them are more germane to family medicine than to surgery, but commonalities among all the interviews are evident. In general, these physicians are confident in their clinical competence and are comfortable with their roles as mentor and teacher. They view learners as collaborators; their approach is to solve patient problems together. They are very supportive of learners, encouraging them to make medical decisions without unnecessary intervention from the attending physician-teacher. Dr. K.B. stresses:

> "The other thing I think is important in a clinical teaching situation is, you have to separate the activity that goes on as pure teaching—with the faculty-student interaction—from patient care. So, in front of the patient we [resident and attending] make observations and discuss findings and try to be reassuring, and usually I tell them [patients] we'll confer and one of us will be back, and usually that's going to be the resident since I like to have the patient and resident have the doctor-patient relationship rather than the patient and me."

The interviewees appear to be comfortable with the fact that they take risks with learners and indeed consider risk taking to be an inherent part of clinical teaching. The learners have to have the opportunity to become fully competent practitioners, and they cannot do so if they are not allowed to take care of patients. Risk taking is defined by the interviewees as letting residents make all patient management decisions—intervening only when it is necessary, questioning learners without "pimping" them, and admitting their own weaknesses in certain clinical areas—even though admitting weakness might threaten their credibility with the learner. Interviewees seem to believe the risk is worth taking. Dr. N.F. asserts that you have to question the learners, although questioning sometimes makes them uncomfortable. He remarks:

> "Questioning is always putting people at risk because people don't like for other people to know what they don't know. They don't have a problem with people knowing what they know.....[Not knowing] embarrasses their ego. They feel they ought to know. They feel that 'I've come this far why shouldn't I know this?' They feel that you ought to tell them things rather than ask them things. But that isn't teaching. Information unchallenged is dangerous."

These physicians are open to learners' opinions. They praise learners for their successes and evince a great deal of respect for them. Nearly every interviewee affirms that excellent clinical teachers are able to admit when they feel vulnerable in a teacher-learner encounter. Dr. C.N. confesses:

> "I think it's appropriate to be vulnerable most of the time as a teacher....That's OK....It's honest. I mean, that's how I interpret it. If you're really honest you are vulnerable. Not unnecessarily so, I think that's sort of a judgment call. None of us are impenetrable, when that impenetrable image is presented I feel like somebody is still fooling themselves."

Dr. C.G. pursues the subject:

> "One [vulnerability] is that I recognize that I may be wrong, or I recognize that I may give an opinion that they can then ask someone else who may or may not be more expert than me and get a different opinion. So...I try to anticipate a wide range of opinions. The other vulnerability is being asked questions...which I simply do not have the answer to. I think we always feel vulnerable about that, but to me there are two ways to deal with that vulnerability. One is to BS your way around it, which I try to avoid doing. The other is just to acknowledge that 'I just don't know. That's an area I'm weak in, or I haven't seen a lot of patients with that kind of situation, or in my practice when I saw those kind of patients, I tended to refer them out.' I try to be very honest about my vulnerability or lack of knowledge and facilitate the resident on to someone else who can provide the answer for them."

Dr. S.T. says:

> "When I say vulnerable, I mean someone who is willing to say, 'I don't know. I'm wrong. Let's find out the answer to this. Let's tackle this problem together.' I had a few experiences where I did let my guard down—being vulnerable—where I actually saw a good outcome from a learning experience. So I decided that this isn't going to be a bad learning experience just because I'm vulnerable to new learning on my own...I don't have to know it all. So, I can express

How Expert Clinical Educators Teach What They Know

surprise. I can express frustration that I don't know the answer to something; so that I can express intense resolve that I'm going to figure this thing out. They [residents] need to see that...And how you do that, rather than just sit back on your heels and wait for everybody else to solve the problem for you...And that's, to me, that's being vulnerable."

Even if teachers do not feel vulnerable, or if they do not verbalize what they feel as "vulnerable," they still are able to admit when they don't know what is going on with a particular patient or when they make mistakes. Dr. T.G. says:

"Especially if it's an area in which I am not necessarily knowledgeable, then I think it's good for the residents to know that I can...learn something about the situation as well as the resident."

The interviewees say they recognize when a learner is having difficulty. Difficulty can manifest itself in many ways: the learner's may speak hesitantly or unintelligibly when she or he presents a patient history; the learner may be frustrated or angry, blaming the patient for not getting better; or the learner may be overly tired or having personal problems. Usually, the teacher knows what to do to help. They know what happens when the clinical teaching encounter goes awry. Dr. K.B. relates that, in most cases, it is not a matter of a learner's knowledge deficit; he cites two specific situations where he was at fault:

"The underlying deficit was my personal lack of interest [not in a teaching mood] or attention to what was going on at the time [being rushed because there were a lot of other things going on]."

Lack of time to do an effective job of teaching was mentioned by several other physicians as a primary constraint in a teaching encounter. Dr. T.G. explains:

"I think it is important to tailor the amount of teaching that you do and the kind of teaching you do to the time that you have, or the time that the students have, otherwise they are just going to be so frazzled they won't get anything that you are talking about."

These physicians try to reflect on the learning that is occurring to understand the learners' frame of reference. They seek ways to involve learners with patients and, when evident from patient encounters, they try to reengage learners who have disengaged from particular patients (a problem particularly germane to family medicine). Finally, interviewees report that excellent clinical teachers are open to constructive criticism and feedback on how they teach.

The "Fit" with Schön's Model

The interviewees describe how they help residents to learn in ways that reflect the stages of Schön's model. Below are quotes taken from interview field notes.

Sonia Crandall

Knowledge-in-Action:

Dr. S.T. says:

"I guess I try to get them [residents] to organize their knowledge like I organize my knowledge. In my mind, I organize my knowledge around—it's almost a visual recognition kind of thing, a pattern recognition kind of thing—what I think I do, in terms of medical knowledge and medical learning is, I organize facts and clues around things I've seen before that are like this [particular problem]. I can't tell you names or give you specific patient examples. I just know I've seen that pattern before."

Dr. K.B. comments:

"I use, sparingly, few facts and percentages. There are some and if it's a surgical discipline—complications rates and chances of success and chances of problems—that sort of thing, come up a fair amount and certainly the surgeon needs to have a pretty good feel for most of those things. I guess it falls back on realizing or trying to realize that so much of what we think are facts today will normally be half-truths or non-facts 5 or 10 years from now and what's important are the principles—to understand why you're doing what you do and thinking the way you're thinking. Hopefully, when those underlying principles get challenged, that's good, that's when new learning takes place or when new ideas come out—you say, 'Why does it have to be that way, or are we sure about that principle?'"

Surprise:

Dr. L.D.:

"I had an inexperienced resident helping with an inguinal hernia this morning. I told him before we started that I had no idea about how many inguinal hernias I had done, it's got to be thousands, and I always find something I've never seen before. And I said, 'I'm just going to show you.' And so we did—I'd never seen anything quite like it—and I said, 'OK, there it is. You may never see this.' So the answer is, we get surprised all the time. I think it's absolutely important to say, 'I didn't expect this.'"

Dr. C.N.:

"So before we went in there [to see the patient] I said, actually to my surprise, 'I was excited about seeing somebody who we didn't understand and who had something chronic.' It was a genuinely, sort of positive interest in seeing this person as opposed to 'Oh no, it's five o'clock and we have to admit her and what a pain in the neck.' The resident was a bit...taken off balance by that. I explained to him that sometimes it's fun to see people that are mystifying because we sometimes get their input in a different way if we think about it as a puzzling case as opposed to a pain in the neck...It dawned on me when you asked me about surprises, that that might be a key question. If I interpret that [surprise] in a negative way on an average day then I'm not having much fun. So surprises that are interpreted as a positive thing tell me about the sort of mind set of anybody...As you asked that, I realized that I really sort of anticipate each day that there will be something I don't know, or don't anticipate that's going to happen and I sort of enjoy that, that's why it's fun: So surprises are equated, to me, with sort of a standard day, and that's not a negative. That's why it's fun...surprises are what make it fun. There are some that are overwhelming and that isn't fun, but that's more to do with content than the fact that they're unpredicted."

Dr. T.G.:

[When asked ifsurprises are good] "Oh, I think so, assuming there's not a horrible outcome as a result of it. But I get very excited about such a thing and I try to make a point of showing the resident that 'Wow, that's really neat. We all missed that, and boy, we will really learn from that and that will be great for us to apply to the next situation that is similar to this!' So I try to be positive and enthusiastic about it."

Reflection-in-Action:

Dr. D.B.:

"The resident who comes in with the, 'Golly, I'm really stuck or I don't know what's going on here.' What I try to do is start back at square zero and move them through and help them try to discover where and why they're stuck. Usually, it's one of those four or five things. They're not relating to the patient, they're not gathering the right data that's there, they got the data but because of a cognitive gap they don't recognize it, or they got the facts but they're having trouble putting it together because they've never seen it before or they overestimated one clue compared to another....Then if we can come to some agreement of where they're stuck, then you make the acute decision. If it's a fact, you just supply it to them. If it's a problem solving thing, you kind of map it out and you demonstrate to them how you came to that conclusion."

Experimentation:

Dr. M.S.:

"Ideally, I would say pose your hypothesis and construct a design to see if it answers your hypothesis....Sometimes you have to do educated experimentation. There will be times when your 'experiment' does not come out like you think it should, but that tells you just as much as when it does come out."

Dr. C.N.:

[In response to: "Is experimenting OK?"] "I would hope so. There are certain limits to that within medical sort of cultures. I think they [residents] need to test themselves to see how much variability they can tolerate and their patients can tolerate in the diagnosis and treatment and understanding of illness. If they want to use one antibiotic instead of another I generally ask them to justify it, and many times there is more than one option. They need to experiment with that and see which option fits them and their mentality and situation the best."

Sonia Crandall

Dr. D.B.:

> "I just never thought about it I guess, I do experiment a little bit because I'll say, 'Well, this person I'll try the new one [approach], this person I'll try the traditional [approach].' I'll start asking people a little bit what they thought about it....I have in the past encouraged residents, I'd say, 'Well why don't you do this? The next three patients you see with such and such, try the new approach. Talk to them, see what you think about it. The other three, stay with the traditional, as long as it's safe.'"

Reflection-on-Action:

(when the experiment works)

Dr. D.B.:

> "I guess I take the 'Little Jack Horner' approach, stick in your thumb and pull out a plum and say, 'My, what a good boy am I.' Ah, what happens? Two things happen, one, you're somewhat impressed—'Geez, maybe they really know what they're talking about, boy, this is really great.' Then I guess the other side of it is, that's the excitement and seduction if you will, and you're tempted to now make this your dogma. You tried it once and it worked, now it becomes fail-safe, then it becomes dogma. Hopefully, the other side of that happens too, and that is 'Okay I'm not turned off by this, let's think about it cautiously.' I think when it works, the temptation is to jump on the bandwagon. I have that temptation to jump on the bandwagon, but I also try to maintain a healthy skepticism, and be careful about not just going with every new thing down the road every time."

(when it doesn't work)

Dr. D.B.:

> "I think what you're alluding to, 'what happens when it doesn't work,' maybe that's going to be the next question—is, 'what happens when it doesn't work?' It's the opposite. You can't be so overcome by the fact that it failed, if you will, that you never try it again. So I think it's a balance between those two things. When it works positively, there's an excitement, you think about it, it makes sense, this is good. But then I think you should also maintain a certain level of skepticism. I think our experiments in the literature show us that."

Discussion

The findings of this study provide some convincing evidence that physicians think like the professionals Schön observed when he established his theory of reflective practice. The stages of his model are apparent in how good physician-teachers help residents learn from their patient care experiences. They reveal the ways they help learners become reflective practitioners. It would follow that they themselves must be reflective practitioners and that they consider being reflective practitioners a valuable outcome of residency education.

What does all of this mean for education within the medical culture? Certainly, Schön's Model of Reflective Practice is applicable and adaptable to medical education along any point in the medical education continuum. It provides educators with a tool to help organize their learners' knowledge and experience in a focused way to help learners become better problem solvers. Using the model has several benefits. Schön's model:

- offers a method for self-assessment, as well as teacher assessment of learners
- helps the learner to recognize learning needs—knowledge gaps—in general or in specific knowledge domains
- focuses the learner on each specific patient problem so she or he can find direction for narrowing the gap or deficiency
- offers the learner immediate feedback on each specific patient problem
- encourages self-directed learning, i.e., gives the learner "control over the exercise of intentions, decisions, and actions in a given situation associated with implementing a plan for learning directed toward altering professional performance"[4]
- prompts episodic memory by helping the learner to reflect on past experiences; episodic memory facilitates more efficient problem solving and learning than the use of declarative knowledge that relies on rote memory

Incorporating the Reflective Practice Model into Existing Curricula

Many medical educators believe it is time to alter the traditional medical education culture from a focus on a basic science curriculum (disease and organ systems of the body) that emphasizes students' rote memorization and test-taking ability, to a focus on a curriculum that encompasses developing clinical expertise in all four years of medical training. This would mean teaching the strategies necessary to solve simple and complex patient problems ethically in an ever changing climate of real-world medicine—the basis for wise action. Many family medicine educators often complain that their "interns" (R1s, PGY1s) have to be reeducated because of the dysfunctional undergraduate training they have received. To avoid this, the educational process that transforms novices into expert clinicians must be a continuum beginning in predoctoral training, continuing through residency education and beyond, during the 40 or so years that physicians continue to learn.

Schön's model provides a tool for professionals in training to critically evaluate their own learning needs. In order to incorporate this model effectively into any undergraduate or residency curriculum, educators must first train clin-

Sonia Crandall

ical teachers in the methods and techniques of guiding learners through the stages of the model to learn how to question learners in ways that get them to think like reflective practitioners. To use the model with practicing professionals, no matter where they are along the lifelong learning continuum, they must be trained to make their thought processes conscious. The model is not mysterious or mystical in nature, it is how physicians frame and solve problems. What we need to impart to physicians—and to physician educators—is how to make what seems to be implicit and unconscious into something that is explicit and conscious. The process is generic, i.e., it is appropriate for all learners at any level or stage of development—predoctoral, residency, or continuing education.

Schön's model blends naturally with the problem-based learning curriculum. Instead of using paper cases, however, the clinical cases are better presented live, using real or simulated patients. Students can also be assigned to primary care clinics and work in concert with other students and residents alongside their attendings/mentors in a clinical setting. To make the model usable will require some overhauling of the traditional curriculum. Evidence is accumulating that it can be done. A number of medical schools have installed, in the first and second year of predoctoral training, year-long courses that focus on establishing the doctor-patient relationship and patient interviewing. Many of these courses use small-group discussion as a primary means of delivering content—not too different from PBL; these courses can be modified to use the model with live case presentations.

Implications for the Continuum of Professional Education

Schön's Model of Reflective Practice is especially relevant to CME, notably focused or self-directed CME, because it provides practicing professionals with a tool to help them learn from the patient problems they see in their practices. This aspect is particularly important in light of Cervero's recent suggestion[3] that physicians learn best from their patients and that CME should become more practice based. Cervero's assertions are supported by what physicians say about lifelong learning as well.

Dr. K.B. describes what he does with the fourth-year students during the last month of medical school. Students are responsible for giving special seminars, and Dr. K.B. gives a written exam covering the topics presented. The last two questions of the exam are: (1) name six strengths and six weaknesses of this medical school, and (2) tell me how you're going to keep up with advances in medical sciences over the next 30 years.

How Expert Clinical Educators Teach What They Know

Dr. K.B. comments:

> "The majority of the time, they talk about reading their journals, and going to meetings, and a lot of them will say they want to be affiliated with the medical school, clinical assistant professor, whatever. Which is all well and good, but that...unfortunately tells me I haven't gotten my message through to them. It's probably not how your average practitioner is going to keep up. In reviewing your own cases and finding your frustrations, I think, is what stimulates you to learn and to do something different. There's always a danger in relying totally on your own experience because...anecdotal things are dangerous. Just because you get six reactions to medication in a row, that may be only six out of ten thousand. They just happen to be yours, anecdotal things anyway. But we try to have our students keep a record of the patients that they interact with in the two months on the rotation....I think practitioners need to do that as well. At the end of every year I, and a resident on the vascular service, go over all the vascular cases for the year. We look at the types of complications we've had and the numbers we've done....It shows us a more global perspective [of] how we're doing. Recognizing frustrations, or problems, or patterns that we hadn't really seen in a day-in-day-out, week-to-week sort of review, stimulates us to look for better ways to do things and to keep up with what's going on. That's what I'd like to get the students to learn how to do."

Findings of the "change study"[9] suggest that felt needs (intrinsic) may be more compelling forces for physicians to implement change than prescribed needs (extrinsic), depending of course on the nature of the prescribed need or the authority of the "prescriber." If continuing medical educators believe in a self-directed curriculum for change, they should provide professionals with the tools they need to critically evaluate their own practices. The reflective practice model is such a tool. CME providers could offer programs in which practitioners are guided through Schön's model and taught how to use it in their daily practice to help them identify gaps in their ability to solve simple and complex patient problems. Practitioners who are able to assess their learning needs should be more likely to focus on areas where learning—and reflection on that learning—may alter practice patterns, improve performance, and, ultimately, improve patient outcomes.

Physicians agree that the medical decision-making process is fraught with uncertainty. Medical facts change at an incredible rate. The advantage of the reflective practice model is that it acknowledges and legitimizes the ubiquitous nature of uncertainty. It makes uncertainty, uniqueness, and surprise a positive part of medical practice, instead of something to dread. It blends the science of medicine with the physician's clinical acumen—a function of his or her repertoire of experiences—to weave the tapestries that frame and solve medical problems. Consciously working through the stages of the process gives

Sonia Crandall

physicians more experience in resolving ambiguous patient problems and ultimately enlarges their zone of mastery. It is a cyclical process that expands a physician's ability to act wisely.

Although this qualitative study had a limited number of participants, it does provide a preliminary look at the phenomenon of educating the reflective practitioner as it occurs in clinical teaching in the medical culture. Further exploration with physician-teachers in other specialties is needed. Quantitative studies also are needed to document the relationships among the stages of Schön's model. Studies like this one can help identify—early in their training—learners who are having difficulties framing and solving medical problems. With early identification, such physicians should be able to acquire strategies that will help them learn what they need to know so as to be prepared for dealing with the medical uncertainties of their professional practices.

Acknowledgements

Portions of this article are drawn from a paper published in the proceedings of the 22nd Annual Standing Conference on University Teaching and Research in the Education of Adults, University of Kent, England.

The author wishes to thank Deborah Cacy, Paul Kleine, and Paul Mazmanian for their support and thoughtful input during the developmental stages of this project and preparation of the manuscript. A special thanks goes to the physicians who participated in the interviews and shared their insights.

References

1. Schön DA. Educating the reflective practitioner. San Francisco: Jossey-Bass, 1987.
2. Fox RD, Mold JW. Clinical teaching—Learning to learn from experience. Presented at the Oklahoma geriatrics education center conference, December 1990.
3. Cervero RM. Professional practice, learning, and continuing education: An integrated perspective. Int J Lifelong Educ 1992; 11:91-101.
4. Fox RD. New research agendas for CME: Organizing principles for the study of self-directed curricula for change. J Cont Educ Health Prof 1991; 11:155-167.
5. Shapiro J, Talbot Y. Applying the concept of the reflective practitioner to understanding and teaching family medicine. Fam Med 1991; 23:450-456.
6. Glaser BG, Strauss AL. The discovery of grounded theory. New York: Aldine DeGruyter, 1967.
7. Flanagan JC. The critical incident technique. Psych Bull 1954; 51:4:327-358.
8. Lincoln YS, Guba EG. Naturalistic inquiry. Newbury Park, CA: Sage Publications, 1985.
9. Fox RD, Mazmanian PE, Putnam, RW. (eds.) Changing and learning in the lives of physicians. New York: Praeger, 1989.

DAVID M. IRBY, PhD

What Clinical Teachers in Medicine Need to Know

Abstract—In order to identify the components of knowledge that effective clinical teachers of medicine need, the author carried out a qualitative study of six distinguished clinical teachers in general internal medicine in 1991. Using data from interviews, a structured task, and observations of each ward team, he identified six domains of knowledge essential to teaching excellence in the context of teaching rounds: clinical knowledge of medicine, patients, and the context of practice, as well as educational knowledge of learners, general principles of teaching, and case-based teaching scripts. When combined, these domains of knowledge allow attending physicians to engage in clinical instructional reasoning and to target their teaching to the specific needs of their learners. The results of this investigation are discussed in relation to both prior research on teacher knowledge, reasoning, and action and faculty development in medicine. *Acad. Med.* 69(1994):333–342.

Attending physicians use many forms of knowledge as they listen to case presentations by medical students and residents. This knowledge base enables them to diagnose patients' problems, assess learners' needs, and provide targeted instruction.[1] What do clinical teachers in medicine need to know in order to teach effectively? Conventional wisdom suggests that knowledge of medicine is all that is necessary to be an excellent teacher. An alternative perspective, articulated most frequently by problem-based learning advocates, is that knowledge of teaching skills is fundamental and that teachers do not have to be content experts.

RELEVANT KNOWLEDGE DOMAINS

In the context of clinical teaching, which of the perspectives just mentioned is accurate? Earlier research on physicians' and teachers' knowledge may provide clues to relevant domains of knowledge for teaching. These might include knowledge of subject matter, knowledge of learners, knowledge of general principles of teaching and learning, and knowledge of content-specific teaching.

A slightly different version of this paper was presented at the annual meeting of the American Educational Research Association in Atlanta, Georgia, on April 22, 1993.

Dr. Irby is professor, Department of Medical Education, University of Washington School of Medicine, Seattle.

Correspondence should be addressed to Dr. Irby, Department of Medical Education, HQ-32, University of Washington, Seattle, WA 98195.

Knowledge of Subject Matter

"If you understand your discipline, then you should be able to teach it." This instructional assumption is translated into an often-cited dictum of clinical education: "See one, do one, teach one." This experiential learning model suggests the close relationship between learning, performing, and teaching. Physicians develop an extensive knowledge base of medicine and its related disciplines through experience with a broad array of clinical cases. As clinical experience increases, clinical knowledge becomes more tightly compiled and interconnected. Clinical knowledge is then retained in memory in the form of *illness scripts* (clinically relevant information on the enabling conditions, causes and consequences of an illness) and *instance scripts* (recollections of specific patients who suffered from a disease).[2,3] Alternative descriptions of this knowledge structure are *semantic structures*,[4] *knowledge representations*,[5] and *reciprocating networks*.[6] Patel and Groen argue that expertise in medicine involves the development of adequate knowledge representations combined with the ability to distinguish between relevant and irrelevant information in a problem—thereby filtering out irrelevant material.[5]

Educational researchers assert that knowledge for teaching requires an in-depth and flexible understanding of subject matter.[7–12] Teachers need to know their content well enough to make connections within the subject, across disciplines, and with their learners.[13] Alternative conceptions of content help teachers switch back and forth between the student's, the discipline's, the textbook's, and their own conceptions.[14] Expert teachers also have richer, more tightly connected subject matter knowledge, and more detailed plans organized around content to be taught, than do novice teachers.[12,15]

Knowledge of Learners

Beyond content expertise, teaching involves connecting learners with subject matter. Teachers need to understand their learners' prior knowledge as well as their conceptions and misconceptions of the subject matter. This includes knowledge of students' typical errors and the normal development path along which students progress in understanding content.[9,16–18] For example, expert math teachers employ this knowledge to elicit typical errors and then use those errors in lessons to teach the correct concepts.[16] Teachers' knowledge of learners' needs, motivations, and abilities also affects their teaching methods. Effective instruction emerges from the interaction between understanding learners and comprehending subject matter.[12]

Knowledge of General Principles of Teaching and Learning

In addition to knowledge of subject matter and learners, teachers possess knowledge of general principles of teaching and learning. Teachers have general conceptions about how students learn and how instruction can enhance learning.[19] These personal theories appear to develop from the apprenticeship of observation (seeing positive and negative examples of teaching) and from the reflective experience of teaching. Experienced teachers also have large repertoires of teaching strategies (e.g., lecturing, leading group discussions, asking questions) that can be combined to teach specific concepts. These are general principles of teaching and learning because they are not embedded in specific content, contexts, and learners.

Knowledge of Content-specific Instruction

When general content knowledge and general teaching methods are transformed into content-specific instruction for a particular group of students, a new form of knowledge results. This is termed *knowledge of content-specific pedagogy*[19] or *pedagogical content knowledge*.[10,20,21] This special form of knowledge unique to teachers develops through the repetitive experience of teaching specific content to specific students. The resulting knowledge becomes organized into teaching scripts. These scripts are analogous to play scripts that dictate the action on stage. Teaching scripts contain general goals of instruction, key teaching points, specific representations of content (explanations, analogies, examples, learning tasks),[9,22] an understanding of the conceptions and misconceptions of learners, and procedures for overcoming learning difficulties.[8–10,13,23,24] The essence of content-specific instruction is content knowledge organized for teaching purposes that makes it comprehensible to particular learners.[20,21] This special form of knowledge is what separates teachers from mere content experts.

Other potentially relevant domains of teachers' knowledge might include knowledge of instructional resources.[14,19,25]

While a host of observational studies have described the complexities and challenges of teaching in clinical settings,[26–32] none of them has at-

tempted to define the several knowledge bases needed for clinical teaching and to develop a model of clinical teachers' knowledge.

DEFINING THE KNOWLEDGE BASE OF CLINICAL TEACHERS

I attempted to create such a model in 1991 by carrying out the study reported in the following pages. The method I used was to investigate the knowledge bases for teaching used by six distinguished clinical teachers in general internal medicine. These are the same six teachers described in my previous study about how physicians make instructional decisions during teaching rounds.[1] I chose a case-study design using these six carefully chosen teachers to illustrate the "wisdom of practice" among the best.[21] I selected outstanding clinical teachers rather than representative ones to identify the knowledge of the best educators, knowledge that is extraordinary, not ordinary. Studying the knowledge of representative teachers could have led to a description of "the unimaginative practices of the uninspired."[33] This research strategy focuses on what is possible rather than what is representative. Thus, my research question was "What is the knowledge base for teaching used by distinguished clinical teachers in medicine in the context of teaching rounds?"

The teachers I studied were all from the Department of Medicine at the University of Washington School of Medicine in Seattle. They had received excellent ratings of their teaching from students and residents,[34] and independent nominations by their department chairman and the program director of their department's residency. Further, I selected those who had distinctly different teaching styles and who were serving as attending physicians during spring quarter. This group of teachers comprised one professor, two associate professors, and three assistant professors (four men and two women).

The context of instruction was teaching rounds in general internal

medicine at two university hospitals. *Teaching rounds* is a case-oriented instructional session held predominantly in a hospital conference room with the ward team and is the teacher's primary opportunity to teach medical concepts in the context of patient care.

Data were derived from in-depth, semistructured interviews,[35] a structured task involving a think-aloud exercise,[36] observations of the ward team, and transcriptions of teaching rounds.[37] My interview questions related to the attending physician's knowledge, instructional reasoning, and actions. The two-hour interviews were audiotaped and transcribed.

The structured task involved a think-aloud exercise in response to a written case describing a medical student's presentation of a patient with diabetic ketoacidosis during teaching rounds. The attending physicians were asked to describe how they would respond to the case, what they would teach, and what problems medical students would typically have with this case. This exercise was designed to elicit their teaching scripts and knowledge of learners. Twelve medical students on the six teams were also given the case, minus the diagnosis and treatment, and asked to determine the problem, diagnosis, and recommended treatment. This was done to validate the teachers' knowledge of the learners.

I observed each team for one week, recording my observations in field notes, and summarizing them immediately afterwards. In order to understand what was happening during teaching rounds, observations began with *work rounds* (when the team consisting of two third-year medical students, two interns, and one senior resident review all patients at the bedside) from 8 to 9 A.M., followed by an X-ray conference from 9:30 to 10:00 A.M., and concluded with teaching rounds with the attending physician from 10:30 to 12:00. In addition, all teaching rounds were audiotaped, and one session per attending physician was transcribed. The observations and transcripts of teaching rounds were used to corroborate the interview and think-aloud statements.

I coded the interview transcripts in order to identify the domains of knowledge needed for clinical teaching, and thus construct a model of such knowledge. Preliminary codes were developed based upon Shulman's theoretical model of teachers' knowledge[20,21] and Schmidt's model of physicians' knowledge.[3] My initial codes were knowledge of clinical medicine, knowledge of basic sciences, knowledge of patients, knowledge of learners, knowledge of general pedagogy, and pedagogical content knowledge. Intercoder agreement was 83% among two doctoral students in education and myself using a sample of the transcripts.[38] The codes were successively revised as analysis proceeded to account for all of the major themes in the data. The codes changed as categories were collapsed (knowledge of clinical medicine and knowledge of basic sciences became knowledge of medicine, because the informants said that these two categories were integrated), titles of codes were changed to make them more understandable (pedagogical content knowledge became content-specific teaching), and codes emerged from the data (knowledge of context and case-based teaching scripts). The final codes were validated by two general internists and myself using selective quotes from the transcripts. Intercoder agreement was 95% among the internists and myself. Final coding categories were knowledge of medicine, patients, context, learners, general principles of teaching, and case-based teaching scripts. The results were then checked against my observations of teaching rounds and the transcripts of rounds.

A MODEL OF CLINICAL TEACHERS' KNOWLEDGE

The model of clinical teachers' knowledge identified by this study is depicted in Figure 1. Below, I discuss each type of knowledge shown in the figure, beginning with a description of the key features of the domain followed by illustrative quotes from the

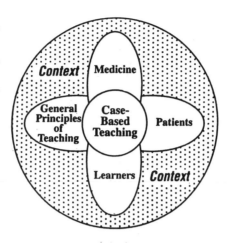

Figure 1. The domains of knowledge needed for clinical teaching in medicine as identified by six distinguished attending physicians in the context of teaching rounds in general internal medicine. In the figure, these domains of knowledge are artificially differentiated for emphasis.

attending physicians. The teachers' names are pseudonyms and their comments have been edited slightly for readability.

Knowledge of Medicine

All of the attending physicians described the importance of general medical knowledge, referring to it as human biology, clinical experience, judgment and insight, clinical skills, pathophysiology, basic sciences, knowledge of psychosocial medicine, and epidemiology. Knowledge of medicine is drawn from a variety of disciplines and incorporates both basic sciences and clinical experience. Dr. Baker describes the medical knowledge base he uses for teaching purposes:

> What I know about human biology that is affirmed by clinical experience is what I selectively use for teaching purposes. My clinical experience is drawn off human biology and allows me to teach people how to use human biology to take care of their patients. There are subsets of human biology — biochemistry, physiology, pathoanatomy — and larger social and environmental issues. There is also a relationship between these elements that determines how well a person with the disease is doing.

Dr. Davis uses a concentric-circle model of the discipline. He begins at the cellular level, then goes to the causes and manifestations of a disease, treatment options, and the psychosocial aspects of the case, and ends with the societal and epidemiologic context for the disease. "I try to get a sense of all these levels, from the cellular level up to the societal level. I use my skills to address the ones that haven't already been addressed."

These statements illustrate the broad scope of medical knowledge, the integrated nature of that knowledge, and the distinct conceptual schemas of these teachers. The teacher's conceptual framework of the discipline is an important determinant of the content that will be taught.[23]

Knowledge of Patients

In addition to medical knowledge, these attending physicians possess knowledge of specific patients that they have seen on their services. This knowledge is used to verify clinical diagnoses, to check on learners' progress, to stimulate the teaching of practical tips on patient care, and to motivate learning. This process ensures quality patient care and quality instruction, and was described as follows by Dr. Able:

> Many of the patients I know because I have seen them before. They are my own patients, and I have a sense of what the story is ... If I know my patients, then I can get at problems in my learners.

Dr. Ellis reported, "I get information about the patient through the trainee. When I go back to talk to the patient, I'm checking up on the trainee to a certain extent."

Knowledge of specific facts about each patient and knowledge of general principles of medicine are closely linked[2] and when combined create the attending physician's clinical credibility in the eyes of the ward team. This credibility is critical to the team members' acceptance of the attending physician's teaching.[28]

Knowledge of Context

All the teachers mentioned that knowledge of context affected their teaching. Context includes the patient population served by the hospital, the social context of the patient, the historical context of therapeutic practices, and the context for encountering the patient's story (case presentation versus direct interaction with the patient). Dr. Charles described the impact of the patient population on teaching:

When you are at Harborview Hospital [a county teaching hospital] certain diagnoses are a lot more common than when you are at University Hospital. I know that a third of the patients that come in may have a history of IV drug use at Harborview and only 5% at Swedish [a private community hospital]. So even if the team doesn't tell me that, I am processing it.

Dr. Baker observed that students encounter patients in the context of an acute illness and frequently fail to appreciate what precipitates the illness and what follows it. Studies of teachers' knowledge in other settings have identified knowledge of context as important as well.[8,10,20,21]

Knowledge of Learners

This domain comprises knowledge of specific learners, knowledge of the ward team as a group, and general assumptions about learners by level of training. Knowledge of learners emerges from teaching experience. Dr. Fagan reported, "It is a lot less work for you as a teacher if you can figure out where your student is — whoever the student happens to be . . . The longer you teach, the easier it is to see where they are." Dr. Ellis agreed: "Every month I attend I go through a period of trying to figure out where the team is, what their needs are, and what their personalities are like so that I can interdigitate with them the best." According to Dr. Davis,

Sometimes with a third-year student you have to go through a problem-ori-ented approach to get them to tie it all together in a coherent picture. By the fourth year you expect them to be able to do that. By the time they're interns and residents, you should expect them not only to identify the problem but to understand the broader issues.

To investigate the accuracy of these teachers' knowledge of learners, I gave each of the attending physicians and each of the 12 medical students a hypothetical case presentation by a third-year medical student of a patient with diabetic ketoacidosis (DKA). All 12 students correctly defined the problem, identified DKA, and made appropriate treatment recommendations. Five of the six attending physicians accurately predicted the student's knowledge and performance; the least experienced attending physician underestimated the students' ability.[1] As is true of teachers in other disciplines, these teachers had an accurate knowledge of their learners' understanding.[10,17,21,39]

In addition to knowledge of learners by level of training, these attending physicians possessed knowledge of particular students. This knowledge is acquired through asking questions and observing performance. "I ask students questions constantly. I've asked the questions enough times that I know mostly what people can say as third-year medical students," said Dr. Baker. This general knowledge of learners combined with particular knowledge of specific learners enables the teachers to efficiently and effectively diagnose learners' difficulties.

Knowledge of General Principles of Teaching

The most commonly articulated general principles of teaching and the numbers of the six attending physicians who described the principles were: actively involve learners and ask lots of questions (6/6), capture attention and have fun (6/6), connect the case to broader concepts (6/6), go to the bedside (5/6), meet individual needs (5/6), be practical and relevant (4/6), be selective and realistic (4/6), and provide feedback and evaluation (3/6). These principles, discussed below, emerged from many readings of the interview transcripts.

1. Actively involve learners (6/6). All of the attending physicians studied conduct highly interactive teaching sessions. "Keeping everyone involved is my ideal," said Dr. Fagan. One way to achieve active involvement and to diagnose learners' difficulties is to ask questions. "I use a lot of questions to get some assessment of the residents' and students' knowledge base," reported Dr. Charles. Similarly, Dr. Baker stated that "the kind of teaching I like to do is Socratic, or kind of probing question-and-answer. I ask them questions constantly."

2. Capture attention and have fun (6/6). In order to make learning memorable, teaching must capture and retain attention. This is accomplished by using humor, dramatic case examples, suspense, and enthusiasm. Dr. Able said, "I always try to suck people into having as good a time as I am having." Dr. Ellis emphasizes the importance of drama in teaching: "I try to dramatize a point. In a sense, it is making teaching into theater — trying to present things in a way that captures people's attention." All six physicians studied seemed to enjoy teaching, and they all made learning fun and memorable.

3. Connect the case to broader concepts (6/6). Clinical teaching connects learners' knowledge of the patient's particular problems to a broader understanding of the relevant disease. This helps learners generalize appropriately from their experience and offers them a conceptual scaffold for building new knowledge. Dr. Baker said: "You draw out something specific from that patient to say [such as] 'When you are taking care of people like this, you can expect that these will be problems.'" All the attending physicians related the case at hand to underlying constructs of the illness and/or to broader health issues.

4. Go to the bedside (5/6). When students are unable to give a coherent case presentation, or the diagnosis does not adequately explain the patient's problems, the attending physicians lead the team to the bedside. Dr. Baker, the only teacher who went to the bedside every day during this study, stated, "If I don't make a point of doing bedside teaching, it is real easy to just talk and the patient is left out." When a case presentation is unfocused, Dr. Charles goes to the bedside. "The easiest way to determine whether it is a patient or student problem is to go talk to the patient." Some of the other attending physicians went to the bedside to validate physical examination findings and to model and observe interactions with the patient. One attending physician stated that he was uncomfortable teaching in front of the patient, and another said that she perceived bedside teaching to be an unproductive experience for the team in most instances. Thus, neither of them routinely went to the bedside as part of teaching rounds—although both of them saw their patients independently from the team.

5. *Meet individual needs (5/6)*. One of the great difficulties with clinical teaching is dealing with the diversity of learners' knowledge and skills. The teachers studied identify the interests of the team members during the first week of the rotation and attempt to meet those interests during the month. Dr. Davis stated: "I tell them my strengths and weaknesses, and I ask them how I can best help them. So up front I find out who they are, what they want to do, and what their needs are." Dr. Fagan indicated that she has the same approach: "My job is to figure out what they want to know this month. People don't learn unless they are ready for it." Identifying learners' interests and needs helps these teachers discover teachable moments.

To meet the diverse needs of learners, these attending physicians use a variety of instructional strategies. "The hardest thing about attending rounds is bridging all those different levels. I try to do it by hierarchizing knowledge," said Dr. Fagan. This involves asking students questions about pathophysiology, asking interns questions about day-to-day treatment, and asking the senior resident questions about broader medical

and health care issues. To meet the unique needs of students, she and the rest of the attending physicians periodically teach the students separately.

Teaching rounds are also adapted to the natural flow of patient care. During this study, four of the six attending physicians participated in work rounds (where the team visits the bedside of each patient and makes work assignments for the day) on post-call mornings and shortened or eliminated teaching rounds on those days. Post-call mornings occurred every four days following all-night work in the emergency room where the physicians treat and/or admit new patients to their service. During the next two days post-call, discussions in teaching rounds emerged out of the most teachable cases. The last day before on-call night was often spent dealing with broader topics and giving more formal presentations.

6. *Be practical and relevant (4/6)*. Clinical teaching must be both practical and relevant. Dr. Baker said that he frames his teaching with this question to himself: "What practical bits of knowledge have been necessary for me to know about taking care of patients like this? What are the real practical bits of knowledge that need to be brought out about a certain case to get the most learning from it?" Part of the process of being practical and relevant is teaching general concepts in the context of specific patients on the service.

7. *Be selective and realistic (4/6)*. These six teachers focused on a few important teaching points per case, prioritized time among cases to deal with a few cases in depth, and established realistic expectations for learning during the rotation. "Realizing that the more you say the less people learn, I try to hit two or three themes really heavily during an hour," reported Dr. Charles. "I try to find out where they are and give them the basic skills . . . to teach them four or five things" during the month", said Dr. Davis. Less is better to begin with.[40]

8. *Provide feedback and evaluation (3/6)*. "I think feedback is real important and labeling it as such is also,

because otherwise they don't know what they are getting," reported Dr. Fagan. "Evaluation is an important part of teaching. If you can find out whether somebody is learning, then you can increase how much teaching goes on," said Dr. Charles. The process of giving feedback should be both constructive and supportive, suggested Dr. Fagan: "You have to respect the needs of learners and their feelings as people. You should not teach by embarrassment, by pressure, or by berating them." Dr. Ellis concurred: "I take it as a principle that criticizing people in front of others is not appropriate."

All of these teachers gave large amounts of feedback to the learners. Since it was routinely embedded in teaching, the students frequently failed to perceive it as feedback. In one instance, I interviewed a medical student immediately following a one-hour meeting with Dr. Charles, who had worked with the two medical students on their case presentations. This had been an intensive teaching session with a great deal of coaching and feedback. When I asked the student whether he received feedback from Dr. Charles, he said that he didn't get much. Since I had just observed a great deal of feedback, I was puzzled. So I asked the student what feedback meant to him. He reported that it was the formal evaluation that he would get at the end of the rotation. Clearly there are differences in perceptions about feedback.

9. *Other general principles of teaching*. Individual teachers in this study identified other general principles of teaching, including using repetition, teaching anecdotally with cases, making things memorable and dramatic, role modeling, and teaching in a style that is right for the teacher. These general principles of teaching offered me initial insights into the next and most important domain of knowledge for teaching, case-based teaching.

Knowledge of Case-based Teaching Scripts

This domain of teachers knowledge, case-based teaching, is concerned with how attending physicians use cases and case content to teach general principles of medicine. Understanding of this domain of knowledge emerged not so much from the interviews as from observations and transcripts of teaching rounds. This form of knowledge involves instructional methods that help learners interpret, reflect upon, and generalize from their cases. For a teacher, this requires knowledge of the patient's illness and life narrative, insight into the learner's representation of the case, and relevant teaching scripts. Through repetitive teaching of similar content and cases, teachers develop teaching scripts.[1,9,22] In this study, the teachers articulated three to five key points that they would teach related to a DKA case.[1] Knowledge of case-based teaching is at the center of teachers' understanding, where it connects all of the other domains.

In the clinical setting, learning begins with a specific patient. In Dr. Baker's words: "The patient is a representation of an illness and has unique features that are examples of a type. There are certain characteristics of the patient that cause you to bring out different points about a person and their reaction to illness." In the context of teaching rounds, several interpretive activities occur. Prior to teaching rounds, the learner elicits the patient's story. Next, the learner summarizes that story, recasts it into medical language, and presents it to the teacher and other team members. The attending physician listens to the case presentation and tries to make sense out of the patient's problem and the learner's representation of the case. Then teacher and learners together develop a coherent explanation for the case. Case-based teaching involves (1) helping learners construct coherent representations of the case, (2) filtering out irrelevant information, and (3) making connections between the specifics of the case and generalizations derived from the medical literature and experience with other patients.

I selected two very different examples of this form of knowledge in ac-

tion to present in this article. Both illustrate how attending physicians use cases for teaching purposes. The first example involves a Socratic or directed-questioning approach to the development of a diagnosis, while the second example was a more presentational style that demonstrates how to communicate with a patient's family. Both come from transcripts of teaching rounds.

In the first instance, Dr. Baker was responding to a medical student's case presentation at University Hospital. After the student gave an extended ten-minute case presentation of a 25-year-old man who had been admitted for persistent epigastric pain, Dr. Baker initiated the following instructional dialogue about this case:

Dr. Baker: Do you think he has acute pancreatitis or do you think he has acute recurrent pancreatitis? Is there a difference between the two?

Student: I think he has an acute recurrent pancreatitis. There are differences between the two . . . Number one is the indolent history of mild epigastric pain, which antacids don't help, and then later the acute and persistent onset.

Dr. Baker: Is that an important distinction?

Student: Yes. I think it is a very important distinction with his history.

Dr. Baker: If it is an important distinction, why?

Student: I looked at the differential diagnosis for epigastric pain . . . For this person with his surgical history, one of the major causes of pancreatitis is pancreatic insult—which he clearly had twice with an insulinoma resection and a later laparotomy.

Dr. Baker: Take a step back to the question: What are two common causes of pancreatitis?

Student: Alcohol.

Resident: Gallstones.

Dr. Baker: Then there is actually a third, which is idiopathic. For the vast majority of cases of acute pancreatitis, it is one of these three. The older the person, the more likely it is obstructive, and the younger the person, the more likely it is alcohol. The minute you get recurrent pancreatitis, though, the differential changes dramatically. Everything in this case points to pancreatitis due to surgical complications. The second possibility is that he may have a tumor. Why is that important in this case?

Dr. Baker continued this interactive teaching process for another 13 minutes. He asked more focused questions, provided brief teaching points, quickly summarized what is known in the literature, and assigned readings on recurrent pancreatitis. Through the questioning process, Dr. Baker drew out of the student the key features of a diagnosis of recurrent pancreatitis, elicited the underlying reasoning of the student, and targeted information from the literature to the learner's point of need.

A second example of knowledge of case-based teaching occurred during Dr. Charles's teaching rounds at Harborview Medical Center (a country hospital managed as a teaching hospital by the University of Washington). An intern presented a case of a 30-year-old man infected with human immunodeficiency virus (HIV), both his mother and his woman companion were asking how long he would live. The following sequence occurred in the midst of a 13-minute discussion of this case:

Intern: His girlfriend wanted to know if he would live to be 60 . . . I'm always tempted to say something like, "Well, he may die tomorrow, but may not." It is hard to know how to respond to that.

Dr. Charles: Sometimes, if they are patients that I know well, I'll be pretty frank with them and just give them the statistics. He has AIDS with probable PCP, so that means life expectancy for him on AZT is probably somewhere between 18 and 22 months. Fifty percent are dead at 18 months.

Intern: . . . Being vague is not bad . . .

Dr. Charles: I think that while he is processing a lot of information, that is very appropriate. But when patients are trying to make life plans on what to do in a couple of years, I basically say that we have patients that are living four or five years with AZT and we don't know what their endpoint will be. They may live eight, nine, or ten years. We don't know. So that gives them hope. But, I add that the average is about two years.

Intern: Actually, I may tell him that. I didn't know those numbers .

The conversation continued, with Dr. Charles offering practical and formal knowledge in the context of dealing with this specific patient. The team was relieved to receive this practical advice, supporting data, and a model of how to share this sensitive information with the patient and his family. This style directly addressed the learners' questions.

In case-based teaching, the teacher discerns both the patient's illness and the learner's representation of the case, and then helps the learner make sense out of the experience. Depending on the circumstances, teachers accomplish this task using Socratic and/or directive styles. The six distinguished teachers made this a highly interactive, engaging, and memorable process.

Researchers of classroom teaching describe this form of knowledge as *content-specific pedagogy,*[19] *pedagogical content knowledge,*[10,20] *curriculum scripts,*[9] and case-based instruction.[41-43] A somewhat similar approach, although oriented towards clinical practice, is the *patient-centered clinical method,* which aims at understanding the unique story of each individual patient.[44,45] While recognizing the uniqueness of each patient, case-based teaching scripts

focus on the question: What is this particular patient a case of? How does this person's unique story relate to stories of other patients with similar diseases and to broader biomedical knowledge?

Other Domains of Knowledge

Individual attending physicians in this study identified communication skills (compassion, sensitivity, intuition) and knowledge of the curriculum (medical school, clerkship, and residency program) as types of knowledge essential to clinical teaching. While knowledge of curriculum is part of classroom teachers' knowledge base,[8,10,20,21,24] this is not generally true for the attending physicians studied.

Sources of Knowledge for Teaching

How did these six clinical educators learn how to teach so well? They acquired their knowledge of teaching primarily from the experience of being a learner (the apprenticeship of observation of good and bad examples) and a teacher (reflecting on what worked and did not work). Dr. Able reported that he had taken no formal courses in teaching methods: "No, none of us have. It's like sex education and parenting, you just do it . . . I think it is an art, and I think you learn it in an apprenticeship sort of way." They all stated that experience was the biggest determinant of their overall teaching styles, and that they taught in ways that they themselves like to be taught and that fostered their own learning. Dr. Davis said, "I draw on my experiences of having been a student and a resident, and try to pick out the things I liked." Several of them said that it took six to seven years to discover a teaching style that they felt comfortable with. Only two of them had read books and articles on teaching and had attended faculty development workshops. Dr. Fagan was unusual in having participated in numerous faculty development workshops, seminars, and short courses.

IMPLICATIONS

Throughout this research, I was impressed with the congruence of what I learned about the six teachers' knowledge, reasoning, and action: what those attending physicians told me in the interviews closely matched what they did in practice. This congruence in turn agreed with what their students reported and what the transcripts of teaching rounds verified. The attending physicians had a rich knowledge base for teaching that accurately reflected their own teaching styles and strategies. They were articulate in expressing their insights into teaching and their struggles to continuously improve. These expert teachers used their knowledge in an encapsulated mode—namely, they could give a concise teaching point but when needed or asked could elaborate on the deeper structure of the knowledge underlying that point. This is similar to the encapsulated knowledge structures of medical experts studied by Schmidt and Boshuizen[46] and the compiled knowledge structures described by Bordage and colleagues.[4,47]

The collective knowledge base for teaching identified in this study has implications for (1) general conceptions of knowledge for teaching, (2) facilitating learning in clinical settings, and (3) knowledge growth and teaching improvement.

Knowledge for Teaching

The knowledge base for teaching the six physicians studied incorporates six domains of knowledge that are tightly connected through the integrative domain of case-based teaching scripts. While knowledge of medicine is foundational, it is inadequate for effective clinical teaching. Over time, knowledge of medicine becomes reorganized for teaching purposes and interconnected with other forms of knowledge.

While all of the domains of knowledge identified in this study are conceptually distinct, they functionally overlap. As Dr. Able commented when asked to diagram the knowledge he uses during teaching rounds: "The domains of knowledge don't exist in my mind when I am teaching . . . For me it is a fairly cohesive mix."

The most elusive and important form of knowledge stored in memory is case-based teaching scripts. While none of the attending physicians spoke directly to this form of knowledge, they demonstrated it during teaching rounds and acknowledged the accuracy of its description in this article. The importance of this component of knowledge is clearly stated by Hunter:

> In the clinical context, teaching and learning begin with the patient.
>
> As an interpretive activity . . . undertaken for the care of a sick person, it (medicine) takes the patient as its text and seeks to understand his or her malady in the light of current biological, epidemiological, and psychological knowledge.[48]

The patient as text is both a unique person and a memorable representation of a general class of disease. After listening to the learner's case presentation of the patient's story, the teacher's task is to diagnose the patient's problem, diagnose the learner's representation of the case, and connect the learner's understanding with broader conceptions of medicine and with other cases. This process aids the learner's development of illness scripts and builds stronger connections among medical concepts. In such an ill-structured domain as medicine, Spiro argues:

> The best way to learn . . . cognitive flexibility . . . for future application is by . . . case-based presentations which treat a content domain as a landscape that is explored by "criss-crossing" it in many directions, by reexamining each case "site" in the varying contexts of different neighboring cases, and by using a variety of abstract dimensions for comparing cases.[49]

Facilitating Learning

Case-based teaching strategies support experiential learning processes of students and residents by encouraging their abilities to reflect upon experience, develop appropriate generalizations, and predict future effects.[50-53] This involves three instructional tasks. First, teachers need to assess learners' knowledge (including errors, misconceptions, or gaps in knowledge) by asking questions. Other research has found deficits in the content of case presentations[54] and the tendencies of residents to slant the presentation to what they think the preceptor expects to hear.[55] Inquiry is essential to overcoming these difficulties. Asking questions also has the side benefit of activating the learners' prior knowledge, which improves subsequent learning.[51,56-58] During this inquiry process, teachers need to have a flexible knowledge base, since learners vary in the ways in which they structure their knowledge.

Second, teachers need to organize and present medical knowledge so that learners can comprehend it and use it to satisfy their learning objectives. This requires knowledge of case-based teaching scripts to present medical knowledge in an understandable and memorable manner. This often takes the form of short teaching points, modeling interactions and reasoning processes, and encouraging learners to elaborate and reflect upon their knowledge. When the latter occurs, subsequent retrieval of the knowledge is enhanced.[57]

Third, teachers can help learners challenge and expand their existing knowledge. In this instance, teachers need knowledge of medicine, patients, learners, general principles of teaching, and case-based teaching scripts. Creative methods may be needed to challenge learners' understanding in a constructive and supportive manner.

The eight general principles of teaching articulated by the teachers studied (e.g., actively involve learners, capture attention, have fun, etc.) facilitate learning, and are congruent with prior research on clinical teaching[59,60] and with constructivist theories of learning.[61-64] The emphasis upon active involvement and the joint construction of meaning in the context of knowledge use capture essential features of constructivism. However, the limited number of teachers mentioning feedback is troubling although not surprising. While these teachers provided a great deal of feedback to their learners, most attending physicians do not. The lack of feedback during clinical rotations appears to be a rather intractable problem in medical education.[34]

Knowledge Growth and Teaching Improvement

Through the apprenticeship of observation and reflective teaching practice, attending physicians and residents may eventually develop a reasonable knowledge base for teaching. However, this process could perhaps be expedited through systematic teaching-improvement programs for residents and faculty members. In studies of residents' teaching, residents frequently fail to take advantage of teaching opportunities during work rounds and tend to favor lecturing over asking questions and actively involving the team in clinical decision making.[31,65,66] Teaching-improvement workshops are effective mechanisms for developing general teaching skills and for increasing teachers' and residents' understanding of learners.[67-70] Knowledge of case-based teaching is best learned in the context of departmental teaching-improvement and mentoring programs where content-specific, case-based teaching scripts and strategies can be shared.[1]

The present study illuminates the wisdom of practice among distinguished teachers in general internal medicine in the context of teaching rounds. Generalizations from this study should be made to theoretical conceptions of teachers' knowledge rather than to the knowledge base of clinical teachers in medicine generally.[38,72,73] To test this framework of professional knowledge for teaching, further research is needed among less distinguished and more novice clinical teachers, in other medical specialties and in other clinical settings.

SUMMARY

The professional knowledge base of clinical teaching in medicine is multi-dimensional. Excellence in clinical teaching requires clinical knowledge of medicine, of specific patients, and of context plus an educational knowledge of learners, general principles of teaching, and case-based teaching scripts. When combined, these domains of knowledge allow attending physicians to engage in clinical instructional reasoning and to target their teaching to the specific needs of their learners.[1]

The author gratefully acknowledges the contributions of many colleagues to the development of this study, in particular, Dr. Lee Shulman of Stanford University for his underlying theoretical work on pedagogical content knowledge, Drs. Pamela Grossman and Samuel Wineburg of the University of Washington for their guidance in qualitative research methods, and Dr. LuAnn Wilkerson of University of California, Los Angeles, for encouraging him to dig deeper into the data. While affirming their contributions, the author accepts sole responsibility for the limitations of this paper.

References

1. Irby, D. M. How Attending Physicians Make Instructional Decisions when Conducting Teaching Rounds. *Acad. Med.* **67**(1992):630–638.
2. Norman, G. R., Brooks, L. R., Allen, S W., and Rosenthal, D. The Development of Expertise in Dermatology. *Arch. Dermatol.* **125**(1989):1063–1068.
3. Schmidt, H., Norman, G., and Boshuizen, H. A Cognitive Perspective on Medical Expertise: Theory and Implications. *Acad. Med.* **65**(1990):611–621.
4. Bordage, G., and Lemieux, M. Semantic Structures and Diagnostic Thinking of Experts and Novices. In *Proceedings of the Thirtieth Annual Conference on Research in Medical Education. Acad. Med.* **66**, Supplement (September 1991):S70–S72.
5. Patel, V. L., and Groen, G. J. The General and Specific Nature of Medical Expertise: A Critical Look. In *Toward a General Theory of Expertise: Prospects and Limits*, K. A. Ericsson, and J. Smith, eds., pp. 93–125. New York: Cambridge University Press, 1991.
6. Feltovich, P. J., Spiro, R. J., and Coulson, R. L. The Nature of Conceptual Understanding in Biomedicine: The Deep Structure of Complex Ideas and the Development of Misconceptions. In *Cognitive Science in Medicine: Biomedical Modeling*, D. Evans, and V. Patel, eds., pp. 113–172. Cambridge, Massachusetts: MIT Press, 1989.
7. Brophy, J., ed. *Teachers' Knowledge of Subject Matter as it Relates to Their Teaching Practice.* Greenwich, Connecticut: JAI Press, 1991.
8. Grossman, P. L., Wilson, S. M., and Shulman, L. S. Teachers of Substance: Subject Matter Knowledge for Teaching. In *Knowledge Base for the Beginning Teacher*, M. C. Reynolds, ed., pp. 245–264. New York: Pergamon Press, 1989.
9. Putnam, R. T. Structuring and Adjusting Content for Students: A Study of Live and Simulated Tutoring of Addition. *Am. Educ. Res. J.* **24**(1987):13–48.
10. Wilson, S., Shulman, L., and Richert, A. 150 Different Ways of Knowing: Representations of Knowledge in Teaching. In *Exploring Teacher's Thinking*, J. Calderhead, ed., pp. 104–124. London, England: Cassell, 1987.
11. Wilson, S. M., and Wineburg, S. S. Peering at History through Different Lenses: The Role of Disciplinary Perspectives in Teaching History. *Teachers College Record* **89**(1988):522–539.
12. Wineburg, S. S., and Wilson, S. M. Subject-Matter Knowledge in the Teaching of History. In *Teachers' Knowledge of Subject Matter as it Relates to Their Teaching Practice*, J. Brophy, ed., pp. 305–347. Greenwich, Connecticut: JAI Press, 1991.
13. McDiarmid, G. W., Ball, D. L., and Anderson, C. W. Why Staying One Chapter Ahead Doesn't Really Work: Subject-Specific Pedagogy. In *Knowledge Base for the Beginning Teacher*, M. C. Reynolds, ed., pp. 193–205. New York: Pergamon Press, 1989.
14. Carlsen, W. S. Subject-Matter Knowledge and Science Teaching: A Pragmatic Perspective. In *Teachers' Knowledge of Subject Matter as it Relates to Their Teaching Practices*, J. Brophy, ed., pp. 115–143. Greenwich, Connecticut: JAI Press, 1991.
15. Leinhardt, G. Math Lessons: A Contrast of Novice and Expert Competence. *J. Res. Math. Educ.* **20**(1989):52–75.
16. Leinhardt, G. Development of an Expert Explanation: An Analysis of a Sequence of Subtraction Lessons. *Cognition and Instruction.* **4**(1987):203–223.
17. Peterson, P. L., Fennama, E., and Carpenter, T. P. Teachers' Knowledge of Students' Mathematics Problem Solving Knowledge. In *Teachers' Subject Matter Knowledge as it Relates to Their Teaching Practice*, J. E. Brophy, ed., pp. 49–86. Greenwich, Connecticut: JAI Press, 1991.
18. Smith, D. C., and Neale, D. C The Construction of Subject-Matter Knowledge in Primary Science Teaching. In *Teacher's Knowledge of Subject Matter as it Relates to Their Teaching Practice*, J. E. Brophy, ed., pp. 187–244. Greenwich, Connecticut: JAI Press, 1991.
19. Reynolds, A. What is Competent Beginning Teaching? A Review of the Literature. *Rev. Educ. Res.* **62**(1992):1–35.
20. Shulman, L. Those Who Understand: Knowledge Growth in Teaching. *Educ. Res.* **15**(1986):4–14.
21. Shulman, L. Knowledge and Teaching: Foundations of the New Reform. *Harvard Educ. Rev.* **57**(1987):1–22.
22. Leinhardt, G., Putnam, R. T., Stein, M. K., and Baxter, J. Where Subject Knowledge Matters. In *Teachers' Knowledge of Subject Matter as it Relates to Their Teaching Practice*, J. E. Brophy, ed., pp. 87–114. Greenwich, Connecticut: JAI Press, 1991.
23. Gudmundsdottir, S. Pedagogical Models of Subject Matter. In *Teachers' Knowledge of Subject Matter as it Relates to Their Teaching Practice*, J. E. Brophy, ed., pp. 265–304. Greenwich, Connecticut, JAI Press, 1991.
24. Marks, R. Pedagogical Content Knowledge: From a Mathematical Case to a Modified Conception. *J. Teach. Educ.* **41**(1990):3–11.
25. Grossman, P. L. *The Making of a Teacher: Teacher Knowledge and Teacher Education.* New York: Teachers College Press, 1990.
26. Adams, W. R., et al. A Naturalistic Study of Teaching in a Clinical Clerkship. *J. Med. Educ.* **39**(1964):164–166.
27. Becker, H., Geer, B., Hughes, E., and Strauss, A. *Boys in White.* Chicago, Illinois: University of Chicago Press, 1961.
28. Mattern, W. D., Weinholtz, D., and Friedman, C. P. The Attending Physician as Teacher. *N. Engl. J. Med.* **308**(1983):1129–1132.
29. Reichsman, F., Browning, F. E., and Hinshaw, J. R. Observations of Undergraduate Clinical Teaching in Action. *J. Med. Educ.* **39**(1964):147–153.
30. Shulman, R. Wilkerson, L., and Goldman, D. Multiple Realities: Teaching Rounds in an Inpatient Pediatric Service. *Am. J. Child.* **146**(1992):55–60.
31. Tremonti, L. P., and Biddle, W. B. Teaching Behaviors of Residents and Faculty Members. *J. Med. Educ.* **57**(1982):854–859.
32. Weinholtz, D. The Socialization of Physicians During Attending Rounds: A Study of Team Learning among Medical Students. *Qualitative Health Research* **1**(1991):152–177.
33. Shulman, L. S. Toward a Pedagogy of Cases. In *Case Methods in Teacher Education*, J. H. Shulman, ed., pp. 1–30. New York: Teachers College Press, 1992.
34. Irby, D. M., and Rakestraw, P. Evaluating Clinical Teaching in Medicine. *J. Med Educ.* **56**(1981):181–186.
35. Spradley, J. P. *The Ethnographic Interview.* Chicago, Illinois: Holt, Rinehart and Winston, 1979.
36. Ericsson, K. A., and Simon, H. A. Verbal Reports as Data. *Psychological Rev.* **87**(1980):215–251.
37. Spradley, J. P. *Participant Observation.* New York: Holt, Rinehart and Winston, 1980.
38. Miles, M. B., and Huberman, A. M. *Qualitative Data Analysis: A Sourcebook of New Methods.* Newbury Park, California: Sage

Publications, 1984

39. Sabers, D., Cushing, K., and Berliner, D. Differences among Teachers in a Task Characterized by Simultaneity, Multidimensionality, and Immediacy. *Am. Educ. Res. J.* 28(1991):63–88.

40. Bordage, G. The Curriculum: Overloaded and Too General? *Med. Educ.* 21(1987): 183–188.

41. Christensen, C. R., Garvin, D. A., and Sweet, A. *Education for Judgment: The Artistry of Discussion Leadership.* Boston, Massachusetts: Harvard Business School Press, 1991.

42. Schon, D., ed. *The Reflective Turn: Case Studies in and on Educational Practice.* New York: Teachers College Press, 1991.

43. Shulman, J. H. *Case Methods in Teacher Education.* New York: Teachers College Press, 1992.

44. Levenstein, J. H., et al. The Patient-Centered Clinical Method: I. A Model for the Doctor/Patient Interaction in Family Medicine. *Fam. Pract.* 3(1986):24–30.

45. McWhinney, I. R. *A Textbook of Family Medicine.* Oxford, England: Oxford University Press, 1989.

46. Schmidt, H. G., and Boshuizen, H. P. On the Origin of Intermediate Effects in Clinical Case Recall. *Memory and Cognition* 21(1993):338–351.

47. Bordage, G., and Zacks, R. The Structure of Medical Knowledge in the Memories of Medical Students and General Practitioners: Categories and Prototypes. *Med. Educ.* 18(1984):406–416.

48. Hunter, K. M. *Doctors' Stories: The Narrative Structure of Medical Knowledge.* Princeton, New Jersey: Princeton University Press, 1991, p. 25.

49. Spiro, R. J., et al. Knowledge Acquisition for Application: Cognitive Flexibility and Transfer in Complex Content Domains. In *Executive Control Processes*, B. C. Britton, and S. Glynn, eds., pp. 177–200. Hillsdale, New Jersey: Erlbaum, 1987.

50. Hewson, M. G. Reflection in Clinical Teaching: An Analysis of Reflection-on-Action and its Implications for Staffing Residents. *Med. Teach.* 13(1991):227–231.

51. Hewson, M. Clinical Teaching in the Ambulatory Setting. *J. Gen. Intern. Med.* 7(1992):76–82.

52. Kolb, D. A. *Experiential Learning: Experience as the Source of Learning and Development.* Englewood Cliffs, New Jersey: Prentice-Hall, 1984.

53. Schon, D. *The Reflective Practitioner: How Professionals Think in Action.* New York: Basic Books, 1983.

54. Kihm, J. T., Brown, J. T., Divine, G. W., and Linzer, M. Quantitative Analysis of the Outpatient Oral Case Presentation: Piloting a Method. *J. Gen. Intern. Med.* 6(1991):233–236.

55. Bucher, R., and Stelling, J. G. *Becoming Professional.* Beverly Hills, California: Sage Publications, 1977.

56. Franks, J. J., Bransford, J. D., and Auble, P. M. The Activation and Utilization of Knowledge. In *Handbook of Research Methods in Human Memory and Cognition*, C. R. Puff, ed., pp. 395–425. New York: Academic Press, 1982.

57. Norman, G. R., and Schmidt, H. G. The Psychological Basis of Problem-based Learning: A Review of the Evidence. *Acad. Med.* 67(1992):557–565.

58. Steward, D. E., and Feltovich, P. J. Why Residents Should Teach: The Parallel Processes of Teaching and Learning. In *Clinical Teaching for Medical Residents: Role, Techniques, and Programs*, J. C. Edwards, and R. L. Marier, eds., pp. 3–14. New York: Springer Publishing Company, 1988.

59. Irby, D. M. Clinical Teacher Effectiveness in Medicine. *J. Med. Educ.* 53(1978): 808–815.

60. Stritter, F. T., Hain, J. D., and Grimes, D. A. Clinical Teaching Reexamined. *J. Med. Educ.* 50(1975):877–882.

61. Bruner, J. *Acts of Meaning.* Cambridge, Massachusetts: Harvard University Press, 1990.

62. Dewey, J. *Experience and Education.* New York: Collier Books, 1938.

63. Lave, J. *Cognition in Practice: Mind, Mathematics and Culture in Everyday Life.* Cambridge, U.K.: Cambridge University Press, 1991.

64. Resnick, L. B. *Education and Learning to Think.* Washington, D.C.: National Academy Press, 1987.

65. Lewis, J. M., and Kappelman, M. M. Teaching Styles: An Introductory Program for Residents. *J. Med. Educ.* 59(1984):355.

66. Wilkerson, L., Lesky, L., and Medio, F. J. The Resident as Teacher During Work Rounds. *J. Med. Educ.* 61(1986):823–829.

67. Edwards, J. C., Kissling, G. E., Plauche, W. C., and Marier, R. L. Long-Term Evaluation of Training Residents in Clinical Teaching Skills. *J. Med. Educ.* 61(1986):967–970.

68. Edwards, J. C., and Marier, R. L. *Clinical Teaching for Medical Residents: Roles, Techniques, and Programs.* New York: Springer Publishing Company, 1988.

69. Skeff, K. M., et al. Assessment by Attending Physicians of a Seminar Method to Improve Clinical Teaching. *J. Med. Educ.* 59(1984):944–950.

70. Skeff, K. M., Stratos, G. A., Berman, J., and Bergen, M. R. Improving Clinical Teaching: Evaluation of a National Dissemination Program. *Arch. Intern. Med.* 152(1992):1156–1161.

71. Shulman, L. S. Autonomy and Obligation: The Remote Control of Teaching. In *Handbook of Teaching and Policy*, L. S. Shulman, and G. Sykes, eds., pp. 485–504. New York: Longman, 1983.

72. Bromley, D. B. *The Case-Study Method in Psychology and Related Disciplines.* New York: John Wiley & Sons, 1986.

73. Glaser, B., and Strauss, A. L. *The Discovery of Grounded Theory: Strategies for Qualitative Research.* Chicago, Illinois: Aldine, 1967.

An Alternative Approach to Defining the Role of the Clinical Teacher

JOHN A. ULLIAN, PhD, CAROLE J. BLAND, PhD, and DEBORAH E. SIMPSON, PhD

Background. A number of studies have attempted to identify the components of the clinical teacher role by examining learners' numerical ratings of items on researcher-generated lists. Some of these studies have also compared different groups' perceptions of clinical teaching, but have not directly compared the perceptions of first- and third-year residents. This study addressed two questions: (1) What do residents consider important components of the clinical teacher role? (2) Do first- and third-year residents perceive this role similarly? **Method.** A content analysis was performed on the comments written on evaluation forms by 268 residents about 490 clinical teachers over a five-year period (1980–81 through 1984–85) at a large family practice residency. Of 5,664 forms completed by the residents, 2,388 (42%) contained written comments; comments were on 1,024 (46%) of the first-year residents' forms, 701 (41%) of the second-year residents' forms, and 663 (39%) of the third-year residents' forms. Themes in these comments were coded into a coding dictionary of 157 categories, within 37 clusters, within four roles. **Results.** The ten highest-ranked categories (Global; Teaching: General; Knowledgeable; Gives Resident Responsibility; Supportive; Miscellaneous; Interested in Teaching; Clinical Competence; Makes Effort to Teach; and Gives Resident Opportunity to Do Procedures) accounted for 41% of the themes coded. The first- and third-year residents differed in the clusters they used to describe their clinical teachers on evaluation forms ($\chi^2 = 149.86$, $df = 36$, $p < .0001$). **Conclusion.** The results suggest that content analysis can be used to validly and reliably study residents' written evaluative comments about their teachers. This study contributes to the definition of the clinical teacher role, showing the relative importances of its components, and also supports Stritter's Learning Vector theory, finding the anticipated differences between the comments made by first- and third-year residents. *Acad. Med.* 69(1994):832–838.

Clinical teaching is the primary method of instruction from at least the last half of medical school through residency, and serving as a clinical teacher is a critical role for medical school faculty.[1] Since roles are defined by the expectations of others,[2] an understanding of the role of the clinical teacher requires an understanding of learners' (students' and residents') perceptions of that role. Clinical teaching has been studied in several ways.[3] One type of study has examined learners' perceptions by presenting students and/or residents with a list of hypothetically important components of clinical teaching, and asking them either to rate a teacher (most recent,

Dr. Ullian is assistant professor and associate director of predoctoral education, Department of Family Medicine, Baylor College of Medicine, Houston, Texas; Dr. Bland is professor, Department of Family Practice and Community Health, University of Minnesota Medical School–Minneapolis; and Dr. Simpson is associate professor, Department of Family and Community Medicine, and director, Division of Educational Services, Medical College of Wisconsin, Milwaukee.

Correspondence and requests for reprints should be addressed to Dr. Ullian, Department of Family Medicine, Baylor College of Medicine, 5510 Greenbriar, Houston, TX 77005.

best, or ideal), or to rate how important the component was to their learning. Results have been presented as factors (to show the underlying structure of clinical teaching), comparisons (to show similarities between groups), or rank-ordered lists (to show the relative importance of the listed components).

The factor-analytic studies[4–16] have resulted in varying numbers of factors, but an examination of these studies suggests that learners perceive that there are four roles within the clinical teacher role:[17] *physician* (models knowledge and skills in performing medical duties); *supervisor* (provides opportunities for performance, observes, gives feedback); *teacher* (selects, organizes, and delivers information); and *person* (exhibits specific interpersonal and intrapersonal characteristics). These roles parallel the four themes of research on clinical teaching identified by Dinham and Stritter[3]: the role model, practice and evaluation, organization of the learning, and the instructor's attitude. They are also similar to the clinical teacher roles suggested by Simon[18]: resource, supervisor, designer of instruction, and role model; and by Irby[19]: role model, clinical supervisor, and instructional leadership; and to the roles suggested for the classroom teacher by

Cooper[20]: learner, manager, teacher, and person.

Comparative studies[7,8,11,15,16,21–26] have typically found no or only limited differences among the perceptions of different groups of individuals, whether comparing students' or residents' perceptions with those of faculty or comparing those of individuals in different institutions, suggesting agreement among the various groups' perceptions of the clinical teacher role. Stritter's Learning Vector theory[27] strongly suggests that, since the nature of clinical teachers' contributions to residents' learning should change with the professional development of the residents, residents at different levels should perceive the clinical teacher role differently. While none of the studies cited above compared first-year with third-year residents' perceptions, Williamson et al.[28] found support for the Learning Vector theory in an observational study that found decreasing consultation rates and durations from first to third year, and increasing clinical independence and assertiveness.

Rank-ordering studies[7–9,14–16,21,23,24,29] are difficult to summarize, since learners responded to different lists of clinical teaching components. However, items representing several components have appeared often in the lists and have typically been ranked highly: enthusiasm, organization/ preparation, feedback, availability, explanations/discussions, clinical competence, answering questions, and interest in students/residents. Highly ranked in at least three of the five studies[7,14,16,23,24] that provided rankings of residents' responses were confidence, enthusiasm, approach to patients, explanations, organization/ preparation, respect for resi-dents, and answering/encouraging questions.

Thus, these studies of learners' perceptions of clinical teaching have required learners to respond to researcher-generated lists of hypothetically important components of the clinical teacher role. This use of these lists of specified clinical teaching components prevents the discovery of other components important to students or residents but not on the lists. Only three studies have examined, all in a limited way, verbal[10,30] or written[7] statements by learners about clinical teachers, despite a call about 15 years ago for a study of learners' written comments about their clinical teachers.[31] What learners write about individual clinical teachers is relevant to the definition of the clinical teacher role, because when individuals describe the holder of a role, they use dimensions or categories they consider salient to the role.[32-33] Thus, learners' written comments about clinical teachers, such as those commonly found on evaluation forms, can be analyzed to identify the components of the clinical teaching role as perceived by those learners.

The present study asked two questions: (1) What do residents consider to be the important components of the clinical teacher role? (2) Do first- and third-year residents perceive this role similarly?

METHOD

A content analysis was performed on the comments written on evaluation forms by 268 residents about 490 clinical teachers over a five-year period (1980–81 through 1984–85) at a large family practice residency located at six affiliated sites. The clinical teachers represented almost all of the medical and surgical specialties, and were either medical school faculty or hospital attending physicians. Most of the rotations were hospital-based, but some were office-based. Residents completed 5,664 evaluation forms: 39% were from postgraduate-year-one (PGY1) residents, 31% from postgraduate-year-two (PGY2) residents, and 30% from postgraduate-year-three (PGY3) residents. Overall, 2,388 (42%) of the forms contained written comments: 1,024 (46%) of the PGY1 forms, 701 (41%) of the PGY2 forms, and 663 (39%) of the PGY3 forms.

Content analysis requires the coding of the recording units into a comprehensive and mutually exclusive set of categories. The recording unit selected for this study was the theme,[34] a single assertion about a subject, i.e., a word, phrase, etc., judged to reflect a single idea. To limit the potential subjectivity of the coding, Miles and Huberman[35] recommend beginning with a coding dictionary of 80–90 categories (developed from the literature, research questions, hypotheses, and key variables), followed iteratively by coding, revising of the dictionary, recoding, etc., until the dictionary allows accurate coding of the data. The coding dictionary for this study began with 80 clinical teaching components suggested by a prior study of evaluation forms used by family practice residency programs.[36] A subset of the database of comments was coded to revise the dictionary, during which it grew to 184 categories aggregated into 42 clusters; this dictionary was then used to code the whole database. Following this, the dictionary was once again revised to fit the comments better, resulting in the final coding dictionary (available from JAU) of 157 categories in 37 clusters, in the four clinical teacher roles identified in the review of factor analytic studies. Two categories and their clusters [Global (e.g., "good") and Miscellaneous] were included to permit the coding of all recording units, although they belong to none of the roles. Several category entries in the annotated version of the coding dictionary are presented in the boxed text ("Sample Categories . . .") elsewhere in the text.

Intercoder agreement was examined to test the reliability of the coding process. The primary coder (JAU), who had developed the coding dictionary, coded 400 randomly selected resident comments. A second coder (DES) received brief training and used the final coding dictionary to code the same comments. This sample size was based on McCall's formula 12.2[37] for sample size estimation to insure agreement beyond chance. The coefficient of reliability [CR = agreements/(agreements + disagreements)][34] was .80, an acceptable level in content analytic research.[38] Combining the categories into clusters resulted in a CR of .85.

Frequency data for each category, cluster, and role were tabulated. The frequency of each category is the number of times that category was used to code a theme in the database. The frequency of each higher level of aggregation is the sum of the frequencies of the categories within it. Chi-square statistics were computed to determine whether the comments made by PGY1s and PGY3s were distributed in the same proportions among the category clusters. Given the large sample size, a conservative value of $\alpha = .001$ was adopted. The contingency coefficient was used to determine the strength of association between PGY1 and PGY3 results.

RESULTS

What do family practice residents perceive to be important components of the clinical teacher role? The ten highest-ranked categories (Global; Teaching: General; Knowledgeable; Gives Resident Responsibility; Supportive; Miscellaneous; Interested in Teaching; Clinical Competence; Makes Effort to Teach; and Gives Resident Opportunity to Do Procedures) accounted for 41% of the total number of themes coded. All four roles were cited substantially in the comments, as evident in the percentage of themes (excluding Global and Miscellaneous from the denominator) coded into each role: *physician*, 22%; *supervisor*, 16%;

mension of Understanding higher than did PGY3s.

DISCUSSION AND CONCLUSIONS

Sample Categories from the Annotated Coding Dictionary of Written Comments on Evaluation Forms of 268 Family Practice Residents about 490 Clinical Faculty, 1980–81 through 1984–85*

22. Knowledgeable—Knowledge of general medicine or specialty. Use 23 (Well-read) for knowing the literature. Use 24 (Current) for current knowledge. [Cluster 4, Knowledge; Physician role.]

59. Teaching: General—General or global statements about teaching, e.g., good teacher, good instruction, taught well. [Cluster 10, Teaching: General; Teacher role.]

99. Supervises—Provides or is available for observation, guidance, backup, assistance, help, direction. Use 184 (Helpful) for general helpfulness. [Cluster 16, Supervision; Supervisor role.]

122. Discussions—Discusses; willing to discuss; spends time discussing; enjoys discussions; good, interesting, enjoyable, etc., discussions. Use more specific categories when possible (e.g., use 100 (Reviews Patient with Resident) for discussion of specific patients; use 123 (Gives Reasons for Decisions) for discussing decisions made by preceptor. [Cluster 18, Dialogue; Teacher role.]

124. Explanations—Explains; willing to explain; spends time explaining; enjoys explaining; good, useful, practical, etc., explanations. Use 18 (Explains Things to Patients) for explanations to patients. Use 123 (Gives Reasons for Decisions) for explaining decisions. [Cluster 18, Dialogue; Teacher role.]

188. Interested in Resident—Cares about residents; enjoys residents; likes to work with residents. Use 67 (Concern for Quality of Rotation) for caring about residents' learning. Use 63 (Interested in Teaching) for likes teaching residents. [Cluster 28, Caring; Person role.]

259. Global—Good preceptor; good guy; wonderful person; good rotation; good experience; good learning experience; enjoyable experience. Use 59 (Teaching: General) for good teacher. Use 4 (Clinical Competence) for good doctor, competent. [Cluster, 38 Global; no role.]

*In all, the dictionary contains 157 categories in 37 clusters in four clinical teacher roles: physician, supervisor, teacher, and person. The residents were first-, second-, and third-year residents at a large residency located at six affiliated sites.

This study used an alternative approach to ratings-based studies of the components of clinical teaching by employing a content analysis of residents' written comments about their clinical teachers to help define the role of the clinical teacher. In addition, the study sought to add to the comparative research data on the clinical teaching role by comparing the perceptions of first- and third-year residents.

The limitations of the study are in three areas: the resident sample, the method of data collection, and the content analysis methodology. Generalizability of the findings may be limited given that all residents were family practice residents affiliated with a single training program. They were, however, at six separate sites, commenting most often on clinical teachers unique to each site, and were in rotations in most medical specialties. Comments were obtained as part of a routine evaluation on a form that did not provide resident anonymity, and this may have limited the comments made, especially negative comments. Since the evaluation form included scaled items on clinical teaching, those items may have had a cueing effect on resident comments. Finally, content analysis necessarily involves some subjective judgments, such as those involved in creating the coding dictionary and aggregating categories into clusters and roles. The use of a research-based coding dictionary and an intercoder reliability analysis attempted to limit some of these problems of subjectivity. Future research could address these limitations more fully by replicating the study in other medical specialties and across institutions, by collecting descriptions of clinical teachers anonymously and independent of the evaluation process, and by testing whether other coders can reliably use the coding dictionary.

What do family practice residents

teacher, 38%; and *person*, 24%. Table 1 lists the 25 highest-ranked categories arranged by role.

Do first- and third-year residents perceive the clinical teaching role similarly? Table 2 lists the rank orders and frequencies of the clusters for all three years of residents combined and for PGY1s and PGY3s separately. As indicated in this table, PGY1s and PGY3s differed in the clusters they used to describe their clinical teachers ($\chi^2 = 149.86$, df $= 36$, $p < .0001$). The contingency coefficient of .17 suggests that the difference, although statistically significant, is relatively weak.

While many of the cluster rankings were very similar for first- and third-

year residents, some differed by three or more places in the rankings. An examination of the latter shows that Didactic Teaching, Rounds, Availability, Dialogue, and Feedback were more important to first-year than to third-year residents. Further, first-year residents wanted the teacher to be a Role Model who demonstrates an Approach to Patient Care. In contrast, third-year residents focused on specific content and on their own learning, as demonstrated by their higher ranking for Topics Taught, Resident's Learning, Readings, and Areas of Interest. The intrapersonal dimension of Calmness was more important to PGY3s, while PGY1s ranked the interpersonal di-

perceive to be important components of the clinical teaching role? The rank-ordered lists of categories and their clusters that resulted from this study indicate the relative importances of those clinical teaching components to family practice residents. Four roles within the role of the clinical teacher were identified in the literature, and the residents found components of all four to be important. The following "thumbnail sketch" describes the clinical teacher who embodies the highest-ranked components of clinical teaching.

As a *physician*, the clinical teacher is knowledgeable and clinically competent, is seen as a role model, has good rapport with patients, and has an appropriate attitude toward family practice. As a *supervisor*, the clinical teacher gives the resident responsibility for patient care and opportunities to do procedures, involves the resident, and reviews patients with the resident. The preceptor is a good *teacher*, interested in teaching and making an effort to teach; although busy, he or she is available and spends time with the resident, explaining, discussing, and answering questions. Finally, as a *person*, the clinical teacher is supportive, easy and fun to work with, helpful, and friendly.

While these results are similar to the findings of ratings-based studies, thus providing some evidence of the validity of both types of studies, there were differences that add to what we know about clinical teaching. Three of the seven highest-ranked clusters in this study (Opportunities Provided Residents, Knowledge, and Support) were not highly ranked in the ratings-based studies. Since the authors typically did not publish the entire list of items used in their studies, it is not known whether the items representing these clusters were not listed or were ranked lower. In any event, the picture drawn from the ratings-based studies did not include these three clinical teaching components that the residents in this study found important.

The importance of practice opportunities, the highest-ranked cluster, seems obvious (as is reflected in the

experiential nature of residency programs), and perhaps the authors of the ratings-based studies considered it too obvious to include in their lists. By making this their highest-ranking cluster, the residents' comments about their clinical teachers in this study thus remind us in medical education (as the earlier studies did not) that residents need to be active, engaged learners, and that the clinical teacher's role includes seeing that residents are allowed and encouraged to *practice medicine.*

The clinical teacher's knowledge was ranked fifth in this study and third in that of Wolverton and Bosworth,[16] but was not among the highly rated items in the other studies. Asking learners to rate their teachers' knowledge has always been controversial, and perhaps it was not included in the lists. Likewise, the clinical teacher's support for the learner was ranked sixth in this study, tenth in that of Wolverton and Bosworth,[16] and not as high on the other studies.

Table 1

Ranks and Frequencies of Highest-ranked Categories Arranged by Role and Cluster, Derived from Written Comments from 268 Family Practice Residents about 490 Clinical Faculty, 1980–81 through 1984–85*

Role	Category and (Cluster)	Rank†	Frequency
Physician	Knowledgeable (Knowledge)	3	312
	Clinical Competence (Clinical Competence)	8	246
	Role Model as a Physician (Role Model)	14	115
	Rapport with Patients (Approach to Patient Care)	16	108
	Attitude toward Family Practice (Attitudes toward Medicine)	20t	91
Supervisor	Gives Resident Responsibility (Opportunities Provided Resident)	4	308
	Gives Resident Opportunity to do Procedures (Opportunities Provided Resident)	10	171
	Involves Resident (Opportunities Provided Resident)	13	119
	Reviews Patient with Resident (Supervision)	18	99
Teacher	Teaching: General (Teaching: General)	2	459
	Interested in Teaching (Commitment to Teaching)	7	270
	Makes Effort to Teach (Commitment to Teaching)	9	191
	Available (Availability)	11	135
	Explanations (Dialogue)	15	109
	Spends Time with Residents (Availability)	19	96
	Answers Questions (Dialogue)	22	90
	Busy (Availability)	23t	81
	Discussions (Dialogue)	25	77
Person	Supportive (Support)	5	290
	Easy to Work with (Preceptor as Co-worker)	12	121
	Fun to Work with (Preceptor as Co-worker)	17	107
	Helpful (Support)	20t	91
	Friendly (Amiability)	23t	81
—	Global (no cluster)	1	567
—	Miscellaneous (no cluster)	6	284

*In all, 2,388 evaluation forms contained written comments, which were coded into 157 categories in 37 clusters in four clinical teacher roles. The residents were first-, second-, and third-year residents at a large residency located at six affiliated sites. The table shows the 25 highest-ranked categories of the total of 157.

†In the rank column, "t" indicates a tie in the rankings.

Table 2

Roles, Ranks, and Frequencies of Clusters of Categories of Written Comments by 268 Family Practice Residents about 490 Clinical Faculty, 1980–81 through 1984–85*

Cluster	Role	Rank†			Frequency		
		For All Residents	For PGY1s	For PGY3s	For All Residents	For PGY1s	For PGY3s
Opportunities Provided Resident	Supervisor	1	1	3	671	324	147
Global	—	2	7	1	567	185	198
Commitment to Teaching	Teacher	3	2	4	548	268	104
Teaching: General	Teacher	4	8	2	497	183	161
Dialogue	Teacher	5	3	7	464	223	87
Knowledge	Physician	6	5	6	416	194	96
Support	Person	7	6	5	399	193	101
Availability	Teacher	8	4	9	387	206	84
Clinical Competence	Physician	9	9	8	366	178	85
Miscellaneous	—	10	10	10	284	141	59
Caring	Person	11	11	11	254	124	56
Clinical Teacher as Co-worker	Person	12	13	12	243	117	53
Amiability	Person	13	15	13	232	92	51
Approach to Patient Care	Physician	14	12	15	214	123	41
Supervision	Supervisor	15	14	14	210	100	47
Attitudes toward Medicine	Physician	16	17	16	161	72	39
Resident's Learning	Teacher	17t	20t	17	134	63	32
Task Orientation	Person	17t	18t	20t	134	66	22
Rounds	Teacher	19	16	22t	131	81	21
Expectations for Resident	Supervisor	20	20t	20t	124	63	22
Role Model	Physician	21	18t	22t	115	66	21
Topics Taught	Teacher	22	26	18	103	40	29
Teaching Clinical Reasoning Skills	Teacher	23	22	22t	94	56	21
Openness	Person	24	24t	25	82	41	20
Feedback	Supervisor	25	23	28	81	52	13
Areas of Interest	Physician	26	30t	19	79	32	23
Experience	Physician	27	27	33t	70	37	8
Readings	Teacher	28	30t	27	69	32	15
Dynamism	Person	29	28t	26	66	33	16
Didactic Teaching	Teacher	30	24t	35	61	41	7
Intelligence	Physician	31	32	29t	56	28	12
Understanding	Person	32	28t	32	55	33	9
Calmness	Person	33	33	29t	46	25	12
Relationships with Others	Person	34	34	31	33	14	10
Confidence	Person	35	35	33t	28	13	8
Specific Teaching Activities	Teacher	36	36	37	16	9	4
Self-criticism	Physician	37	37	36	15	8	5

$X^2 = 149.86$ (df = 36); $p < .0001$; contingency coefficient = .166

*A total of 2,388 evaluation forms contained written comments, which were coded into 157 categories in four clinical teacher roles. The forms were completed by postgraduate-year-one (PGY1), postgraduate-year-two (PGY2), and postgraduate-year-three (PGY3) residents at a large program located at six affiliated sites. In all, 1,024 PGY1 forms and 663 PGY3 forms contained written comments.

†In the rank column, "t" indicates a tie in the rankings.

Of the clinical teaching components typically ranked among the most important in the ratings-based studies but not in this study, feedback stands out. Its importance in clinical teaching is without question, but the term was not among those most often used by the residents in their evaluative comments. The term "feedback" may suggest to residents an external control, a corrective action, and therefore manipulation. From the perspective of the resident who sees himself or herself as a professional responsible for patient care as well as for his or her own education, feedback may be expressed in terms more suggestive of receiving needed information in a way that allows the resident to maintain control. Thus residents may prefer to think of discussing or reviewing patients, an swering questions, making suggestions, or other forms of teacher–resident dialogue, which ranked higher in this study than did feedback itself. This is consistent with Bucher and Stelling's[39] conclusions regarding residents' control over the resident–preceptor interaction, and is also supported by the higher ranking of the Feedback cluster by PGY1s than by PGY3s, since the latter are typically more independent and control-oriented than the former.

Do first- and third-year residents perceive the clinical teaching role similarly? Rankings of most clusters were similar, but there were differences, which resulted in a statistically significant chi-square test. The differences found between first- and third-year residents' perceptions are consistent with Stritter's Learning Vector theory.[27] That theory suggests that as residents develop professionally during their years in training, their perceptions regarding the nature of their clinical teachers' contributions to their learning should also change, with residents developing from passive learners to independent, collegial learners. The results of this study suggest that PGY1s define the clinical teacher as the expert who is available and provides didactic instruction, feedback, and one-to-one discussion with the resident. In contrast, PGY3s seem to perceive their clinical teachers more as colleagues than as their teachers, and these residents assume greater responsibility for their own learning.

This study also supports Bucher and Stelling's[39] findings regarding residents' control over resident–teacher interactions. From this viewpoint, the clinical teacher's primary responsibility should be to provide, or at least allow, practice opportunities for the resident, and then to remain available with explanations and answers for the resident, and to be knowledgeable, helpful, and supportive in doing so. One specific comparison highlights this control issue: the category for the clinical teachers' *asking* questions was used only 24 times in the database, while the category for their *answering* questions was used 90 times. While clinical teachers may feel a bit uneasy

with this portrait of residents' control, the scenario may appear more appropriate when cast in terms of the resident as a goal-directed adult learner, as discussed by Knowles.[40] Residents' perceptions of the role of the clinical teacher (and, by inference, of their own role as learners) are very consistent with Knowles' theory of adult learning. That theory suggests that teachers are role models, resources, and facilitators, and that learners are self-directed, learn from their own increasingly richer individual experience bases, and learn in order to solve problems within the demands of their own roles. The results of this study support Knowles' concepts, with third-year residents matching the adult learning pattern more than first-year residents.

Methodologically, this study has brought a new perspective to the study of the components of the clinical teacher role. Its content analysis of residents' written comments on preceptor evaluation forms provides an alternative to the ratings-based approach prevalent in this line of research. It has shown that such a content analysis can be performed with reliability and validity. In doing so, it has shown that comments written by residents about their teachers have validity, at least when considered over a large number of residents and teachers. (The accuracy of individual comments about a teacher was not studied here.) The coding dictionary created during iterative passes through the database is a comprehensive classification system for the components of the clinical teacher role. It is more inclusive than any of the lists of clinical teaching characteristics used in prior, ratings-based studies.

The results of the study can be used to improve the evaluation and performance of clinical teachers. Highly ranked categories and clusters should be considered for inclusion on evaluation forms used by residents to evaluate their preceptors. Faculty development programs can use the results first to show the complexity of the clinical teaching role, and then to set the agenda for addressing the more important areas of clinical teacher performance. Just as the knowledge of

teachers' implicit theories of students has been used to help improve college teaching,[41] knowledge of residents' implicit theories of clinical teaching (their expectations of clinical teachers) can be used to improve clinical teaching.

In summary, this study has contributed to the definition of the clinical teaching role by performing a content analysis of written evaluative comments made by residents about their clinical teachers. Its resulting rank-ordered lists of categories and clusters show the relative importances of the various components of the clinical teaching role. Stritter's Learning Vector theory[27] was supported in the comparison of PGY1 and PGY3 comments. This comparison produced results that were also consistent with Bucher and Stelling's[39] views regarding residents' control over the teacher–resident interaction and with Knowles'[40] concepts of the adult learner. Finally, this study has demonstrated that written evaluative comments can be a valuable source of research data, and can be reliably and validly analyzed.

References

1. Bland, C. J., Schmitz, C. C., Stritter, F. T., Henry, R. C., and Aluise, J. J. *Successful Faculty in Academic Medicine: Essential Skills and How to Acquire Them.* New York: Springer, 1990.
2. Stryker, S., and Statham, A. Symbolic Interaction and Role Theory. In *The Handbook of Social Psychology*, Vol. I, 3rd ed, G. Lindzey and E. Aronson, eds., pp. 311–378. New York: Random House, 1985.
3. Dinham, S. M., and Stritter, F. T. Research on Professional Education. In *Handbook of Research on Teaching*, 3rd ed, M. C. Wittrock, ed, pp. 952–970. New York: Macmillan, 1986.
4. Cotsonas, N. J., Jr., and Kaiser, H. F. A Factor Analysis of Students' and Administrators' Ratings of Clinical Teachers in a Medical School. *J. Educ. Psychol.* 53 (1962):219–223.
5. Cotsonas, N. J., Jr., and Kaiser, H. F. (1963). Student Evaluation Of Clinical Teaching. *J. Med. Educ.* 38(1963):742–745.
6. Elliott, D. L., and Hickam, D. H. Medical Students' Evaluations of Their Preceptors' Teaching in an Introductory Course. *Acad. Med.* 66(1991):243–244.
7. Irby, D. M. *Clinical Teacher Effectiveness in Medicine as Perceived by Faculty, Residents*

and Students. PhD diss., University of Washington, 1977.

8. Irby, D. M. Clinical Teacher Effectiveness in Medicine. J. Med. Educ. 53(1978):808–815.

9. Irby, D. M., and Rakestraw, P. Evaluating Clinical Teaching in Medicine. J. Med. Educ. 56(1981):181–186.

10. Irby, D. M., Ramsey, P. G., Gillmore, G. M., and Schaad, D. Characteristics of Effective Clinical Teachers of Ambulatory Care Medicine. Acad. Med. 66(1991):54–55.

11. McLeod, P. J., James, C. A., and Abrahamowicz, M. Clinical Tutor Evaluation: A 5 Year Study by Students on an In-Patient Service and Residents in an Ambulatory Care Clinic. Med. Educ. 27(1993):48–54.

12. Miller, M. D. Factorial Validity of a Clinical Teaching Scale. Educ. Psych. Meas. 42(1982):1141–1147.

13. Shellenberger, S., and Mahan, J. M. A Factor Analytic Study of Teaching in Off-Campus General Practice Clerkships. Med. Educ. 16(1982):151–155.

14. Stritter, F. T., and Baker, R. M. Resident Preferences for the Clinical Teaching of Ambulatory Care. J. Med. Educ. 57(1982):33–41.

15. Stritter, F. T., Hain, J. D., and Grimes, D. A. Clinical Teaching Reexamined. J. Med. Educ. 50(1975):876–882.

16. Wolverton, S. E., and Bosworth, M. F. A Survey of Resident Perceptions of Effective Teaching Behaviors. Fam. Med. 17(1985):106–108.

17. Ullian, J. A. Family Practice Residents' Perceptions of the Role of Preceptor: A Content Analysis of Written Evaluative Comments. PhD diss., University of Minnesota, 1989: pp. 26–31 and Appendix A.

18. Simon, J. L. A Role Guide and Resource Book for Clinical Preceptors. DHEW Publication No. HRA 77-14. Washington, D.C.: U. S. Department of Health, Education, and Welfare, 1976.

19. Irby, D. M. Clinical Teaching and the Clinical Teacher. In Clinical Education of

Medical Students. J. Med. Educ. 61, part 2 (September 1986):35–45.

20. Cooper, C. R. Different Ways of Being a Teacher: An Ethnographic Study of a College Instructor's Academic and Social Roles in the Classroom. J. Classroom Interaction. 16(1981):21–37.

21. Calkins, E. V., Arnold, L. M., Willoughby, T. L., and Hamburger, S. C. Docents' and Students' Perceptions of the Ideal and Actual Role of the Docent. J. Med. Educ. 61(1986):743–748.

22. Fallon, S. M., Croen, L. G., and Shelov, S. P. Teachers' and Students' Ratings of Clinical Teaching and Teachers' Opinions on Use of Student Evaluations. J. Med. Educ. 62(1987):435–438.

23. Gjerde, C. L., and Coble, R. J. Resident and Faculty Perceptions of Effective Clinical Teaching in Family Practice. J. Fam. Pract. 14(1982):323–327.

24. Hilliard, R. I. The Good and Effective Teacher as Perceived by Pediatric Residents and by Faculty. Am. J. Dis. Child. 144(1990):1106–1110.

25. Hitchcock, M. A., Lamkin, B. D., Mygdal, W. K., Clarke, C. M., and Clarke, S. O. Affective Changes in Faculty Development Fellows in Family Medicine. J. Med. Educ. 61(1986):394–403.

26. Irby, D. M., Gillmore, G. M., and Ramsey, P. G. Factors Affecting Ratings of Clinical Teachers by Medical Students and Residents. J. Med. Educ. 62(1987):1–7.

27. Stritter, F. T., Baker, R. M., and Shahady, E. J. Clinical Instruction. In Handbook for the Academic Physician, W. C. McGaghie and J. J. Frey, eds., pp. 98–124. New York: Springer Verlag, 1988.

28. Williamson, H. A., Glenn, J. K., Spencer, D. C., and Reid, J. C. Development of Clinical Independence: Resident-Attending Physician Interactions in an Ambulatory Setting. J. Fam. Pract. 26(1988):60–64.

29. Calkins, E. V., and Wakeford, R. Perceptions of Instructors and Students of Instructors' Roles. J. Med. Educ. 58

(1983):967–969.

30. Lewis, B. S., and Pace, W. D. Qualitative and Quantitative Methods for the Assessment of Clinical Preceptors. Fam. Med. 22(1990):356–360.

31. Patridge, M. I., Harris, I. B., and Masler, D. S. Towards Effective Clinical Teaching: Suggestions for Research. Paper presented at the Annual Conference of the American Educational Research Association, San Francisco, California, April 1979.

32. Beach, L., and Wertheimer, M. A Free Response Approach to the Study of Person Cognition. J. Abn. Soc. Psych. 62(1962):367–374.

33. Schneider, D. J. Implicit Personality Theory: A Review. Psych. Bull. 79(1973):294–309.

34. Holsti, O. R. Content Analysis for the Social Sciences and Humanities. Reading, Massachusetts: Addison-Wesley, 1969.

35. Miles, M. B., and Huberman, A. M. Qualitative Data Analysis: A Sourcebook of New Methods. Beverly Hills, California: Sage, 1984.

36. Ullian, J. A., and Bland, C. J. Characteristics of Effective Clinical Teaching: Evaluation Items Used in Family Practice Residence Programs. Paper presented at the Annual Conference of the Society of Teachers of Family Medicine, Boston, Massachusetts, April 1983.

37. McCall, C. H. Sampling and Statistics Handbook for Research. Ames, Iowa: Iowa State University Press, 1982.

38. Krippendorff, K. Content Analysis: An Introduction to its Methodology. Beverly Hills, California: Sage, 1980.

39. Bucher, R., and Stelling, J. G. Becoming Professional. Beverly Hills, California: Sage, 1977.

40. Knowles, M. The Adult Learner: A Neglected Species. 2nd ed. Houston, Texas: Gulf Publishing, 1978.

41. Carrier, C. A., Dalgaard, K., and Simpson, D. E. Theories of Teaching: Foci for Instructional Improvement Through Consultation. Rev. Higher Educ. 6(1983):195–206.

Clinical Teaching is More Than Evaluation Alone!

Susan Flagler, DNS, RN
Sue Loper-Powers, MN, RN
Ada Spitzer, Phc, RN

ABSTRACT

Gaining self-confidence as a nurse is an essential aspect of the nursing student's professional development. The purpose of this study was to determine clinical instruction behaviors that students perceived as important in promoting their self-confidence. One hundred thirty-nine baccalaureate students rated 16 clinical teaching behaviors as to the degree each helped or hindered their self-confidence as nurses. Factor analysis of these behaviors revealed five dimensions of clinical teaching that characterized the instructor as: resource, evaluator, encourager, promoter of patient care, and benevolent presence. Behaviors contributing to the dimensions of clinical instruction other than evaluation were rated by students as helpful in the development of their self confidence as nurses. Students' responses to open-ended questions provided further evidence of the importance of the nonevaluation dimensions. Focusing on evaluation to the exclusion of other aspects of clinical teaching may impede nursing students' professional development.

Introduction

At a time when the recruitment and retention of students is occupying the minds of most educators in schools of nursing, why give any attention to clinical instruction?

SUSAN FLAGLER, DNS, RN, Postdoctoral Research Fellow, Robert Wood Johnson Foundation, Clinical Nurse Scholars Program, University of Rochester; **SUE LOPER-POWERS, MN, RN; ADA SPITZER, Phc, RN,** Doctoral Candidate, School of Nursing, University of Washington.

The first two authors were faculty in the School of Nursing at the University of Washington when this study was conducted.

The first author gratefully acknowledges the encouragement of Anne Loustau to investigate this topic.

Clinical teaching strategies deserve attention since the character of the students' clinical experiences may well contribute to the problem of student retention. A teacher's focus on evaluation to the exclusion of the aspects of clinical instruction, which promote the students' self-confidence as nurses, may contribute to the problem by adversely affecting the students' professional development. If identity as a nurse and identification with the nursing profession is not developed, there is little incentive to stay in nursing.

Self-confidence as a nurse is defined as the person's trust or belief in his or her ability to function as a professional nurse. The authors view this attribute as an essential component of professional role development and clinical competency. Self-confidence appears to influence both the student's and the graduate nurse's experience. Wiedenbach (1969) indicated that students' sense of security in their ability to function was a necessary prerequisite to the provision of effective and comprehensive nursing care. Carpenito and Duespohl (1985) discussed the favorable influence of a positive self-view on a person's ability to apply energy in creative endeavors and goal achievement. Kramer (1974) reported that head nurses identified the lack of self-confidence as a primary cause of new graduates' inability to function effectively.

Self-confidence as a nurse cannot be learned in the classroom. Therefore, gaining self-confidence as nurses is an important aspect of students' clinical experience. Only by trying and mastering new role skills can students overcome commonly experienced feelings of incompetency and begin to identify themselves as professional nurses (Cotanch, 1981). Students build confidence in their ability to function by experiencing successes in the clinical area.

Literature Review

Mager (1968) indicated that teachers can promote successful experiences and increase the student's confidence. Clinical teaching behaviors that enhance the nursing student's self-confidence as a nurse are our specific focus.

eaching strategies used by the clinical instructor may have a profound effect on the students' learning and professional role development. Although not typically the main focus of the literature about clinical teaching, faculty behaviors that influence the student's self-confidence as a nurse have been reported.

The instructor's display of confidence in the student has been described as helpful to learning in the clinical area. Komorita (1965) surveyed 56 junior and senior nursing students, asking them to list what they "liked" and "disliked" with regard to the teaching methods used by their clinical instructors. Displaying confidence in the student's ability was one of the most frequently reported behaviors that students liked. Fischbach (1977) described the characteristics of a clinical experience that promote the student's learning and personal growth. Two essential components of this approach are the development of student confidence and reinforcement of the expectation of success. Wong (1978) used the critical incident technique to explore the effect of clinical instruction behavior on student's learning. Her findings are based on the analyses of the incidents reported by the 14 participating nursing students. Students identified the teacher's display of confidence in him/herself and in the students as helpful to student learning.

Griffith and Bakanauskas (1983) discussed attributes of nursing student-instructor relationships. Drawing upon the work of Carl Rogers, they stressed the importance of fostering the student's positive self-concept for professional socialization. Griffith and Bakanauskas (1983) also stated that the instructor's expectation of the students' success creates a positive learning environment where students will be more likely to succeed. Success, in turn, promotes the students' self-confidence in their ability as nurses. Brown (1981) surveyed 82 senior nursing students and 42 faculty members about the characteristics of an effective clinical instructor. More than any other item, students ranked the item "conveys confidence in and respect for students" as very important. On the average, faculty ranked this item as important, but five other items received higher faculty ratings. Faculty rated items reflecting the instructor's ability to relate theory to practice and to communicate knowledge to the student as more important than conveying confidence in the student.

The references to self-confidence in the literature cited above support the premise that developing the students' self-confidence is an important consideration in clinical instruction. Low self-confidence appears to impede professional role development and performance. The authors wanted to learn from the student perspective the clinical instructor behaviors that enhance the student's self-confidence as a nurse.

Purpose and Method

The purpose of this study was to determine baccalaureate nursing students' perceptions of clinical teaching behaviors that help or hinder the student's self-confidence as a nurse.

A survey method was used to collect data. The questionnaire devised for this survey consisted of two parts. The first part contained 16 clinical instructor behaviors (e.g., gives positive feedback) that respondents were asked to rate on a five-point scale as to the degree each behavior helped or hindered the student's self-confidence as a nurse. The midpoint of the scale was to be marked if the item was neutral or unrelated to self-confidence (see Table 1). The items were selected from the literature on clinical instruction (Blainey, 1980; Brown, 1981; O'Shea & Parsons, 1979) and from the authors' experiences with clinical supervision. The items included in the first part of the questionnaire were judged to be relevant by faculty members' involved in clinical instruction. The second part of the questionnaire consisted of two open-ended questions in which the respondent was requested to identify additional clinical instructor behaviors or attitudes that helped or hindered his or her self-confidence as a nurse.

The questionnaires were distributed to baccalaureate nursing students attending a university in the Pacific Northwest. Over a period of two years, 155 students received the questionnaire at the completion of their maternity nursing course. Questionnaires were distributed to students at the end of a class period at the same time course evaluation forms were given to the students. The voluntary nature of completing the questionnaire was emphasized. Students were told that this survey was not a part of the course evaluation and that they should draw upon all of their experiences with clinical instruction in responding to the items.

The data on instructor behaviors from the first part of the questionnaire were summarized using descriptive statistics. These 16 instructor behaviors were also submitted to a factor analysis to identify the principal components. Orthogonal factors were produced using the varimax rotation technique available in SPSS/PC software. The students' written responses from the second part of the questionnaire were reviewed to identify and categorize key words and phrases that described instructor behaviors that enhanced or hindered the student's self-confidence as a nurse. The initial categorization was completed by one investigator, then reviewed and discussed with the other investigators. Only when total agreement occurred as to the category of an individual response was that response viewed as contributing to the specific category.

Limitations of the study are related to the utilization of a non-random sample and questionnaire without previously established validity and reliability. Some degree of content validity was established by selecting the items from literature on clinical teaching and submitting the items to judges to verify applicability of each behavior to clinical teaching. Replication of the findings with additional samples would increase the generalizability of our results.

Results

Of the 155 students who received the questionnaire, 139

TABLE 1

STUDENTS' RATING OF CLINICAL TEACHING BEHAVIORS THAT HELP OR HINDER SELF-CONFIDENCE AS A NURSE

	Percent of Responses				
	Helps			Hinders	
Instructor behavior	Very Much	Some	Does Not Apply	Some	Very Much
Gives positive feedback (III)	94	6	1	0	0
Accepting of students' questions (I)	86	10	0	1	0
Encourages students to ask questions (I)	86	12	1	0	0
Creates a climate in which less than perfect behavior at new skills and application of knowledge is acceptable (III)	83	13	0	1	3
Provides opportunities for student's independent actions (IV)	81	17	0	2	0
Encourages discussion of patient care (IV)	77	21	1	1	0
While observing student providing care, instructor is present for support (V)	66	29	4	1	0
Instructor is readily available to student on the clinical unit (I)	64	27	4	4	1
Assists students in answering their own questions (I)	63	32	2	1	1
Instructor clarifies purpose of his/her presence in observing student providing patient care (V)	46	43	8	2	1
Holds students responsible to seek help (Reversed, V)	27	42	3	22	1
Expects report of patient care at specified time each day (IV)	16	22	24	32	7
Asks questions re: patients and patient care at random times (II)	14	39	9	32	3
While observing students providing care, instructor is present for evaluation (II)	12	25	7	42	13
Unannounced, the instructor observes student providing patient care (II)	1	16	9	52	21
Gives mostly negative feedback (Reversed III)	1	2	9	20	68

NOTE: N = 139. Items have been reordered from most to least helpful. Total percentages less than 100 reflect missing cases and/or cases that responded in two categories. Totals greater than 100 reflect error due to rounding numbers. The Roman numeral in the parentheses indicates the factor for which the item had the highest loading.

---

students (89%) completed the first part. One hundred twenty-three students (80%) wrote additional comments in the second part. At the time the questionnaires were completed, these students had received from five to seven quarters of clinical instruction and were in their junior or senior year of nursing school.

The students' ratings of the 16 instructor behaviors from the first part of the questionnaire are displayed in Table 1. The behaviors have been reordered from the most frequently rated as "helpful" to the most frequently rated as "hindering self-confidence as a nurse." "Gives positive feedback" received the most favorable rating and "gives mostly negative feedback" received the least favorable rating.

One hundred eight students (78% of the sample) responded to the open-ended question in the second part of the questionnaire about instructor behaviors that enhanced the student's self-confidence as a nurse. The major categories of response were giving positive reinforcement, showing confidence in the student, encouraging and accepting questions, providing support, and giving specific feedback (see Table 2).

One hundred eleven students (80% of the sample) responded to the open question regarding instructor behaviors that hinder the student's self-confidence as a nurse. The responses were more varied and did not cluster to as great an extent as the responses about enhancing behavior. The categories that reflect the greatest number of responses about instructor behaviors that hinder the student's self-confidence were no feedback or negative feedback only, intimidation, and distress about student's lack of knowledge or performance (see Table 3).

Factor analysis of the 16 instructor behaviors from the first part of the questionnaire revealed five factors that were responsible for 59% of the total variance (see Table 4). When the individual items that contribute to each factor are examined (see Table 5), a picture of the different dimensions of clinical instruction emerges. Five aspects of clinical instruction are evident: instructor as resource (Factor I); instructor as evaluator (Factor II); instructor as encourager (Factor III); instructor as promoter of patient care (Factor IV); and instructor as benevolent presence (Factor V).

TABLE 2

MAJOR CATEGORIES AND EXAMPLES OF STUDENTS' WRITTEN COMMENTS
ABOUT INSTRUCTOR BEHAVIORS THAT ENHANCE SELF-CONFIDENCE[1]

Giving Positive Reinforcement[2] (90)
   Gives good, useful positive feedback.
   Praise for what I did correctly. Recognition that I was making a good effort.

Giving Specific Feedback[3] (21)
   Giving feedback about skills observed and about comments from staff or patients.
   When after procedure or other observations instructor sits down *away* from situation and tells what was good about observed acts and what
   could be improved.

Showing Confidence in Student[2] (90)
   States that she has confidence in my abilities to give patient care and she knows I can handle the situation.
   Conveyed to me that they had confidence in my ability (already) *and* in my ability to learn.
   Showing confidence in me by allowing me to perform a skill without the instructor present.
   Expects competence, assumes I am responsible. Trusts me.

Encouraging/Accepting Questions[4] (32)
   Encourages questions and helps me answer them myself.
   Allowed me to ask questions without making me feel like my grade would suffer.

Providing Support[2] (26)
   Taking a personal interest in me, ie, desiring that I learn; assessing where I am and works with me form there.
   By being understanding and concerned about my stress level and personal situation.
   When I was insecure and unsure of myself, built up my self-esteem—brought up some of my accomplishments.

---

1 Values in the parentheses indicate the number of responses contributing to the category from the 108 students who reponded.
2 Related to instructor as encourager (Factor III).
3 Related to instructor as evaluator (Factor II).
4 Related to instructor as resource (Factor I)

The students' ratings of the degree each behavior helped or hindered their self-confidence reveal that the behaviors contributing to the resource (I), encourager (III), promoter (IV), and benevolent presence (V) factors were rated as helpful by more than 70% of the sample. Conversely, the majority of the behaviors that contribute to the evaluator factor (II) were rated by the students as hindering self-confidence as a nurse.

Discussion

Factor I, instructor as resource, depicts the availability of the instructor to the student and a willingness to address their questions. The contribution of this aspect of clinical teaching to the promotion of self-confidence gains support from the students' written comments in the second part of the questionnaire. More than 30 comments addressed the importance of being encouraging and accepting of questions. (Table 2)

Although not comprising a major category of responses, additional written comments indicated the student's self-confidence as a nurse was enhanced when the instructor acted as a resource person and assisted students with problem solving.

Being encouraging and accepting of student's questions was viewed as very helpful to the development of self-confidence, both in the instructor behaviors rated and the students' written comments. Layton (1969) and Wong (1978) identified the instructor's willingness to answer questions and offer explanations as attributes of effective clinical teaching. Jacobson (1966) surveyed 961 nursing students as to effective and ineffective teaching behaviors. Her respondents indicated that learning in the clinical setting was facilitated when the instructor made them feel free to ask questions or to seek help. Conversely, not being available for students or being unable to provide answers or to assist the student in seeking answers was viewed by the students Jacobson surveyed as ineffective clinical teaching.

The items that comprise Factor II, instructor as evaluator, received ratings indicating that this dimension of clinical instruction is the least helpful in building the students' confidence as nurses. (Table 1) Evaluation of students is, however, a necessary part of clinical instruction. In one sense, the clinical instructor is the first level of quality control to ensure the standards of clinical practice are maintained in the nursing profession, not a light responsibility. Where evaluation is an essential component of clinical teaching, clearly, focusing on evaluation alone is not desirable. Attention to the other dimensions of clinical instruction identified in this study can assist instructors in achieving an equally important aspect of their role, development of the student's self-confidence as a nurse.

At times, clinical faculty may feel as though they are in a double bind, wanting to encourage and teach students while feeling the responsibility to evaluate. Facilitative

---

TABLE 3

MAJOR CATEGORIES AND EXAMPLES OF STUDENTS' WRITTEN
COMMENTS ABOUT INSTRUCTOR BEHAVIORS THAT HINDER SELF-CONFIDENCE[1]

No Feedback or Negative Feedback Only[2] (24)
 No feedback after procedures—whether positive or negative.
 Always pointed out how to do better—never what was good already.
Intimidation[3] (21)
 "Some of you may never make it as nurses."
 Belittling, confrontations; reprimanding me in front of staff or patients.
 Made me afraid to ask questions; taking points off for asking questions.
 Quizzed, grilled me; intimidated me with question after question without explaining the importance of why knowledge of it was important.
 They demoralized me and made me feel like I was going to be a worthless nurse who knows a little but never enough to be competent.
Distressed About Student's Lack of Knowledge or Performance[3] (7)
 Non-verbal expressions of agitation and frustration with any performance of procedure or explanations of medications
 Scolded us for not knowing how to do a specific skill.
 Was angry or acted like she was in response to inadequate knowledge on student's part.

---

1 Values in parentheses indicate the number of responses contributing to the category from the 111 students who responded.
2 Related to instructor as evaluator (Factor II).
3 Inversely related to instructor as encourager (Factor III).

---

behaviors give way to evaluative behaviors, and evaluative strategies are too often based on what is wrong or omitted rather than what is correct. In these situations, students are likely to feel threatened by the instructor rather than assisted as evidenced by student comments such as "we would hide from her whenever possible," and "she wrote down what I said wrong then brought her 'black book' to the final evaluation." A solution to this double bind is for the instructor to make a distinction between teaching time and evaluation time as suggested by Morgan, Luke, and Herbert (1979). By clarifying for students the time when questions are welcome, and the instructor is present to assist learning, the student can focus on learning without the additional and often overwhelming anxiety of being graded. Morgan et al (1979) suggested that, whenever possible, evaluation should occur at the end of the clinical experience to allow for maximum learning before the student is evaluated.

The students' written comments from the second part of the questionnaire provide information as to how instructors can be more effective in the evaluator role. "Giving specific feedback" was a major category, which emerged from the responses addressing instructor behaviors that help build student self-confidence. (Table 2) Feedback from the instructor indicating whether or not the student is "on the right track" and how the student can improve, were described as helpful. Providing students with no feedback or giving only negative feedback were instructor behaviors respondents indicated as hindering self-confidence in the written comments (Table 3) as well as in the ratings of instructor behaviors in the first part of the questionnaire.

With regard to Factor III, instructor as encourager, the high ratings of the individual items contributing to this factor in promoting the student's selfconfidence (Table 1) and the great number of written comments, attest to the

importance of this dimension of clinical instruction. Three major categories of responses as to behaviors that enhance the student's self-confidence as a nurse represent aspects of the instructor as encourager. The most frequent responses referred to showing confidence in the student and giving positive reinforcement. (see Table 4) Providing emotional support through actions such as taking a personal interest in the student and understanding the student's stress level were also described by students as helpful to the development of self-confidence as a nurse. Intimidating instructor behaviors described by students could represent the opposite end of continuum of encouragement. (see Table 3)

The importance of the instructor's support of, and interest in, the student as a person for the student's learning has been addressed in the nursing literature on clinical instruction. Of the junior and senior nursing students surveyed by O'Shea and Parsons (1979), the clinical instructor's personal characteristics identified most frequently as facilitating learning were being supportive and showing concerned understanding. The personal characteristic most frequently identified by these students as interfering with their learning was criticizing the student in the presence of others. The findings of this survey on clinical teaching behaviors that help or hinder the students' self-confidence as nurses closely parallel the findings of O'Shea and Parsons. Jacobson (1966), Komorita (1965), Layton (1969), and Wong (1978) also found that clinical instruction was more effective when the instructor conveyed a sense of support to the student.

Rogers (1969) wrote that the student's learning is facilitated by attitudinal qualities that reflect the teacher's genuineness, acceptance and trust of the learner, and empathetic understanding of the student's reactions and internal responses. Many of the students' written comments related to the instructor as encourager echo the importance of these qualities. The respondents identified the instructor's willingness to take a personal interest in them and to discuss their feelings about clinical situations as enhancing behaviors. Based on the number of written responses, the instructor showing confidence and trust in the student was equal in importance for enhancing self-confidence only to the instructor giving positive feedback.

The students' written comments and their rating of the instructor behaviors in the first section of the questionnaire clearly indicate the importance students place on positive reinforcement for their development of self-confidence as nurses. The signficance of positive reinforcement for enhancing learning has been identified in numerous works (de Tornyay & Thompson, 1982; Jacobson, 1966; Komorita, 1965; O'Shea & Parsosn, 1978). In pondering why nursing instructors often fail to reinforce desired behaviors in the face of the substantial evidence that supports the use of positive reinforcement, de Tornyay and Thompson (1982) suggest that instructors believe nursing students are intrinsically motivated and, therefore, do not need to be told when they are doing well. Even though the majority of students are intrinsically motivated, they still may benefit from positive reinforcement. Mager (1968) suggested that positive reinforcement leads to success and the acknowledgement of success increases the student's self-esteem and confidence. Our findings support this view.

Factor IV, instructor as promoter of patient care, consisted of instructor behaviors that facilitate the student's discussion of and active involvement in patient care. (Table 5) The emergence of this dimension of clinical instruction as a major factor is not surprising as patient care is the business of nursing. That this dimension of clinical instruction helps to develop the student's self-confidence as a nurse is central to the thesis of this article. The student gains self-confidence as a nurse by successfully providing patient care. Self-confidence as a nurse cannot be developed without active involvement in clinical practice.

To develop confidence in their ability to act independently, students need the opportunity to act independently. Layton (1969) recommended giving students increased responsibility when they are ready. Similarly, Wong (1978) indicated that the appropriate amount of supervision is an important element of effective clinical instruction. Students in our survey felt hindered by the instructor who hovered and helped by the instructor who was present when the student was facing a new and complex situation. What the student perceives as hovering or helping is likely to vary with the student and the character of the situation and is probably best determined by simply asking the student.

Factor V, was labeled the instructor as a benevolent presence because the items that load on this factor depict the instructor as "being there" for the student and not holding the student responsible for seeking help. (see Table 5) Of interest is a difference in this dimension of clinical instruction as compared to other dimensions. One can note from Table 1 that the behaviors rated by more than 75% of the respondents as "helps very much" contribute to the encouarger (III), resource (I), and promoter (IV) factors.

TABLE 4

SUMMARY OF FACTOR EXTRACTION RESULTS

Factor	Eigenvalue	Percentage of Variance Explained	Cumulative Percentage of Variance Explained
Characterizes instructor as:			
I Resource	2.87	17.9	17.9
II Evaluator	2.47	15.4	33.3
III Encourager	1.65	10.3	43.7
IV Promoter of Patient care	1.33	8.3	52.0
V Benevolent presence	1.14	7.1	59.1

These three factors require active interaction between instructor and student. Where the items contributing to the benevolent presence factor (V) were rated as helpful (Table 1), this more passive dimension of clinical instruction does not appear to help the students' development of self-confidence to as great an extent as the dimensions involving more active instructor-student exchange.

Conclusion

The findings from this study lend further support to earlier work on clinical instruction: the importance of showing confidence in the student, being accepting of questions, and giving positive reinforcement. This study has made a new contribution to the literature on clinical instruction by identifying dimensions of clinical instruction and indicating how each dimension contributes to the development of the student's self-confidence as a nurse. The identification of four factors that describe dimensions of teaching other than evaluation underscores the importance of not viewing clinical instruction as unidimensional or primarily evaluative. If the student's professional development is to be fostered, teaching behaviors that encourage the student, promote action and discussion about patient care, and provide resources for carrying out effective care must be integral parts of clinical instruction.

Replications are needed to substantiate and increase the generalizability of our findings. Future research could identify additional dimensions of clinical instruction and further explicate instructor behaviors, which express each dimension. Additional studies could also determine differences in the importance of a given dimension related to the level of student experience. As this study focused on the students' pespective, research that explored instructor behavior and student performance rated by an outside observer would provide additional insights.

The factor structure of clinical instruction identified here

CLINICAL TEACHING

TABLE 5

ROTATED FACTOR MATRIX

Instructor behavior	Factor				
	I	II	III	IV	V
Accepting of students' questions	.91	−.05	.03	.11	−.12
Encourages students to ask questions	.86	.02	−.24	.13	.11
Instructor readily available to student on the clinical unit	.53	.16	.34	−.13	.39
Ask questions re: patients and patient care at random times	.04	.84	.08	−.08	−.05
Unannounced, the instructor observes student providing patient care	.08	70	−.33	.21	.06
While observing students providing care, instructor is present for evaluation	−11	.64	−.08	.23	−.04
Creates a climate in which less than perfect behavior at new skills and application of knowledge is acceptable	−.13	−.01	.75	−.02	−.29
Gives mostly negative feedback	.10	.38	−.58	.05	−.25
Gives mostly positive feedback	.18	−.01	.57	.11	.20
Expects report of patient care at specified time each day	−.10	.13	−.32	.72	−.01
Encourages discussion of patient care	.20	.33	.21	.56	.03
Provides opportunities for student's independent actions	.37	−.02	.34	.51	−.32
Holds students responsible for when to seek help	.06	.05	.18	.18	−.68
While observing student providing care, instructor is present fo support	.08	.03	.18	.12	.66
Instructor clarifies purpose of his/her presence in observing student providing care	.08	−.10	.13	.54	.60

could be useful for the evaluation of clinical teaching. Clinical instruction is expensive for schools and, in terms of time, for the faculty. In some schools, clinical hours are being reduced and pressure mounts to ensure the most effective use of clinical time. The dimensions of clinical instruction, which emerged from this study, could serve as a basis for evaluating clinical teaching. An objective measure of effectiveness would provide valuable information to both the individual instructor and the school toward the goal of improved, cost-effective clinical instruction.

Clinical experiences have an important impact on nursing students. The clinical setting is not only a laboratory in which to learn but an interpersonal environment, where the students receive cues from patients and staff as well as the clinical instructor regarding their capabilities as nurses. These experiences influence not only the students' acquisition of knowledge and skills, but their professional development as well. Clearly, the instructor cannot control all the variables in this complex environment. The instructor can, however, attend to the multiple dimensions of clinical teaching and use teaching strategies that enhance the students' self-confidence and ability to make effective use of clinical experiences.

References

Blainey, C.G. (1980). Anxiety in the undergraduate medical-surgical clinical student. *Journal of Nursing Education, 19*(8), 33-36.

Brown, S.T. (1981). Faculty and student perceptions of effective clinical teachers. *Journal of Nursing Education, 20*(9), 4-15.

Carpenito, L.J., & Duespohl, T.A. (1985). *A guide for effective clinical instruction* (2nd ed.). Rockville, MD: Aspen.

Cotanch, P.H. (1981). Self-actualization and professional socialization of nursing students in the clinical laboratory experience. *Journal of Nursing Education, 20*(8), 4-14.

de Tornyay, R., & Thompson, M.A. (1982). *Strategies for teaching nursing* (2nd ed.). New York: John Wiley & Sons.

Fischbach, F.M. (1977). Professional growth and learning of students in an open-ended clinical experience: A motivational philosophy. *Journal of Nursing Education, 16*(2), 30-33.

Griffith, J.W., & Bakanauskas, A.J. (1983). Student-instructor relationships in nursing education. *Journal of Nursing Education, 22*(3), 104-107.

Jacobson, M.D. (1966). Effective and ineffective behavior of teachers of nursing as determined by students. *Nursing Research, 15*, 218-224.

Komorita, N.J. (1965). Student's opinions toward methods of guidance and evaluation of clinical nursing. *Nursing Research, 14*, 163-167.

Kramer, M. (1974). *Reality shock.* St. Louis: C.V. Mosby.

Layton, M.M. (1969). How instructor attitudes affect students. *Nursing Outlook, 17*, 27-29.

Mager, R.F. (1968). *Developing an attitude toward learning.* Belmont, CA: Fearon.

Morgan, B., Luke, C., & Herbert, J. (1979). Evaluating clinical proficiency. *Nursing Outlook, 27*, 540-544.

O'Shea, H.S., & Parsons, M.K. (1979). Clinical instruction: Effective/and ineffective teacher behaviors. *Nursing Outlook, 27*, 411-415.

Rogers, C. (1969). *Freedom to learn.* Columbus, OH: Merrill.

Widenbach, E. (1969). *Meeting the realities in clinical teaching.* New York: Springer.

Wong, S. (1978). Nurse-teacher behaviors in the clinical field: Apparent effect on nursing students' learning. *Journal of Advanced Nursing, 3*, 369-372.

Teaching Techniques

Clinical Teaching by Video-enhanced Study Club Discussion Sessions

Douglass B. Roberts, D.D.S., M.S.; Robert L. Kinzer, D.D.S.; Shirou Kunihira, Ph.D.

Key Words: *clinical teaching, video, study club, operative dentistry education*

One challenge faced in clinical teaching is finding a method that allows students to receive important feedback about their progress without affecting student-patient relationships. An answer to this challenge is the use of video recording equipment combined with small group discussions as an adjunct to clinical teaching. Video recordings have been used in a variety of applications in dental and medical education, such as reducing fear in dental patients[1,2] and teaching interpersonal skills.[3-6] Television also has been used in teaching the technical aspects of dentistry.[7] Brown reported the use of interactive live television,[8] where it was possible to ask questions as the procedure progressed. However, Stevens[9] suggested that recordings were better than live television because the important stages and sequences could be shown without the lengthy sequences of routine procedures. He also emphasized the importance of a good quality recording to properly illustrate the procedure presented.

In small group discussions of clinical procedures, it is important that discussion be centered on problem solving,[10] not just facts. To enhance a problem-solving discussion, a video recording can be used to provide a more objective record of a situation than is allowed with a verbal description.[11] Not only is the timing of these discussions or feedback sessions important,[12] but it has been noted that the more specific the feedback is, the more it will stress a specific aspect of the procedure, which in turn leads to additional emphasis on the point in question.[13] Therefore, the use of clinical video recording together with small group discussions is used to enhance clinical teaching by providing students with rapid feedback about their performance and involving them in problem-solving group discussions.

Dr. Kinzer is chairperson, Department of Restorative Dentistry, and Drs. Roberts and Kunihira are also in the Department of Restorative Dentistry; all are at Loma Linda University, Loma Linda, CA 92350. Send correspondence and reprint requests to Dr. Kinzer.

Procedure

A "study club" method of teaching operative dentistry in a clinical setting has been used by the Loma Linda University School of Dentistry for the past 14 years. The "study club" consists of two clinical instructors and 12–14 students. The format consists of a four-hour clinical operating session and a one-hour discussion period immediately following the clinical session. The procedures performed during these sessions include direct gold restorations, inlay and partial coverage cast restorations, and complex amalgam restorations. Although most procedures are performed on patients, manikins are also used due to limited patient availability for these specific procedures. Students are encouraged during these sessions to employ unique procedures and techniques, with instructors available to provide help as needed.

During the clinical sessions each student's preparation and completed restoration are made known to the entire group so the other participants may observe the product, thus exposing the student to multiple operative procedures during a single clinic session. However, the time constraint and the students' reluctance to leave their own patients indicated a need to develop an alternative system of observation and recall. The capabilities of the portable, self-contained, and light-weight video recording equipment provided such an alternative.

A video recording is made of the preoperative situation (including radiographs), any significant steps of the preparation procedure, and the completed restoration. In addition, any unique or unfamiliar situation, procedures, or products can be recorded as they are encountered. Using video equipment allows for immediate availability of the recording for recall at the discussion session.

The equipment used is a Sony Video 8 Auto Focus camera recorder with a zoom lens and a 4 diopter close-up attachment. This allows a field of view ranging from approximately 8 inches in width to about ¾-inch at a focal length of approximately 8 inches, which enables instructors to record the whole mouth, placing the procedure in perspective, and then to zoom in on the

Figure 1. Large TV Monitor Provides Good Visualization of the Operating Session during Postoperative Discussion Period

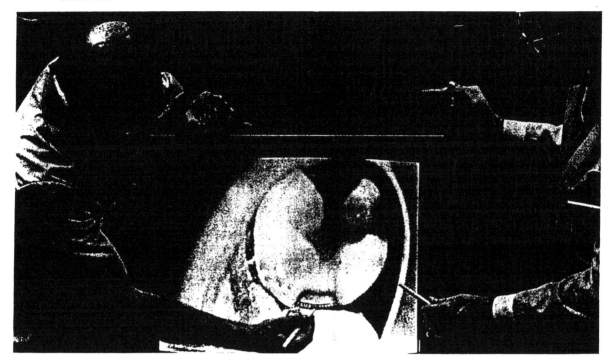

Figure 2. Results of Student Survey

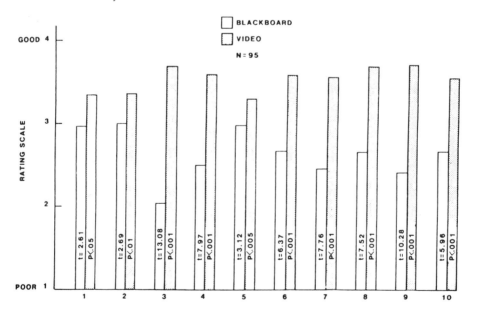

1. Precise understanding of details and important points.
2. Understanding instructor's explanation and discussion.
3. Interest in and learning from fellow students' cases.
4. Stimulation to think and evaluate your techniques, skills, and improve performance.
5. Understanding of rationales, principles, and criteria involved to improve performance.
6. Practical application and help in future performance.
7. Remembering what was pointed out and discussed.
8. Effectiveness as an instructional tool.
9. Level of interest and stimulation for learning.
10. Effectiveness in changing and improving future performance.

specific tooth being operated. The high resolution obtained from the use of this particular camera allows for viewing of very detailed aspects of the procedure. The field of view may be either direct or in a mirror. In the case of a mirrored view, it is usually necessary to use a front surface mirror to avoid·a double image effect. When using the mirror, the camera is held in a relatively stationary position and directed at the mirror, which is moved to pan around the tooth for multidirectional viewing of the subject. A built-in microphone records audio simultaneously when the camera is in operation. This allows for on-the-spot comments and questioning of the student performing the procedure.

During the postoperative discussion period held in a small classroom, the tape of the operating session is replayed on a large color TV monitor (Figure 1) with the instructor using the "stop action" mode by pressing the pause button. This allows students and instructors to discuss specific points of interest and concern while viewing the picture of the procedure under discussion. A water-soluble felt-tipped pen is used to draw directly on the video screen superimposing alternative designs or procedures graphically over the visual image.

Evaluation

Prior to the use of the video recorder, discussion periods were conducted using the chalkboard to illustrate points of interest. The relevancy of the discussion depended largely upon what the individual student had been able to observe personally during the operative session and the instructor's ability to reconstruct the session verbally and using a chalkboard.

A group of senior dental students (N = 95) who experienced "study club" sessions under both "chalkboard" and video recording conditions were asked to compare the two methods, evaluating them for ten factors listed in Figure 2. The students rated the video recording method significantly higher (p<.05 to <.001) in all ten areas of comparison. They gave the new meth-

od highest ratings for being more stimulating and interesting and also being helpful in learning from fellow students' cases.

Because of the demonstrated usefulness of video recording for revisualization of procedures during feedback discussions, as well as the students' enthusiastic involvement in these programs, on-the-spot video recording should be considered as a valuable tool in dental education. Present technology has some limitations, particularly in regard to adequate lighting. However, as more advanced equipment with greater resolution is developed, it is anticipated that the use of video procedures will become even more effective.

REFERENCES

1. Melamed BG, Weinstein D, Hawes R, Katin-Borland M. Reduction of fear-related dental management problems with use of filmed modeling. J Am Dent Assoc 1975;90:822-6.
2. Gatchel RJ. Impact of a videotaped dental fear-reduction program on people who avoid dental treatment. J Am Dent Assoc 1986;112:218-21.
3. Cassata DM, Conroe RM, Clements PW. A program for enhancing medical interviewing using video-tape feedback in the family practice residency. J Fam Pract 1977;4:673-7.
4. Kahn G, Cohen B, Jason H. Teaching interpersonal skills in family practice. J Fam Pract 1979;8:309-16.
5. Green TG, O'Connor P, Starks DD, Eddlemon CL. Improving clinical teaching by videotaping performance. J Dent Educ 1983;47:118-19.
6. Kotz CA. Use of video vignettes in empathy training. J Dent Educ 1983;47:115.
7. Stevens L, Pratley M. Teaching dental prosthetics using television. Aust Prosthodont Soc Bull 1980;10:27-30.
8. Brown CPM. Interactive live television in clinical dental teaching. Br Dent J 1984;156:371-2.
9. Stevens L. A comparison of two methods of demonstrating an exercise in dental technology. Aust Dent J 1977;22:280-3.
10. Foley R, Smilansky J, Konke A. Teacher-student interaction in a medical clerkship. J Med Educ 1979;54:622-6.
11. Konrad HR, Hopla DM, Bussen J, Griswold FC. Use of videotape in diagnosis and treatment of cancer of larynx. Ann Otal 1981;90:398-400.
12. Black NMI, Harden RM. Providing feedback to students on clinical skills by using objective structured clinical examination. Med Educ 1986;20:48-52.
13. Edwards WS, Morse PK, Mitchell RJ. A practical evaluation system for preclinical restorative dentistry. J Dent Educ 1982;46:693-6.

Medical Teacher, Vol. 15, No. 4, 1993   283

Twelve tips for using role-plays in clinical teaching

YVONNE STEINERT, *Department of Family Medicine, Sir Mortimer B. Davis Jewish General Hospital and McGill University, Montreal, Quebec, Canada*

Role-plays have been defined as dramas in which a number of participants are asked to portray a particular character, but no lines are learned (McKeachie, 1986). The individuals involved temporarily adopt a specified role and try to behave in ways characteristic of a person in that role (Whitman, 1990), improvising their responses to a particular situation. A role play typically involves two or more people. In medicine, it usually involves a doctor-patient interaction. It can, however, also be used to portray a family interview, a teacher-student exchange, or a multidisciplinary team meeting.

Role-plays differ from 'simulated' patients (Barrows, 1993; Coonar *et al.*, 1991; Stillman *et al.*, 1990) in that the role of the patient is not standardized and not scripted as carefully. Role-plays are generally more flexible and more spontaneous. They are also a powerful, but often neglected, teaching technique.

The goal of this article is to outline ways in which role-plays can be conducted more effectively (see Table I). This description will hopefully enable clinical teachers to use role-plays constructively and to adapt them to the individual needs of teachers and students.

Prior to the role-play

Tip 1   Consider the varied uses of role-plays in clinical teaching.

Role-plays are an effective method to promote skill acquisition. They enable students to define a problem, to develop solutions to a problem, to try out new behaviours, and to receive feedback (Simpson, 1985). Because role plays generally provoke less anxiety in students than real life situations, students may be able to use newly acquired skills more easily and to attend to what is going on in the situation with fewer distractions and concerns (Talbot *et* al., 1991). Role-plays

TABLE I. Guidelines for effective role-plays

Prior to the role-play
(1)   Consider the varied uses of role-plays in teaching.
(2)   Recognize the limitations of role-plays and work to overcome them.
(3)   Design the role-play with care and use prepared scripts whenever possible.

During the role-play
(4)   Convene the group and create an environment for learning.
(5)   Outline the goals and objectives of the teaching session.
(6)   Assign roles and change the players' identities.
(7)   Set the stage for the role-play.
(8)   Conduct the role-play.
(9)   Discuss the role play.
(10) If appropriate, try again.
(11) Debrief the players.
(12) Summarize and evaluate the teaching session.

generally represent a simplified version of reality. Because of this, students can experience many facets of the real life setting without some of its complexities, and they can try to master learning that might otherwise be overwhelming (Plunkett & Olivieri, 1989). Role-plays afford an excellent opportunity for rehearsing professional behaviours in a relatively safe environment before trying them out in the real world (Cox & Ewan, 1982).

Role-plays also allow students to gain a sense of how others feel in a certain situation. By participating in a role-play, medical students or residents can discover their own feelings about a particular situation and gain insight into the patient's presenting problems or life situation. Taking on a different role helps students to experience new feelings and reactions and to develop empathy.

> John D. was asked to 'play' Mrs C. who was coming to his office at least twice a week with frequent complaints of chest pain and difficulty breathing. Her husband had recently been hospitalized for investigation of a newly diagnosed cardiac problem, and her son was moving to another city. It was only after he role-played Mrs C. that John D. began to understand why she was coming to his office as frequently as she did, and what role he was playing in her life.

Role-plays can also be used creatively to demonstrate 'expert' behaviour or to illustrate particular principles under discussion. They are particularly useful for making theoretical issues more practical and to illustrate the difference between thinking and doing. In my own setting, residents often state that they know how to take a sexual history from patients, and they easily tell me what questions they would ask. However, when they are asked to pose a question directly to a co-teacher or resident, playing the role of patient, they often run into difficulty. The difference between knowing what to ask—and asking—is well illustrated by role-play situations.

Role-plays are generally useful for teaching interpersonal and communication skills, medical history-taking, and clinical problem solving (Collins, 1988; Koh *et al.*, 1991; Smilansky *et al.*, 1978; Yaffe, 1989). They can also help to promote the integration of biomedical and psychosocial aspects of medical care, and to encourage active learning.

Tip 2   Recognize the limitations of role-plays and work to overcome them.

Role-playing depends heavily on the student's imagination and capacity to project himself into another situation. This attribute can be both a strength and a weakness. Role plays are often anxiety-provoking for the student and the teacher alike. At times, students feel 'on the spot' in front of their colleagues. At other times, they may overidentify with their roles and develop strong feelings and reactions. Observers can also attribute the characteristics of a role-play to the person playing a particular role.

> Sam K., a clinical teacher in family medicine, was playing the role of a 'problem' resident in a session on *How to Give Effective Feedback*. In discussing the role-play afterwards, one of the teachers called Sam a 'turkey' and asked him why he always made such 'dumb' remarks. The teaching session ended abruptly after that, and Sam K. left the session not knowing whether he was being called a 'turkey' in his role as a resident or as a teacher.

Role-playing requires skill on the part of the teacher. The teacher must be sensitive to the participants' feelings and must be sufficiently perceptive as to recognize when someone is having difficulty. Because of the skill required to use this technique, teachers often avoid it. Role-playing can also become artificial, and therefore, not real or relevant. Teachers do not want to hear from students that they would *finally* like to see a *real* patient. Role-playing can be overused. It can become a game—fun in and of itself but not pertinent to the resident's real world. Clinical teachers must work to overcome this problem, which is more likely if the players do not view the role-play as life-like, or if what they practice is not applicable to real situations (Talbot *et al.*, 1991).

Tip 3   Design the role-play with care and use prepared scripts if possible.

The degree of formality or 'structure' of a role-play can vary significantly from situation to situation. Often, the most influential and useful role-plays are those that arise spontaneously out of a group discussion. Whenever possible, however, try to design a role-play before the teaching session and use prepared scripts, based on *real* clinical examples. Be careful, however, not to choose a situation that is too difficult or overwhelming. Teachers and students are often tempted to choose the most complex case for discussion. Try to avoid this temptation and work to ensure that the role-play situation does not resemble the students' own personal circumstances too closely.

> In our own setting, one student was asked to tell a patient that she had breast cancer during a teaching session on *Giving Bad News*. After two minutes, the student became weepy, and had difficulty continuing. It soon became evident that the student's mother had just recently been diagnosed with cancer. Although this event was handled in the teaching situation, it was an emotionally draining and difficult session.

Unfortunately, teachers cannot always predict how a role-play will proceed. Whenever possible, however, try to take appropriate precautions. Work to build the role-play for success and make sure that the teaching method meets the intended goals and objectives.

Written scripts help to give the players some security in their roles and to ensure that the teaching goals will be met. To be useful, scripts should provide students with a brief but realistic description of their role. This description should include who the person is as well as a number of background details to help the actor flesh out his or her role (van Ments, 1983). Depending on the role play, the teacher might wish to include the actor's emotional status (e.g. the patient is very frustrated with the lack of progress in making a diagnosis; the patient is very depressed by his current life situation) as well as how the patient relates to others in the script (e.g. when the doctor tells you that nothing can be found, become angry; when your spouse starts to nag about your physical condition, withdraw). Although the amount of details may vary, some structure is necessary in order to give direction to the players. Role-players can also be instructed to "make-up" what they don't know. One of the interesting aspects of role-plays is the similarity with which people play out their roles, even when detailed information is lacking.

The one person who may not be scripted is the 'doctor' in a doctor-patient interaction, or the 'teacher' in a teacher-student interaction. Role-plays are generally most beneficial if these people 'play themselves' and then get feedback on their own behaviour. However, if students are not comfortable playing themselves, brief scripts can be used, especially if they are vague enough so that they allow students to rely on their own repertoire of behaviours.

Videotape reviews also lend themselves well to role-play situations. For example, a group may be watching a family interaction on tape, and then chose to continue the interview in a role-play, trying an alternate approach to care. In this situation, the role-players know who the family members are and how they present to the physician. Little preparation is needed for the role-play to succeed.

Role-plays often work best when they arise spontaneously out of a discussion. Although the teacher or student may have prepared a script, the teacher should be prepared to abandon the script if necessary. Whenever possible, the role-play should try to meet the needs of the medical student and resident. It is also important for the role-play to have some 'structure' and for the students to feel that the teacher is in 'control'.

During the role-play

Tip 4   Convene the group and create an environment for learning.

For role-plays to succeed, it is essential to create as relaxed and supportive an environment as possible. Teachers can facilitate a cooperative atmosphere by personal example and by reinforcing appropriate student behaviours. As in all teaching situations, the learner must be respected and no one should be forced to do something with which he or she is not comfortable.

Tip 5   Outline your goals and objectives.

The goals and objectives of the teaching session should be clarified to all of the participants. For example, the teacher might explain that: "in the following role-play we would like you to understand the influence of the family on the patient's presenting problem". Although the teacher might not specify which aspects of family functioning he or she wants the students to examine, it is essential to explain the more general goals and objectives of the session.

In another situation, the teacher might say that: "the goal of this role-play is to focus on the doctor's history-taking skills rather than on his problem-solving strategies". Such a directive will focus the students' attention to what is required of them and alleviate potential concerns about the role-play going "out of control".

The advantages of a role-play in a particular situation should also be made explicit. For example, teachers may tell the group that "in today's role-play, we will try out different ways of asking the patient about his family. Although we cannot do this with 'real' families, we have the advantage of stopping the role-play at any time, and of asking the 'family members' how they feel about the questions that you ask".

Acknowledging potential resistance to the role-play is also beneficial at this stage. Recognizing how difficult it is to 'perform' in front of one's colleagues often helps to decrease potential anxiety and the reluctance to participate actively. Checking out the participants' experiences with role-plays can also be helpful to achieve this goal.

Tip 6   Assign roles and change the players' identities.

To select the 'actors', some teachers prefer to ask for volunteers; others prefer to give out the roles at random. Although my philosophical preference is to ask for volunteers, I have often had more success when I have given out the roles to group members, either as a deck of cards, or by holding the scripts upside down 'like a fan' and asking the participants to choose. The deadly silence following my request for volunteers has, at times, altered my behaviour.

If the teacher is using written scripts, they should be given to the participants before the role-play so that the players can think about their roles. It is preferable to ask the players not to tell each other what is written on the paper. When a written script is not available, try to take the students out of the room and briefly describe their role to them. They can also be told to improvise what they don't know.

For a role-play to succeed, it is essential that the students change their identities and their names. Often students say that they can use their own names; it won't bother them. It is essential, however, to change names—and identities—because of the problems resulting from students overidentifying with their role, or observers attributing characteristics to the players that are not theirs. Using nametags or labels to identify each player is particularly helpful. In this way, everyone can see that the role-player's identity has been changed. Nametags also help group members remember who is playing what role, and they can be very useful in the debriefing process; students can take off their names—and their identities—in a 'dramatic' way.

As we mentioned before, the only person who does not usually change his or her identity is the 'doctor' in a doctor-patient interaction, or the 'teacher' in a teacher-student interaction. Group facilitators should also not take on a role as this might reduce their objectivity and their ability to be helpful to the group.

In larger groups, it is preferable to assign a role to all of the participants so that everyone feels involved. Group members who will not be taking on a particular part can be asked to be observers or to take on the role of the 'Greek chorus'. In addition, they can be instructed to consider particular behaviours or aspects of the interview, with or without a predefined grid for analysis. It is also important to remember that observers should stay in the background and remain as uninvolved as possible. Laughter from the observers has influenced the outcome of many a role-play.

Tip 7   Set the stage for the role-play.

In introducing the role-play, the teacher should describe the situation as clearly as possible and outline who the key players will be. For example, the teacher might specify that the group will now meet the Cross family: "This includes Mr and Mrs Cross, the grandmother Mrs Bens, and two teenagers, Jamie and Joan. Dr T. will now meet with the Cross family to discuss placement issues". This context should be given to all the participants and observers, at least verbally. Sometimes, if there are many players involved, a written 'programme' of key players can be helpful.

To make the role-play as realistic as possible, it is worthwhile to bring in 'props'. I often bring in a white coat for the doctor, a stethoscope, some charts, and my daughter's toy telephone. It is also preferable to set up the role-play in a separate part of the room, away from the other participants who will become the observers. Try to arrange the chairs as realistically as possible, organize the props, and ask the 'patient' to knock and walk in. Setting up the scene in this way, as a group, often helps to alleviate anxiety and to make the role-play more fun. Humour and a sense of play is important in role-plays, and yet, when overdone, can undermine the goals and objectives of the teaching situation.

Tip 8   Conduct the role-play.

Although many teachers feel that role-plays are time-consuming, role-plays can be brief to make their point. One of the most common problems in observing role-plays is that they continue for too long. Whereas all the actors can get quite involved in the role-play, watching a lengthy role-play can become tedious.

It is advisable to let the role-play go on long enough so that the players get 'into role' and acquire a sense of what the play is about. Five to ten minutes is usually just right; fifteen to twenty minutes can be too long. At times it is preferable to conduct two scenes of five to ten minutes each, rather than one long one. The main focus of discussion is often forgotten after ten minutes of acting, or else there are too many issues to discuss.

The advantage of a role-play, compared to real life, is that the interview can be stopped at any time. Some role-plays end themselves. More frequently, however, the leader has to stop them. This can often be done with humour: "Dr John, there is a call for you on line 1". It is also important to give permission to the players in the role-play to stop. This gives them an increased sense of control and an opportunity to ask for help.

Tip 9   Discuss the role-play.

Discussion of the role-play is essential. Without discussion, the role can quickly become irrelevant and important issues can become lost. Role-plays can also elicit many different themes and it is often difficult to remain focused. Try, therefore, to direct the discussion according to the session's original objectives.

The discussion of a role-play can focus on a number of themes: the doctor-patient relationship; the physician's interviewing style; the management of the interview; history-taking and problem solving strategies. Whenever possible, however, the 'actors' should be asked to comment on their reactions and feelings to the role-play first, starting with the person in the 'hot seat'. Participants generally feel more protected when they are allowed to comment first on their role and the role-play. These comments will also set the tone for the discussion that follows.

To lead the discussion, open-ended, non-interpretive questions are most useful. What were you thinking when you played the role of Mr T.? What were you feeling? How did you react when Dr D. asked you about your daughter's illness? What would you have liked him to say differently? Questions like this will help to clarify the feelings and thoughts behind the players' actions, and will encourage participants to more easily understand another person's perspective. Comments from group members are also often more effective than the teacher's. For example, the person who played the patient can usually make comments and observations about the doctor's behaviour that are far more pertinent—and easily understood—than anyone else's because only he can say how he truly felt.

Group participation should be encouraged so that everyone feels involved, but value judgements and speculation on 'what ifs' should be avoided. One could have always done something better—and in a different way. Drama critics should also be discouraged. The role-play is not about acting skills. Teachers and group members should remember that it is very easy to slip from a discussion of skills (usually most valuable in a role-play) to a discussion of the patient's issues and problems, during which both the patient and the doctor are lost. The strengths and merits of role-plays as a teaching method should not be forgotten.

Tip 10 If appropriate, try again.

As we have mentioned before, one of the benefits of role-plays is the opportunity to try out professional behaviours. Teachers or students may wish to replay the role-play, keeping the same roles, changing roles, altering the situation, or playing a follow-up scene. Often, there is no lack of volunteers at this time. Participants often see the value of role-playing after the first attempt, and they now want to benefit from it as well. Whereas I always point out that the person in the 'hot seat' benefits the most from the role-play, residents and students do not usually believe me before the role-play activity begins. Now they do.

Tip 11 Debrief the players.

This is probably the most important step in conducting role-plays, and yet, it is often overlooked. Players who become involved in role-plays collect feelings and emotions which may persist for a long time (Cox & Ewan, 1982) and they need to talk about them. It is the teacher's responsibility to make sure that these feelings are brought to the surface. Even when players do not have any feelings to report, it is important to go through this process, which need not be difficult, especially if it is done routinely. The identification and clarification of feelings is usually enough to provide resolution. Problems arise if this process does not occur and if the role-players do not have an opportunity to disengage from the role-play.

To debrief the players, I generally go around the room and ask everyone who played a role to comment on how they felt about being that person. What was it like? Is there anything they want to say about having played an 'aggressive person' ·or 'a wimp'? Is there anything they want to say about having been Mr Smith? I then ask them to 'take off' their identity and to return to themselves. Whenever possible, I try to ensure that the person in the 'hot seat' is the first and the last to speak. They have the most to gain—and the most to lose.

Debriefing is essential to the success of the role-play. No matter how limited the available time, the teacher cannot avoid this very important part of the process.

Tip 12   Summarize and evaluate.

Although the role-play may have been lively, and the participants were all involved, an effective summary is still necessary. So is a discussion of whether the session was helpful or not. What did you learn today? What can you take away from the teaching session? What was useful and what was not? Student feedback is essential in determining whether the objectives were met and in planning follow-up sessions.

Conclusion

Whereas role-plays are most commonly used for re-creating the doctor-patient relationship, they can be used creatively for many purposes including giving 'bad news' to patients and their families, experiencing what it is like to be a patient and going through the health care system, improving multi-disciplinary team meetings or committee meetings, and teaching teachers to teach.

As with most other novel techniques, the effectiveness of role-playing depends to a large extent upon the confidence of the teacher and the students' feelings that the experience is going to be valuable (McKeachie, 1986). Like any other technique, it can be used to such an extent that it becomes repetitious. It can, however, be an extremely rewarding experience if it is used to accomplish definite goals, and if the students perceive their progress towards these goals. The best way to learn to use role-plays effectively is to apply them in different situations and to request feedback from students and colleagues.

Correspondence: Dr Yvonne Steinert, Herzl Family Practice Center, Sir Mortimer B. Davis Jewish General Hospital, 5757 Legare Street, Montreal, Quebec, Canada H3T 1Z6.

REFERENCES

BARROWS, H.S. (1993) An overview of the uses of standardised patients for teaching and evaluating skills, *Academic Medicine*, 68, pp. 443–450.

COLLINS, J.A. (1988) The effectiveness of role playing in cardiac care rehabilitation education, *Military Medicine*, 153, pp. 464–468.

COONAR, A.S., DOOLEY, M., DANIELS, M. & TAYLOR, R.W. (1991) The use of role play in teaching medical students obstetrics and gynaecology, *Medical Teacher*, 13, pp. 49–53.

COX, K.R. & EWAN, C.E. (1982) *The Medical Teacher* (New York, Churchill Livingstone).

McKeachie, W.J. (1986) *Teaching Tips: A Guidebook for the Beginning College Teacher* (Boston, DC Heath and Company).

Koh, K.T.C., Goh, L.G. & Tan, T.C. (1991) Using role play to teach consultation skills—the Singapore experience, *Medical Teacher*, 13, pp. 55–61.

Plunkett, E.J. & Olivieri, R.J. (1989) A strategy for introducing diagnostic reasoning: Hypothesis testing using a simulation approach, *Nurse Educator*, 14, pp. 27–31.

Simpson, M.A. (1985) How to use role plays in medical teaching, *Medical Teacher*, 7, pp. 75–82.

Smilansky, J., Foley, R., Runkle, N. & Solomon, L. (1978) Instructor plays patient: An alternative to the case presentation method, *Journal of Family Practice*, 6, pp. 1037–1040.

Stillman, P.L., Regan, M.B., Philbin, M. & Haley, H.L. (1990) Results of a survey on the use of standardized patients to teach and evaluate clinical skills, *Academic Medicine*, 65, pp. 288–292.

Talbot, Y., Christie-Seely, J., Dussault, R., Steinert, Y. & Turcotte, R. (1991) *Family Systems Medicine: A Faculty Development Curriculum* (Montreal, Publicola Reg'd).

van Ments, M. (1983) *The Effective Use of Role Play: A Handbook for Teachers and Trainers* (London, Kogan Page).

Whitman, N. (1990) *Creative Medical Teaching* (Salt Lake City, University of Utah School of Medicine).

Yaffe, M.J. (1989) The medi-drama as an instrument to teach doctor-patient relationships, *Medical Teacher*, 11, pp. 321–329.

Leadership development through clinical education

Jane Mazzoni, M.S., R.R.A.
Instructor and Clinical Education Coordinator

Valerie J.M. Watzlaf, M.P.H., R.R.A.
Assistant Professor
Health Records Administration
University of Pittsburgh
School of Health Related Professions
Pittsburgh, Pennsylvania

DEFINING the word "leader" is not an easy task. Referring to a dictionary may provide as many as 130 definitions. Being a leader and practicing leadership is not a science; it is an ability, a process. Leadership is often defined as the process of influencing others.

Being a leader requires certain characteristics—some innate, some developed. An individual may develop leadership characteristics through processes such as mentoring or through the influence of others, such as parents, teachers, and employers. It is an ongoing developmental process that can be enhanced by certain experiences, clinical education, for example. Clinical educators (persons who work with students in a clinical health care setting) can greatly influence student development in terms of leadership and management capabilities. Clinical educators can also help students develop more self-confidence. Arranging activities and providing a mentoring, role model atmosphere are ways that clinical educators can assist in developing leadership traits in students. Development of these traits will

Top Health Rec Manage, 1989, 9(3), 35–41
© 1989 Aspen Publishers, Inc.

better prepare students for the situations they will be involved in during their professional lives.

Students in the Health Records Administration (HRA) Department at the University of Pittsburgh spend five weeks in a management internship in an acute care hospital's medical record department. This internship involves one-on-one communication between the clinical educator and the student. Shortly after returning from this internship, the students graduate and within a few weeks to a few months, are in management positions as supervisors, assistant directors, or directors of medical record departments.

In discussions between HRA instructors and senior students prior to their management internship, many students expressed concern regarding their leadership skills. Thus, a pre- and post-management internship survey was conducted to ascertain whether the students' perception of their leadership skills strengthened after their management internship.

METHODOLOGY

A three-part questionnaire followed by a comment section was designed. In section A, students were asked to rate themselves on prominent leadership characteristics from the literature[1-3] and personal experiences. A Likert-type rating scale (very weak, weak, moderate, strong, very strong) was used to measure the students' perception of their leadership characteristics. In Section B, students were asked to note their qualifications in assuming certain job positions in medical record departments. In Section C, students were asked to note their capability of performing certain job activities. The questionnaire was pilot-tested by two graduate assistants in the health records

department in measure clarity. The questionnaire was then distributed to 27 HRA senior students three weeks before the start of the management internship. The students were told to complete the questionnaire based on their current self-image. They were given five minutes to complete the questionnaire in order to force spontaneity of response. The same questionnaire was administered to the same 27 HRA students the day they returned from their management internship. The same instructions and time constraints were given. The completed questionnaires were collected, compiled, and analyzed.

Limitation of the survey included small sample size and absence of random selection of the sample. Patterns of response may therefore result from sampling variability or chance. Thus, results of the survey cannot be generalized to other samples or populations. Another limitation of the survey was that definitions of the leadership characteristics were not provided to the students, nor was clarification of these terms given during administration of the questionnaire. Because of the unfamiliarity with the terms, some students did not respond to some questions or may have chosen an inaccurate response to some of the questions. It is suggested that future research be conducted with a larger sample size and that students be strongly encouraged to complete all questions. A more rigorous statistical analysis such as pairing the responses and performing a Wilcoxan Signed Rank Test will also be done.[4] This nonparametric test for paired data will determine whether the differences seen before and after the internship are significant. It is also suggested that future researchers attempt to control for external factors that may influence the students' perceptions of their leadership capabilities.

ANALYSIS

Table 1 shows pre- and post-survey mean results for each of the leadership characteristics in section A of the questionnaire. The mean was computed for each of the response categories. It can be seen from this table that the majority of characteristic means increased after the internship. Tables 2 and 3 report frequencies for responses to questions in sections B and C of the questionnaire related to job positions and activities.

Table 4 demonstrates that overall, before the management internship, 75% of the HRA students believed they could work in various management positions, while after the internship, almost 78% believed they could work in these positions. The supervisor and the assistant director of a community hospital were positions all students believed they could hold before and after the internship. The amount of

uncertainty in working in these positions decreased from 13.3% before the internship to 6.9% after the internship. Before the internship, 11.7% did not believe they could work in these positions, and after the internship, this percentage increased to 15.3%. Part of this increase may be due to the types of positions included, for example, technical employee (most students want a management position after graduation) and director of a medical record department in a large teaching hospital (most students do not feel capable of assuming the position immediately after graduation). Overall results, as demonstrated in Table 5, show that students perceive themselves more capable of assuming managerial responsibilities after the management internship (85.6%) than before (68.2%).

In addition, student comments were collected from the questionnaire. These comments reflect more self-confidence in some of

Table 1. Pre- and post-survey means on leadership characteristics (N = 27)

Characteristic	Pre-survey $\overline{X}$	Post-survey $\overline{X}$	Characteristic	Pre-survey $\overline{X}$	Post-survey $\overline{X}$
Delegator	3.2	3.3	Manipulative	2.8	3.1
Planner	4.0	4.2	Mature	4.2	4.4
Organizer	4.5	4.4	Realistic	4.1	4.3
Goal-oriented	4.1	4.5	Listener	4.2	4.4
Accountable	4.0	4.4	Dreamer	3.3	3.2
Director	3.7	4.0	Initiator	3.4	3.8
Problem-solver	4.0	4.1	Aggressive	3.4	3.5
Role model	3.8	4.2	Powerful	3.0	3.2
Motivator	4.0	4.0	Perceptive	3.9	4.0
Ethical	4.2	4.4	Honest	3.8	4.4
Sincere	4.2	4.4	Knowledgeable	3.9	4.1
Creative	4.0	4.2	Self-motivated	4.1	4.4
Visualizer	3.7	4.0	Mentor	4.0	4.0
Manager	3.7	4.1	Concerned	4.2	4.5
Communicator	3.7	4.1	Self-confident	3.7	4.2
Assertive	3.5	3.7	Fair	4.2	4.5
Charismatic	3.5	3.7			

Table 2. Pre- and post-survey self-evaluation of qualification for positions (N = 27)

Position	Would be qualified Y	Would not be qualified N	Uncertain
Director—large teaching hospital			
Pre-survey	1 (3.7)*	17 (63.0)	9 (33.0)
Post-survey	1 (3.7)	18 (66.7)	8 (29.6)
Director—community hospital			
Pre-survey	17 (63.0)	3 (11.1)	7 (25.9)
Post-survey	21 (77.8)	5 (18.5)	1 (3.7)
Assistant Director—large, teaching hospital			
Pre-survey	24 (88.9)	0	3 (11.1)
Post-survey	22 (81.5)	2 (7.4)	3 (11.1)
Assistant Director—community hospital			
Pre-survey (1 missing)	26 (100.0)	0	0
Post-survey	27 (100.0)	0	0
Manager			
Pre-survey	24 (88.9)	0	3 (11.1)
Post-survey	27 (100.0)	0	0
Supervisor			
Pre-survey	27 (100.0)	0	0
Post-survey	27 (100.0)	0	0
Technical employee			
Pre-survey	22 (81.5)	2 (7.4)	3 (11.1)
Post-survey	22 (81.5)	4 (14.8)	1 (3.7)

*Percent in parentheses

the students after the internship. Typical student comments before the management internship are "I'm scared about entering the 'real' world, but I do think I could handle it" and "I feel that I do not know enough sometimes, but hopefully once I will be out and getting experience, I will get more confidence." After the management internship, students had the following to say: "The internship had a positive effect on many of these areas"; "I feel the internship greatly increased my confidence in my knowledge and myself"; "I feel after the internship that I have gained valuable skills and traits which will help me in my career and life"; and "The internship helped tremendously with these managerial skills."

DISCUSSION

During and after the management internship, the clinical education coordinator and students identified some activities that may have helped increase the students' perceptions of their leadership characteristics and management capabilities. The following activities are presented to enable clinical educators to plan projects and activities:

• A student documented a series of mock informal counseling sessions conducted with an employee who was persistently late; the student also completed a series of corrective action forms that described the circumstances of the tardiness and the

Table 3. Pre- and post-survey responses to job activities performed (N = 27)

Activity	Capable of performing	Not capable of performing	Uncertain
Conducting job interview			
Pre-survey	24(88.9)*	1(3.7)	2(7.4)
Post-survey	26(96.3)	0	1(3.7)
Conducting performance evaluation			
Pre-survey	20(74.1)	2(7.4)	5(18.5)
Post-survey	26(96.3)	0	1(3.7)
Evaluating employee productivity			
Pre-survey	23(85.2)	0	4(14.8)
Post-survey	27(100.0)	0	0
Chairing a committee			
Pre-survey	14(51.9)	3(11.1)	10(37.0)
Post-survey	18(66.7)	0	9(33.3)
Conducting in-service educational seminars for physicians and administration			
Pre-survey	16(59.3)	6(22.2)	5(18.5)
Post-survey	24(88.9)	0	3(11.1)
Terminating an employee			
Pre-survey	14(51.9)	8(29.6)	5(18.5)
Post-survey	20(74.1)	1(3.7)	6(22.2)
Counseling employee with history of tardiness			
Pre-survey	22(81.5)	2(7.4)	3(11.1)
Post-survey	25(92.6)	0	2(7.4)
Facilitating major departmental change			
Pre-survey	15(55.6)	2(7.4)	10(37.0)
Post-survey	24(88.9)	0	3(11.1)
Handling employee grievance in union hospital			
Pre-survey	13(48.1)	3(11.1)	11(40.7)
Post-survey	15(55.6)	0	12(44.4)
Maintaining positive employee morale in setting of constant change			
Pre-survey	23(85.2)	0	4(14.8)
Post-survey	26(96.3)	0	1(3.7)

*Percent in parentheses

subsequent action taken by the student acting as supervisor.

- A student shared the results of a new quality assurance procedure with the involved employees and collected input from them regarding the new procedure.
- A student presented a report to the oncology committee.

- A student supervised the file clerks and chart retrieval area in the absence of the actual supervisor; she examined productivity and offered suggestions for improving productivity. The student commented that she noticed some patterns in her management style beginning to develop.
- Another student supervised the clerks in

Table 4. Pre- and post-survey self-evaluation of qualification for management positions; percentage by category (N = 27)

Category	Pre-survey	Post-survey
Yes	75	77.7
No	11.7	15.3
Uncertain	13.3	6.9

the medical record department in the absence of the supervisor. The employees came to the student with their day-to-day problems, concerns, and questions.

- Many students observed their field instructors conducting performance evaluations and interviews; students were then asked their opinions of the sessions and were encouraged to formulate ideas as to how they will handle such activities when they are managers.
- Many students conducted inservice education seminars for employees; topics included Medisgroups, an automated quality monitoring and utilization management system using microfilm equipment, and release of information.
- Two students were sent to an off-site storage area for medical records and instructed warehouse employees on the

Table 5. Pre- and post-survey self-evaluation of capability in handling job responsibilities; percentage by category (N = 27)

Category	Pre-survey	Post-survey
Yes	68.2	85.6
No	10.4	0.3
Uncertain	21.9	14.1

proper filing, purging, and destruction of the medical records.

- One student performed a preliminary review of resumes and applications received for a position in the department; she made recommendations to her clinical educator based on her review.

None of these situations were created for the student; they were drawn from real world experiences occurring in the departments at the time of the students' presence. They represent some very good methods used by these clinical educators to involve their students in the day-to-day tasks of the medical record director. They are activities that can help students identify their own strengths and weaknesses in leadership and management and might enable students to begin developing their own leadership and management styles. These activities can help students begin to develop these capabilities while strengthening their self-confidence.

• • •

The results of this survey suggest that clinical educators have a great deal of responsibility for the students they work with during management internship. Under the guidance and direction of clinical educators, students are given the chance to work independently, which may help them develop their own leadership characteristics and management styles. Clinical educators have a responsibility to help develop student leadership and management capabilities, and they should attempt to involve their students in actual situations and experiences that will enhance this development. Their responsibilities may also include increasing the competence of students by adding to their technical skills and educating them in the formal and informal organization and its political framework; including the students in confidential matters; sharing or delegating challenging assignments; making students 100% responsible for a project; allowing students to independently make contacts with necessary individuals to complete a project; providing praise, encouragement, feedback, and constructive criticism in order to help build self-confidence in not only student skills but also in themselves; complimenting and recommending them and their work to others; and providing networking, career, and educational opportunities.

The leaders and managers of today's medical record departments must play a pivotal role in developing the leaders and managers of tomorrow's medical record departments. The results of this survey, although very preliminary, sug-

gest the importance of that role. Future longitudinal surveys subjected to more rigorous statistical measurements may more strongly demonstrate the importance of a clinical educator's influence in designing internship activities. Future studies may provide some answers to the following questions: Can leadership characteristics be developed or strengthened through clinical education? Can internship activities contribute to the development of students' self-confidence and managerial skills? Future studies may also better demonstrate the importance of the clinical educator's role and influence. As the role of the medical record director continues to change and strengthen in today's health care environment, the clinical education of our future leaders has greater significance.

REFERENCES

1. Culp, L. "1988—A Year of Influence." *Journal of AMRA* 59, no. 1 (1988): 9.
2. Moskal, W.F. "Leadership for the Future: Things Your Mentor Never Told You about Change in the Health Care Industry." *Topics in Health Record Management* 8, no. 3 (1988): 73-76.
3. Koontz, H., and O'Donnell, C. *Management: A Systems and Contingency Analysis of Managerial Functions.* 6th ed. New York: McGraw-Hill, 1976.
4. Bourke, G.J., Daly, L.E., and McGilvay, J. *Interpretation and Uses of Medical Statistics.* 3d ed. Boston: Blackwell Scientific, 1985.

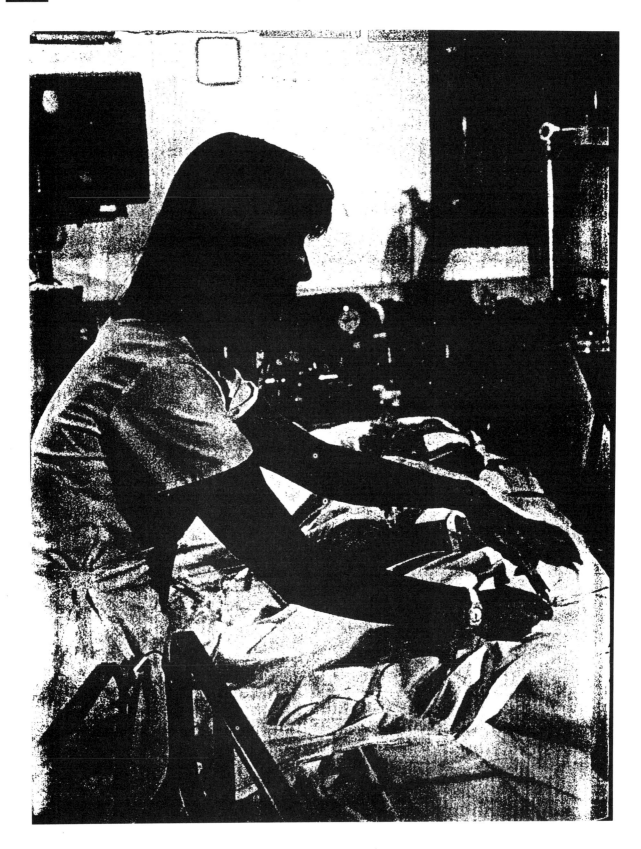

Leadership Theory Lets Clinical Instructors Guide Students toward Autonomy

MARY J. KEENAN
PATRICIA S. HOOVER
ROBERT HOOVER

*A*ccountability, participation, and *decentralization* are among today's managers' buzzwords. Employees who aren't willing or ready to do their part in helping an organization meet its goals may find that, at the very least, their chances for advancement will be limited. Therefore, to do right by their students, nurse educators have to ready them to step into participatory roles.

Nursing faculty members also have to bear in mind the effects the teacher-student relationship may have on the learning process, help students progress toward more self-directed learning, and adapt teaching strategies to students' learning style preferences [1-4]. To meet these challenges, nursing faculty members must find ways to prepare students to function responsibly and accountably as active, contributing members of participatory, decentralized nursing systems. To do so, they have to examine their teaching strategies and be willing to be flexible in their interactions with students.

We believe that, by applying Hersey and Blanchard's Situational Leadership Theory within clinical learning settings, clinical instructors can help students participate more responsibly in their learning experiences [5].

Mary J. Keenan, PhD, RN, is an associate professor in the School of Nursing at the Medical College of Ohio in Toledo and developed the Mid-Management Track in the Graduate Program in Nursing there. Patricia S. Hoover, MSN, RN, is an assistant professor of nursing at the Medical College of Ohio. Robert M. Hoover, MSN, RN was a psychiatric nurse clinician at Riverside Hospital in Toledo and an instructor of nursing at the Medical College of Ohio. Currently he is enrolled as a full-time doctoral student at the University of Toledo.

Situational leadership theories are based on the premise that an effective leader's decisions are consistent with the needs and demands of the environment and of the individuals who are to be led. This view moves beyond previous singular conceptions of leadership styles, which characterized a leader as autocratic, democratic, or laissez-faire. According to situational leadership theories, a leader's activities should be judged based on the demands of the particular situation [6]. Lewin said that individuals' perceptions and motivations are inextricably tied to their environments [7]. He held that individuals' goals result from their need systems as well as from their perceptions about the goals to which they might aspire. Because of this relationship, Lewin believed that behavior cannot be separated from the situation or the environment in which it occurs.

Hersey and Blanchard have built on these ideas by describing effective leadership as the relationship between the style the leader adopts for a particular situation and the maturity level of the followers to accomplish a specific task. They call the four leadership styles telling, selling, participating, and delegating. The four maturity levels are M1, M2, M3, and M4, and Hersey and Blanchard consider a follower's maturity level to be the level of knowledge, skill, and motivation he or she has to perform a specific task.

Figure 1 shows the relationship among the four styles of leadership behavior and the four maturity levels. The telling style of leadership, in which the leader sets goals and the ways to meet them, is most appropriate when followers lack the knowledge and skill to accomplish the task and the motivation to do so. Previous leadership theories labeled this type of directive leadership as autocratic and often cast it in a negative light. Hersey and Blanchard consider it appropriate when the follower's maturity level is quite low.

Using the selling style of leadership, a leader offers ideas to the followers and directs them toward accomplishing the task. The leader assumes that followers have a moderate maturity level, and, although they lack the competence to perform the task without help, they are motivated enough to move forward to learn and accomplish it. Hersey and Blanchard suggest that, when using the first two leadership styles, the leader should display limited socioemotional support, which the follower could misconstrue as permissiveness or see as a reward for poor behavior. We suggest that the leader give socioemotional support as the individual progresses in competence and motivation. Withdrawing support could interfere with the individual's progress, and an educator should not ignore the fact that learning is both a cognitive and a social process.

Using the participatory leadership style, a leader assumes a supportive, non-directive style with followers who have shown that they have the necessary knowledge and competence to perform the task but who are unwilling to move forward on their own. Such unwillingness, often the result of a lack of confidence on the followers' part, indicates the need for the leader to create a supportive atmosphere.

A leader who is using the delegating style keeps a low profile and provides little if any direction for followers who have reached a high maturity level. At this point, there is no need for a great deal of socioemotional support because the individuals have shown that they can provide it for themselves [8].

To help students function more independently, faculty members must choose the right leadership style for the situation. Therefore, they have to be able to assess the students' maturity levels at any given time. In Figure 2,

we compare the behaviors educators may observe in students. The teachers may see these behaviors, which reflect the maturity level for a specific clinical situation, in any student and at any point in the nursing program. A student with a high maturity level in one clinical situation may revert to a low or moderate level in another due to anxiety, lack of experience, lack of interest, or personal stress at the time. Performance evaluations in other clinical areas may give the educator an idea of the student's growth potential, but the educator should use them cautiously, if at all, when doing an initial assessment for a new clinical area. In terms of specific task-relevant maturity, the past does not necessarily apply.

Although the behaviors at the M4

level are ideals to work toward, it is unlikely that a student will be at this level at the beginning of a clinical experience. If he or she is, the educator should question whether he needs the course. Students at the M2 or M3 level display varying degrees of ability and motivation to perform the tasks required of them, and they show areas of knowledge, skill, and motivation they can develop in the course. In these intermediate stages of maturity, students' awareness of their learning needs is growing and they are beginning to take actions to meet those needs.

Case Example

To see how educators can apply Hersey and Blanchard's Situational Leadership Theory to a clinical teaching situation, consider this example. A clinical teaching faculty member gave students in a beginning level course patient assignments the day before they were to begin care. She distributed an outline that contained specific requirements so the students could plan for the clinical experience. On the day they were to begin care, she expected them to come with written and verbal evidence that they had done so.

One student came to the clinical site without having met the requirements the faculty member had listed on the guide. Although the student asked her peers for help, she did not ask the faculty member. In a private conference, the teacher told the student that she was inadequately prepared for the clinical experience and asked what kind of help she thought she needed. The student said she didn't need help, but that she had to spend more time preparing for clinical work. She said she would meet the guidelines for the next clinical experience.

However, she was again unprepared the following week and she gave the same rationale she had used the first time. The educator informed her in writing that her performance was unsatisfactory, and the student and faculty member arranged a conference during which they could talk about strategies for change. At the conference, the student said she felt overwhelmed by the amount of information in the patients' charts and that she was unable to organize the data. She also said she was frustrated by having to prepare a day in advance of providing

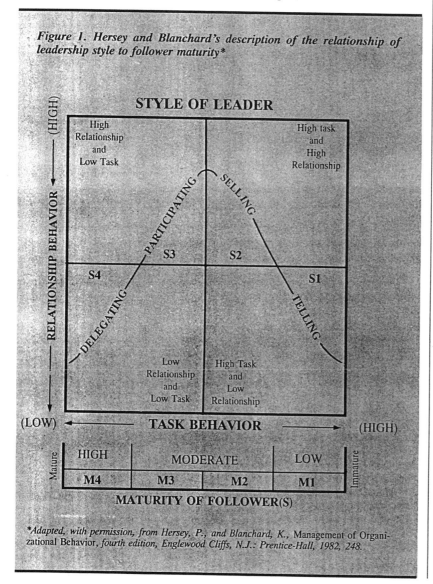

Figure 1. Hersey and Blanchard's description of the relationship of leadership style to follower maturity*

STYLE OF LEADER

(HIGH)

RELATIONSHIP BEHAVIOR

High Relationship and Low Task

High task and High Relationship

PARTICIPATING   SELLING

DELEGATING   TELLING

S3   S2

S4   S1

Low Relationship and Low Task

High Task and Low Relationship

(LOW) ◄——— TASK BEHAVIOR ———► (HIGH)

Mature	HIGH	MODERATE		LOW	Immature
	M4	M3	M2	M1	

MATURITY OF FOLLOWER(S)

*Adapted, with permission, from Hersey, P., and Blanchard, K., Management of Organizational Behavior, fourth edition, Englewood Cliffs, N.J.: Prentice-Hall, 1982, 248.

care because the client's status could change. The faculty member next asked herself what she could do to change the student's behavior.

Hersey and Blanchard developed a Leader Effectiveness and Adaptability Description (LEAD) for assessing leadership styles across varying situations, and the educator put the two versions of this instrument to use [9]. With the LEAD Self, leaders indicate how they would respond in a given situation, and with the LEAD Other, followers indicate how they think the leader would respond in the same situation. Table 1 shows an example of an item on the LEAD Self instrument.

Using the LEAD Self, the educator determined that her primary leadership style was the selling style. The students, who completed the LEAD Other, concurred that this was her primary style of leadership.

Using the Maturity Scale developed by Hambleton, Blanchard, and Hersey, the educator further determined that the student's maturity level was low [10]. And, after considering the concepts of the Situational Leadership Theory, the faculty member decided that a telling rather than a selling leadership style would be more appropriate for work with this particular student.

The faculty member then guided the student toward improving her organizational skills and helped her think through her frustration with the constant change that is inherent in clinical settings. Using the telling style of leadership, the educator repeatedly involved the student as she analyzed her organizational plan and gave the student explicit directions for planning and carrying out patient care. Subsequently, the student came to clinical experiences prepared. Throughout the course, the faculty member periodically reinforced desired behaviors and eventually reduced her supervision as she increased her socioemotional support. Through this process, the educator helped the student increase her maturity level.

All too often, an educator will consider an inconsistency between his or her leadership style and a student's maturity level to be the student's problem, and the student pays the price. Instead, it is the teacher's responsibility to adapt his or her leadership style to the student's maturity level. In this case, the educator changed to the ap-

---

Figure 2. Behavior observed in students at the different maturity levels

M1 student behaviors:
- demonstrates inability to initiate care activities, such as standing outside the patient's door or spending more time with the chart than with the patient
- demonstrates a lack of knowledge of the subject matter required for a given task
- turns in assignments late or not at all
- may engage in distracting tactics, such as bringing up topics unrelated to the task
- demonstrates inability to ask the questions necessary for learning in a given situation
- demonstrates inability to set goals
- overestimates his or her competence to achieve goals

M2 student behaviors:
- asks appropriate questions
- demonstrates increased cognitive and psychomotor skills for specific tasks
- expresses feelings when asked to
- asks for help in setting goals
- seeks approval from faculty members

M3 student behaviors:
- determines the answers to task-relevant questions
- demonstrates the cognitive and psychomotor skills needed to perform specific tasks
- suggests learning activities
- seeks approval and suggestions for improvement from faculty members
- demonstrates increased ability to motivate himself or herself to complete the task

M4 student behaviors:
- asks for help when needed
- functions independently most of the time
- gets assignments done on time
- expresses enjoyment while working independently
- asks for extra projects or suggests appropriate alternate experiences
- tells classmates about thoughts and feelings
- offers help and encouragement to students with lesser competence
- demonstrates ability to set goals

---

propriate telling style, even though she tended to value a high-relationship style in her interactions with students.

Although increasing student participation in finding ways to meet learning objectives is a goal to which most student and faculty members ascribe, it is not without risks. By allowing a student to participate fully, the educator assumes that the student has the knowledge, skills, and motivation to accomplish a task unaided.

Educators must accurately assess students' learning needs as well as their abilities to accomplish a task. Inappropriate use of participatory involvement can lead students to see the faculty member as lacking in expertise, initiative, or self-confidence. Individuals may consider a leader who uses participation extensively to be weak and

ineffective. This can create a problem for faculty members, because their desire to increase students' chances to exercise autonomy can result in student perceptions that they are unprepared or incompetent.

To prevent this, faculty members can remind students that they will ask for student input before they give specific directions. They should also seek specific feedback from students to find out how the students are progressing in developing participatory skills. These actions can prevent students from becoming confused about appropriate role responsibilities for themselves and for the faculty member.

Allowing students to participate in learning takes more time than directing them does. In cases in which there isn't enough time, or when a critical situa-

Table 1. Example of situation from LEAD Self assessment tool*	
Situation	**Alternative Actions**
Your subordinates are no longer responding to your friendly conversation and obvious concern for their welfare. Their performances are declining rapidly.	a. Emphasize the use of uniform procedures and the necessity for task accomplishment.
	b. Make yourself available for discussion, but don't push your involvement.
	c. Talk with subordinates and then set goals.
	d. Intentionally do not intervene.

from Hersey, P., and Blanchard, K., Management of Organizational Behavior: Utilizing Human Resources, fourth edition, Englewood Cliffs, N.J.: Prentice-Hall, 1982, 99, with permission.

tion requires immediate action, participatory involvement is inappropriate and risky. Faculty members have to be able to accurately assess not just the students' learning needs but also the demands of the situation to determine how much participation to look for from students.

On the plus side, students' participation in setting and putting in place their own learning goals and activities can help them better understand and accept the goals for the course. It can also lead them to evaluate their progress toward meeting goals and to develop ways to achieve them. This process enhances students' responsibility and accountability for meeting their learning needs and for showing that they have met course objectives.

As students work more closely with faculty members to set learning goals and to find the right activities to meet them, they take more interest in the learning process. This increased interest means that they see the course objectives as their own. They are also able to evaluate their progress more accurately and to seek out remedial or additional activities as needed. They take responsibility and accountability for their progress, work with faculty members to achieve their learning goals, and do not have to blame others for any lack of achievement. At this point, students understand and can participate in setting and meeting goals.

We encourage faculty members to explore further the possible applications of the Situational Leadership Theory to teaching and to research. As educators become adept at incorporating this theory into their teaching methods, students will reap the benefits of participatory learning and will be prepared to take their positions in organizations that demand participation and accountability.

References

1. Rogers, C., *Freedom to Learn,* Columbus, Ohio: Charles E. Merrill, 1979.
2. Carkhuff, R., *Helping and Human Relations,* New York: Holt, 1969.
3. Knowles, M., *The Adult Learner: A Neglected Species,* second edition, Houston: Gulf, 1978.
4. Merritt, S.L., Learning style preferences of baccalaureate nursing students, *Nursing Research,* 32 (6), 1983, 367-372.
5. Hersey, P., and Blanchard, K., *Management of Organizational Behavior: Utilizing Human Resources,* fourth edition, Englewood Cliffs, N.J.: Prentice-Hall, 1982.
6. Yukl, G., *Leadership in Organizations,* Englewood Cliffs, N.J.: Prentice-Hall, 1981.
7. Lewin, K., *A Dynamic Theory of Personality,* translated by Adams, D.K., and Zener, K.E., New York: McGraw Hill, 1935 (original work published in 1933).
8. See note 5, above.
9. Hersey, P., and Blanchard, K., *Leader Effectiveness and Adaptability Description (LEAD Scales),* Escondido, CA: Center for Leadership Studies, 1973.
10. Hambleton, R.K., Blanchard, K.H., and Hersey, P., *Maturity Scales: Manager Rating Form,* Escondido, CA: Center for Leadership Studies, 1977.
11. See note 6, above.

Professional Development for Clinical Faculty

Long-Term Evaluation of Training Residents In Clinical Teaching Skills

Janine C. Edwards, Ph.D., Grace E. Kissling, Ph.D., Warren C. Plauché, M.D., and Robert L. Marier, M.D.

Abstract—In the present study, the authors examined the long-term effectiveness of a course for residents on how to teach students, patients, and peers. Residents of various specialties attended a mandatory short course on clinical teaching skills in the middle of their first year of postgraduate medical training. Three types of evaluation data were collected at three times during a two-year period: self-ratings by the residents, questionnaires completed by the residents, and ratings completed by students taught by the residents. Complete data for 18 residents indicated that the residents rated their teaching skills significantly higher after the course (at the end of both the first year and the second year) than before it. At the end of the second year, 94 percent of the residents stated that the course was helpful, 67 percent could recall and explain specific principles of teaching, and 61 percent reported using principles from the course in their teaching. Students' ratings of these 18 residents were too scanty to be interpreted validly. The study suggests that residents of varying specialties can profit from an introductory course on teaching skills and that the effects endure for at least one and a half years.

Residents hold a middle position in the medical education hierarchy, for they are trainees of the clinical faculty but trainers or teachers of medical students. Broad economic and political changes in the United States are directing increased attention to graduate medical education. The U.S. government has attempted to contain federal health care costs by establishing diagnosis-related groups (DRGs) for determining reimbursements for

Dr. Edwards is coordinator, Office of Educational Development and Evaluation, Dr. Kissling assistant professor, Department of Biometry and Genetics, Dr. Plauché professor, Department of Obstetrics and Gynecology, and Dr. Marier professor. Department of Medicine. Louisiana State University School of Medicine in New Orleans.

health care under the Medicare program. The full effect of DRGs on graduate medical education is not known yet, but it is likely that major changes in financing such education will be made. Medical school faculties also are feeling economic pressures that will affect residents. For example, the maintenance and growth of many medical schools are becoming dependent on faculty members generating more revenue through patient care and extramural funding of research (1). This dependence will allow faculty members less time to teach. The role of residents in teaching medical students, then, can be expected to take on added importance.

A number of institutions are attempting to train residents in teaching skills (2,

967

Reprinted with permission from the *Journal of Medical Education.* Edwards JC, Kissling GE, Plauché WC, Marier RL. 1986;61(12):967-970. The *Journal of Medical Education* was renamed *Academic Medicine* in January 1989.

968 *Journal of Medical Education*   VOL. 61, DECEMBER 1986

3), but little is known about the effectiveness of these programs. Furthermore, relatively little evaluation has been done in the area of faculty development (4). Only one study (5) has evaluated both short- and long-term effects of a teacher-training workshop in a medical school. That study reported that significant improvement in teaching skills endured for two years. In the present study, the authors address the question of how effective a short course on clinical teaching skills is for residents.

Methods

Sixty-one of the 93 first-year residents at the Louisiana State University (LSU) Medical Center attended a short course on clinical teaching midway through the 1983–84 academic year. This half-day course is mandatory for first-year residents; however, emergency room duty and off-campus rotations preclude 100 percent attendance. The course has been offered and taught by a team comprising the authors and senior residents during the middle of each academic year since 1982–83. A complete description of this course has been published elsewhere (6). From the 61 residents attending the course in 1983–84, data were requested three times during the first two years of their postgraduate training: before the course, at the end of postgraduate-year one (PGY-1), and at the end of PGY-2. The data following PGY-1 and PGY-2 were collected by mail. Complete data were obtained on 18 residents (30 percent) with the following specialties: medicine, family medicine, pediatrics, obstetrics-gynecology, surgery, orthopedics, urology, and neurology.

At each of the three times, the residents were asked to rate their teaching skills on Irby's inventory of teacher behaviors (7). The inventory consists of 54 items concerning the following characteristics: organization/clarity, enthusiasm/stimulation, instructor knowledge, rapport, instructional skill, clinical supervision, clinical competence, and professional characteristics. An average or summary score was computed for each resident from the ratings of these eight characteristics. At the end of PGY-2, they also were asked to complete an eight-item questionnaire about the course and teaching. Four questions concerned the course (including recall of specific points taught), two queried interest in additional teacher training, and two inquired about teaching ability and opportunity to teach in PGY-2 as compared with PGY-1. All questions allowed residents to add personal comments. Nonrespondents were encouraged to respond by a follow-up mailing and a verbal reminder by their chief residents. Anonymous student ratings of the residents' teaching were routinely collected at the end of each required third-year clerkship. The students used a short version of the inventory of teaching behaviors (8) to assess the residents' teaching skills.

Paired t-tests were used to analyze the residents' self-ratings. The students' ratings of each resident were averaged, and paired t-tests compared these ratings at the three different times. The students' ratings and the residents' self-ratings were also compared with t-tests.

Results

The residents rated their teaching skills significantly higher ($p < 0.001$) on six of the eight characteristics measured by the inventory (organization, enthusiasm, knowledge, skill, supervision, and competence) and on the summary score of the inventory at both times after the course than before it. The ratings at the end of the first year did not differ significantly from the ratings at the end of the second year.

The residents' responses at the end of the PGY-2 to the questionnaire about the half-day course were generally positive (Table 1). Ninety-four percent thought that the course was helpful. A frequent comment was that the course had raised the residents' awareness of their teaching role. At the end of PGY-2, 67 percent could still recall specific points presented. These points included giving positive and negative feedback appropriate to the situation, using generic techniques for teaching clinical and/or surgical procedures, specifying teaching objectives, using questioning techniques, and setting a climate conducive to learning. Furthermore, 61 percent of the respondents reported at the end of PGY-2 using ideas from the course in their teaching. These ideas included but were not limited to the following: communicating more effectively with patients and students, recognizing their own areas of weakness, being stimulated to make more active efforts to teach, being thorough in discussing patients' cases, giving feedback, supervising the performance of procedures, explaining their expectations, correcting errors as soon as they are made, and improving supervision of students while they perform procedures.

Two questions were asked about the residents' ability and opportunity to teach in PGY-2 compared with PGY-1 because the authors are interested in determining the optimum time to deliver training in teaching skills to residents. A majority of the residents stated that their teaching ability had improved and that they had more opportunity to teach during the second than the first year. This information may indicate that the most opportune time to provide teacher training is late in the first year or early in the second year—in tandem with the residents' growth in ability and need to teach.

The students' ratings ($n = 108$) of these 18 residents were too scanty to be interpreted validly. The students' ratings were collected at the end of each clerkship and were grouped by dates for analysis. As the study was designed, each resident had to have been rated by at least three students at each of three times: before the course, in the first year after the course, and during the second year. Only six of the residents, however, were evaluated by the requisite number of students for each period; therefore, the analyses of these ratings could not be interpreted.

TABLE 1

Numbers and Percentages of 18 Second-Year Residents Responding to Questions on a Half-Day Course in Teaching Skills That Was Taken 18 Months Previously, Louisiana State University Medical Center, 1985

Questions	Responses*			
	Yes		No	
	No.	Percent	No.	Percent
Consider course beneficial	17	94	1	6
Recall principles taught in course	12	67	6	33
Have used principles taught in course	11	61	7	39
Want more training early in PGY-2	8	57	6	43
Want more training late in PGY-2	7	50	7	50

* Number of responses vary because not all residents answered all questions.

Discussion and Conclusions

In the study reported here, a group of residents rated their teaching skills significantly higher after attending a half-day course on clinical teaching than before the course. These assessments endured without decay for at least a year and a half. The residents could still recall and explain major teaching points and reported that they had used these teaching points 18 months after the course. Prior findings (9) about the effectiveness of short faculty development courses indicated increased awareness and knowledge of teaching principles among faculty members after such courses. The present study not only confirms these findings for residents but also gives evidence of behavior change, albeit self-evidence. In addition, this study shows that residents of various specialties can profit from an introductory course. Prior studies (2, 3) of teaching by residents have included residents in only one specialty.

The low response rate of 30 percent was, in the authors' opinion, probably attributable to the heavy demands on and accumulated fatigue of the second-year residents rather than antipathy to teaching. Further evidence of the effectiveness of training in teaching skills with larger numbers of residents is necessary, and the authors are conducting a two-year study using experimental and control groups of residents.

References

1. Perry, D. R., Challoner, D. R., and Oberst, R. J. Research Advances and Resources Constraints: Dilemmas Facing Medical Education. *N. Engl. J. Med.*, **305**:320–324, 1981.
2. Camp, M. G., Hoban, J. D., and Katz, P. A Course on Teaching for House Officers. *J. Med. Educ.*, **60**:140–142, 1985.
3. Jewett, L. S., Greenberg, L.W., and Goldberg, R. M. Teaching Residents How To Teach: A One-Year Study. *J. Med. Educ.*, **57**:361–366, 1982.
4. Stritter, F. T. Faculty Evaluation and Development. In *Handbook on Health Professions Education*. C. H. McGuire, R. P. Foley, A. ,Gorr, and R. W. Richards (Eds.). San Francisco, California: Jossey-Bass, 1983.
5. Mahler, S., and Benor, D. E. Short and Long Term Effects of a Teacher-Training Workshop in Medical School. *Higher Educ.*, **13**:265–273, 1984.
6. Edwards, J. C., and Marier, R. L. (Eds.). *Resident Teaching: Roles, Techniques, and Programs.* New York: Springer, (in press).
7. Irby, D. M. Clinical Teacher Effectiveness in Medicine. *J. Med. Educ.*, **53**:808–815, 1978.
8. Irby, D., and Rakestraw, P. Evaluating Clinical Teaching in Medicine. *J. Med. Educ.*, **56**:181–186, 1981.
9. Bland, C. J. *Faculty Development Through Workshops.* Springfield, Illinois: Charles C Thomas, 1980.

Design and Implementation of a Problem-based Continuing Education Programme:
A guide for clinical physiotherapists

ANGELA C TITCHEN MSc MCSP

Professional Adviser (Post-registration Education)
Chartered Society of Physiotherapy, London

Key words: Problem-based learning, self-evaluation, self-initiated learning, peer-group teaching and learning, facilitator, unconventional use of experts.

Summary: This paper has been written as a tool to help clinical physiotherapists to set up and run a problem-based continuing education programme for themselves and their colleagues in their work-place. The programme model is based on small group work, self-evaluation, self-initiated and self-directed learning, group learning and peer-group teaching and has been developed from the evaluations of innovatory CE programmes for therapists and general practitioners. This approach is designed to enable physiotherapists to take responsibility for their own education. It is suggested that the skills required for planning and implementing a problem-based initiative are already possessed by physiotherapists, and that these skills will be refined through the education process. The five stages of setting up and running a programme are described. A check list and suggestions for further reading are presented for potential programme planners.

Biography: Having qualified at St Mary's Hospital School of Physiotherapy, Angela Titchen worked at University College Hospital, Nether Edge Hospital, The Western Infirmary, Glasgow, and Vancouver General Hospital. She was a research physiotherapist at Mary Marlborough Lodge until taking up her current post as a CSP professional adviser (education). Her interest in problem-based learning was kindled on an MSc course in rehabilitation studies at the University of Southampton. She has recently returned from visiting a Dutch school of physiotherapy in The Hague, and a continuing education programme in Maastricht, where problem-based curricula are being implemented.

Introduction

THE need for continuing education (CE), to ensure that physiotherapists maintain their competence to practise, has long been recognised by the Chartered Society of Physiotherapy (CSP, 1983). However, CE still lags behind pre-registration education and the development of validated post-registration courses in the national priorities for physiotherapy education. This is understandable, in view of the limited resources available and the infancy of our post-registration education structure. Nevertheless, the CSP is aware that the maintenance and improvement of standards of the physiotherapy service are dependent largely on individual physiotherapists' commitment to lifelong learning. The World Health Organisation (WHO, 1977) states that this commitment involves individuals taking responsibility for their own CE. However, in a pilot study, Titchen (1987) found that although physiotherapists recognised the importance of CE, and were well-motivated to participate in it, there was some evidence to suggest that they had not been adequately prepared by their basic professional education to take responsibility for it, ie to initiate and direct it themselves. They tended to view CE predominantly as something that was arranged for them.

This paper seeks to help all clinical physiotherapists to participate actively in their own education, by giving guidance on how to set up and implement a problem-based CE programme for colleagues in their department, practice or District/Area. This innovative approach is based on small group work, and aims to promote self-initiated and self-directed learning, peer-group teaching and learning and self-evaluation, which are factors recognised as essential for the CE process (Richards, 1978; Knowles, 1970; Laxdal, 1982).

It has been reported (Trent Regional Health Authority, 1984) that many experienced physiotherapists have a lot to offer to junior colleagues, but that they do not always possess the skills to 'plan and implement educationally viable courses' However, this author suggests that the planning and teaching skills that physiotherapists use in the treatment and management of their patients are similar to those needed to set up a problem-based programme. It is hoped that this article will help physiotherapists recognise that they already possess these skills, and that involvement in such a programme will refine them.

Problem-based Learning

Problem-based learning focuses on the problems met by physiotherapists in their daily work. These could be patient management, managerial or educational problems. In a small group, physiotherapists identify what they need to know to solve the problem. They share with each other what they already know and then allocate information collection tasks. Information is sought from a variety of sources, including books, journals, case studies and senior staff. This is presented to the group and then used to tackle the problem. Using this approach physiotherapists find things out for themselves, and they do not rely on being 'told' by experts or specialists. These experts are used in different ways, either to set problems in areas identified by the group, or to give feedback on the group's conclusions and solutions (this is termed 'unconventional use of experts').

The argument for this format is that while enhancing the problem-solving process that physiotherapists use every day, it matches their individual needs. It is also based on features which physiotherapists perceive help them to learn, that is relevance to patients, active involvement, talking to colleagues, receiving feedback on their performance, and practice at presenting their work and ideas (Titchen, 1985). Educational arguments for the approach are discussed in the following paper for interested readers to pursue.

Conventional CE in-service programmes very often focus on individual disciplines, for example pathology or psychology, or on fields of knowledge, such as physiotherapeutic techniques. Many of the sessions are didactic (Titchen, 1987), with opportunities for application of the knowledge by the learners, usually at the end of the session. In a problem-based approach a reversal has taken place. The problem or application comes first and knits together the disciplines and fields of knowledge, thus helping people to integrate and apply multidisciplinary knowledge.

Fig 1: The five stages of a problem-based programme

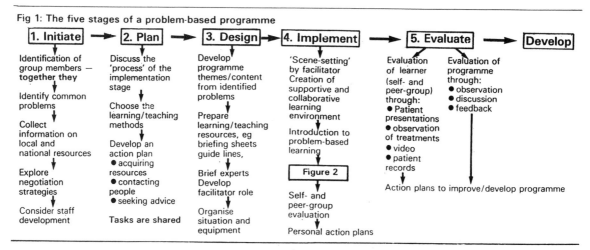

Setting up the Programme

The following guide lines are intended to provide a framework for setting up a problem-based programme. Considerable flexibility can be exercised.

The five stages are presented separately for clarity (fig 1), however, in reality there is considerable overlap between respective stages.

1. Initiation

(a) Consider appropriateness and feasibility: Discuss the arguments in support of problem-based learning with your colleagues and your manager, and decide together whether this type of programme is appropriate and feasible in your department.

(b) Identify common problems: To give a focus for planning, the common problems that you and your colleagues experience should be identified through discussions in your own department, meetings with representatives of the physiotherapy departments or experts in your District/Area, or questionnaires.

(c) Collect information: Find out what resources are available in your District/Area that you and your colleagues may find useful later on. Lists of resource people should be compiled, for example bio-engineers, statisticians, physiotherapy researchers and health education officers. You may want to discover what distance learning opportunities are available in your field, or the resources that your medical library, learning resource centre or health education department can offer you.

(d) Explore negotiation strategies: You may find that you need to explore strategies to negotiate with your manager for study time. In Titchen's (1983) study of physiotherapists, it is reported that a superintendent physiotherapist had introduced one study afternoon per month for staff to use in any way they chose. These physiotherapists spent the time doing library research, attending clinics, working on small research projects or peer-group teaching. Some managers, who feel that it is their responsibility to organise the in-service education, may need to change their attitude if self-initiated learning is to thrive, and this change may need to be negotiated.

(e) Consider staff development: Some of your colleagues may hold attitudes that do not match the educational methods you are proposing. Physiotherapists in Titchen's (1987) study reported that they lacked the confidence to participate actively in small group discussions or patient presentations. A typical comment was: 'You feel that people are going to trip you up and find you out.'

Your colleagues who view key features of problem-based learning as new and intimidating may require staff development, ie they need an opportunity to explore their attitudes, and to see that their fears are unfounded — in the same way that you help a patient view his/her condition in a new light. For example, physiotherapists who think that they do not possess skills for peer-group teaching should be helped to recognise that such skills are not dissimilar to those which they use when teaching their patients.

2. Planning

In a problem-based approach, a process model of planning is adopted. This means that the participants in the programme have a responsibility for planning the programme equal to that of the initiators. This has been tried by general practitioners and found to be successful (Savile, 1982). You may decide to seek the help and advice of a physiotherapy teacher at this stage.

The main task at planning meetings is to select the most suitable methods for learning rather than deciding on the content. Schmidt (1983) and McKenzie et al (1985) considered that it is often the process of learning that determines whether learning is retrievable and useful in professional practice, rather than the content of the learning. Does this reflect the old song, 'It's not what you do, but the way that you do it'? Physiotherapists in Titchen's (1987) study cited lectures as the most useful form of CE, probably because this was their previous experience of education. However, comparative studies have shown that although the lecture is as effective as participatory methods for transmitting information, it is not as effective as other methods for stimulating thought and for changing people's values and attitudes (Bligh, 1972). As problem-based learning aims to stimulate critical thinking, problem-solving and attitude change, as well as to transmit information; participatory small group methods are adopted. Many different group methods are available, some of which are described in appendix A. Although it appears that physiotherapists have had very little experience of small group work (Titchen, 1987), those who have reported that it was very useful (Gray, 1985). Participants on CSP workshops have also valued this method. So the formal lecture is reserved either for areas beyond the resources of the group, or to give structure where people are having difficulties.

Once the learning methods are selected, the planners are able to establish what sort of facilities, resources and resource people (for giving advice, information or demonstrating skills) they will require. The planners should divide up the tasks of making contacts and asking for help and co-operation.

3. Design

This stage involves the design of a theme, the development of learning resources and teaching materials, and organisation and action in the learning/teaching situation.

Once you have established the common problems, you will be able to design a framework on various themes. This suggestion arises from a study of a problem-based programme by Bouhuijs (1985), who concludes that 'a systematic curriculum containing key topics for GPs is a better way to ensure the effectiveness of CE'. This supports Bruner's (1960) conclusion that knowledge requires a structure.

The development of learning resources and teaching materials includes:

(a) Briefing experts: When using experts unconventionally, it will be necessary to prepare them. You may find it easiest to develop a briefing sheet describing the philosophy of your programme and what you expect them to do, ie they are not to give formal lectures or demonstrations, but they are to allow the group members to define their own requirements and to clarify, extend and elaborate the group's knowledge (*see* appendix A — Question and answer). The specialists may need your support and encouragement, but most will probably accept the challenge with enthusiasm.

(b) Developing the role of facilitator: It is envisaged that the role of group facilitator would be taken up by senior physiotherapists, as they are probably already responsible for teaching junior colleagues. The facilitator creates a social structure in which they can draw out colleagues' problems, and also help them to transfer what they are learning to their own situation. Physiotherapists may need help in developing this role (*see* 'Further reading'). They might consider finding someone with this kind of experience who is prepared to listen, talk and guide them, for example a health education officer. They could also read about group dynamics. Gray (1985) reports that therapy tutors on the EDURP course were 'generally found to be excellent facilitators and co-ordinators who developed this style as the course ran on'

(c) Preparing learning/teaching materials: Preparing guide lines, check lists, handouts and reference lists will help participants in the programme with both content and process. For example, guide lines may be useful to help group members when they are going to present a patient or lead a discussion (the notes in appendix A may be useful), and an action plan handout may help participants to fulfil their learning goals (appendix B). The production of such materials may prompt the development of similar aids for patient and carers.

(d) Learning to use a library: It will probably be necessary to ask the librarian to organise a session on 'How to use a library', since many physiotherapists are unfamiliar with the procedures involved in locating specific papers or books.

The layout of the room is an important consideration when organising the space for group work. For task-oriented groups a large table will be needed for writing. For other small group methods the chairs should be arranged in a circle. This is far less threatening to a presenter than rows of faces, and it reflects and reinforces the group's cohesion and the equality of its members. It also aids discussion. For practical sessions plenty of space will be required.

Finally, audio-visual equipment may be needed. If your department does not possess a flip-chart and stand, or slide or over-head projector, you could contact your nearest librarian, audio-visual aids department (usually situated in District general hospitals), postgraduate medical centre or health education department to find out where they can be borrowed.

All of these preparation and development tasks are themselves part of the CE process, and should therefore be shared by the group members. While learning to set up educational events, physiotherapists are refining the organisational, group, management, interpersonal and teamwork skills that they already possess, and that they need in professional practice.

Fig 2: An example of the problem-based approach

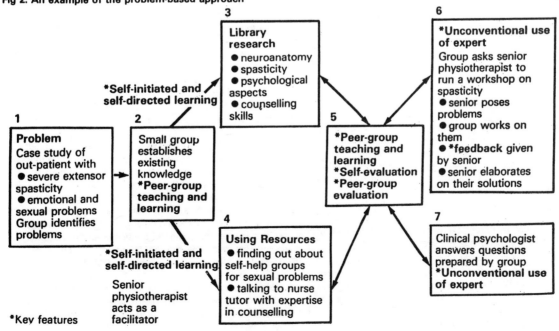

4. Implementation

The model devised by the author (Titchen, 1985), and elaborated in figure 2, forms the core of the implementation stage. The figure represents one example of the problem-based approach. It is stressed that there are many possibilities open to a creative, self-determining group.

The programme begins when the group considers a case study and identifies the patient's problems (box 1). Having established and shared existing knowledge between themselves (box 2), the physiotherapists decide what they need to know to solve the problem and how they are going to find it out (boxes 3 and 4). They allocate tasks, for example library research on particular aspects of the problem, or seeking advice or information from local resources or resource people. The physiotherapists work individually or in pairs as they choose. The group comes back together (box 5), and new information or skills are shared and used to solve the patient's problems. In this way, physiotherapists learn from each other and are able to evaluate themselves and their peers. They may now decide to continue with library research and using resources, or to use experts unconventionally (boxes 6 and 7). The group then decides to undertake a project to evaluate the treatment and management of patients with extensor spasticity. As the group members are unsure how to go about this, they go back to the processes described in boxes 2 to 7, but this time they establish and share existing knowledge about evaluation, undertake library research on various methodologies, and use experts to give feedback on their evaluation design and data analysis. These groups go on re-forming and regenerating through self-motivation and self-direction as the physiotherapists encounter new problems.

Some group members may share the experience of the physiotherapists in Titchen's (1987) study. They reported infrequent participation in professional reading and difficulty with learning from books. However, they did say that it was easier if the information was relevant to their patients. This approach will provide that relevance. Learning will also be optimised, because the programme will enable therapists to *do* something with the information, for example teach it to others, present patients, lead discussions, solve problems or evaluate practice. Using knowledge results in better understanding and remembering information (Anderson and Reder, 1979).

Such a programme should give therapists confidence that they seem to lack when presenting patients or contributing to small group discussion (Titchen, 1987). In turn, this will enhance their communication and interpersonal skills when working with the multidisciplinary team. It will also help them to evaluate themselves and others critically, and to accept criticism and act on it.

Group members may find it helpful to draw up personal action plans, with dates for their goals to be achieved (appendix B). It is stressed that the emphasis of the programme is always on collaboration and not competition. This can be achieved by the social structure created by the facilitator.

5. Evaluation

Evaluation has two prongs — evaluation or assessment of the learner, and evaluation of the programme itself.

(a) Evaluation of the learner: Self-directed learning requires self-evaluation (Knowles, 1970), and peer-group evaluation, and in problem-based learning is achieved through the group process. For example, at the beginning of a programme theme, participants present to the group their written assessment and treatment of a patient. When the theme is drawing to a close, they present the same, or a similar case, and a comparison with the original is made. Alternatively, physiotherapists in two or threes look at each other's patient records (Laxdal, 1982), observe each other treating patients, or make video recordings of themselves treating patients. With all these methods it is important to establish criteria beforehand, so that standards have been defined. These criteria are set by the peer-group, and allow the individual to make comparisons of her/his own performance against the standard. The facilitator's role is crucial in this process.

(b) Evaluation of the programme: Evaluation of continuing education programmes is rare in all professions, including physiotherapy. This is probably because a complex network of variables surrounds the effect an educational programme has upon a professional's practice. It is not easy to establish whether an educational event has enhanced a physiotherapist's competence, and changed her/his behaviour in some aspect of patient care. Systematic evaluation would involve looking at the whole complex scene and all the variables. This is not feasible for busy clinicians. However, it is possible to weave evaluation into the fabric of the programme, and to use what is already happening. For example, evaluation of the learner, as described above, gives some indication of the value of the programme. The action plan (appendix B), too, not only enables self-evaluation, but can also be used for programme evaluation. Open and frank discussion can be built in to consider whether the programme is useful and relevant, and where there are strengths and weaknesses. The facilitator should ensure that time is available at all the sessions for feedback from the participants. Observation of the group will help to validate what people say. Using these methods, the group will be able to make informed judgements and decisions on how the programme can be developed. This mirrors the constant observation, evaluation and subsequent modification of treatment that all physiotherapists carry out in their daily work.

To help physiotherapists through these five stages a check list is presented in appendix C.

Conclusion

In summary, it has been established that although few resources are allocated nationally to physiotherapy CE, lifelong learning is considered essential by the CSP and practitioners alike. It is argued that the skills required to set up and implement a problem-based CE programme parallel the skills physiotherapists use in their treatment and management of patients. These planning, organisational, interpersonal, negotiating and team-work skills are enhanced, because the programme is developed by all group members. Thus, the process as well as the content of the programme benefits patient care.

A problem-based programme will also provide opportunities for physiotherapists to develop confidence in presenting their ideas and work in a context that will facilitate learning and integration and retrieval of knowledge.

Planning and implementing such a programme is time-consuming, as it involves much more than deciding on the content, choosing speakers and organising venues. However, there is evidence from clinical physiotherapists and their managers that this time can be found. Nearly two-thirds (63.6%) of physiotherapists in Titchen's (1983) study were willing to spend more time continuing their education and 98 (60.5%) felt that they could make more time by better self-organisation. Graveling (1984) recognised the responsibility that physiotherapy managers have in ensuring that their staff continue their education.

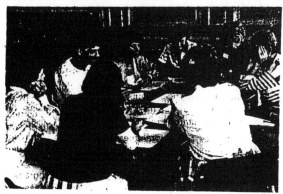

Task-oriented group work at the CSP post-registration education workshop 'Teaching and assessment skills', Loughborough, 1986

Physiotherapy managers may like to consider supporting their staff in the setting up and running of a problem-based programme, and providing them with study time in which to do it. Physiotherapists in Titchen's investigation were more willing to use their own time for CE if their manager allocated time as well.

In addition, physiotherapy managers could reflect on the notion of sharing the tasks described by Graveling (1984), namely those of assessing the training needs of staff, and planning and implementing training. The author proposes that managers move towards the role of overall facilitator, guiding their staff towards a matching of CE and service needs. They may help their staff to identify the gaps in their competencies, but they should allow staff to take responsibility for their own education. If a problem-based approach is to work, the physiotherapy manager must adopt this new role.

Finally, physiotherapy departments that set up a problem-based programme should undertake to write up and publish their programme evaluations, so that other physiotherapists may benefit from their experiences. This may also lead to an increase in resources being invested in CE by employers.

Problem-based learning is an exciting alternative way to enhance competence to practise. The author hopes that physiotherapists will experiment and accept the challenge.

ACKNOWLEDGMENT

The author would like to thank Antoinette Thomas for typing this paper.

REFERENCES

Anderson, J R and Reder, L M (1979). 'An elaborative processing explanation of depth of processing', in: Cormak, L S and Craik, F I M (eds) *Levels of Processing in Human Memory*, Erlbaum, Hillsdale.

Bligh, D A (1972). *What's the Use of Lectures?*, Penguin, Harmondsworth.

Bouhuijs, P A T (1985). 'Planning continuing medical education for general practitioners: A case study from the Netherlands', *Studies in Higher Education*, **10**, 269-275.

Bruner, J S (1960). *The Process of Education*, Harvard University Press, Cambridge, USA.

Chartered Society of Physiotherapy (1983). 'Report of the Review Committee', *Physiotherapy*, **69**, 3, supplement 1-16.

Gray, S (1985). *An Evaluation of the EDURP Pilot Year Care of the Elderly Course*, EDURP, Bristol.

Graveling, B M (1984). 'Post-registration training: The physiotherapy manager's role', *Physiotherapy*, **70**, 5, 189-191.

Knowles, M S (1970). *The Modern Practice of Adult Education: From pedagogy to andragogy*, Cambridge Book Company.

Laxdal, O E (1982). 'Needs assessment in continuing medical education: A practical guide', *Journal of Medical Education*, **57**, 827-834.

McKenzie, J, O'Reilly, D and Stephenson, J (1985). 'Independent

study and professional education', *Studies in Higher Education*, **10**, 187-197.

Richards, R K (1978). *Continuing Medical Education: Perspectives, problems, prognosis*, Yale University Press, London.

Savile, C W (1982). 'Continuing education — A new approach', *Journal of the Royal College of General Practitioners*, **32**, 342-347.

Schmidt, H G (1983). 'Problem-based learning: Rationale and description', *Medical Education*, **17**, 11-16.

Titchen, A C (1983). *Continuing Education: A Study of Physiotherapists' Perceptions, Attitudes and Participation*, MSc dissertation, University of Southampton.

Titchen, A C (1985). 'Innovative continuing education: An in-service model', *Physiotherapy*, **71**, 11, 464-467.

Titchen, A C (1987). 'Continuing education: A study of physiotherapists' attitudes', *Physiotherapy*, **73**, 3, 121-124.

Trent Regional Health Authority (1984). *Towards a strategy for post-registration physiotherapy training*. Unpublished report.

WHO Regional Office for Europe (1977). *Continuing Education of Health Personnel: Report on a Working Group*, IPC/HMD 029, World Health Organisation, Copenhagen.

FURTHER READING

Beckett, C and Wall, M (1985). 'Role of clinical facilitator', *Nurse Education Today*, **5**, 259-262.

Collier, G (1983). *The Management of Peer-group Learning: Syndicate methods in higher education*, Society for Research in Higher Education, University of Surrey, Guildford.

Cox, K R and Ewan, C E (1982). *The Medical Teacher*, Churchill Livingstone, Edinburgh.

Heron, J (1977). *Dimensions of Facilitator Style*, University of Surrey, Guildford.

Keeley-Robinson, Y (1986). 'Teaching adults: Some issues in adult education for health education', *Physiotherapy*, **72**, 1, 49-52.

Knowles, M S (1978). *The Adult Learner: A neglected species*, Gulf Publishing Co, Houston, Texas, USA.

Newble, D and Cannon, R (1983). *A Handbook for Clinical Teachers*, MTP Press Ltd, Lancaster.

Rogers, C (1983). *Freedom to Learn in the 80s*, Charles E Merrill, London.

Rudduck, J (1978). *Learning Through Small Group Discussion*, Society for Research in Higher Education, University of Surrey, Guildford.

RESOURCES

Distance learning course, *Teaching Nurses*, available from the 'Managing Care' series, designed by the Distance Learning Centre, Polytechnic of the South Bank, Manor House, 58 Clapham Common North Side, London SW4 9RZ.

'Adult Education Issues for Health Education' is a review and annotated bibliography written by Yvonne Keeley-Robinson. It is very relevant for physiotherapists who are setting up CE programmes, workshops and courses. The review is available from Yvonne Keeley-Robinson, Health Education Unit, School of Hospitality Management and Home Economics, Leeds Polytechnic, Calverley Street, Leeds LS1 3HE. Copies are free of charge, but requests should be accompanied by a large (A4) SAE: 1 issue 34p, 5 at £1.13, 10 at £1.72, and 20 at £2.30.

CSP post-registration education workshops, run annually in July, are advertised in *Physiotherapy*. There is no fee.

APPENDIX A: Types of Groups

Free discussion: This is not the same as the informal discussion that might occur in the staff room, which is often fairly superficial and annecdotal. It provides learning situations in which the topic and the way of exploring it are determined by the group members. The basic principle is to place the resources available within the group at the disposal of all the individuals within it. The group must feel that everyone's needs count. This method enables people to learn how to work together and become aware of their strengths and weaknesses, and their roles and responsibilities within the group.

Peer-group teaching: A member of the group has expertise in a particular area which she shares with the group by presentation, perhaps with audio-visual aids and demonstration. The peer-group and facilitator provide feed-back to the presenter.

Task-oriented or syndicate work: This can involve many different types of activity over a short or long-term. For example, a specialist may set practical problems for the group members to work on. They

Combined Clinical Visits and Regional Continuing Education for Clinical Instructors

Bella J May, EdD, PT, FAPTA
Harold G Smith, EdD, PT
Jancis K Dennis, MAppSci, PT

ABSTRACT: The academic coordinators of clinical education of the Medical College of Georgia regionalized clinical visits and presented continuing education programs for clinical instructor development in response to increasing numbers of clinics and students and decreasing travel budgets. We visit all affiliating clinical facilities in one geographic area during the same trip and present a clinical instructor development program on one or more evenings. One of the local center coordinators of clinical education provides the needed meeting and audiovisual support and responds to local questions. We invite practitioners within 2 hours driving time of the meeting. The system has been used since 1989, and 18 continuing education programs have been presented to date. All have been very well-received. The system has allowed us to visit more facilities with the same budgetary allocation and to reach about 436 therapists in clinical education-oriented programs.

INTRODUCTION

Academic coordinators of clinical education (ACCEs) must communicate effectively with center coordinators of clinical education (CCCEs) to properly administer the clinical education program. Written correspondence, telephone contact, and personal visits are used to share information and resolve clinical placement problems. The importance of personal communications between education programs and clinical facilities, the value of clinical visits both for new and established

Dr May is Professor and CoACCE, Department of Physical Therapy, School of Allied Health Sciences, Medical College of Georgia, Augusta, GA 30912. Dr Smith is Associate Professor and CoACCE, Department of Physical Therapy, School of Allied Health Sciences, Medical College of Georgia. Ms Dennis is Associate Professor and Director, Center for the Study of Physical Therapy Education, Department of Physical Therapy, School of Allied Health Sciences, Medical College of Georgia. She was CoACCE when the described program was initiated. This article was adapted from a poster presented at the American Physical Therapy Association Combined Sections Meeting, San Francisco, CA, February 1992.

clinical sites, and the need for clinical instructor development has been well-supported in the literature.[1-5] The system described in this article is based on the philosophy that it is the responsibility of the ACCE to maintain close contact with each CCCE, to be familiar with each clinical site, and to contribute to development of clinical instructors.

MEDICAL COLLEGE OF GEORGIA CLINICAL EDUCATION PROGRAM

The Medical College of Georgia is a state-supported health sciences university. The Physical Therapy Department has three education programs: an associate (AS) degree program for physical therapist assistants, with 18 students; a baccalaureate (BS) degree program for physical therapists, with 80 students; and a master's in health education (MHE) degree with 4 to 6 students attending part time. The two entry-level programs integrate clinical experiences and academic courses throughout the curriculum. Graduate clinical experiences are individually scheduled for each student.

The AS degree program has four clinical courses, the BS degree program has six, and the master's degree program has two courses. The ACCEs schedule approximately 100 different students into 12 clinical courses each year. The Medical College has clinical education agreements with 180 clinical sites, located primarily but not solely within the southeastern United States.

Background

Until the early 1980s, ACCEs scheduled clinical site visits each time a student was assigned to a long-term (4- to 6-week) clinical affiliation. This process proved expensive and time consuming and was revised to include a personal visit to each clinical site when first developed, once every 2 years after that, and when a student was affiliating. Depending on the distance between clinics, this meant an ACCE could visit one or

maybe two facilities in one day and spent considerable time traveling between locations because not all facilities in one locale necessarily had students scheduled at the same time.

Over the years, the ACCEs used several different methods to provide for clinical faculty development. Included were week-long and weekend courses, in-services while on clinical visits, recommending attendance at national conferences, consortium meetings with other schools of physical therapy education programs, and one-on-one mentorship. Each of these methods had varying degrees of success, but in recent years attendance at week-long and weekend continuing education courses on clinical education decreased; the last scheduled program of the Georgia Consortium for Clinical Education was canceled for lack of attendance.

Problems

Several factors led the ACCEs to review the clinical education program and, in 1988, the following specific problems were identified:

1. The cost of travel was increasing while our travel budget was decreasing.

2. The number of students in each class was increasing, leading to a greater number of clinical placements.

3. ACCE classroom teaching loads were increasing; thus decreasing the time available for clinical travel.

4. Many clinical instructors were young, relatively inexperienced clinicians with little or no background in clinical education.

We reviewed our philosophy of clinical education and decided that the major purposes of the clinical visit were (1) the interchange of information between the ACCE and the CCCE; (2) the opportunity to explore philosophies of education; (3) the ability to see the clinical facilities firsthand; interact with the director and other staff members; and gain information on ambiance, patient care activities, and interest in clinical education; and (4) the opportunity to provide some clinical instructor development. Routinely visiting students while on clinical affiliation was less important because faculty advisors telephone each clinical instructor (CI) right after mid-evaluation to ascertain the student's progress and respond to any issues or questions. These calls are made for each long-term clinical affiliation.

The ACCEs designed a system that organized clinical facilities into geographic regions and developed a travel schedule where all affiliating sites in a geographic region were visited on one trip. Overnight stays were arranged in communities with several clinical facilities whenever possible so that a continuing education program, relevant to clinical education, was presented at night. This system has proven to be both cost-effective and educationally effective.

METHOD
Planning Clinical Visits

The sequence of activities involved in planning regionalized clinical visits is outlined in Figure 1. Clinical visits for the academic year are planned in the fall. The computer generates a list of (a) facilities that have not been visited for at least 2 years; (b) newly developed facilities that have never been visited; and (c) any facilities identified as needing to be visited for any reason. A facility may need to be visited if there have been major staff changes or if assigned students report some problems. The listed facilities are prioritized, with frequently used clinics or those identified as needing a special visit having a higher priority than those used less often. The facilities are grouped geographically, and tentative travel schedules are developed. Early consultation with our travel agent and detailed study of state and city maps are very helpful in deciding the best sequence from city to city.

One of the more difficult aspects of scheduling clinical visits is determining how much time is needed for each facility. Two visits usually are scheduled each day; three may be scheduled if the facilities are close together and not large. Our experience indicates that we need about 2 hours to visit the average facility if no student is present, and 3 hours if a student is affiliating. More time is allocated if there is more than one student in the facility or if it is a large, multi-program institution. We try to arrange the schedule to maximize visit time and minimize travel time, although we have a number of facilities in small towns or rural areas. We sometimes use a large community as a hub, making day trips to more remote sites and returning each

FIGURE 1
Selecting facilities to visit.

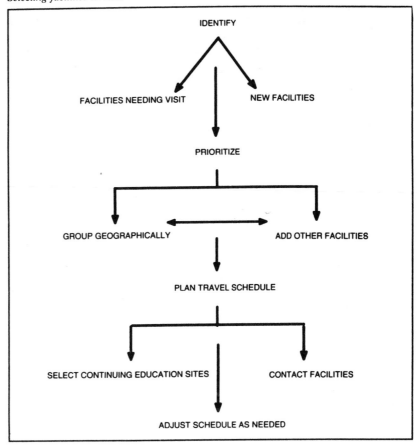

night. This allows us to combine flying and driving for better time efficiency.

Because the clinical visit no longer is tied to the student's presence in the clinic, it can be scheduled at any time during the academic year. Visits are made in late fall and mid spring and occasionally in late summer according to the ACCEs' teaching schedules. We limit a visit sequence to one week because paying per diem costs over a weekend is not efficient. Generally we have been able to schedule from 9 to 12 visits in a week, depending on the distance between major locations. The travel schedule has benefited from our policy of developing new facilities only in areas where we already have affiliating facilities. Obviously, some facilities are close enough to Augusta to be visited in one day without an overnight stay. Local facilities also are visited once every 2 years. After a tentative schedule has been developed, the clinical facilities are contacted to ensure that the day and time of the visit is convenient. Scheduling several visits in one locale gives us some flexibility, and CCCEs have been most cooperative with our logistical efforts.

Planning Continuing Education Programs

Visiting several facilities in an area requires an overnight stay, so we plan the continuing education program for a convenient evening. The sequence of planning activities is outlined in Figure 2 and begins 6 to 8 weeks before the actual trip. We ask one of the CCCEs to host the program and to arrange the exact time by local convenience. Most programs are scheduled from 5:30 to 7:30 PM. We prepare a flyer announcing the program and send it to all affiliating facilities within 100 to 150 miles of the location. We also encourage the host CCCE to send flyers to other facilities and practitioners with an interest in clinical education. Participants are not limited to physical therapists or physical therapist assistants; occupational therapists, occupational therapy assistants, and other health professionals have attended. The host CCCE serves as the local contact and provides the meeting place, refreshments, and audiovisual support. Sometimes a local vendor supplies refreshments.

Continuing Education Program

The first program developed was entitled "Teaching Clinical Decision Making in the Clinic (Fig. 3). The emphasis is on the role of the CI in planning the learning experience, clinical teaching strategies, and the use of stimulus questions. Stimulus questions can best be answered by explanation, discussion, justification, or amplification. They are used to guide learning in a particular direction, to help the learner discover salient data, and to make links between pieces of information to form a clinical picture. Handouts accompany the program and provide a reference for future use. Participants are encouraged to raise questions or items for discussion. The formal presentation takes about 1½ hours, depending on the extent of participant interaction; we try to allow about ½ hour of open discussion on topics of interest to the audience. The Medical College of Georgia sends certificates of attendance to each participant. Both ACCEs have been presenting the same program; a second program entitled "Working with the Exceptional Student" is in development and clinical facilities will be given a choice of programs in the future.

Program Evaluations

"Teaching Clinical Decision Making in the Clinic" has been presented 18 times since 1989 to audiences ranging in size from 12 to 60. Evaluations have been very positive, with

Figure 2

Planning the continuing education program.

    I. Select Host Facility
        A. Provide appropriate meeting room
        B. Provide audiovisual support
        C. Serve as contact person for local
           facilities
        D. Provide refreshments
        E. Copy handouts
   II. Select Program Time with Host
       Facility
        A. Schedule to meet local needs
        B. Consider driving distances
  III. Develop and Disseminate Flyer
        A. Master flyer in the computer
        B. Fill in time, place, and contact
           person
        C. Send to all contract clinics within
           150 miles
   IV. Implement Program
    V. Return from Trip
        A. Review program evaluations
        B. Send certificates of attendance
        C. Thank-you letter to host center
           coordinator of clinical education.

both new and experienced CIs commenting on the value of the program, the benefit of having an opportunity to discuss problems with other CIs, and the value of the handouts. Some program areas most often cited as most valuable included presentation of stimulus questions, discussion of different teaching strategies for use in the clinic, discussion of specific student issues, learning the difference between novices and experts, and the handouts for future reference.

Other frequent positive comments included: "The time of day was good for this program (5:00 PM)," "I understand more how to create a positive environment for learning," "Realized the importance of guiding the student versus giving answers," "It [the program] allows discussion between facilities in the community," and "Learning the progression from novice to expert was helpful."

There also were some suggestions for improving the program: "Participant interaction is sometimes hard to follow," "The teaching and planning suggestions seem rather ideal," "There was not enough time for the content," and "There was too much audience participation."

BENEFITS

One of the major benefits is the opportunity for CI development to a large number of CIs. A 2-hour program is more effective than a 30-minute lunchtime inservice squeezed in during a clinical visit. The program is free and attendance requires little traveling for most CIs. It provides an opportunity for recent graduates to learn about clinical education before being involved with students and allows uninterrupted time for discussion and explorations of issues. The evening continuing education program also provides an opportunity for the Medical College of Georgia to do something for the clinical facilities and creates a positive image of our educational institution. It also helps validate our valuing of the clinical education program and of the importance of CIs in the total preparation of students.

Evening programs allow for interchange between the staff of different facilities in the community and have led to some networking. One program was reported to have become the catalyst for the eventual development of a clinical education consortium. The discussions encourage interaction between academic and clinical faculty and between experienced and new CIs. Inviting all facilities in an area has led to the establishment of new clinical facilities. This is important as we strive to cluster our clinical facilities geographically for financial reasons.

Figure 3

Teaching clinical decision making in the clinic: program outline.

    I. Introduction
        A. The Medical College of Georgia
           Physical Therapist/Physical
           Therapist Assistant Curriculum
           1. Philosophy of education
           2. Sequence of learning activities
           3. Integration of clinical courses
   II. Role of Clinical Education
        A. Integral part of total education
           program
        B. Provide application experiences
        C. Professional socialization
        D. Illustrate the breadth of the
           profession
        E. Interaction between clinic and
           academe
  III. Clinical Decision Making
        A. The decision-making process
        B. Characteristics of an expert
           decision maker
        C. Characteristics of a novice
           decision maker
        D. Developing clinical expertise
   IV. Educational Implications
        A. Characteristics of the adult learner
        B. Structuring the clinical learning
           experience
        C. Teaching/learning strategies
        D. Use of stimulus questions
        E. Assessing decision-making skills
    V. Issues in Clinical Education

Initially, we only invited facilities in the immediate area but found that some CIs were willing to drive up to 2 hours to attend the program. Now we send flyers to facilities as far as 150 miles and have had good attendance from the more distant clinics. The value of the program was summarized by one participant who wrote on the evaluation, "Regional continuing education programs are very valuable as they are more readily available for a greater number of people."

Financially it is difficult to determine the impact of the regional visits or the continuing education program, because our financial resources and travel costs have changed in the last several years and accurate records of clinics visited were not kept until we started the computer data base in 1990.[6] In the 1990–1991 academic year, the second year of regional visits, we visited 65 facilities; during the 1991–1992 academic year, we either have visited or plan to visit 56 facilities on a budget that is 50% smaller.

There are no records of inservices that may have been presented for individual facilities before the 1989–1990 academic year. During the 1989–1990 academic year, we presented six continuing education programs to approximately 95 participants. In the 1990–1991 academic year, we presented six programs to 145 participants, and for the current academic year (1991–1992) we have presented six programs to 196 participants and plan to present five additional programs.

LIMITATIONS

The major limitation is the short time span for the program and the demands on the traveling ACCE. Depending on the number of different regions visited in one trip, the ACCE may present two or three programs in a week and visit 8 to 12 facilities. This can be very tiring, and travel arrangements sometimes can be difficult. The only costs of the continuing education program are the hand-

outs, overheads, and postage. In many instances, original handouts can be sent to the host CCCE, who can provide the needed copies. Travel costs are the same because the ACCE must spend the night regardless of whether a continuing education program is given. The other difficulty is scheduling a program at a time and place that is convenient to all facilities being visited. We have some excellent facilities that are more than 150 miles from other facilities.

The regional continuing education programs are not designed to eliminate the longer weekend program we schedule every other year either alone or with some other education programs in Georgia. The regional programs supplement and enhance our total CI development activities.

REFERENCES

1. Moore ML, Perry JF. *Clinical Education in Physical Therapy: Present Status/Future Needs.* Washington DC: American Physical Therapy Association, Section for Education; 1976.
2. *Leadership for Change in Physical Therapy Clinical Education.* Washington DC: American Physical Therapy Association, Department of Education; March 1986.
3. Perry JF. Who is responsible for preparing clinical educators. In: *Pivotal Issues in Clinical Education: Present Status/Future Needs.* Washington DC: American Physical Therapy Association, Section for Education; 1988:22–31.
4. Deusinger SS, Cornbleet SL, Stith JS. Using assessment centers to promote clinical faculty development. *Journal of Physical Therapy Education.* 1991; 5:18–23.
5. Gwyer J. Resources for clinical education: current status and future challenges. *Journal of Physical Therapy Education.* 1990; 4:55–58.
6. Dennis JK, May BJ. Computer-assisted student clinical placements. *Journal of Physical Therapy Education.* 1990; 4:87–92.

Faculty Status for Clinician–Educators: Guidelines for Evaluation and Promotion

Michael B. Jacobs, MD

By 1989, at least 74% of our 126 U.S. medical schools had separate clinician-educator tracks, almost all of which were formal, full-time, salaried, nontenure-track appointments for physician faculty primarily engaged in patient care and teaching.[1,2] Many of these were created recently; more are soon to follow. Explicit and widely accepted criteria by which these faculty can be judged for appointment and promotion have yet to be defined and disseminated. The purpose of the present document is to begin a process of consensus building about these criteria by crafting a statement reflective of the collective aspirations of clinician-educators and endorsed by academic leadership. In so doing, a pivotal question must be addressed; how should faculty spend their time? The answer will depend on the faculty reward system in place. Moreover, if appointments and promotions are to require scholarship, how is this to be defined? I hope that this document will foster debate on these ques-

tions. Out of such broad discussions among university faculty, meaningful evaluation guidelines and policy decisions can emerge.

SURVEY

To draft a statement that would be representative of and responsive to the concerns of clinician-educators at other academic institutions, I mailed a questionnaire to the chiefs of divisions of general medicine at 133 medical centers (identified through the Society of General Internal Medicine Central Office). The purpose was to assess how these physicians spend their time and how they are evaluated. From this informal survey, several points emerge. First, separate clinician-educator faculty tracks are prevalent at our teaching institutions. Among the institutions represented in the survey, 73 (83%) had faculty clinician-educators, two-thirds of whom occupied a separate academic track distinct from the

tenure-line faculty. Second, scholarship is typically considered necessary for promotion in these tracks; in three-fourths of the responding institutions it was required for promotion. Third, there is little time free from patient care commitments for clinician-educators to engage in research or written scholarship. Only one-fourth of the institutions provided three or more half-days free for scholarship, yet three-fourths of the division chiefs indicted that at least three half-days would be necessary to make a meaningful scholarly contribution. Finally, there is a need not only for widely accepted criteria by which clinician-educators may be fairly evaluated but also for a reconsideration of how scholarship is defined.

Given this need for both explicit evaluation criteria and a broader, more explicit definition of scholarship, I formulated a set of guidelines, presented below. These are based on results from (1) a small-group session–Academic Promotion for Clinician Teachers: Developing a Na-

Reprinted with permission from *Academic Medicine*. Jacobs MB. 1993;68(2):126-128.

tional Strategy — at a 1991 national meeting of the Society of General Internal Medicine (SGIM), (2) written feedback from 17 newly appointed clinician-educators in the Stanford Medical Center Professoriate, (3) discussions with selected Stanford University and SGIM leadership, and (4) a review of the relevant literature.

PROPOSED GUIDELINES

Scholarship constitutes the cornerstone of the guidelines for evaluation and promotion of clinician–educators. Accorded a broader definition, scholarship should be a requirement for promotion. This new, expanded definition[3] should include

1. The Scholarship of Application, i.e., building bridges between theory and practice, applying knowledge to consequential problems
2. The Scholarship of Teaching, i.e., communicating knowledge, inspiring trainees, transforming the difficult-to-understand to the easy-to-assimilate
3. The Scholarship of Integration, i.e., creative synthesis or analysis, looking for connections across disciplines, bringing new insights to bear on original research, "horizontal" scholarship
4. The Scholarship of Discovery, i.e., the elucidation of new knowledge, research in its traditional sense, "vertical" scholarship

Regardless of the type of scholarship used to judge the clinician–educator, it should satisfy two criteria: first, excellence, and second, the capability for review by peers and dissemination in the public domain. Examples of activities rightfully considered scholarly and suggested means of evaluating their quality follow. The degree of detail is not meant to be all-inclusive or prescriptive; rather it is intended to begin the process of defining a practical evaluation scheme and one that lends itself to peer review.

The Scholarship of Application

The best example of this type of scholarship is the scientific practice of clinical medicine. A method of evaluation could include the selection of an ad hoc committee on clinical excellence (for example, composed of senior clinicians, head nurses, and a social worker)[4] that would assess clinical, communication, and interpersonal skills; availability; and humanistic qualities. A clinical portfolio could be

created and might include a patient questionnaire (to judge counseling skills and overall patient satisfaction) and a review of a sampling of charts (to judge diagnostic, therapeutic, and monitoring strategies). Clinical care awards and the intensity of clinical activity could also be considered.

The Scholarship of Teaching

Examples of teaching scholarship include education in any setting (bedside to classroom) but in addition encompass a variety of other activities: for example, developing a new and innovative course, shaping a core curriculum, or creating educational software or video cassettes. Evaluation might include the contemporaneous compilation of a teaching portfolio[5-7] composed of a description of the faculty member's teaching environment and responsibilities; examples of course outlines, syllabi, and annotated bibliographies; and outside evaluations from learners at all levels (students to peers). In addition, there should be an ad hoc "clinician–educator" committee to observe teaching (ideally against a set of explicit criteria) and to review the teaching portfolio. Teaching awards and teaching intensity could also be considered.

The Scholarship of Integration

Examples of this type of scholarship include the publication of subject reviews, editorials, chapters, and popular writing. Evaluation could involve the use of existing standards and procedures for assessing written work by peer review.

The Scholarship of Discovery

Examples of this type of more traditional scholarship include research in medical education, epidemiology, decision analysis, social sciences, ethics, and resource utilization. Evaluation could involve usual and existing criteria for assessing the quality of original research by a panel of peers.

PRINCIPLES OF APPLICATION

In applying this concept of an expanded definition of scholarship to promotion decisions, several fundamental principles should be honored. Diversity among a university faculty should be encouraged. We should not insist on identical activities and accomplishments for all faculty. Diversity of institutional, departmental,

and division missions requires diversity of faculty.[2,3] Thus, some clinical–educators may be largely evaluated on their Scholarship of Application and Teaching and others on their Scholarship of Application and Integration, for example. At all times, scholarship would be a criterion for evaluation.

Although the emphasis operating in the evaluation may depend upon the institution, the department, the individual, and his or her career stage, I suggest that clinician–educators be evaluated under the following point system: A weighted importance of 3 each should be given to the Scholarship of Application and the Scholarship of Teaching, while a weighted importance of 2 each should be given to the Scholarship of Integration and the Scholarship of Discovery. In this manner the relative importances of the different types of scholarship would be emphasized and thus the success of this faculty line ensured. I would further propose that reappointment as an assistant professor would require a minimum score of 6, promotion to an associate professorship a minimum score of 7 as well as evidence of regional activities (beyond the candidate's parent institution), and promotion to a professorship a minimum score of 8 with evidence of some national activities. This type of scoring requirement thus acknowledges that for promotion to more senior faculty ranks, outstanding clinicians and teachers should be expected to share their knowledge, expertise, and special talents beyond their own institutions.

There are two other fundamental principles that should be operative. Specific criteria for evaluation should be both discipline-determined and institution-determined and should reflect each institution's unique history, culture, mission, and environment.[2] Finally, individual performance should be judged in the context of resources and time made available to the faculty member. This fact should be explicitly stated at the time of initial appointment and at all subsequent performance reviews.[3]

CONCLUSION

The evaluation scheme proposed here is meant to serve as a framework only. It is not intended to be interpreted rigidly; rather, its strength lies in its flexibility. It is expected that institution to institution, department to department, and perhaps even division to division and individual to individual, there will be modifications or "subweights" applied to activities within each category. In that way academic medical centers, their subunits, and their individual faculty members will be able both to explicitly define their goals and activities and to have a means of assessing them.

Dr. Jacobs is professor of medicine and head, Section on Primary Care Medicine, Stanford University School of Medicine, Stanford, California.

Correspondence and requests for reprints should be addressed to Dr. Jacobs, Section on Primary Care Medicine, Stanford University School of Medicine, 300 Pasteur Drive, A381, Stanford, CA 94305.

References

1. Jones, R. F. Clinician–Educator Faculty Tracks in U.S. Medical Schools. *J. Med. Educ.* **62**(1987):444–447.
2. Bickel, J. The Changing Face of Promotion and Tenure at U.S. Medical Schools. *Acad. Med.* **66**(1991):249–256.
3. Boyer, E. L. *Scholarship Reconsidered: Priorities of the Professoriate.* [The Carnegie Foundation for the Advancement of Teaching.] Princeton, New Jersey: Princeton University Press, 1990.
4. Ramsey, P. G., Carline, J. D., Inui, T. S., Larson, E. B., LoGerfo, J. P., and Wenrich, M. D. Predictive Validity of Certification by the American Board of Internal Medicine. *Ann. Intern. Med.* **110**(1989):710–726.
5. Edgerton, R., Hutchings, P., and Quinlan, K. *The Teaching Portfolio: Capturing the Scholarship in Teaching.* Washington, D.C.: American Association for Higher Education, 1991.
6. Wolfe, K. *The School Teacher's Portfolio: Practical Issues in Design, Implementation, and Evaluation.* [Teacher Assessment Project, School of Education. Stanford, California: Stanford University, 1991.
7. Shulman, L. S. A Union of Insufficiencies: Strategies for Teacher Assessment in a Period of Educational Reform. *Educ. Leadership* **46**(November 1988):36–46.

FACULTY PERSPECTIVES OF A VALID AND RELIABLE CLINICAL TUTOR EVALUATION PROGRAM

P. J. McLEOD
*McGill University and
Montreal General Hospital*

Evaluation of clinical tutors by students is potentially useful for tutor feedback and to assist administrators in decisions about tenure and promotion. At most universities, there has been inadequate attention paid to clinical tutor evaluation. McGill University in Canada designed an evaluation system adhering rigidly to accepted psychometric standards of reliability and validity and has used it successfully for the past 5 years. When researchers investigated its credibility with McGill tutors, they found significant ambivalence and some hostility toward the process. Apparently, these tutors are suspicious of the credibility of student ratings of their teaching skills. Part of the explanation for this lies in their own self-doubts as reflected in lower self-ratings. Much of the ambivalence relates to lack of recognition of clinical teaching by administrators and lack of impact of teaching evaluations on promotion and tenure decisions.

EVALUATION & THE HEALTH PROFESSIONS, Vol. 14 No. 3, September 1991 333-342
© 1991 Sage Publications, Inc.

Medical educators have long recognized the usefulness of student evaluations of their teachers. Much of the education literature deals with evaluation of teachers in lecture and large group settings, but tutor evaluation in the clinical setting differs from that done in other settings (Jolly & MacDonald, 1987) in that clinical instruction involves multiple instructors and a small number of students (Irby, 1978). Since no consensus has emerged on how to accurately identify the best clinical tutors (Fallon, Groen, & Shilow, 1985), it is not surprising that evaluations of clinical tutors have not been actively studied. Nor have the results been widely accepted for use in promotion and tenure decisions. It is understandable if clinical tutors are skeptical about the results of evaluation of their teaching and reluctant to invest valuable time and energy in an activity if it has little formal recognition by administrators.

In 1984, we felt the need for formal clinical tutor evaluation in our department and set out to establish a system that would have credibility among our tutors and administrators. To enhance the likelihood of its acceptance, we sought to assure rigid standards of reliability, validity, generalizability, and durability (Rippey, 1981). This report outlines the features of our evaluation system and compares tutor self-evaluation with student evaluation, using our ratings questionnaire. It also outlines the results of an attitude survey of the undergraduate clinical tutors who have been regularly evaluated over the past 5 years.

METHOD

In 1984, we developed a clinical tutor rating form based on the tutor self-assessment inventory used at the University of Washington (Irby & Rakestraw, 1981). The form was modified following consultation with all active clinical tutors at our hospital and with educators at the McGill Centre for Medical Education and was pilot-tested for a year. After minor modifications, we put into use a questionnaire form containing 25 items, each listed as a statement reflecting a single descriptive teaching characteristic which a student could be expected to validly observe (see appendix). These 25 items reflect seven dimensions of teaching effectiveness: attitude to teaching (Items 1, 11, 17, 22, and

25), humanistic orientation (Items 2, 8, and 14), perceived subject matter expertise (Items 3, 9, and 13), teaching skills (Items 4, 10, 12, 18, and 19), problem-solving emphasis (Items 5, 21, and 24), student-centered teaching strategy (Items 7, 15, and 23), and active student participation (Items 6, 16, and 20). Students rate each of the 25 items on a 6-point scale, with descriptors ranging from *very strongly agree* to *very strongly disagree*. For tutor feedback, each item is categorized with others reflecting the same teaching dimension, so tutors receive an individual "profile" of their strengths and weaknesses (Mulholland, 1988).

Since 1985, all tutors in a 10-week undergraduate clinical course in internal medicine have been regularly evaluated by students in their clinical tutorial groups. Of the 35 individuals active in this course a core group of 15 do most of the teaching and all have been evaluated on at least five occasions since the study began. On average, each tutor has been evaluated by 50 students over the 5-year period. Analysis of those evaluations using principal components factor analysis revealed that students reliably differentiate between the teaching abilities and the personality characteristics of their tutors. Comparison of between-student tutor evaluations using the Wilcox rank sum statistic showed that students predictably evaluate tutors over time, with between-tutor differences being highly significant ($p < .008$). Details of the reliability studies have been submitted for publication elsewhere. We are assured of reasonable validity of the evaluation instrument by the expert input judgments contributing to the evaluation format and by the long-term stability of the evaluations. Furthermore, the factor analysis indicating that students are discriminating judges of teaching skills strongly supports the instrument's validity.

Having convinced ourselves and the administrators that we had developed a valid and reliable tutor evaluation system, we decided, after 5 years of experience with it, to assess how the faculty view the process and the information it provides. To do so, we developed a seven-item closed-response questionnaire, with questions related to the usefulness of the assessment results, the impact of the assessments on tutor teaching practices, and the usefulness of breaking down the dimensions of teaching effectiveness into seven categories. We also questioned tutors about what use should be made of the assessments after they are received in the teaching office. Respondents indicated their agreement or disagreement by checking yes or no, respectively, for each question. Finally, the questionnaire included an open-ended section requesting comments and suggestions. Each mailed questionnaire was accompanied by a clinical tutor evaluation from (see appendix) and a request that each do a candid self-evaluation of his or her own teaching skills by rating the 25 items on the form using the 6-point scale.

To compare student and self ratings of the teaching effectiveness of each tutor, the average global evaluation received by each over 5 years' time was compared with the global rating that each gave him- or herself. Similarly, comparisons were made between student and self evaluations in each of the seven dimensions of teaching effectiveness. In both cases, a paired t test was used to compare differences. The Kruskall-Wallis test was used to compare tutor rankings among their peers as derived from student and self ratings.

RESULTS

Of the 35 active undergraduate clinical tutors, 24 (71%) returned completed questionnaires, and all were suitable for analysis. Eighteen completed the self-evaluation form. Table 1 outlines the respondents' agreement or disagreement with the seven closed-response statements on the questionnaire. It is apparent that many feel that evaluation results are useful and should be used in promotion and tenure decisions, but most would be reluctant to have the results made public. Although many agree that the seven teaching categories appropriately represent the important dimensions of clinical teaching, only 13 of the 24 agreed that the categorization is useful to them. Only half felt that feedback from the students during the 5 years of study has led to a change in the way they teach, and only 11 of the 24 agreed that the ratings accurately reflect their teaching skills.

The disquieting ambivalence apparent in the closed-response section of the tutor questionnaire was more apparent in the comments section. Nearly all respondents wrote comments. Although the language used was subtle and not overly critical, widespread negativity

TABLE 1
Clinical Tutor Responses to Questionnaire Statements Regarding Student Ratings of Their Teaching Skills

Questionnaire Statement	Number of Tutors Agreeing or Disagreeing	
	Agree	Disagree
Results of student evaluations are useful to me.	20	4
Results of student evaluations of tutors should be used in promotion and tenure decisions.	20	4
Results of student evaluations of tutors should be made public.	5	19
The seven categories of teaching indicated on the rating form are representative of the important dimensions of clinical teaching.	23	1
The breakdown of teaching skills into seven categories is useful in my teaching.	13	11
The results of student evaluations of my teaching have led me to change the way I teach.	12	12
Student ratings accurately reflect my teaching skills.	11	13

of attitudes was easily discernible. Comments such as "The rating system emphasizes personality and approachability and may not reflect my teaching skills" and "The evaluations are popularity contests! A pleasant dumb teacher may get better evaluations than a demanding smart teacher!" were common. One tutor felt that the ratings categories are "vague with significant overlap"; another said that it is common for "student and resident evaluations to miss obvious weaknesses of the tutors." The most common theme involved the use or nonuse of the evaluations by the administrators. Many indicated that there is a difference between the policies and the practices of university administrators when deciding on the value of clinical teaching. One respondent's comment reflected the feeling of many: "Academic promotion should be available to clinician-teachers as much as to clinician-researchers."

Comparison between the global rating that each of the 18 tutors accorded him- or herself and the average global rating that each

TABLE 2
Average Student Rating of Tutors, by
Teaching Dimension, and Average Tutor Self-Rating, by Dimension

Teaching Dimension	Average Tutor Rating (±SD) by Students Over 5 Years	Average Tutor Self-Rating (±SD)
1. Attitude to teaching	5.22 (±.36)	4.86 (±.65)
2. Humanistic orientation	5.19 (±.31)	4.96 (±.57)
3. Perceived subject matter expertise	4.94 (±.47)	4.57 (±.64)
4. Teaching skills	5.09 (±.33)	4.51 (±.53)
5. Problem-solving emphasis	5.23 (±.39)	4.77 (±.71)
6. Student-centered teaching strategy	5.29 (±.28)	4.67 (±.66)
7. Active student participation	5.19 (±.35)	4.61 (±.68)

received from the students over the 5-year period of the study showed that 3 tutors rated themselves higher than did the students and 2 gave themselves an identical rating; the other 13 rated themselves lower than did the students. The differences were statistically significant ($p < .002$). Table 2 outlines the average tutor rating over the 5 years in each of the seven teaching dimension categories compared to the rating in each category from the self-evaluation. For each of the five categories which predominantly reflect clinical teaching skills (Categories 3 through 7), students evaluated tutors more favorably than tutors rated themselves (p value range: .001-.04). For items in the "personality categories" (attitude toward teaching and humanistic orientation), there were no significant differences between student and self ratings ($ps < .06$ and $.19$).

Comparison of student ratings of their tutors over the 5 study years using the Kruskall-Wallis statistic revealed that different students rated tutors consistently in repeated evaluations ($p < .008$). Ranking of tutors compared to their peers was therefore highly predictable. An attempt to correlate these rankings with how tutors evaluated themselves showed no significant relationship. That is, the tutors' perceptions of how their teaching is valued compared to that of their peers are at variance with what students feel. Furthermore, whether or not the variance will be positive or negative cannot be predicted for an individual tutor.

DISCUSSION

Having satisfied ourselves that we had in place a clinical tutor evaluation system that is valid and reliable, we assumed that it would be heartily embraced by our clinical tutors. We were therefore dismayed at the ambivalence which teachers showed toward the usefulness of the system after 5 years of its use. Fewer than half feel that the students' ratings accurately reflect their teaching skills, and there was limited evidence that the evaluation results led to any changes in teaching practices. Some of the lukewarm questionnaire responses, such as "The results are useful in a limited way," imply that respondents are unenthusiastic but are reluctant to downplay the efforts of the evaluation organizers.

We were less surprised that almost 70% of teachers rate themselves lower than do students, although it is surprising that tutors rate their own personality-related teaching characteristics more highly than they do those practices reflecting their pedagogic skills. Perhaps there are self-doubts about teaching effectiveness related to a lack of formal education in how to teach. Widespread reluctance to have evaluation results made public may also reflect self-doubts. Of course, there are precedents for lower self-ratings than those given by other evaluators. Studies comparing self- and supervisor evaluations among trainees often indicate a lack of congruence between the two sets of ratings (Kolm & Verhulst, 1987), and students often rate themselves lower than do tutors (Morton & MacBeth, 1977). In a recent study, students' global ratings of their instructors were higher than the instructors gave themselves (Fallon, Groen, & Shelov, 1987).

There appear to be numerous reasons for the tutors' lack of enthusiasm for our evaluation system. Among these is the feeling that the evaluations are popularity contests reflecting the instructor's wit and personality more than his or her teaching skills. Our study and others (Abrami, Leventhal, & Perry, 1982; Marsh & Ware, 1982) showed that personality and "expressiveness" matter but not independently of content considerations. This message must be more forcefully transmitted to our teachers. Tutors' self-doubts and concerns about comparing unfavorably to their peers probably play a role. The perceptions that students' ratings probably miss some weaknesses and that feedback has little impact on teaching practices may also contribute. In all likelihood, the major cause of tutors' ambivalence is their skepticism about the impact of evaluation results on the chances of academic recognition and promotion. Perhaps many of our clinical tutors feel like those at another North American medical school — "disenfranchised relative to established educational policies" and convinced that the administration's activities relative to undergraduate teaching are "arbitrary and ill-informed" (Rothman & Cleave-Hogg, 1990, p. 19).

Although the evaluation system is educationally and statistically sound, the finding that large numbers of the clinical teaching faculty do not give it credence means that the process must be changed. It would make no sense for us to abandon clinical tutor evaluation, as students' attitudes toward their instructors are a vital factor in the total learning situation. The first step in our attempt to improve its credibility will be to provide more detailed personal explanation of the evaluation results, as tutors may not correctly interpret them (Baggott, 1987). Second, a valuable way to involve the tutors in the entire educational process and to enhance their confidence is to insist on attendance at faculty development courses specifically designed for clinical tutors. Finally, we must continue to pursue the tutors' concerns about linking clinical teaching success with academic promotion. There is evidence that McGill is leaning in that direction, and there are encouraging signs from elsewhere (Rothman, Poldre, & Cohen, 1989). Not until clinical teaching and student evaluation of clinical teaching have a significant impact on promotion and tenure can we expect to have more than limited credibility of our evaluation system. In short, psychometric "purity" alone cannot assure the success of a clinical tutor evaluation system.

APPENDIX
Clinical Tutor Evaluation

1. Is enthusiastic and stimulating
2. Seems interested in social and psychological aspects of illness
3. Inspires confidence in his/her knowledge of subject
4. Emphasizes concepts rather than factual recall
5. Poses problems for me to solve
6. Provides opportunity for discussion
7. Encourages me to think
8. Attitudes to patients fit my concept of professional behavior
9. Occasionally challenges points presented in texts and journals
10. Is usually well prepared for teaching session
11. Conveys enjoyment of associating with me and my colleagues
12. Provides feedback and direction
13. Displays good judgment in decision making
14. Deals with colleagues and staff in a friendly manner
15. Teaching is suited to my level of sophistication
16. Invites comments rather than providing all the answers
17. Is interested in helping students to learn
18. Presents divergent viewpoints for contrast and comparison
19. Is clear and understandable in explanations
20. Encourages me to ask questions
21. Emphasizes problem-solving approach rather than solutions per se
22. Dependability of attendance is good
23. Encourages me to take responsibility for my own learning
24. Emphasizes clinical skills, not lab tests for patient management
25. Is usually readily available for discussion

NOTE: Each of the 25 evaluation items was rated on a 6-point scale, ranging from 1 = *very strongly disagree* to 6 = *very strongly agree*. Students were also asked to provide their name, the tutor's name, date of the evaluation, and any comments they might have.

REFERENCES

Abrami, P. C., Leventhal, L. & Perry, R. (1982). Educational seduction. *Review of Educational Research, 52,* 446-464.

Baggott, J. (1987). Reactions of lecturers to analysis results of student ratings of their lecture skills. *Journal of Medical Education, 62,* 491-496.

Fallon, S., Groen, L., & Shelov, S. P. (1987). Teachers' and students' ratings of clinical teachers and teachers' opinions on the use of student evaluations. *Journal of Medical Education, 62,* 435-438.

Fallon, S., Groen, L., & Shilow, S. (1985). Measuring teaching excellence in clinical medicine: A faculty perspective. *Proceedings of the Annual Conference on Research in Medical Education, 24,* 257-262.

Irby, D. M. (1978). Clinical teacher effectiveness. *Journal of Medical Education, 53,* 808-815.

Irby, D. M., & Rakestraw, P. (1981). Evaluating clinical teaching in medicine. *Journal of Medical Education, 56,* 181-186.

Jolly, B., & MacDonald, M. M. (1987). More effective evaluation of clinical teaching. *Assessment and Evaluation in Higher Education, 12,* 175-190.

Kolm, P., & Verhulst, S. J. (1987). Comparing self and supervisor evaluations: A different view. *Evaluation & the Health Professions, 10,* 80-89.

Marsh, H. W., & Ware, J. (1982). Effects of expressiveness, content coverage and incentive on multidimensional student rating scales. *Journal of Educational Psychology, 74,* 126-134.

Morton, J. B., & MacBeth, W.A.A.G. (1977). Correlations between staff, peer and self assessments of fourth year students in surgery. *Medical Education, 11,* 167-170.

Mulholland, H. (1988). What is . . . A profile? *Medical Teacher, 10,* 277-282.

Rippey, R. M. (1981). What standards characterize the quality of measures of teaching? In R. M. Rippey (Ed.), *The evaluation of teaching in medical schools* (pp. 32-55). New York: Springer.

Rothman, A. I., & Cleave-Hogg, D. M. (1990). A medical school learning environment: Views from the trenches. *Teaching and Learning in Medicine, 2,* 12-19.

Rothman, A. I., Poldre, P., & Cohen, R. (1989). Evaluating clinical teachers for promotion. *Academic Medicine, 64,* 12.

CLINICAL ENVIRONMENT AND RESOURCES

Constructs, Principles, and Structure for the Clinical Learning Environment

Participatory Clinical Education

Reconceptualizing the Clinical Learning Environment

**Elaine Tagliareni,
Susan Sherman,
Verle Waters, and
Andrea Mengel**

Health care is shifting emphasis from acute care centers to chronic care services. Within the next 30 years, the nursing home client population is expected to double. Care of nursing home clients differs significantly from that of clients in communities and in hospitals because nursing home clients have greater functional and cognitive disabilities. On the average, they have four or more chronic illnesses and frequent episodes of acute illness.

In 1986, in an effort to respond to changes in health care and in the nation's demographics, the W. K. Kellogg Foundation funded The Community College–Nursing Home Partnership Project. This project promised to show how 778 associate degree nursing programs dispersed throughout urban and rural America could influence present and future care in the country's 16,000 nursing homes. A wide array of activities were undertaken at each of the six demonstration sites to meet the two major partnership project goals: (1) to develop nursing potential in long-term care settings through inservice education, and (2) to influence the redirection of associate degree nursing education to prepare graduates for roles in both long-term and acute care settings. The demonstration sites are Community College of Philadelphia, Pennsylvania; Ohlone College, California; Shoreline Community College, Washington; Triton College, Illinois; Valencia Community College, Florida; and Weber State College, Utah. Four years have passed since the project was funded, and in the six demonstration sites, faculty and their nursing home partners have shown how changes can occur in nursing education and nursing homes.

As a result of the project, new alliances and shifting paradigms have occurred. The Community College–Nursing Home Partnership caught the crest of an already formed wave, swelled by recent literature regarding a paradigm shift in nursing education (Bevis & Watson, 1989; Diekelmann, 1988) and a growing awareness of epidemiological reality, where older individuals with multiple, chronic health problems and concomitant functional disabilities are the primary seekers of health care (Olshansky & Ault, 1986). Dissatisfied with the current "sick care system" (Quinn, 1989), nurses were eager to explore opportunities to be healers within a care-oriented system.

Moving into the nursing home setting provided project faculty with the opportunity to examine themselves as teachers and to re-think student-teacher relationships. Project faculty have given themselves permission to move beyond an insistence on behavioral objectives, to work phenomenologically, to recognize that knowledge is interpreted reality, and to reflect on the lived experiences of students. During the 4 years of the project, faculty moved from focusing on the need to

Elaine Tagliareni, MS, BSN, is an assistant professor, Department of Nursing, Community College of Philadelphia. Susan Sherman, MA, RN, is head and professor, Department of Nursing, Community College of Philadelphia. Verle Waters, MA, BS, is project consultant, The Community College–Nursing Home Partnership, and dean emeritus, Ohlone College, Fremont, California. Andrea Mengel, PhD, MSN, BS, is a professor, Community College of Philadelphia.

significantly change attitudes toward older adults—their own as well as students'—to creating learning environments that empower both teachers and students in caring for frail older adults. Faculty have acknowledged new models of learning and embraced as colleagues nurses in the nursing home. They have moved from seeking the right answers to becoming aware of the need to ask the right questions. This article highlights the outcomes of The Community College–Nursing Home Partnership project in three areas: faculty development, curriculum innovation and collaborative relationships.

Faculty development

Early in the project, a vigorous approach to faculty development occurred at each college. Workshops, retreats, and other faculty development activities focused on dealing with knowledge deficits; stereotypical thinking; and legal, ethical, and cultural issues associated with aging. At the start, faculty firmly believed that a solid foundation of knowledge about gerontological nursing in general and frail older adults in particular would adequately prepare them for teaching roles in long-term care settings. Despite an updated and expanded knowledge base, as they moved into clinical teaching in the nursing home, faculty found themselves unprepared for the role changes they experienced.

Accustomed to teaching in the acute care setting, faculty found the familiarity of staff support, the stimulation of rapid client change, and the structure of medically driven care replaced by fewer staff, barely measurable client changes and faint medical support. The nursing home environment was unfamiliar, and faculty were outside of their comfort zone. The major issue, they began to realize, was not updated or expanded knowledge in gerontological nursing; rather, it was confrontation of the long-established traditions of hospital-based learning and the search for value, opportunity, and comfort as a teacher in the nursing home. Only after faculty came to terms with the new practice setting did real integration of gerontology content occur. Before this happened, teachers in the nursing home moved through observable stages of change.

Most faculty enter the nursing home setting ambivalent about its value as a learning site but ready to share knowledge about current nursing practice. After all, the nursing instructor reasons, the nursing home is a deprived environment eager for input from an educator. There is a small staff, few professional role models, and minimal opportunities for staff to keep abreast of emerging trends in health care. Faculty will make things better; they will bring enlightenment. This is the first stage—the stage of idealism.

Next, faculty are quickly immersed in the expert practitioner–expert teacher dilemma. Because the nursing home setting is less focused on cure-oriented technology and more focused on maintenance and rehabilitative interventions, nursing practice is less structured. The technically focused, acute care practitioner is no longer the expert. Rules that work in the acute care hospital for experience-based clinical judgment and traditional clinical teaching methodologies are no longer valid. Benner explains the dilemma by noting, "... students are not the only novices; any nurse entering a clinical setting where she or he has no experience with the patient population may be limited to the novice level of performance if the goals and tools of patient care are unfamiliar" (1984, p. 21). Nonetheless, instructors realize they must plunge in and structure learning experiences for students. The faculty quickly discovered that the reactive model of clinical teaching, where the clinical instructor responds to available learning situations (dry IVs, a need for pain medication, crisis situations), does not work in the nursing home. Furthermore, faculty were accustomed to working in acute care where

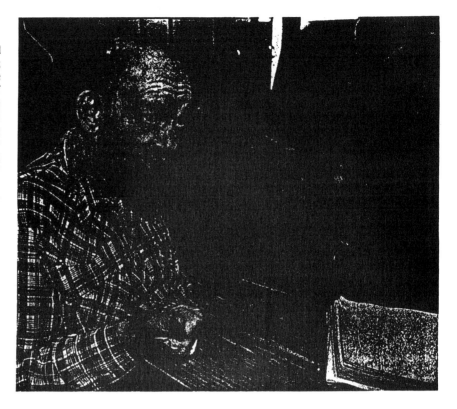

Tagliareni, Sherman, Waters, and Mengel report on an important associate degree program effort to incorporate nursing home care and geriatrics into the education program. Educators and practitioners found out that they had a lot to learn and a lot to share.

Key words: nursing home, geriatrics, long-term care, skilled care, nursing education

the instructor and students engage in parallel play—selecting a set of activities to carry out alongside the hospital nursing staff. In parallel play, the assigned client is often viewed by staff as being the responsibility of the faculty member and the nursing student. In this scenario, the staff refers all clients' needs to the student. A second scenario involves fragmentation of clients according to students' skills, learning needs, and time available. Either way, mutual care planning between student and staff is limited. Fortunately, parallel play is unsuited to the nursing home. Because nurses in nursing homes know the residents and their families intimately and because the residents

value highly their relationships with familiar staff members, the faculty member must teach with, rather than next to, nursing staff.

The paradigm shift from a reactive to a proactive stance and from parallel play to collaborative care giving can threaten faculty, giving rise to a stage characterized by anger, frustration, and resistance. Feeling the loss of expert status as both teacher and practitioner, instructors commonly assume the extremely limited and inflexible rule-governed behavior of the novice role (Benner, 1984). Without administrative support and nurturance during this stage, faculty would, most likely, abandon the nursing home as a clinical setting and return to the more comfortable, and seemingly more rewarding, acute care setting.

Resolution of the expert practitioner–expert teacher dilemma for project faculty came when they began to value the practitioner role in the nursing home and to develop new practice patterns. At this point, the nursing challenge is to find ways to improve the resident's life, not merely to intervene in the illness process. Resolution of the teacher role followed as faculty created learning environments that applauded creativity, individualization of care, and collaborative practice.

In the process of resolving the practitioner–teacher role in a new setting, faculty began to reexamine their philosophy about how the teacher teaches and how the student learns. Tanner (1988) writes, ''We have much to learn from practice and from experts in practice. Now when I think of curriculum revolution, I do not think of developing more elegant and detailed formal models to be passed on to the next generation of nurses for them to take and apply in their practice. Rather, I am struggling with ways in which the concerns of practice can truly be addressed by our educational activities'' (p. 430). Nursing practice in the nursing home stimulated faculty to ask:

How will we assist students and staff to individualize care to residents? Does the nursing process, the analytical step-by-step method, help or hinder?

What clinical teaching strategies enhance the development of caregivers who actively pursue the rehabilitation potential of aged clients?

How can we assist students and faculty to be empowered by their experiences with older adults?

Dissatisfaction with the written care plan surfaced during the nursing home experiences. Instructors were troubled by students who wrote detailed care plans without addressing factors most relevant to the individu-

al resident. One day, a project faculty member correcting care plans for fourth-semester students during the nursing home experience wrote in bold letters across the top of a voluminous care plan, ''Where is the person?'' The limitations of the linear nursing process for addressing individual needs within the holistic perspective needed in the nursing home setting became apparent. Understanding the lived experiences of illness and frailty escapes the formalizations of the traditional nursing care plan approach (Tanner, 1988). Faculty began to search for ways to individualize nursing care in the nursing home. As a result, student teams wrote care plans together for their group of residents, and critiqued care plans by peers in postconference. Faculty commended unique interventions not described in a textbook.

Also, faculty began to realign power relationships between student and teacher. It was time to encourage collegiality: to share care planning, for example, rather than asking students to invent a care plan each week. Students were assigned the same group of clients for the entire nursing home experience and shared at least one client with the instructor. Together student and faculty conducted assessments, co-lead reminiscing or activity groups, and brainstormed about creative approaches to care.

The nursing home became an environment where students could truly begin to grasp the concept of holistic care and where students, staff, and faculty could participate in a nursing model that encourages an individualized, caring approach. The nursing home experience has provided a paradigm to generate active, collaborative teaching approaches that are applicable in a variety of settings. Faculty are compelled to create alliances ''for active engagement of students, for collaboration with expert practitioners, for a commitment to reality and lived experiences and for phenomenological

teaching methods'' (Bevis & Watson, 1989, p. 127).

Curriculum

When the project began in 1986, the prevailing faculty attitude about curriculum development was that since the majority of patients in the acute care setting are elderly, gerontology was integrated. In truth, it has taken 4 years to develop gerontology curriculum content, to understand healthy aging, and to appreciate the needs of older adults in both acute and long-term care settings. Project faculty have developed learning activities for well-elderly experiences in the community and incorporated these in the first nursing course. Students gain a broader perspective of the aging process and learn general concepts of normal growth and development, health, and communication with older adults before caring for the frail elderly (Eddy, 1986; Hogstel, 1988; Ross, 1985). They come to understand that actual or anticipated aging changes have relevance for people in all stages of life and begin to accept aging as one more stage in a continuum of life events (Strumpf & Mezey, 1980). Aging is viewed as a change process, rather than as a decline (Dye, 1985). Emphasis is placed on the needs of the older adult to be treated as a unique person and to be acknowledged for his or her strengths and wisdom.

The signal innovation in curriculum within the project is in the nursing home clinical experience for second-year students. A nursing home experience at an advanced level of student development is based on the premise that the ambiguity and complexity of providing health-promoting, holistic nursing care to frail older adults with multiple chronic disabilities necessitates a well-developed knowledge base in assessment, intervention, evaluation, management, and psychomotor skills. Initially, many project faculty considered gerontological nursing as primarily custodial. There is now agreement that a well-designed, second-year clinical experience in the nursing home not only teaches the student about the care of frail older adults but also empowers students to provide new ways of caring.

The decision to incorporate a

*N*ursing homes have been at the bottom of the nursing totem pole, afforded a status below that of acute care facilities, and largely ignored by nursing education.

(continued on p. 261)

Health care is shifting emphasis from acute care centers to chronic care services.

second-level clinical experience in the nursing home, when the student would be close to graduation, led to the question of essential curriculum content for the associate degree program. Although the literature offers lists of suggested gerontological nursing content (Brower, 1985; Hogstel, 1988), it seemed important to look closely at the nursing home practice setting for information about essential practice knowledge.

The Developing a Curriculum (DACUM) process was employed to bring together 12 directors of nursing from nursing homes affiliated with project schools in 1988 to identify systematically the competencies required for RN practice in long-term care settings. Their list included over 300 competencies within the 18 categories of essential clinical skills listed in Table 1. As a second step toward definition of essential curriculum content, faculty in project schools identified the salience of each of the over 300 competencies for the associate degree program.

There was agreement about competencies that cannot be taught within the four semesters of the associate degree curriculum, such as staff supervision, equipment maintenance, and long-term planning for inservice offerings. Faculty also agreed that a large number of the DACUM competencies dealt with general nursing knowledge and only a small percentage dealt specifically with the care of the frail older adult in the nursing home.

Further refinement of the DAC-UM list was needed. While each of the DACUM competencies was seen as important in providing care to older adults, some are specific to the nursing of frail older adults with multiple chronic health problems and potential or existing functional and cognitive impairments. These were named as specific competencies to be mastered by associate degree nursing students in order to be effective caregivers of frail elders in both the acute and long-term care setting.

In addition, a new question was asked: Of these specific competen-cies, which ones are best taught in long-term care? There was agreement among the faculty members at the six project schools that the 22 competencies shown in Table 2 are essential to care of the frail older adult and are best taught in the long-term care setting. Superficially, the 22 practice competencies appear common to all settings. On closer examination, however, it is clear that the nursing home setting, where prevention, rehabilitation, and maintenance of quality of life for residents are primary considerations, provides a special opportunity for mastery of these competencies. Obviously, the 22 competencies listed in Table 2 cannot be taught only during the nursing home experience. Clinical education about assessment, rehabilitation, and management must be introduced prior to the nursing home experience and threaded throughout acute care content. For students, the nursing home experience provides a rich environment for focusing on these competencies.

Refining the DACUM list of competencies resulted in the addition of three competencies seen as essential to the care of older adults in the nursing home setting, but not identified in the DACUM exercise. They were val-

---

Table 1
Initial DACUM Categories

Communicate effectively
Continue professional and personal growth
Exhibit management skills
Perform assessment of resident
Develop plan of care
Implement plan of care
Administer medication to a large group of residents within a limited time
Perform technical skills
Practice rehabilitation nursing skills
Document resident care data
Practice risk management
Practice infection control
Manage the living environment
Practice within legal parameters
Practice code of ethics
Respond to emergency situations
Educate others
Manage resident and family stress

---

uing goals that maintain functional ability, facilitating residents' choices to decrease learned helplessness, and providing opportunities for expression of ethnic and cultural practices of residents. Together with the 22 "best taught" competencies in Table 2, these form the basis for curriculum decisions and clinical education in project schools.

In the nursing home, students have the opportunity to be healers and to create therapeutic environments. Students graduating today must be competent caregivers for older adults. The recently revised Statement of Educational Outcomes of Associate Degree Nursing Programs Roles and Competencies (NLN, 1990) describes a graduate who promotes rehabilitation and serves as a client advocate. These behaviors can be learned in the nursing home and transferred to the acute care setting. For faculty in project schools, supporting students in generalizing from the nursing home to other settings has become a major curriculum focus. The key is assisting students to recognize the value of prevention, maintenance, and rehabilitation in both settings.

Collaborative relationships among faculty and nursing home staff

Formal and informal mechanisms to foster collegiality among faculty and nursing home staff have emerged. The process of bringing together the unique cultures of nursing faculty and nursing home nurses has created participatory strategies that enhance a caring, educative environment. These relationships take time to nurture and evolve. One of the outcomes of this convergence has been the development of a new community of nurses concerned with the health care needs of the elderly.

Nursing homes have been at the bottom of the nursing totem pole, afforded a status below that of acute care facilities, and largely ignored by nursing education. Nurses associated with the care of the elderly were seen stereotypically as passive, powerless, and on the periphery of nursing. That shabby image persists in our attitudes and values. It is much easier to recognize intellectually the aging of the U.S. population and the growing number of clients in nursing homes

I*nitially, many project faculty considered gerontological nursing as primarily custodial.*

than it is to change the way nurse educators feel about what is valuable and important in the work of the nursing home nurse.

Respect for nurses who choose to work in these settings has grown among project faculty. Faculty have moved from telling and critiquing nursing home staff to listening and responding. They have learned to appreciate the unique culture of the nursing home and value their nursing home partners as colleagues and mentors.

To elicit ideas about the essential ingredients of a successful partnership, a Delphi study was conducted by project staff (Mengel et al., 1990). Respondents were faculty, administrators, and staff associated with the six community colleges and 27 nursing homes participating in the partnership. The study revealed that both the community college and the nursing home wish to remain autonomous while collaborating on management of the partnership. One partner, most likely the community college, needs to assume responsibility for doing the majority of the work to maintain the partnership, as respondents felt that the benefits and responsibilities need not be equal. The basis for a solid partnership includes mutual respect and understanding, a commitment to high-quality education for students and high-quality service to patients, and clear communication.

As project faculty began to appreciate the benefits of the nursing home setting and to understand the characteristics of a successful partnership, collaboration between the nursing home and the nursing program increased. Another study, conducted in fall 1989, examined the effects of partnership activities on caregiving in partnership nursing homes (Carignan, 1990). Directors of nursing were asked, What do you see as the major benefits of your relationship with your project school? Responses included increased educational opportunities for nursing home staff, enhanced image of nurses in nursing homes, and positive interactions between students and nursing home staff.

It became clear that learning objectives and strategies for nursing students were also well suited to the sometimes urgent needs of nursing home staff. Over time, participatory models of learning evolved. Bevis (1989) calls these relationships among teachers, clinicians, and students tripartite alliances, a partnership forming the backbone of educative care. Faculty and staff have generated exciting participatory learning activities involving students, faculty, and nursing home staff. Two examples illustrate this activity:

A director of nursing expresses concern that the staff sees only the resident's decubiti and does not address nutritional, hydrational, or mobility factors that may contribute to poor healing. Also, they look only at the medical diagnosis and do not address nursing outcomes. In a planning conference, the instructor suggests that the nursing assistants participate in student learning activities for decubitus care. Students discuss assessment findings with the nursing assistants at the bedside and jointly develop goals.

The director of nursing expresses concern that most required inservice activities are primarily didactic and content-laden. College faculty initiate informal exchanges with staff about other teaching strategies. Inservice classes begin to include techniques to foster participation and experiential learning.

Summary

Bringing together the unique cultures of nursing faculty and nursing home staff, and fostering tripartite alliances can create a caring, educative environment. The shared experiences of faculty, students, and nursing home staff give rise to a new community of nurses concerned with the health care needs of the elderly. The nursing

---

Table 2
Competencies "BEST TAUGHT" in the Nursing Home

Exhibit management skills
  Adopt leadership style appropriate to situation
  Delegate appropriately
  Resolve problems utilizing problem-solving skills over an extended
    period of time
  Update plan of care

Perform assessment of resident
  Assess current mental status
  Assess ADL (functional) abilities
  Differentiate normal aging process from disease process
  Recognize age-related differences in disease processes
  Value goals that maintain functional ability

Practice rehabilitation nursing skills
  Define restorative goals
  Elicit active participation of resident in restorative program
  Facilitate choices to decrease learned helplessness
  Promote independence of ADLs
  Initiate bowel and bladder training
  Implement contracture prevention methods
  Evaluate effectiveness of restorative programs
  Implement group therapies (e.g. reality orientation, memory
    enhancement, reminiscing)

Manage the living environment
  Allow resident to continue previous lifestyle to degree possible
  Provide comfortable homelike environment for socialization
  Plan room arrangement to facilitate resident needs
  Reduce environmental stress (e.g., noises, isolation, lighting,
    roommate)
  Provide opportunities for expression of ethnic and cultural practices for
    residents
  Provide for sexual expression of residents
  Initiate interventions to deal with combative residents
  Assist families to cope with unrealistic expectations, guilt, anger

home is now seen as a unique environment where students can truly promote the rehabilitation potential of older adults and where students, nursing home staff, and faculty can collaborate within a nursing model to achieve a caring approach. Clients who need caring, regardless of their cure potential, must be reclaimed by all of nursing. Project activities highlighted the commonalities of the two unique environments, and those shared values are the basis for collaboration.

To share results of the demonstration phase, the project schools have been funded by the W. K. Kellogg Foundation for an additional 3 years. In a series of workshops jointly sponsored by the National League for Nursing, and through a number of publications and a videotape, faculty in other associate degree nursing programs will have the opportunity to explore the following questions: How can faculty develop participatory, educative-caring models of clinical learning with students? What learning strategies can be developed collaboratively among nursing home nurses and faculty for both students and staff? What collaborative activities can assist students and staff to feel empowered by their experiences with older adults? What essential content regarding gerontological nursing should be integrated into the associate degree nursing curriculum? How can faculty assist students to value rehabilitation potential and maintenance? What specific experiences with the well elderly in the community provide the foundation for care of the frail elderly?

Wide-ranging discussions around these questions with faculty across the country will, we believe, provide exciting new ways to educate nurses in managing caring environments for both well and frail elderly.

References

Benner, P. (1984) *From novice to expert: Excellence and power in clinical nursing practice*. Menlo Park, CA: Addison-Wesley Publishing Co.

Bevis, E. O., & Watson, J. (1989). *Toward a caring curriculum: A new pedagogy for nursing*. New York: National League for Nursing.

Brower, T. H. (1985). Knowledge competencies in gerontological nursing. In *Overcoming the bias of ageism in long-term care*. New York: National League for Nursing.

Carignan, A. (1991) Partnership impact on nursing home care. Unpublished.

Dye, C., A. (1985). *Assessment and intervention in geropsychiatric nursing*. Orlando, FL: Grune & Stratton, Inc.

Diekelmann, N. (1988). Curriculum revolution: A theoretical and philosophical mandate for change. In *Curriculum revolution: Mandate for change*. New York: National League for Nursing.

Eddy, D. M. (1986). Before and after attitudes toward aging in BSN program. *Journal of Gerontological Nursing, 12*, 30-34.

Educational outcomes of associate degree nursing programs: Role and competencies (1990). New York: National League for Nursing.

Hogstel, M. (1988). Gerontological nursing in the baccalaureate curriculum. *Nursing Education, 13*(3), 14-18.

Mengel, A., Simpson, S., Sherman, S., & Waters, V. (1990). Essential factors in a community college-nursing home partnership. *Gerontological Nursing, 16*(11), 26-31.

Olshansky, S. J., & Ault, A. B. (1986). The fourth stage to the epidemiologic transition: the age of delayed degenerative diseases. *The Milbank Quarterly, 64*, 355-391.

Quinn, J. (Dec. 1989). On healing, wholeness and the Haelan effect. *Nursing & Health Care, 10*, 553-556.

Ross, M. (1985). The impact of client selection on clinical teaching. *Journal of Advanced Nursing, 10*, 567-573.

Strumpf, N. E., & Mezey, M. D. (1980). A developmental approach to the teaching of aging. *Nursing Outlook, 28*, 730-734.

Tanner, C. (1988). Book Special: Curriculum revolution: the practice mandate. *Nursing and Health Care, 9*, 427-430.

SPECIAL ARTICLE

GORDON T. MOORE, MD, MPH, THOMAS S. INUI, MD, ScM, JOHN M. LUDDEN, MD, and STEPHEN C. SCHOENBAUM, MD, MPH

The "Teaching HMO": A New Academic Partner

Abstract—Health care reform is a potential threat to the academic missions of medical schools and academic health centers. But managed care, the source of much of their concern, may also represent a way for medical schools to improve their future academic outcomes. Harvard Medical School and the Harvard Community Health Plan, a large health maintenance organization (HMO) in greater Boston, recently formed the first medical school department to be based in a freestanding HMO. This arrangement is an example of a model that replicates, in a managed care organization, the long-standing and highly successful teaching hospital academic structure in academic medical centers. The authors describe this model in detail, show how the Harvard collaboration works, and explain the benefits each institution saw in creating a joint entity, the rationale for making that new entity an academic department, and the implications for other academic health centers. They conclude that the Harvard experience shows that alliances between medical schools and large HMOs can create vibrant practice settings for teaching and research in academic areas (such as prevention and primary care medicine) that have been relatively neglected in recent times, and that the "teaching HMO" may have the potential to transform academic medicine in the next century just as the teaching hospital transformed it in this century. *Acad. Med.* 69(1994):595–600.

Many academic health centers (AHCs) are feeling imperiled by health care reform.[1-3] In particular, they see the growth of managed care as a threat to their patient bases, their incomes, and even the academic enterprises of teaching and research. But managed care represents opportunities as well as problems. Some of the predicaments now facing AHCs might actually be resolved by drawing health maintenance organizations (HMOs) into the academic arena. In this article we explore the demonstrated benefits of one such arrangement and the arrangement's implications for academic medicine.

In late 1992, Harvard Medical School (HMS) and the Harvard Community Health Plan (HCHP, or "the Plan"), a large HMO in greater Boston, established the first medical school department to be based in a freestanding HMO: the Department of Ambulatory Care and Prevention. We explain how this new model fits into the spectrum of collaborations between medical schools and HMOs, analyze the advantages and risks of such a close linkage, and draw the implications for other AHCs by analogy with the development of teaching hospitals in the United States.

BACKGROUND

Until now, most HMOs and AHCs have maintained arm's-length relationships.[4,5] The two kinds of organizations have often entered into contractual agreements involving hospital services, diagnostic and treatment technology, and specialist care—arrangements in which each party has a clear business interest. But, despite possible benefits cited by some authors[4-6] and the argument by others[7] that HMOs (self-interest notwithstanding) have a moral obliga-

tion to help medical schools, less than 15% of surveyed HMOs participate in graduate medical education (GME).[8] Considerably fewer undertake academic research or medical student teaching, which is generally considered more intrusive and of less value to HMOs than is GME.

Nevertheless, there are scattered examples of close relationships between HMOs and AHCs. Kaiser Permanente, for example, which has sponsored GME at its hospitals for years, has more recently developed interlocking faculty appointments with several California medical schools to facilitate the placement of students in its health centers.[9] The University of Washington has long contracted with Group Health Cooperative to teach medical students[10] and has forged a fruitful relationship with that HMO's research institute. And one academically owned HMO at George Washington University now serves as an active academic unit for teaching and research.[11]

The AHCs and HMOs in these examples generally share a common feature: they carefully maintain administrative and organizational distance. The HMO and the medical school typically remain peripheral to

Dr. Moore is director, Teaching Programs, Harvard Community Health Plan (HCHP), and associate professor of ambulatory care and prevention, Harvard Medical School (HMS), Boston, Massachusetts; Dr. Inui is professor and chairman, Department of Ambulatory Care and Prevention, HCHP and HMS; Dr. Ludden is corporate medical director, HCHP; and Dr. Schoenbaum is medical director, HCHP, and associate professor of medicine, HMS.

Correspondence and requests for reprints should be addressed to Dr. Moore, Director, Teaching Programs, Harvard Community Health Plan, 126 Brookline Avenue, Suite 202, Boston, MA 02215.

each other, compared with the closeness of most medical schools and their teaching hospitals. This closeness is created largely through joint academic and clinical departments whose unique culture, overlapping appointments, and shared budgets create a high level of interaction, interdependence, common values and goals, and shared products in teaching and research.

Yet until the end of the nineteenth century, hospitals and medical schools also maintained their distance. In 1893, in an attempt to improve the clinical education of its medical students, The Johns Hopkins School of Medicine first created the full model of what has come to be known as the teaching hospital[12] by merging academic departments with a clinical practice site. The teaching hospital model—which links education, research, and clinical service—now dominates clinical medical education and has been responsible for many of the great advances in research applied to clinical practice.

Academic clinical departments benefited both medical schools and their hospital partners. These departments fused the medical schools' academic strengths with the capacity for clinical care that, in the late 1800s, was becoming more scientifically based. Merging created a new structure in which care, teaching, and research could be done efficiently in a shared culture. Clinicians could do research and teaching and be rewarded for the quality of their academic work. Through this structure, medical schools expanded their clinical teaching sites, enlarged their research faculties, gained access to clinical populations for research, and derived new academic income from clinical activities. The teaching hospitals gained in stature and reputation, drew university scientists to their research, acquired academic recognition as an incentive to attract and retain high-quality staffs, and combined academic and clinical experiences to produce better trained physicians and important research.

ADVANTAGES OF CLOSER COLLABORATION

The joint departmental structure was the model used to cross institutional boundaries between hospitals and medical schools. In that model, medical schools delegate academic authority to clinical sites that undertake teaching and research. A shared department has the capacity to satisfy each institution's particular needs for control and accountability while allowing sufficient independence to foster innovation. The same model has both theoretical and practical organizational advantages for AHCs and HMOs. Specifically, having a common academic department can solve several problems both these organizations face, as we now explain.

The Medical School Perspective

Among the many difficulties that medical schools will face in the coming decades, perhaps the most critical will be the need for schools to direct research and teaching to the changing needs of society while maintaining their preeminent position in biological research and tertiary clinical services.[13] Two of these adaptive challenges are to enhance teaching and research in preventive medicine and provide effective primary care teaching.

Preventive medicine. Since the Rockefeller Foundation encouraged the association of academic preventive medicine with schools of public health[14] after the First World War, this discipline has been held relatively separate from clinical practice in the world of biotechnical medicine. This separation has had adverse effects. Gottlieb and Holman, for example, reported[15] that 91% of surveyed deans and chairmen of departments of medicine and preventive medicine considered preventive medicine "underdeveloped." The majority of schools considered research quality in preventive medicine to be inadequate, yet only one-eighth of the units surveyed reported giving high priority to

research training. Further, 55–63% of medical school graduates now say they have had inadequate teaching in preventive medicine.[16]

Poor teaching of preventive medicine has significant consequences. Among the most obvious, it fosters poor practice[17,18] and, by so doing, certainly accounts for a portion of the more than 12 million years of potential life lost from preventable conditions in 1990.[19] The Department of Health and Human Services underscored the need to improve this situation by stressing change in undergraduate medical education as one of its prevention objectives for the nation.[20] Leaders in the field have responded by challenging medical schools to promote preventive medicine and adopt a population-oriented approach to medical care.[21,22] To these ends, foundations have provided funding[23] and new curricula have been proposed.[24]

But change will be insignificant until academic preventive medicine develops links with clinical practice and successfully bridges the gap between the community orientation of public health and the individual orientation of clinical preventive medicine. The keystone in this bridge is access to practice sites—such as HMOs—that deliver large-volume primary care, have definable populations for whom they are responsible, and emphasize a delivery model that expressly includes clinical preventive services. Such an organization enhances a medical school department's ability to teach and carry out excellent research in preventive medicine.

Teaching in ambulatory care settings. The time for more teaching in ambulatory care settings has not only arrived, it is long overdue. Hospitals are inappropriate as sole sites for the clinical education of physicians and other health professionals. Hospital stays have become so brief that students and graduate trainees are often unable to appreciate patients' antecedent histories, their social contexts, and the courses of their illnesses. Sophisticated diagnostic and therapeutic technologies now make it possible to provide excellent care for serious illnesses in ambulatory care settings and have virtually banished certain disorders from inpatient populations. And medical schools have been exhorted to teach students in office settings so that more graduates might choose primary care careers.[25]

These circumstances make it imperative to teach in ambulatory care settings. But a variety of barriers exist. Most important have been the perceived extra expense and inadequate financial support for such teaching[26] as well as shortfalls in numbers and quality of patients, teachers, and practice settings.

The HMO Perspective

Like academic medical centers, HMOs confront many serious challenges. Among the most significant: maintaining a strategic advantage in the face of increasing competitive pressure. For most HMOs, this means differentiating their product favorably while maintaining low premiums — in other words, offering high value to their members. The challenges currently facing HMOs include recruiting and retaining primary care physicians; assuring that these doctors can practice efficiently and effectively in the office; improving relevant research and development in the performance of primary care; and enhancing high-quality practice and reputation while squeezing down the costs of care.

As the pool of primary care physicians shrinks, HMOs encounter difficulty in recruiting enough doctors to match their growth.[27] In response to this problem, HMOs have developed aggressive recruiting programs and raised starting salaries. Many of the physicians recruited in this manner lack appropriate training. The competencies that medical directors most desire their physicians to have (i.e., ability to provide cost-effective care, to maintain quality of care, to perform effective referrals, and to demonstrate experience with ambulatory

care, skill in group dynamics, and knowledge of preventive medicine)[28] are among those least frequently achieved in hospital-based teaching programs.[29] Officials at most HMOs now believe that a close affiliation with educational programs may improve physician recruitment, training, and retention and give an edge in hiring clinical staff.[27]

To be successful in its marketplace, an HMO must constantly improve its medical care, develop new products, and lower costs. By developing a medical school relationship in the form of an academic department, an HMO acquires a new capacity for fresh thinking and innovation. An academic department, by studying current practice and developing and testing new approaches to prevention and primary care, assumes an internal research and development (R & D) function. Finally, in a competitive world, a reputation for quality is an advantage. Because effective teaching is widely believed to improve the quality of practice, a medical school's reputation for educational excellence could enhance an HMO's image as a high-quality organization.

INGREDIENTS OF THE JOINT VENTURE

In the late 1980s, Harvard Medical School and the HCHP decided to explore a more intense relationship — through developing a new medical school department that would be located at the HCHP, thus creating a "teaching HMO" equivalent to the teaching hospital. The two institutions had laid the groundwork for close collaboration over many years. The Plan had been started two decades earlier by the then-dean of HMS, Robert Ebert, who later had signed an affiliation agreement between the HCHP and HMS. The two organizations evolved a deepening working relationship through a number of stages: the HCHP created a research institute (subsequently closed), led the development of a new ambulatory care clerkship, partici-

pated in a school-wide division of primary care, contributed widely to the teaching of medical students and postgraduates, and funded an HCHP foundation to support teaching, research, and community service. The organizations' leaders were positively disposed to cooperate: the Plan's president, Thomas Pyle, spearheaded placing teaching, research, and community service in the HCHP's mission statement, while the medical school dean, Daniel Tosteson, had proposed a type of divisional affiliation as early as 1981.[30]

Creating a joint department was a logical next step. It drew upon the best traditions and values of each partner and emulated six characteristics of effective departments in teaching hospitals that made them strong models. These were that such a department (1) created a high-status entity with a unified new mission that valued clinical and academic excellence; (2) increased participation by clinical faculty, whose quality of work and commitment were stimulated by the potential for academic recognition; (3) intensified interactions of faculty and trainees in clinical settings that were appropriate for apprentice teaching and role modeling; (4) increased access to relevant populations for research, program development, or demonstrations; (5) created reliable sources of funding; and (6) were administratively simple. Below, we use these characteristics as a framework to explore some of the implications of the new HMS–HCHP departmental partnership.

1. A high-status entity with a new mission. The development of a department creates a unified, integrated entity with a new mission, values, and goals that merge the academic traditions of the medical school with the orientation toward the customer, service, management, and patient populations of an ambulatory health care delivery system. The increasing sophistication of ambulatory and primary care and the shifting of health care delivery to managed care create an environment that academics should find desirable. In our case, the new department has already become a venue for drawing together the academic leadership of the school and the management of the HCHP.

2. Enhanced effectiveness in faculty recruitment and career development. The affiliation is expected to help the Plan recruit and retain staff while it increases the pool of ambulatory-care–based teachers and preventive medicine researchers available to the medical school. By ceding control of faculty appointments to an academic unit imbedded in an office practice setting, the medical school enables promotion criteria to be applied with attention to the teaching and research needed in preventive medicine and ambulatory care. With a department that can academically recognize their work, more of the HCHP's over 1,500 physicians and allied health personnel are likely to teach and do research. The new department already figures in the HCHP's recruitment strategy, and more than a dozen of the existing staff have indicated interest in career development and academic promotion.

3. Intensified interactions between trainees and faculty in primary care and clinical prevention settings. Students learn best when they interact with role models and participate in authentic clinical work. In the new partnership, these elements are amplified for the teaching of primary care and clinical prevention as they have been for many years for biomedical teaching in the hospital. The best place to learn clinical prevention is at a site that practices it. Preventive medicine and health promotion are inseparable parts of an HMO staffs' day-to-day provision of care. The Plan offers several hundred prevention courses each year, has developed worksite health promotion programs, and, through its foundation, sponsors numerous health promotion and community service programs.

The HCHP already contributes substantially to the opportunities for students to come in contact with clinical populations relevant to the teaching of prevention and primary care; it is New England's largest

HMO, with 565,000 members who receive ambulatory care at 19 HCHP health centers and other affiliated practice sites. One-fourth of HMS students already undertake course work at the HCHP each year. The presence of students and housestaff also benefit the Plan's staff. On-site trainees are a source of stimulation, variety, and continued learning. On a recent survey at the HCHP, teaching was the highest-cited source of physicians' satisfaction.

4. Providing skilled investigators with access to suitable populations for research. The joint HMS–HCHP department should make it easier to recruit new researchers and tap into a pre-existing network of HMS faculty already conducting excellent research in preventive medicine and primary care. One of the attractions is the opportunity to conduct relevant research on the Plan's members and staff. Although the HCHP has been the site of clinical research projects since its founding in 1969, it has never fully exploited its research and development potential. Some features of the HCHP that expand the research opportunities available at the medical school include a large defined membership, which provides the means to follow information on a substantial population over a long time; an electronic medical record system database for 350,000 members; hundreds of primary care and specialty office practitioners, who are a potential population for study; and the existence of a teaching center (a set of mock clinical offices with observation and videotape facilities) that can be used as a laboratory for research and development in teaching. These unique resources for research have already attracted academic talent. The department has had little difficulty recruiting qualified academics to its available positions from both inside and outside the medical school.

5. Reliable sources of funding. Clinical income now provides at least 45% of the revenues of medical schools, virtually all of which comes from hospital sources.[31] The HMO alliance creates a new partner that benefits

from research and teaching in prevention and primary care and can help finance these activities. For more than ten years, the HCHP has contributed between .5% and 1% of its now billion-dollar annual revenues to its own foundation, which supports teaching, research, and community services. The Plan has contributed space and the majority of core funding for the new department, with HMS providing the rest, largely through support for the major academic staff positions.

6. Administrative simplicity. Consolidating academic activities in a large, well-organized HMO should streamline administrative tasks. Recruiting clinicians to teach and populations to study can be a nightmare, especially in the cases when independent community-based primary care clinicians and their patients are dispersed and thus may be hard to recruit, difficult to communicate with, and complicated to organize. The new department's position as part of the HMO management structure simplifies matters considerably. The department chairman now sits on the executive committee of the HCHP's medical management with the title of Medical Director for Teaching and Research. This one committee coordinates policies, procedures, and communications relevant to the Plan's teaching and research.

DISCUSSION

We have described an example of the kind of academic departmental structure that has potential benefits for medical schools and HMOs. In this new type of academic partnership, office practice in the HMO becomes an active, applied arm of preventive medicine and primary care in much the way that hospital-based clinical medicine is the major avenue for applying, studying, and teaching biotechnical medicine.

The heart of this structure is a reciprocal and mutually beneficial relationship between primary care practice and preventive medicine. Robust teaching and research in prevention depend on a new view of preventive medicine as a clinical discipline based in primary care practice. The other side of the coin is that the field of primary care benefits from a stronger foundation in preventive medicine. The scholarly study of the phenomena that constitute substantial threats to health (such as genetic, economic, social, environmental, and political factors) will enhance the scientific basis for the practice of primary care and generate interventions that will guide effective primary care practice in the future.

By examining the HCHP–HMS collaboration, one can begin to discern the major elements that each party must bring to the table. For example, the medical school must be prepared to offer to large group practices or HMOs — which have not traditionally had academic affiliations — an opportunity for full partnership in the academic establishment, including appropriate academic recognition. In turn, the HMO must endorse teaching and research as important organizational goals.

Attitudes must change on both sides. HMO professionals must overcome their suspicion of AHCs. To be sure, teaching and research could create costs, distract clinical staff from their work, or dissatisfy patients. Our experience with the HCHP, however, supports the idea that teaching and research can benefit HMOs. Medical schools will need to modify the view, held by some faculty, that ambulatory care teachers are inferior to — not merely different from — their hospital counterparts. Research must shift to include issues relevant to managed care.

The HMO and the medical school must commit resources to the venture. Debates about funding for ambulatory care teaching have persistently identified the host site as the major source of support,[32] causing HMO administrators to be nervous about teaching medical students. While those who run HMOs and other community-based sites must appreciate that it is both an obligation and in their best interest to support medical education, the medical schools must prove that they are not

seeking a free lunch. If a medical school finds preventive medicine and primary care education important, it must help provide support for these activities.

The model that we have described is more suitable for large group practice HMOs than for managed care organizations consisting of small, independent practice associations (IPAs). The latter are too dispersed and administratively decentralized to facilitate the organizational structure or the work of a teaching department. Fortunately, large group practice HMOs are present in many cities with medical schools.

Finally, several financial and logistical issues remain to be explored in the teaching HMO. One is how to eliminate or pay for lost patient care productivity while teaching. Another is how to gain patients' acceptance. Studying and solving such problems is critical if the nation's enlarging managed care sector is to be opened fully to medical students and residents.

At the moment when reform is shaking the financial foundations of the teaching hospital, much can be found for medical school leaders to worry about. Perhaps most feared is whether their historic missions of teaching and research can survive. The prospect that managed care might breach the academic walls need not be entirely negative. Instead, as this article indicates, alliances between medical schools and HMOs can create vibrant practice settings for teaching and research in academic areas that have been relatively neglected in recent times. Perhaps a school that can harness the energy of an HMO setting where primary care and preventive medicine are practiced can add a vital and valuable dimension to its core mission. The teaching hospital transformed academic medicine in the twentieth century. Does the teaching HMO have the potential to do the same in the twenty-first?

The authors thank the Harvard Community Health Plan Foundation for its generous support and acknowledge the contributions of Thomas O. Pyle, Daniel C. Tosteson, and S. James Adelstein to this endeavor.

References

1. Fox, P. D., Wasserman, J. Academic Medical Centers and Managed Care: Uneasy Partners. *Health Aff.* 12(Spring 1993): 85–93.
2. Blumenthal, D., and Meyer, G. S. The Future of the Academic Medical Center under Health Care Reform. *N. Engl. J. Med.* 329(1993):1812–1814.
3. Brody, H., et al. The Mammalian Medical Center for the 21st century. *JAMA* 270(1993):1097–1100.
4. Hoft, R. H., and Glaser, R. J. The Problems and Benefits of Associating Academic Medical Centers with Health-maintenance Organizations. *N. Engl. J. Med.* 307 (1982):1681–1688.
5. Moore, G. T. HMOs and Medical Education: Fashioning a Marriage. *Health Aff.* 5(1986):147–153.
6. Moore, G. T. Health Maintenance Organizations and Medical Education: Breaking the Barriers. *Acad. Med.* 65(1990): 427–432.
7. Swanson, A. G. HMOs Have an Educational Obligation. *HMO Practice* 2(1988): 125–128.
8. Corrigan, J. M., and Thompson, L. M. Involvement of Health Maintenance Organizations in Graduate Medical Education. *Acad. Med.* 66(1991):656–661.
9. Eliot Wolfe, Kaiser Permanente Health Plan, Northern California. Personal communication, September 1993.
10. Kirz, H. L., and Larsen, C. Costs and Benefits of Medical Students' Training to a Health Maintenance Organization. *JAMA* 256(1986):734–739.
11. Ott, J. E. Medical Education in a Health Maintenance Organization: The George Washington University Health Plan Experience. *HMO/PPO Trends* 5(1992):6–11.
12. Ludmerer, K. M. *Learning to Heal. The Development of American Medical Education.* New York: Basic Books, 1985, pp. 219–233.
13. Schroeder, S. A., Zones, J. S., and Showstack, J. A. Academic Medicine as a Public Trust. *JAMA* 262(1989):803–812.
14. Fee, E. *Disease and Discovery: A History of the Johns Hopkins School of Hygiene and Public Health.* Baltimore, Maryland: Johns Hopkins Press, 1987.
15. Gottlieb, L. K., and Holman, H. R. What's Preventing More Prevention? Barriers to Development at Academic Medical Centers. *J. Gen. Intern. Med.* 7(1992): 630–635.
16. August Swanson, Association of American Medical Colleges, Personal communication, April 1992.
17. Lewis, C. E. Disease Prevention and Health Promotion Practices of Primary Care Physicians in the United States. *Am.*

J. Prev. Med. **4**, Supplement (1988): S9–S16.

18. Belcher, D. W., Berg, A. O., and Inui; T. S. Practical Approaches to Providing Better Preventive Care: Are Physicians a Problem or a Solution? *Am. J. Prev. Med.* **4**, Supplement (1988):S27–S48.

19. Years of Potential Life Lost before Ages 65 and 85—United States, 1989–1990. *MMWR* **41**(1992):313–315.

20. *Healthy People 2000: National Health Promotion and Disease Prevention Objectives.* Washington, D.C.: Government Printing Office (stock number 017-001-00474-0), 1990.

21. Greenlick, M. R. Educating Physicians for Population-based Clinical Practice. *JAMA* **267**(1992):1645–1648.

22. Amos, A. Health Promotion in Medical Education: A Challenge for the 1990s. *Med. Educ.* **25**(1991):97–99.

23. Showstack, J., et al. Health of the Public: The Academic Response. *JAMA* **267**(1992):2497–2502.

24. Altekruse, J., Goldenberg, K., Rabin, D. L., Riegelman, R. K., and Wiese, W. H. Implementing the Association of Teachers of Preventive Medicine's Recommendations into the Undergraduate Medical School Curriculum. *Acad. Med.* **66**(1991): 312–320.

25. Council on Graduate Medical Education. *Third Report: Improving Access to Health Care through Physician Workforce Reform: Directions for the 21st century.* Rockville, Maryland: Health Resources and Services Administration, October 1992.

26. Schroeder, S. A. Expanding the Site of Clinical Education: Moving beyond the Hospital Walls. *J. Gen. Intern. Med.* **3**, Supplement (1988):S5–S14.

27. Palsbro, S. E., and Sullivan, C. B. *The Recruitment Experience of Health Maintenance Organizations for Primary Care Physicians. Final Report.* Health Resources and Services Administration. Project ID# HRSA 92–190, May 1993.

28. Jacobs, M. O., and Mott, P. D. Physician Characteristics and Training Emphasis Considered Desirable by Leaders of HMOs. *J. Med. Educ.* **62**(1987):725–731.

29. McPhee, S. J., Mitchell, T. F., Schroeder, S. A., Perez-Stable, E. J., and Bindman, A. B. Training in a Primary Care Internal Medicine Residency Program: The First Ten Years. *JAMA* **258**(1987):1491–1495.

30. Tosteson, D. C. Competition in the Medical Marketplace: The Boston Story. In *Health Maintenance Organizations and Academic Medical Centers: Proceedings of a National Conference,* J. I. Hudson and M. M. Nevins, eds., pp. 269–279. Fulton, Missouri: The Ovid Bell Press, 1981.

31. *American Medical Education: Institutions, Programs, and Issues.* Washington, D.C., Association of American Medical Colleges, 1992, p. 4.

32. Delbanco, T. L., and Calkins, D. R. The costs and Financing of Ambulatory Medical Education. *J. Gen. Intern. Med.* **3**, Supplement (1987):S34–S43.

Financial/ Productivity Aspects of Clinical Education

Clinical Education — Funding and Standards

ALAN WALKER MA

Director of Education, Chartered Society of Physiotherapy

IT is likely that a Department of Health working group will shortly be making recommendations on the future funding of clinical education for the health care professions. The working group, chaired by Giles Duncan, Regional personnel director of South West Thames Regional Health Authority, does not have direct representation from the Chartered Society of Physiotherapy, though we have submitted our views in writing.

In its reponse, the Society has welcomed the establishment of the working group, as the funding of clinical education placements has become an anomalous area in health care education since the publication of Working Paper 10.

Several educational developments have combined to highlight organisational problems in clinical education. First, placements have largely changed from the 'half-day' to 'block' model. Instead of being based in only a few hospitals for half a day at a time, alternating with attendance at the school of physiotherapy, students are now based in a very wide range of units, both hospital- and community-based, for weeks at a time. This requires far more organisational commitment from the host unit than the previous system, though it provides a wider range of clinical experience.

The second change is linked to the first. The rapid move to three-year degree-based education in physiotherapy has increased awareness that the clinical component is an integral aspect of the overall education programme. Clinical staff are therefore expected to contribute to the planning, development and evaluation of the course as full members of the course team.

Another development has been the increasing range of placements offered by schools of physiotherapy, especially the 'elective' system of specialist placement, at a time when the actual provision of placements by provider units is becoming scarcer. The development of self-governing Trusts may also affect the provision of specialist placements, if the particular specialism no longer forms part of the Trust's business plan.

For the above reasons, many placement providers have concluded that the increasing resource commitment of clinical education demands that a charge be made for their provision. Some providers have actually attempted to do so, but have been prevented by the NHS Management Executive's ruling that no charges should be made in respect of clinical placements during the 1991/92 financial year. There is no doubt that schools of physiotherapy can no longer rely on the goodwill of providers for the future supply of clinical education.

At present the only form of payment made for clinical education placements is the allowance paid to clinical educators. This payment is currently organised by District management, and schools of physiotherapy have no input into the distribution or quantity of allowances available. This can lead to problems in so far as allowances are often distributed on an irregular and even haphazard basis. Several potential sites of clinical education are therefore closed to schools of physiotherapy if no allowances are paid there. Placements are also vulnerable if a host unit decides to reallocate funds internally.

The increased responsibility of clinical educators points to a continuing need for the existing allowance to be paid in the future, and the Society supports a specific allowance for the clinical teaching of students. If various elements are to be considered for inclusion in charges for clinical placements, it is inconceivable that the allowance for clinical educators should not be among them. There is, however, evidence that the transfer of the budget for student training allowances to schools of physiotherapy would benefit the increased supply and provision of clinical education. Money would effectively follow the student, and schools would no longer need to be constrained in the possible location of placements.

The above arrangement would not, however, resolve the problems of placement provision as perceived by provider units. It is evident that providers of clinical education placements require sufficient resources to ensure students' fulfilment of educational objectives. In addition to allowances for clinical supervisors, which should continue to be paid, other required resources include accommodation, administrative, information resource, and liaison costs, together with the expense of training clinical educators for their work. Perhaps the greatest cost to providers is in the loss of treatment time arising from the use of clinical educators.

The Society is concerned at evidence that the Department of Health working group may be regarding students in physiotherapy and other areas as making a service contribution during their clinical education. In its response, the Society has stressed that students do not, and should not, make such a contribution. Physiotherapy students receive bursaries, not salaries, are trained under supervision, and should be considered as supernumerary to establishment throughout their education.

It is evident that a variety of costs need to be considered in the provision of clinical placements, and these far exceed the present student training allowance. What is less clear is how these costs can be defrayed. It is obviously possible for clinical placements to be calculated on a full-cost basis, and made subject to contracting arrangements between schools of physiotherapy as 'purchasers' and host units as 'providers' of placements. This would satisfy providers that the real costs of placements were being met, and effectively removed from their existing budgets, but would raise the question of where schools of physiotherapy would obtain the funding for full-cost placements.

Since the implementation of Working Paper 10, the vast majority of funding for schools of physiotherapy is from Regional Health Authorities, on the basis of agreed contracts. It is quite unreasonable and impossible for schools of physiotherapy to absorb the total cost of placement provision, and subvention from Regional Health Authorities, as part of an agreed overall contract, would be required to meet these costs.

It has to be asked, however, where Regions would in turn obtain additional money, and the likeliest outcome would be the top-slicing of District or Unit budgets for this purpose. There is thus a prospect of money travelling in circles without any benefit to clinical education or patient care, though involving greatly increased administrative costs. The position of self-governing Trusts must also be considered in this equation, as Regions would not be able to top-slice their budgets for training purposes. The Society therefore believes that if clinical education placements are to be charged on a contracted full-cost basis, then additional funding is required to meet these very real costs.

The Society's new Curriculum of Study states that 'clinical education is an essential and indispensable course element which provides the focus for the integration of the knowledge and skills learnt at the college base'.

To underpin this essential role, and to promote the importance of clinical education at a time when it is threatened by external developments and possibly subject to change, the Society has published a new document 'Standards for Clinical Education Placements'.

These standards form the basis for the selection of clinical education placements by schools. They also provide guidance for managers of physiotherapy services both on what they themselves should be able to offer, and also on what they should expect of schools.

The standards should be used in conjunction with the Chartered Society of Physiotherapy's booklet, 'Standards of Physiotherapy Practice'.

The standards themselves may be summarised as follows:

1. The organisation and development of clinical education placements should involve liaison between the clinical education providers and the schools.

2. The school provides the clinical education placement with relevant information on the course, the placement and the students.

3. The physiotherapy manager provides the appropriate structure for the effective conduct of the clinical placement.

4. The clinical educator has sufficient experience and expertise to fulfil the objectives of the placement.

5. The student receives sufficient inform- ation to allow him/her to comply with the objectives of the placement.

6. The clinical educator undertakes preparation to fufil the objectives of the placement.

7. There is evidence of the student being fully integrated into the physiotherapy department.

8. Within the first week, a learning contract is negotiated between the student, clinical educator and clinical tutor, which takes account of the particular needs of the individual student and the given parameters of the clinical education placement.

9. There is evidence that the clinical educator fulfils the objectives of the learning contract.

10. The clinical tutor fulfils the role as liaison person between the placement and the school.

11. An evaluation of the placement will be carried out by the student, the school, the clinical educator and the physiotherapy manager.

12. There is evidence of a programme designed to review annually the appropriate- ness, applicability and suitability of the clinical education placements.

A copy of the 'Standards for Clinical Education Placements' document, detailing the criteria which apply to the above standards, is available from the Professional Affairs Department, Chartered Society of Physiotherapy, 14 Bedford Row, London WC1R 4ED.

THE FUNDING OF CLINICAL EDUCATION — THE OPTIONS

M. K. Lamont

INTRODUCTION

The professions involved in the delivery of health care all require, as part of their education, some practical or "hands on" clinical training. The present system evolved differently for each profession.

The reforms of the health system announced in the 1991 Budget papers[1] heralded a different approach to health delivery systems. In reviewing the present system it was clear that there were major inefficiencies and inequalities, resulting in funding problems. The Budget papers dealt with "fairness" — ". . . the system must treat people fairly"[2]. Also with "fragmentation" both in funding and delivery — ". . . the funding system is fragmented"[3]. There is little co-ordination between the various provider groups in either the funding system or in the actual delivery of care. There is a duplication of care in a number of instances.

Major reform was needed. The first step was to abolish the Area Health Board system and replace the 14 smaller boards with four larger regional health authorities. Next was to develop a system whereby the funders of health care could be separated from also being the providers. The theory being to improve efficiency and fairness and resolve conflict (all within a capped budget). The funders would determine the range of health services needed in any particular area and then buy services under contract from the providers. Central Government would set the minimum levels of service required and determine the classes within the population who would require various levels of health subsidy.

To seek competitive contracts, the Regional Health Authorities need to know, reasonably accurately, the cost of services. However, included in the cost of some services and in some areas are the costs involved in educating/training health care providers. It could be argued that this is not a legitimate expense in delivering competitive health services. On the other hand, the education programmes must be undertaken so the funding needs to be borne by somebody.

THE PROFESSIONS

The development of the educational systems for health care providers is wide and varied. It has developed without any apparent overall strategy — often it would seem that ad hoc decisions were made to resolve individual problems as they arose. Medical and dental education was at Otago University as was physiotherapy (Footnote 1). Only a few years after its establishment at Otago University the Physiotherapy School was transferred to the Otago Hospital Board. It joined a raft of other emerging health care provider groups (medical laboratory technologists, radiographers, orthotic and prosthetic technicians, occupational therapy and nursing) all of whom were educated from budgets within the hospital board system.

In the early 1970s Government decided that hospital boards were inappropriate organisations to provide education. The decision was to move the health groups to educational facilities — the Technical Institutes or Community Colleges. The split was logical although some professions were consigned to educational facilities which were bereft of clinical facilities (Footnote 2). Little recognition was given to the need to have available a varied and often prolific supply of clinical "material".

The Central Government funding of hospital boards was altered on a number of occasions — most recently to a population basis, but further enhanced to accommodate the extra costs of "teaching hospitals". On some occasions the cost of building hospital facilities was supplemented with funding from the University Grants Committee in recognition of the need to design and build facilities which would be suitable for teaching students.

FINANCIAL CONSTRAINTS

The late 1970s and through the 1980s brought financial constraints on many groups in the health sector. Staffing was reduced because of firm financial constraints from Government via the hospital boards. The numbers of health care providers being educated, however, remained unchanged thus causing some severe pressure upon the clinical facilities within hospitals. The emerging problem of whose responsibility it was to fund clinical education continued to provide some discontent. On the one hand the health providers were being asked to "teach" or provide "teaching material", but there was no reimbursement for cost. This was particularly so with nursing and physiotherapy whose programmes had moved away from hospital based education, but needed hospital input for clinical education. Medical clinical education was funded differently with a recognition by the Universities that clinicians needed a dual role (as health care providers and as teachers) so many hospital positions were "dual funded" (Footnote 3).

OTHER ON-THE-JOB TRAINING

Health clinical training can be compared to other training which requires on-the-job experience. The trades apprenticeship scheme is an example. The employer recognises the need to train the workforce and also accepts that there will be both costs and benefits. The cost is that in the initial years while an apprentice is employed there will be significant job training from senior members of their workforce. To compensate for that "loss" the employer pays a reduced wage as scheduled in Orders made by the Industrial Court of New Zealand (Appendix 1). Additionally, there is a contractual agreement between the employer and the Department of Labour (on behalf of the apprentice) to meet certain conditions pertaining to gaining the requisite trade experience.

There is also an example in the teaching profession when a student teacher is seconded to a school for actual classroom experience. The Department of Education recognises that in assisting and maintaining the student teacher there is a cost and a small additional hourly payment is made to the host teacher. Only teachers who have had at least two years' full-time teaching experience will be considered as hosts.

THE PRINCIPLES

The important principles are that:
1. The trade/profession has a responsibility to provide appropriate on-the-job training.
2. There are costs and benefits for the industry and the individuals.
3. There needs to be co-operation between the industry and the training/education facilities.

4. There are obligations for both parties, which can be defined in a contract.

The medical model which provides clinical education still has significant costs which are "transferred" to the health budget. Apart from the physical (building/furnishing) needs of education there are all of the extra associated costs of laboratory investigations; additional examinations; time in teaching rounds which disrupt the day-to-day running of a hospital ward or clinic; the length of stay in theatre when procedures are being undertaken by junior doctors or supervised as part of "teaching". Research is also a cost and is being met in part by the health budget. Specialist medical training is largely hospital based; however, some private clinical work is undertaken particularly orthopaedics because there is, at some hospitals, insufficient "cold" or elective surgery.

THE UNBUNDLING

The funding requirements of clinical education clearly needed review. An additional complicating factor is the perceived need for the Department of Health to "determine", at least for some professions, the numbers to be accepted for undergraduate courses — the entry numbers. This was a distinct function when health education was via Vote Health and when the Department (through the Hospital Boards) was a significant (and sometimes the only) benefactor of the educational programme. The Department was specifically charged with advising its Minister in this regard. Following the transfer of funding for undergraduate education to the Department of Education the requirement to give this advise to the Minister of Health was somewhat obscure. Nevertheless Health still had the belief that it must make determinations and advise its Minister in this area. The health delivery need and the educational need became confused with Health apparently being unable to relinquish its earlier role. Indeed workforce planning is a most difficult exercise and if based upon perceived needs of a public health system, will invariably be wrong. Dr Alistair Scott the Chairman of the New Zealand Medical Association was recently reported as saying that national manpower policy predictions are "notoriously wrong"[4]. Manpower planning is not about filling jobs in hospitals — it is about providing health services which the community need. It involves an international perspective; the linkage to central Government fiscal and monetary policy particularly in relation to health and welfare; the aspirations and directions of the professional groups themselves — their educational needs and their changing scope of practice; the demands of consumers which can be driven by a multitude of factors; the mix of private and public and the growth of health insurance, are but some of the determinants of manpower needs.

The Department of Health would seem to be the least suitable agency to determine these needs. An independent group with wide skills and independent thinking would be better suited to, conduct the necessary studies in this area. In the end it is probably the market which will determine the size of the health education intakes. The competition for placings will remain high when there is job certainly (either in New Zealand or worldwide) at the end of the education programme (Footnote 4). If the new graduates remain unemployed the personal and financial cost of the programme will lessen its value so the pressure to train will reduce. Defections within the term of the programme will also take place. The programme administrators need to compete for finance so will need to evaluate the direction of the programme and the need of the profession. Reducing intake size is one step, but others may include increasing the postgraduate opportunities; the present facilities (changing the programme to a research school) may increase; attracting overseas students — are some of the options.

THE ADVISORY GROUP

The health reforms directorate of the Department of the Prime Minister and Cabinet appointed Professor David Stewart to "develop policies and a structure for funding clinical education and training in the health sector through explicit contracting for the provision of clinical experience for undergraduate students and postgraduate trainees" (Appendix 2). This appointed committee (five members) received submissions and issued a preliminary options paper entitled "the Clinical Training of Health Professionals: Options for Funding" (Appendix 3). The paper sets out three questions and six options (Footnote 5).

The criteria listed in the draft report are consistent with the criteria being used to drive the health reforms changes, viz: — effectiveness, efficiency, quality assurance, accountability, continuity, adjustability.

The options display a variety of funding mechanisms through the involved Departments:

Option 1: Minimum Change

In this option, identified funding from Vote: Health would continue to be administered by the Department (Ministry) of Health and that from Vote: Education by the Ministry of Education. Payments could be made directly to providers, through RHA's.

Option 2:

A block grant from Vote: Health to teaching hospital CHE's.

Option 3:

Fund clinical training through RHA's from their population based allocation, by allowing or requiring them to pay a premium on the price of certain services purchased from providers with training programmes.

Option 4:

Establish a purchasing agency for Vote: Health funded education and training.

Option 5:

Transfer the funding of all education and training of health professionals to Vote: Education.

Option 6:

Some combination of two or more of the above.

The health sector reforms are based upon the principle of funder — provider split. It is intended that there be a contractual relationship between the two. The contract will specify the services and nominate the cost of those services. The contractual system will be competitive — between providers from both the "public" and "private" systems. It is clear that the "old way of doing things" will not meet the criteria of effectiveness, efficiency, quality assurance etc. A system for funding health education needs to be similarly focused. Within the health reform there is a recognition that a variety of delivery systems can be accommodated — from the development of health plans; to community trusts and the competition between various private and public suppliers. The clinical placement of health professionals is therefore likely to be much wider than the present predominant public system. More community based facilities are likely to be used. To a large degree the need to obtain the appropriate clinical experience will be determined by the educational facility. That need will change as the student progresses through any particular course and may well change as the clinical service itself changes as it contracts for its own funding.

The need will change in relation to either the undergraduate or postgraduate requirements; and to the degree of "specialisation" within any particular programme.

THE MAXIMS

To meet the criteria of the Clinical Review Committee the funding systems will need to be:

— "Transparent" — that it will be clear as to the terms and conditions of funding.
— Contractible — between the purchaser and the provider.
— Variable — over time and between different providers.
— Needs based — that is determined by the educational facility and programme.
— Without "political" interference between competing Government Departments.
— Without linkage to departmental based manpower predictions.

For those reasons option 1 (maintaining status quo) will fail. The present system must change. Likewise Option 2 of funding CHE's from Vote: Health fails to recognise the varied nature of the future clinical placements of students. Option 3 links clinical training to the RHA's by ". . . requiring them to pay a premium on the price of certain services purchased from providers with training programmes"[5]. The option begins to address the need for contractibility between funder and provider, however, there is still the illogical funding mechanism through the health system — the RHA (and presumably the CHE). It is the educational facility which needs to "buy" the clinical experience — diectly with the provider and not through an intermediary.

The 4th option still has funding through Vote: Health although "devolved" into a separate and autonomous agency within the Department (Ministry) of Health. The "political" interference to conform to the Department's policy will continue. This is an education issue and not one of health delivery.

A direct simile can be used by observing the Registration Board's unit — an autonomous unit within the Department of Health. After many years of anxiety over workforce statistic collection various Health Registration Boards decide not to send out the Departments "survey" forms with 1992 annual practising certificate renewal requests. The Department reacted by emphasising that even though the Unit was autonomous it MUST confirm and obey Departmental directives!

Option 5 provides for the transferring of all education funding to the Department of Education. The funding within and access to programmes would be contestable. The educational facility would buy (contract) the exact clinical experience it needed — directly from the provider. The provider has the ability to submit and contest for the available funding. The links with the present workforce planning would certainly be weak, however, they are now so that will not impede the system. As discussed earlier workforce planning is not a logical function of the Department of Health.

The final option is a proposal for combinations with respect to some funding via Vote: Health (postgraduate) and some via Vote: Education (undergraduate). Once again there is the opportunity of Departmental bias in offering funding to only those programmes which the Department, in its wisdom, thinks it needs. It is the profession and the educational facility with perhaps input from the Department, which will ultimately determine the needs of each professional group.

SUMMARY

The transference of all funding to Vote: Education is most appropriate (Option 5). It allows the educational facility the flexibility to purchase the services it requires. It gives adequate flexibility and adaptability. Through contractual arrangements it can give accountability and have pre-determined quality assurance systems. The linkage between the purchaser (the educational facility) and the provider can be very specific and need not be via an RHA or CHE, but directly to a service. Whether or not the service is public or private will not be an issue. Option 5 gives the greatest consistency within the total health reforms package.

REFERENCES

1. Upton, S. Your health and the Public Health; Minister of Health Parliament Buildings, Wellington, July 1991.
2. Ibid. P. 18.
3. Ibid. P. 14.
4. Scott, Alistair. New Zealand Doctor, New Zealand Doctor Newspapers Ltd. 21 May 1992. P. 64.
5. "The Clincial Training of Health Professionals: Options for Funding": Health Reforms Directorate: Department of Prime Minister, Wellington. P. 8.

FOOTNOTE 1: Dental nurse education was developed post Second World War to deal with a dental caries problem in children. It was funded directly by the Department of Health and a number of dental clinics (educational) were established. All except one have now been closed.

FOOTNOTE 2: The Central Institute of Technology (CIT) set out to become a "Health Science" institution and was allocated Occupational Therapy; Orthotics and prosthetics, podiatry, radiotherapy and pharmacy. The nearest clinical facility was the Hutt Hospital and the nearest basic anatomy facility was Palmerston North (being a "teaching" hospital). Today only podiatry remains at CIT.

FOOTNOTE 3: At the end of the financial year there was a "swapping" of cheques to balance the books with respect to work done for each party. There was a recognition that clinical training took time and had to be paid for.

FOOTNOTE 4: There are about 1,000 applicants for the 120 physiotherapy student placements in New Zealand each year. Similar demand is experienced in medicine.

FOOTNOTE 5: Question 1: Should the funding of clinical training be linked with other aspects of workforce development, for example ongoing workforce planning?

Question 2: How should those excess costs of teaching hospitals not attributable to clinical training be funded in the new health system?

Question 3: Which of the proposed options is most likely to provide a structure which meets the criteria listed in Section 8.1?

APPENDIX I

NEW ZEALAND CARPENTRY AND JOINERY INDUSTRY — APPRENTICESHIP ORDER

Dated 20/12/74

Published and issued by the New Zealand Government Department of Labour

(e) For the purpose of this order an employer who himself works substantially at the branch of the industry to which the apprentice is to be apprenticed shall be entitled to count himself as a journeyman. An employer shall be deemed to work substantially at the branch of the industry if he devotes sufficient time to train and supervise apprentices, even if he may not devote half his time to actual work at the trade.

(f) For the purposes of this order "journeyman" shall mean a worker who has completed a contract of apprenticeship or who has had sufficient experience in the relevant branch of the industry to satisfy the employer and the local committee of his competence.

(g) The powers and discretions provided for in section 29 of the Apprentices Act 1948 may be exercised by the District Commissioner and the local committee notwithstanding that the employer to whom it is proposed to transfer an apprentice is already employing the full quota of apprentices as determined by the apprenticeship order.

WAGES

11. (a) (i) With the exception of the provisions contained in subclause (e) of this clause, as from 13 January 1975 the minimum weekly rates of wages payable to apprentices shall be the undermentioned percentages of the minimum weekly wage rate for journeymen (or if no weekly wage is prescribed, then of an amount equal to 40 times the minimum hourly wage rate for journeymen) in the branch of the industry to which the apprentice is apprenticed, as prescribed by the award or agreement relating to the employment of such journeymen in the establishment in which the apprentice is employed and in force for the time being and from time to time.

	For apprentices serving an 8,000-hour term Per Cent	For apprentices serving 7,000-hour term Per Cent
First 1,000-hour period	46	52
Second 1,000-hour period	52	57
Third 1,000-hour period	57	62
Fourth 1,000-hour period	62	67
Fifth 1,000-hour period	67	75
Sixth 1,000-hour period	75	85
Seventh 1,000-hour period	85	95
Eighth 1,000-hour period	95	

(ii) Where by virtue of the application of the provisions of subclause (b), (c), and (d) of this clause, there ceases to be any prescribed minimum weekly wages payable to an apprentice who has not completed his term of apprenticeship, such apprentice shall for the remainder of his term of apprenticeship be paid for not less than 100 percent of the minimum rates for journeymen.

(b) An apprentice who in the School Certificate Examination has obtained not less than 50 percent of the possible marks in mathematics and any two of the following subjects — English, woodwork and technical drawing — shall be paid as if he had served 1,000 hours of his apprenticeship.

APPENDIX II

FUNDING OF CLINICAL EDUCATION AND TRAINING PROJECT

Terms of Reference

The proposed Terms of Reference for the consultant, Professor David Stewart are:

To develop policies and a structure for funding clinical education and training in the health sector through explicit contracting for the provision of clinical experience for undergraduate students and post graduate trainees.

To achieve this objective the principal consultant shall:

(i) review and assess models for funding and provision of clinical experience in New Zealand and overseas countries with close health service links to New Zealand;

(ii) develop policy options for the funding of clinical experience in a restructured health service, including consideration of the funding source, required administrative structure or agency, a contracting framework, and any issues relating to the wider health reforms. This will take the form of a discussion paper.

(iii) assist the NIPB in identifying and estimating present health sector costs of providing clinical experience in New Zealand;

(iv) consult with affected parties including the Universities, Polytechnics and Professional Colleges offering health professional qualifications, health service managers, relevant occupational licensing bodies, professional associations, and the Department of Health concerning these options;

(v) consult with officials in the Department of Health, Health Reforms Directorate, the National Interim Provider Board and the Ministry of Education to ensure that the proposed arrangements are consistent with Government policy in health and education; and

(vi) recommend policies and a structure for funding clinical experience in the health sector from July 1993, including a proposed contracting framework, the roles and responsibilities of participating agencies, and legislative measures required to implement the proposals.

In undertaking these tasks, the principal consultant shall be responsible to the Director, Health Reforms Directorate.

Exploring the Costs and Benefits Drivers of Clinical Education

Susan K. Meyers

Key Words: education • fieldwork, occupational therapy, level II • qualitative method

Objective. *This study was designed to identify monetary and nonmonetary costs and benefits, as well as their drivers, to assist persons in clinical sites who are implementing clinical education to minimize costs and maximize benefits.*

Method. *Qualitative research methodology involved students, student supervisors, administrators, and patients in a hermeneutic dialectic process of identifying costs and benefits of Level II fieldwork in three clinical sites.*

Results. *Different costs and benefits were identified by the different groups of respondents. Drivers, or causes, of these costs and benefits reflected unique environmental factors in each site of data collection as well as common factors across the sites.*

Conclusion. *Clinical education may be enhanced and stress reduced for all persons involved in clinical education through improved communication, structure, education, and support.*

Susan K. Meyers, EdD, MBA, OTR, is Associate Professor and Chair, Department of Occupational Therapy, College of Health and Human Services, Western Michigan University, Kalamazoo, Michigan 49008.

This article was accepted for publication January 4, 1994.

Occupational therapy students are dependent on practitioners in clinical environments to provide them with experiences necessary to integrate and apply theory to practice. The monetary costs and benefits associated with clinical education have been identified in the literature (Chung & Spelbring, 1983; Page & MacKinnon, 1987; Porter & Kincaid, 1977; Schauble, Murphy, Cover-Patterson, & Archer, 1989; Shalik, 1987). The net monetary cost benefits to facilities that provide clinical education to students are (a) revenue generated by students who provide treatment to patients and (b) increased revenue generated by therapists who are freed by students from performing clerical and administrative tasks. However, changes in health care environments, including increases in the number of students seeking clinical education and in the demands for productivity in patient treatment, have created new demands for practitioners responsible for the clinical education of occupational therapy students.

In previous cost-benefit analyses, the use of an a priori theory limited costs and benefits to those that could be monetarily quantified. The rigor required for generalization of conventional research has negated the relevance of factors that may be contextually meaningful, such as nonmonetary costs and benefits of therapists, students, patients, and administrators who have a stake in clinical education. This study was designed to identify monetary and nonmonetary costs and benefits, as well as the drivers of these costs and benefits. Identifying the drivers of costs and benefits may assist persons in clinical sites who are implementing or planning to implement clinical education to minimize costs and maximize benefits to all of the stakeholders in the clinical site.

Methodology

This study used the qualitative research methodology of naturalistic inquiry to collect and analyze data from three clinical education sites over a 6-month period. Study participants included 19 administrators and student supervisors; 14 occupational therapy students who were completing first, second, or third rotations of clinical education; and 6 patients who were being treated by the students.

The major methods of data collection were observation, individual and focus group interviews, and documents review. Data collection and analysis were done simultaneously with a constant comparative method (Glaser & Strauss, 1967; Lincoln & Guba, 1985; Strauss & Corbin, 1990). Each piece of data was grouped with similar pieces of data until clear categories that were salient to the research concern emerged. These categories provided the skeletal shape of the information needed to understand the costs and benefits drivers of clinical education. The data led to additional questions and responses that gave flesh to the skeletal shape by providing a collaborative understanding of costs and benefits drivers of clinical education.

Trustworthiness techniques used to establish rigor for the qualitative research were prolonged engagement, persistent observation, peer debriefing, negative case analysis, progressive subjectivity, and member checks (Guba & Lincoln, 1989). Prolonged engagement was achieved by spending 6 months, or two rotations of clinical education, at each site in order to build a rapport with respondents and gain an understanding of the culture of the setting. Persistent observation, which gave depth to the study, was achieved by multiple observations and interviews with each respondent. This technique led to improved understanding of costs and benefits drivers affecting stakeholders of the clinical education process.

Two peer debriefers, disinterested parties with knowledge of the methodology and understanding of the research questions, were used throughout this study. By posing questions and suggestions, the debriefers helped focus the inquiry and kept my work consistent with the methods of naturalistic inquiry.

Negative case analysis involved looking for alternative constructions, or views, to those most often stated by respondents. As respondents generated these alternative views and discussed them with me and each other, respondents either modified their views as a result of new knowledge, or continued to hold their different views; in either case, they acknowledged that other views were also valuable in understanding the costs and benefits associated with clinical education.

Progressive subjectivity occurred when my own construction changed as a result of being better informed by respondents. Member checks provided the mechanism to ensure that a construction was in fact that of the respondent as he or she reported it. At the end of each observation or interview, data that I recorded were reviewed with the contributing respondent. Respondents either verified the accuracy or elaborated on their concerns and clarified their viewpoints. At the conclusion of the study, drafts of the final constructions of costs and benefits drivers of clinical education were distributed to all respondents for their agreement regarding data accuracy. This procedure led to additional clarification, which continued until all respondents agreed that the final construction was accurate, regardless of whether they agreed with the views of others. An audit trail referenced each piece of data reported by respondents to its source. The sources of all data have been kept anonymous.

Results

The results of the analysis indicated that students, student supervisors, administrators, and patients constructed costs and benefits drivers differently. Summaries and comparisons of costs and benefits drivers appear in Table 1.

The costs and benefits drivers were considerably dif-

Table 1
Level II Fieldwork Costs and Benefits Identified by Respondent Groups

Costs and Benefits	Students	Student Supervisors	Administrators	Patients
Monetary costs				
Cost of treatment			•	•
Travel to site	•			•
Space for students		•	•	
Supplies used by students		•	•	
Loss of income from work	•			•
Loss of revenue		•	•	
Potential liability			•	
Clothing	•			
Housing	•			
Tuition	•	•		
Failure	•	•		
Nonmonetary costs				
Stress	•	•		•
Frustration	•	•		•
Loss of esteem	•	•		•
Responsibility		•		
Annoyance to staff members	•		•	
Illness from stress	•			
Failure	•			
Monetary benefits				
Revenue		•	•	
Recruitment		•	•	
Cost savings	•		•	•
Nonmonetary benefits				
Learning	•	•	•	•
Relationship formation	•	•	•	•
Stay current in practice		•	•	•
Satisfaction		•	•	
Self-esteem	•	•		
Excitement	•	•		
Peer support	•		•	
Attention				•
Professional commitment		•	•	
Prestige	•			
Decreased patient load		•		

ferent among student supervisors both across the three clinical sites and within each site. Stress was a nonmonetary cost for all student supervisors, but this stress was driven by different situations indigenous to each site. In some sites, student supervisors identified external pressures to lower standards for student performance so that students who performed poorly would pass the clinical education experience. In two sites, student supervisors reported feeling stressed by organizational structure over which they believed they had little control. In two sites, there were conflicting constructions of nonmonetary cost drivers among student supervisors and their administrators in the organization, which created additional stress for therapists, students, and patients in the sites. When these types of conflicts existed, students identified them as contributors to a stressful clinical education experience.

There were some similarities among student supervisors' constructions of nonmonetary cost drivers. Students' egocentrism and dependence on their supervisors drove costs in all three clinical sites. Some students' behaviors, such as delayed response to treatment team members (especially when this was mentioned by other health care providers), contributed to the student supervisors' negative image of the profession. Student supervisors had to take their own work home in the evenings as a result of the time they spent supervising their students during the day. Although student supervisors from all sites agreed on these drivers of nonmonetary costs, administrators did not identify these drivers. However, administrators agreed that students might be a cause of frustration to student supervisors.

All student supervisors identified the same monetary costs. Student supervisors and administrators agreed that there was minimal cost associated with providing students materials such as manuals and supplies in the clinics. Greater costs were associated with space needed for students in the sites, especially when space was scarce. Another cost was lost revenue driven by the need for student supervisors to spend time educating students instead of treating patients. When students were assigned the task of preparing patients' charges, they missed some of the charges due to inexperience with the billing process.

Student supervisors and administrators agreed that monetary benefits were gained from students treating patients, especially after students completed the first half of a clinical education rotation. Cost savings resulted from hiring students to become staff therapists in the sites studied.

Identification of nonmonetary benefits of clinical education was similar across sites. Student supervisors said they experienced satisfaction and increased knowledge because of their work with students. Students gave their supervisors positive feedback, and supervisors believed that they were doing a service to the profession by educating future clinicians. Student supervisors kept current in treatment techniques and research related to patient care so that they would be better able to teach their students. Students brought new ideas with them to the clinics and completed projects and assignments that were beneficial to their supervisors. When students were performing well, their supervisors had additional time to spend with patients or in other related activities. Students were credited with bringing a freshness and new enthusiasm for clinical practice, which some of the student supervisors identified as a benefit. Administrators in the three sites also tended to be in agreement with these benefits of clinical education.

Students at the three sites identified similar monetary costs drivers, including housing, utilities, and food. All had to pay tuition to their academic institutions for credit hours they received for clinical education. These costs were driven by the requirement to complete assigned clinical education as part of their academic programs. Transportation was another monetary cost, because most students lived a distance from the clinical sites

and incurred local transportation expenses. Some students traveled from another city or state for clinical education. Some students needed to purchase clothing to wear in the clinics because the clothes they owned were not suitable for the clinic. A few students lost revenue from jobs they either gave up or reduced hours for in order to devote their time and energy to their clinical education experience.

Students across the three sites also identified similar nonmonetary costs. Students experienced considerable stress as a result of their clinical education. This stress resulted in symptoms of illness and some absences from the clinic. As some students became more stressed, their performance worsened. This set in motion a vicious cycle in which the students' stress led to poor performance, which in turn resulted in negative feedback from their supervisors. The negative feedback exacerbated the students' stress and, in at least one case, was identified as the cause of student failure. Some of the drivers of stress identified by the students included being watched by supervisors; having trouble with critical thinking, time management, and communication; lacking skills in specific treatment techniques; fearing failure; having heard negative comments about the clinical education site or the supervisors in the site; dealing with the reality of very sick patients; and adjusting to the role of worker. Adapting from a student role to a worker role was especially difficult for students during a first clinical education experience. Just getting to work through morning traffic and working an 8-hr day were identified as being highly stressful. In addition, most of the students said they took large amounts of work home in the evenings.

Some students were more satisfied than others with their clinical education sites, and this satisfaction mitigated the stress they experienced. Students who were in a site that they had requested as their first choice for clinical education were more satisfied than students who were not placed in their first choice sites. Students who were in a site in which they were fairly certain they wanted to continue working after completing their clinical education were the most satisfied and the least stressed.

All of the student respondents agreed that they experienced no monetary benefits from being in the clinical sites studied. They did not identify future monetary benefits that would result from this education process. They did identify cost savings because they did not have to buy textbooks for clinical education. Several students said that their parents were supporting them through clinical education—another form of cost savings.

Nonmonetary benefits were similar for all students who participated in this study. Students learned skills necessary for clinical practice; they also learned more about themselves. Learning in the clinics was driven by exposure to patients and supervisors. Application of theories and techniques learned in school were integrated and given relevance in the clinic settings. Students increased their confidence in their abilities when they were successful in treating patients and received positive feedback from supervisors. Students identified contact with supervisors as helpful in shaping both a professional image and a sense of belonging to a professional group. Some of the drivers decreasing stress identified by the students were receiving a good orientation to the site; having other students with whom to share the clinical education experience; and receiving manuals and handouts that specified expected performance in the sites. Almost anything that increased the structure of the clinical education experience was considered a stress reducer by students.

Costs and benefits identified by the patients were different from those of the other groups of respondents. Patients discussed major monetary costs due to illness and treatment that were not specifically related to treatment in a clinical education environment. They identified nonmonetary costs associated with separation from families and loss of functional abilities due to their illnesses. However, patients identified benefits resulting specifically from the services they received in a clinical education environment. They learned about their illnesses or injuries from supervisors' explanations to students about the treatment process. Patients said that if a supervisor trusted a student, the student must be capable of doing a good job and that the treatment he or she received from that student was of good quality. Patients saw little difference in skill levels between students and student supervisors. Some patients identified differences in attitudes between students and student supervisors. In the sites where student supervisors were more stressed by their working conditions, patients identified students as more enthusiastic than student supervisors about work.

Students and student supervisors identified different reasons for student failures. Student supervisors said that students were not adequately prepared for the work in clinic sites; that students had difficulty because of poor technical, problem-solving, and communication skills; and that students demonstrated inadequate self-awareness. Students said that failures were a result of inadequate supervision, poor communication, inadequate feedback, lack of structure, and personality clashes with supervisors. Students accepted responsibility for contributing to their own failures. Some of the student supervisors shared responsibility for student failures, saying that they could have intervened sooner to prevent failures.

Conclusion

Although the results of this study are not generalizable, information about costs and benefits drivers of clinical education may be useful to other clinical education sites.

Bureaucratic organizational structures of the three sites contributed to nonmonetary costs of clinical education for students and student supervisors. Decisions

made at high levels of the organization were transmitted to persons at lower levels for implementation; however, persons providing direct services to patients believed that high-level decision makers were not adequately informed to make those decisions. The discrepancy between student supervisors and administrators regarding the drivers of costs and benefits appeared to be a result of inadequate communication across hierarchical lines.

When student supervisors were not satisfied with administrators of their work units, there was a direct effect on the clinical education of students; students who heard their supervisors talking about their dissatisfaction became stressed. Student supervisors who were the most stressed seemed to be the least satisfied with the responsibility of educating students. When student supervisors were cohesive with other supervisors in their work units, clinical education was a positive experience for students. Student supervisors' report of satisfaction with autonomy in their work and with their relationships with each other and with their administrators seemed to result in the best environment for providing clinical education to students.

As data collection for this study progressed, respondents began to make changes in their environments. Communication improved among respondents, and more structure was provided for students in some sites. Administrators' concerns with what was occurring in clinical education sites appeared to increase. Some of the changes that were made to improve clinical education appeared to be the result of the interactive nature of the research methodology used in this study. Naturalistic inquiry seemed to be the catalyst for turning ideas expressed by respondents into actions that would maximize benefits and minimize costs of clinical education.

Recommendations

The goals of cost-benefit analysis are to maximize benefits and minimize costs. On the basis of this study, the following six guidelines are recommended to facilities that want to establish or improve existing clinical education programs and reduce stress to all persons involved.

1. Establish effective communication between administrators and student supervisors related to worker satisfaction. Informal and consistent communication between administrators and subordinates lessens stress in the work environment and enhances clinical education.
2. Decentralize decision making related to task performance within the clinic sites, including decisions related to clinical education. Persons with direct contact with students in the work environment have the greatest information with which to make decisions about scheduling, supervising, and terminating students. Decentralized decision making allows decisions to be made quickly and

to be made in response to changes in the environment. If decentralized decision making is not possible, the administrator responsible for making decisions should spend time in the clinic site and be willing to discuss and negotiate decisions with those subordinates responsible for carrying out the tasks of clinical education.

3. Offer education and support to supervisors. Student supervisors in clinics that have well-established, successful education programs, in which student supervisors and students have satisfying experiences, should share their methods with student supervisors in other sites who have less satisfying experiences. This sharing of information may be accomplished through supervisor support groups or individual mentoring of a new supervisor by a more experienced supervisor who enjoys working with students.

4. Provide students with a structured learning experience. A clearly defined structure for clinical education assists students in adapting to a work environment and maximizes their performance. Such a structure includes frequent formal evaluation of students so that the students know how they are performing. Students should also be accountable for tasks in the site; a checklist of performance expectations would be helpful to both students and their supervisors.

5. Establish criteria for student performance. Academicians who send students into clinical education sites should be aware of the requirements for student performance in each site. Students should be prepared to adequately perform tasks required in the clinic sites. Additional course content, including training in assertive behavior, critical thinking, and time management, may need to be added to improve student success. (In this study, students had more difficulty with general behaviors than with specific treatment techniques.)

6. Limit some clinical education sites to students who are in a second or third rotation of clinical education. (In this study, when a clinical site required specialized skills, students on a first rotation had great difficulty performing while adjusting to the new role of worker.) ▲

References

Chung, Y. I., & Spelbring, L. M. (1983). An analysis of weekly instructional input hours and student work hours in occupational therapy fieldwork. *American Journal of Occupational Therapy, 37,* 681–687.

Glaser, B., & Strauss, A. (1967). *The discovery of grounded theory: Strategies for qualitative research.* Chicago: Aldine.

Guba, E. G., & Lincoln, Y. S. (1989). *Fourth generation evaluation.* Newbury Park, CA: Sage.

Lincoln, Y., & Guba, E. (1985). *Naturalistic inquiry.* Beverly Hills, CA: Sage.

Page, S. S., & MacKinnon, J. R. (1987). Cost of clinical instructors' time in clinical education: Physical therapy students. *Physical Therapy, 67,* 238–243.

Porter, R. E., & Kincaid, C. B. (1977). Financial aspects of clinical education to facilities. *Physical Therapy, 57,* 905–908.

Schauble, P. G., Murphy, M. C., Cover-Paterson, C. E., & Archer, J. (1989). Cost effectiveness of internship training programs: Clinical service delivery through training. *Professional Psychology: Research and Practice, 40*(2), 17–22.

Shalik, L. D. (1987). Cost-benefit analysis of level II fieldwork in occupational therapy. *American Journal of Occupational Therapy, 41,* 638–645.

Strauss, A., & Corbin, J. (1990). *Basics of qualitative research: Grounded theory procedures and techniques.* Newbury Park, CA: Sage.

Clinical Education Costs and Benefits: Application of a Fiscal Analysis Model

Doris R. Kling
Joyce A. Bulgrin

ABSTRACT: A model for analyzing the costs and benefits of clinical education through active data collection was developed and implemented in an associate degree medical laboratory technician program. Five years later the model was retested and results of the study were compared to the original findings. In each case, data were generated by students over a two-semester period. Differences between the total cost of clinical education and the value of student service work, in terms of labor produced and revenue generated, were calculated. Evaluation of the data indicated that it is not possible to calculate a value for the net cost of clinical education representative of all participating hospitals because of a large variance in factors affecting costs. The data were also useful in evaluating other aspects of clinical education, such as the relationship of instruction time to total assignment time (instruction ratio); the percentage of service work performed by students; and the types of laboratory procedures most frequently performed by students.

Concern for health care cost containment, the lack of information about the cost of the clinical component of medical laboratory science programs, and a state-level recommendation to review the cost of allied health clinical education were the factors that influenced the development of a model for analyzing the cost of the clinical component of clinical laboratory science programs. Ori-

Doris R. Kling, MT(ASCP), PhD, is dean of the Career Education Division, and Joyce A. Bulgrin, MT(ASCP), MSA, is an instructor in the MLT-AD Program at Illinois Central College in East Peoria, Illinois 61635.

Manuscript received December 29, 1986; accepted Febuary 13, 1987.

Reprinted with permission from the *Journal of Allied Health.* Kling DR, Bulgrin JA. 1987;16(5):135-145.

ginally conceived and tested in 1979-80 for an associate degree medical laboratory technician program, the methodology was retested in 1984-85, using the same program and its affiliated hospitals.

This model for fiscal analysis, however, is not limited to associate degree education. It is applicable to any level of clinical laboratory science education that incorporates learning experiences in a service laboratory. Moreover, the technique may be adapted to other health profession education programs that have a clinical component.

Review of the literature revealed that little has been published about clinical education cost analysis in medical laboratory science at the associate degree level. A few articles did, however, focus on medical laboratory science education at the baccalaureate level. Wiebe, for example, described the cost-benefit analysis performed in the twelve-month clinical component of a "3 + 1" baccalaureate medical technology program. Her study found that this program cost the hospital $5,000 in 1981-82, but that several other "identifiable benefits help offset this expense and contribute to the quality of health care."[1]

Smith and Malcolm designed a cost inventory document that was completed appropriately by four out of five hospitals providing the clinical component of the medical technology program of Louisiana State University.[2] This study used estimates of the annual work load that each employee devoted to the instruction of students; average annual cost for extra laboratory supplies; and average annual purchase, repair, and maintenance of equipment required because of the education program. Subtracting estimated student contribution to cost reduction resulted in a $5,100 clinical education cost per student annually.

A study of ten allied health education programs, including medical technology, was reported by Harper and Gonyea at The Ohio State University in 1977.[3] This research resulted in a method for cost analysis, which took into account the costs related to an entire program, including both university and clinical expenses. Information was gathered by questionnaire and estimates were made about the 1974-75 school year. The average yearly cost per student was calculated at $4,078.

In contrast, Pobojewski found an estimated benefit of $46,186 to a hospital that provided the clinical experience for a two-year, college-based radiologic technology program.[4] Examining estimated educational cost, material cost, overhead cost, and the revenue-producing activities performed by the students, Pobojewski concluded that this benefit was probably conservative as no value had been assigned to the anticipated increase in productivity of staff members whose time was freed up by students performing some activities.

Similarly, Carney and Keim collected productivity information on radiologic technology students through interviews with hospital administrators, clinical instructors, students, and graduates.[5] Participants in the study agreed that the work load carried by students equaled or excelled the time staff members devoted to teaching activities. Minor significance was assigned to capital cost and consumable items. The fact that students kept staff alert and facilitated "an influx of new ideas" was cited as an intangible benefit.

In 1982, Hammersberg reported the results of an analysis of costs and benefits in health care facilities that affiliated with allied health programs at Miami-Dade Community College.[6] This study used a questionnaire to determine estimates of the time involved in teaching students and the costs related to educational supplies. These estimates were considered the cost or debit of the affiliation while the work contributed by students was used as the benefit or credit. The study found the debits were greater than the credits in all programs under consideration. Moreover, there was a wide variation in cost per student between programs. Hammersberg expressed concern about the variation in the reported cost of supplies and indicated that some figures might have been "wild guesses." This is one of the disadvantages of gathering data on a retroactive basis.

Selecting activities to include in a cost measurement is a problem that several researchers have addressed. Koehler and Slighton stated that the cost of all activities that affect the educational process directly and indirectly must be measured.[7] Others, like Johnson and Eady[8] and Haggart,[9] disagreed. On this point, Haggart wrote that it is increasingly acceptable not to allocate indirect costs in program budgeting "because it reduces the danger of unknowingly biasing the cost of individual programs." She reasoned that biasing can occur because there are many logical rules for allocation and each can produce different results under identical circumstances.

METHOD

The medical laboratory technician program selected for study was a two-year community-college-based program that combined campus class work with part-time clinical experience in four local hospitals. Hospitals A and B were community hospitals, each with about a 350-bed capacity, while Hospitals C and D were larger, complex teaching institutions, each with its own baccalaureate-level medical technology program. Because of the diversity in clinical affiliate size and test volume, students were assigned on a rotation basis to different sections at each hospital for a total of 480 hours per student during the last three semesters of the program.

The first study began in January 1979 when the twenty-five enrolled students were asked to keep track of all practice and service tests that they performed on forms specifically designed for this purpose.[10] The forms were categorized by laboratory section and were color-coded to differentiate the practice from the service functions. Students recorded the type and number of tests performed in each assigned rotation on a daily basis.

In addition, students recorded the amount of daily instruction time received from clinical personnel. This was categorized as preparation time, direct instruction, demonstration, and supervision. Students were asked to record the amount of teaching time received from laboratory personnel in hours and minutes after each daily assignment. Information about preparation time, used for preliminary tasks, such as special sample preparation and organization of material, was requested directly from the instructors. Students and instructors were assured that lack of preparation time would not be viewed as neglect of professional responsibility because in many cases special preparation was not necessary.

Criteria for categorizing instruction time were carefully explained to the students. Additionally, they were given sheets that defined each type of instruction. Direct instruction was defined as the occasion when the instructor presented new information to the student in an organized manner. Time during which the instructor performed an activity that the student merely observed was to be recorded as demonstration time. Lastly, time during which the instructor monitored student progress while the student performed an activity, for which necessary knowledge had been acquired previously, was classified as supervision. In this situation, direct or constant interaction with the student did not necessarily occur and the instructor was usually able to perform other tasks at the same time.

Recording continued to the end of the spring semester in May 1979 and resumed again in August 1979 for the fall semester. During the spring semester, the thirteen freshmen and twelve sophomores were placed in a total of 125 assignments. Reports were received on 109 of these assignments for a response rate of 87.2%. Twelve of the thirteen freshmen continued as sophomores in the fall semester and again the response rate on assignments was excellent (86.6% for instruction time data and 76.7% for test data). Interviews with selected hospital personnel confirmed that students had recorded their work and that the types and numbers of tests seemed reasonable.

Each hospital was asked to supply the financial data needed for cost calculation: gross number of tests performed per laboratory and per individual section; the average hourly salary of medical technologists, medical technicians, and technical specialists; the average labor costs per test; average supply costs per test; and the costs allocated per test for building depreciation, plant operation and maintenance, housekeeping, employee benefits, and administration, including fiscal services, personnel, and purchasing (allocated indirect costs)

Hospitals A, B, and C provided all the necessary data for both semesters. Hospital D, however, submitted only partial information for the spring semester and ultimately withdrew from the study without returning any data for the fall semester. Therefore, complete calculations were limited to Hospitals A, B, and C while only partial calculations were made for Hospital D.

Through the use of a computer program written especially for this purpose, instruction time was tallied according to preparation, direct instruction, demonstration, and supervision for each hospital section. The second portion of the program compiled test data for each hospital section and calculated costs related to test numbers.

Calculations were based on the following equation that took into account the variables affecting net cost:

$$\begin{array}{c}\text{Total} \\ \text{Instruction} \\ \text{Cost}\end{array} + \begin{array}{c}\text{Total} \\ \text{Supply} \\ \text{Cost}\end{array} + \begin{array}{c}\text{Indirect} \\ \text{Cost}\end{array} - \begin{array}{c}\text{Cash value of} \\ \text{labor for ser-} \\ \text{vice produced} \\ \text{by students or} \\ \text{revenue generated} \\ \text{by student service work}\end{array} = \begin{array}{c}\text{Net} \\ \text{clinical} \\ \text{education} \\ \text{cost}\end{array}$$

For comparative purposes the equation was also applied with the exclusion of indirect cost:

$$\begin{array}{c}\text{Total} \\ \text{Instruction} \\ \text{Cost}\end{array} + \begin{array}{c}\text{Total} \\ \text{Supply} \\ \text{Cost}\end{array} - \begin{array}{c}\text{Cash value of} \\ \text{labor for ser-} \\ \text{vice produced} \\ \text{by students or} \\ \text{revenue generated} \\ \text{by student service work}\end{array} = \begin{array}{c}\text{Net} \\ \text{clinical} \\ \text{education} \\ \text{cost}\end{array}$$

Instruction time, which is assigned to cost, was calculated by adding the total preparation, direct instruction, and demonstration time and including one-half of the supervision time. Because supervision time is used to monitor student progress and does not require constant interaction with the student, only half of it was assigned cost in the final calculation. Due to the lack of complete reports, data on instruction time and test totals were adjusted to reflect the full complement of students assigned to the section. Total instruction cost was then determined by multiplying the grand total by the average hourly salary rate for laboratory personnel.

Supply and indirect costs for all hospitals were calculated on the basis of the adjusted practice test data. The total adjusted number of practice tests was multiplied by the average cost of supplies per test to arrive at total supply cost. Multiplying the total adjusted number of practice tests by the average indirect cost per test yielded the total indirect cost.

Because student service work provides a benefit for the hospital, the net clinical education cost was determined by off-setting the total costs with either the cash value of student labor or the revenue generated by them. The cash value of labor produced by students was derived from the adjusted number of service tests performed and the average labor costs per test. The revenue generated by student service work was based on the per-test revenue multiplied by the adjusted test total.

In addition to financial information, the collected data provided a means for evaluating several other aspects of clinical eduction. Specifically, the relationship of instruction time to total assignment time was established as the instruction ratio (IR). Moreover, it was possible to determine the percentage of practice and service tests assigned to students and to assess the types of laboratory procedures students were performing most frequently.

In 1983, one of the clinical affiliates requested reimbursement for some of the reagents that the students were using for practice procedures. While the money involved was not a sizable sum, program officials became concerned about future requests of this nature. It was concluded that another study of clinical education costs was warranted. Thus, the original data collection process was once again implemented during the fall of 1984 and spring of 1985. Repeating the original model confirmed the usefulness of the technique and provided a means of establishing a comparison of costs as well as the auxiliary parameters, such as the instruction ratio, types of tests performed, and amount of service work assigned to students.[11]

RESULTS

The data in both studies indicated that the total cost of clinical education was influenced by instruction time, supply costs, indirect costs, numbers of students assigned to a hospital, and the length of assignment. Revenue generated by student service work was found to be substantially higher than the cash value of labor produced. A comparison of total and net costs of clinical education is presented in Table I.

The net costs of clinical education per hour of student assignment are shown in Table II. In most cases, these costs showed a marked increase in the second study, although in both studies, when revenue generated was considered, excluding indirect cost, only one hospital showed net costs and they were very low.

The studies also produced data on the educational aspects of student assignments including the relationship of instruction time to length of student assignments and the number and types of tests performed by students (Tables III and IV, respectively). Review of the test data indicated that the students were performing approximately the same number of tests per hour at all four hospitals. Concurrently, similar test principles were being taught at all hospitals even though test methodology varied.

CONCLUSIONS

Overall, the latter study revealed that Hospital A had the highest costs while Hospital D had the lowest. Of the three factors considered in calculating total costs, indirect cost in Hospitals A and C was the largest expense followed by supply cost and instruction cost. On the other hand, indirect cost was secondary to instruction cost in Hospital D during both semesters. Wide variation was seen in Hospital B, with instruction time being the largest expense in the first semester and the lowest expense in the second semester.

The value of labor produced by student service work offset total costs to some degree at all hospitals. Total educational costs were completely negated in only one instance, the fall semester in Hospital B when the value of student labor was applied to total costs without indirect cost.

TABLE I

A Comparison of Total and Net Costs of Clinical Education
1979/1984-85

Hospital	Total Cost		Value of Labor	Revenue Generated	Total Net Costs Per Semester According to Methods of Calculation			
	With Indirects	Without Indirects			Value of Labor with Indirects	Value of Labor without Indirects	Revenue Generated with Indirects	Revenue Generated without Indirects
Hospital A								
Fall								
1979	$ 3453.02	$ 2356.82	$ 476.00	$ 2199.45	$ 2977.02	$1880.82	$ 1253.57	$ 157.37
1984	14822.48	8464.40	1221.66	2405.75	13600.82	7242.74	12416.73	6058.65
Spring								
1979	4924.95	2950.23	1016.88	3259.65	3908.07	1933.35	1665.30	(309.42)[a]
1985	20690.14	12047.59	7447.19	12854.70	13242.95	4600.40	7835.44	(807.11)[a]
Hospital B								
Fall								
1979	2782.52	1775.02	576.81	2308.08	2205.71	1198.21	474.44	(533.06)[a]
1984	9079.27	6360.75	6463.25	23079.45	2616.02	(102.50)[a]	(14000.18)[a]	(16718.70)[a]
Spring								
1979	2218.68	1299.65	618.12	2699.84	1600.56	681.53	(481.16)[a]	(1400.19)[a]
1985	8465.31	5496.75	2786.15	7907.70	5679.16	2710.60	557.61	(2410.95)[a]
Hospital C								
Fall								
1979	7596.58	4549.90	2122.98	12625.69	5473.60	2426.92	(5029.11)[a]	(8075.79)[a]
1984	11101.60	6016.60	3104.40	11151.96	7997.20	2912.20	(50.36)[a]	(5135.36)[a]
Spring								
1979	7878.15	5282.43	2688.42	12352.00	5189.73	2594.01	(4473.85)[a]	(7069.57)[a]
1985	19801.22	11075.72	6770.40	18866.80	13030.82	4305.32	934.42	(7791.08)[a]
Hospital D*								
Fall 1984	5349.11	3986.92	2612.94	13943.82	2736.17	1373.98	(8594.71)[a]	(9956.90)[a]
Spring 1985	7124.05	5593.60	4716.56	20384.70	2407.49	877.04	(13260.65)[a]	(14791.10)[a]

[a] Financial benefit to hospital

* Financial data for this year only; Hospital D withdrew from the earlier study and no comparisons can be made.

When evaluating total costs with respect to revenue generated by student service work, Hospital D realized financial benefits both semesters even when indirect cost was included, while Hospital A showed no benefits gained in the fall semester, but realized a financial benefit in the spring semester when indirect cost was excluded from analysis. Hospitals B and C also demonstrated a benefit in all cases when indirect cost was excluded and even in most cases when it was not.

As expected, the latter study confirmed that costs had increased in all hospitals and especially in Hospital A. Here, the low number of student assignments and the lack of student service work contributed to this increase, particularly in the fall semester.

TABLE II

A Comparison of the Net Cost of Clinical Education Per Hour of Student Assignment
1979/1984-85

	Test Number with Indirect Cost and Value of Labor	Test Number without Indirect Cost and Value of Labor	Test Number with Indirect Cost and Revenue Generated	Test Number without Indirect Cost and Revenue Generated
Hospital A				
Fall 1979	$ 7.75	$ 4.89	$ 3.26	$ 0.41
1984	34.35	18.29	31.36	15.30
Spring 1979	6.39	3.16	2.72	None (309.42)*
1985	22.98	7.93	13.60	None (807.11)*
Hospital B				
Fall 1979	6.33	3.44	1.36	None (533.06)*
1984	4.96	None (102.50)*	None (14,000.18)*	None (16,718.70)*
Spring 1979	3.65	1.55	None (481.16)*	None (1,400.19)*
1985	11.27	5.38	1.11	None (2,410.95)*
Hospital C				
Fall 1979	7:36	3.26	None (5,029.11)*	None (8075.79)*
1984	11.30	4.11	None (50.36)*	None (5,135.36)*
Spring 1979	5.11	2.56	None (4,473.85)*	None (7069.57)*
1985	10.76	3.56	0.77	None (7,791.08)*
Hospital D				
Fall 1979	NA	NA	NA	NA
1984	3.86	1.94	None (8,594.71)*	None (9,956.90)*
Spring 1979	NA	NA	NA	NA
1985	3.57	1.30	None (13,260.65)*	None (14,791.10)*

* Benefit to Hospital provided by students

Hospital B, on the other hand, exhibited large increases in the value of student labor and the revenue generated from student service work. This was attributed for the most part to the complete automation of the chemistry department. During the first study, a large portion of chemistry procedures were performed manually and student service involvement was minimal. Students were permitted to use the automated instruments exclusively in the last study.
ξ Hospital C appears to have controlled student costs reasonably well in the five-year interval between studies. Since Hospital D did not submit financial data in the earlier study, no comparisons were made. However, the low rates

TABLE III

A Comparison of the Relationship of Instruction Time to Length of Student Assignment
1979/1984-85

		Number of Student Assignments	Average Clock Hours Per Student Assignment	Average Clock Hours Instruction Time Per Student Assignment	Instruction Ratio*	Instruction Time Cost Per Hour of Student Assignment
Hospital A						
Fall	1979	9	42.7	41.0	0.96	$ 4.74
	1984	9	44	40.3	0.92	6.07
Spring	1979	23	26.6	43.1	0.49	2.42
	1985	22	26.2	24.45	0.93	6.54
Hospital B						
Fall	1979	9	38.7	31.6	0.82	3.81
	1984	14	37.7	36.5	0.97	6.24
Spring	1979	17	25.8	12.4	0.48	2.24
	1985	15	33.6	22.13	0.66	4.26
Hospital C						
Fall	1979	24	31.0	22.7	0.73	3.55
	1984	22	32.2	14.5	0.45	3.14
Spring	1979	36	28.2	19.9	0.71	3.84
	1985	55	22.0	11.95	0.54	3.76
Hospital D						
Fall	1979	18	38.0	39.1	1.03	NA
	1984	20	35.4	26.1	0.74	4.86
Spring	1979	37	22.5	19.8	0.88	4.20
	1985	37	25.0	20.9	0.84	5.39

* Represents percentage of available assignment time devoted to instruction. Includes instructor preparation time.

found here during the second study indicate that this institution is able to function cost-effectively as an affiliate.

The total and net costs of clinical education in the selected medical laboratory technician program were affected by many variables, producing diverse results. In view of the influences imposed by these variables, it was concluded thata value for the net cost of clinical education uniformly applicable to all hospitalscould not be calculated. Instead, each hospital had to be considered as an individual entity for which separate calculations were required. Moreover, such cost calculations are not exact but rather represent reasonable estimations predicted on knowledge and experience.

It was also concluded that the amount of instruction time devoted to students affected the total cost of clinical education. Therefore, the cost of in-

TABLE IV

A Comparison of the Average Number of Practice and Service Tests Performed by Students Per Assignment
1979/1984-85

	Number of Tests Per Student Assignment	No. Service Tests Per Student Assignment	Total Tests Per Student Assignment	Percent Service Tests	No. Tests per Hour of Student Assignment
Hospital A					
1979 Fall	90	53	143	37.1	3.3
1984	131	22	153	14.4	3.48
1979 Spring	41	36	77	46.8	3.0
1985	73.4	54.9	128.3	42.8	4.9
Hospital B					
1979 Fall	86	55	141	39.0	3.6
1984	73	89	162	54.9	4.3
1979 Spring	71	39	110	35.5	4.1
1985	74.4	36.1	110.5	32.7	3.29
Hospital C					
1979 Fall	70	36	106	34.0	3.4
1984	51.4	27.1	78.5	34.5	2.44
1979 Spring	37	34	71	47.9	2.5
1985	32.25	23.67	55.92	42.3	2.68
Hospital D					
1979 Fall	37	98	135	72.6	3.6
1984	38	61	99	61.6	2.8
1979 Spring	19	58	77	75.3	3.4
1985	23.11	59.68	82.79	72.1	2.39

struction was higher for freshmen and first-semester sophomore students who required more attention than for students completing the second year of the program.

The instruction ratio (IR) provided yet another measure of program quality. Students who have little or no hospital experience require more attention from the clinical instructors, while students nearing the end of the program are expected to work somewhat independently. The IR can therefore quantify these instructional relationships and highlight problem areas.

Furthermore, it was concluded that net cost results can be skewed to show benefit or cost for a hospital, depending on the method of calculation used and the factors considered. The educational program did create direct costs. On the other hand, students provided service work and added to laboratory productivity. The value of this service as a potential offset to these costs was contingent upon whether the value of labor produced by students or the revenue generated by them was considered. In view of the reimbursement policies currently affecting hospitals, the usefulness of the revenue-generating method of determining benefits to a clinical affiliate is questionable and requires further study.

Finally, these studies brought out several policy implications:

1. Affiliated hospitals must be reviewed individually to establish clinical education costs if it becomes necessary for the college to negotiate payment for the use of the facilities.

2. The amount of instruction in the clinical area can vary from semester to semester and must be monitored on a continuing basis if program quality is to be maintained.

3. To assure equality of clinical experiences, the number and types of laboratory procedures performed in each of the affiliated hospitals must be periodically reviewed.

REFERENCES

1. Weibe MF: How much does an MT program cost the hospital? *MLO* 1984;3:105-111.
2. Smith S, Gray M: Education costs for medical technology programs in hospital laboratories. *Am J Med Technol* 1974;40:273-276.
3. Harper RL, Gonyea MA: *Cost Analysis of Ten Allied Health Education Programs.* Columbus, OH, The Ohio State University, 1977.
4. Pobojewski TR: Case study: Cost/benefit study of clinical education. *J Allied Health* 1978;7:192-198.
5. Carney MK, Keim ST: Cost to the hospital of a clinical training program. *J Allied Health* 1978;7:187-191.
6. Hammersberg SS: A cost/benefit study of clinical education in selected allied health programs. *J Allied Health* 1982;1:35-41.
7. Koehler JE, Slighton RL: Activity analysis and cost analysis in medical schools. *J Med Educ* 1973;48:531-550.

8. Johnsen GN, Eady CM: How much does diploma nursing education really cost? *Nurs Outlook* 1972;20:658-664.

9. Haggart SA (ed): *Program Budgeting for School District Planning.* Englewood Cliffs, NJ, Education Technology Publications, 1972.

10. Kling DR: Cost of Clinical Education in an Associate Degree Medical Laboratory Technician Program, doctoral dissertation. Illinois State University, Normal, IL, 1980.

11. Bulgrin J: Cost of Medical Laboratory Technician Training to the Hospital: A Comparative Study, thesis. Central Michigan University, Mount Pleasant, MI, 1985.

Research Report

The Impact of the Prospective Payment System: Perceived Changes in the Nature of Practice and Clinical Education

Michael J Emery

Background and Purpose. *Health care financing for teaching hospitals has undergone significant change in the past decade. This report describes changes in physical therapy practice and clinical education in three New England hospitals from 1984 to 1988.* **Subjects.** *Hospital administrators, physical therapy managers, and clinical educators (N=18) from the three teaching hospitals participated in this descriptive study.* **Methods.** *Demographic, environmental, and participant interview data were gathered and examined to identify changes during this period.* **Results.** *Perceived changes in practice include growth in specialized knowledge; increased emphasis on health care quality, efficiency, and accountability; new ethical dilemmas for practitioners; and a changing physical therapy role with new professional development opportunities. Perceived changes associated with clinical education were increased student performance expectations, unchanged resources for clinical education, greater emphasis on student self-directedness, and continued high valuing of this setting for physical therapy clinical education.* **Conclusion and Discussion.** *These results indicate significant change in the role of the physical therapist within these settings and suggest how these changes influence the clinical education of physical therapy students in these teaching hospitals. [Emery MJ. The impact of the prospective payment system: perceived changes in the nature of practice and clinical education. Phys Ther. 1993;73:11–25.]*

Key Words: *Education: physical therapist, clinical education; Hospitals, teaching; Physical therapy profession, professional issues; Prospective payment system.*

Teaching hospitals have undergone significant change in recent years as a result of new health care reimbursement policy. Beginning in 1984, Medicare adopted a prospective system of health services payment for hospital care. The diagnosis-related group (DRG) system changed the hospital payment mechanism from fee-for-service to a prepaid, capitated payment by diagnosis for patients receiving federal funds for their health care.[1] Many states have also adopted prospective payment systems (PPSs) implemented through state-appointed hospital budget review groups to assist private insurers in achieving similar cost control. This combined federal and state prospective payment initiative has had a substantial impact on hospital environments.

Policymakers have predicted numerous changes in the teaching hospital as a result of PPS. These systems were expected to influence physician choice of treatment options based on cost, rate of hospital budget growth, and patient length of stay.[2] With shorter hospital stays, the teaching hospital was expected to be caring for

MJ Emery, EdD, PT, is Associate Professor and Academic Coordinator of Clinical Education, Department of Physical Therapy, School of Allied Health Sciences, University of Vermont, 305 Rowell Bldg, Burlington, VT 05405-0068 (USA).

This article is the result of Dr Emery's dissertation research at the University of Vermont and was supported in part by a grant from the Physical Therapy Fund of the Associates in Physical and Occupational Therapy Inc, Burlington, VT.

This work was approved by the University of Vermont's Committee on Human Subjects.

This article was submitted July 9, 1991, and was accepted July 16, 1992.

patients with more acute illness; experiencing an increase in hospital readmissions; and referring more patients to low-cost environments at discharge, such as home health agencies, nursing homes, and outpatient settings.[3] These predicted changes in the delivery of acute hospital care have been accurate in large part. Studies have documented decreased lengths of hospital stay, increased rates of readmission, more complex case mixes, and increasing numbers of patients discharged in unstable condition.[4-7] Early efforts to assess the quality of health care in the face of these changes have suggested that the quality of health care, as measured by 30-day post-hospitalization mortality rates, has not diminished, although many questions remain to be answered.[8]

The teaching hospital has been particularly vulnerable to these health policy changes. The case mix of patients with more complex diagnoses, the inefficiencies produced by the teaching function of these institutions, the increasing volume of uninsured patients, and the proliferation of technology have contributed to the comparatively high cost of care in these settings.[9,10] Historically, Medicare has allowed for these additional costs by providing an extra payment to teaching hospitals, an indirect medical education adjustment. This extra payment, determined by Congress, has varied each year since 1984 and in 1990 was paid at a rate of 7.7%.[11]

Documented changes in physical therapy practice patterns within the teaching hospital environment have been limited. Physical therapy utilization data under PPS suggest that the rate of patient referral to physical therapy may have increased,[12] the mean number of visits per referral has decreased slightly,[13,14] and patients are functioning at a greater level of dependence at discharge,[7] leading to increases in referrals to aftercare settings.[5,15,16] Patients' length of stay has decreased with 7-day physical therapy coverage, although length of stay varies considerably with diagnosis.[17]

These changes in the teaching hospital have influenced physical therapy practitioners and students within this setting. Practitioners have been encouraged to understand the changes that are under way and to participate in the change process so as to position the profession most effectively within a new health care delivery system.[18] Physical therapy practitioners are also making more difficult decisions regarding the availability of resources and the distribution of these resources in an equitable and efficient manner.[19] Health science students within this practice environment have found that Clinical Instructors (CIs) may have less control of the environment in providing special instructional opportunities for students having difficulty.[20]

Changes in the teaching hospital in recent years seem clear from this literature. This study addressed specific questions regarding these changes: (1) In what ways has the practice of physical therapy in acute care teaching hospitals in northern New England changed following the initiation of PPSs in these settings? and (2) In what ways have these changes in the practice of physical therapy influenced the physical therapy clinical education process for students in these settings?

An environmental assessment approach was used in this study because the introduction of PPSs can be seen as a macrosystem adjustment that affects organizations and individuals. Two frameworks of environmental assessment were utilized in this study: the organizational structure framework and the environmental climate framework.[21] These frameworks of analysis expose environmental shifts early in the change process, which is suitable to this study of recent change in health care finance policy.

The combination of these two frameworks or perspectives on environmental assessment allows examination of both the organization and the interaction between the organization and individuals within it. An organizational structure perspective examines

change through demographic differences in the environment and relies primarily on objective, quantifiable data. An environmental climate perspective examines change through the interaction between organization and individual. This approach relies heavily on perceptions about the organization and how people function within it, producing data of a more subjective nature.[21]

The combination of these frameworks offers an evaluation of how the teaching hospital physical therapy environment has changed quantifiably and how that change is perceived by those in the environment. Different vantage points for these perceptions have been sought by using CIs, Center Coordinators of Clinical Education (CCCEs), department managers, and hospital administrators to increase the richness of the study results rather than to compare perspectives.

Method

Sites

Hospitals in northern New England with teaching as a primary function were sought for this study. Four criteria were used to select these sites. Sites were (1) to function as a primary and tertiary medical center in their state or region, (2) to have a primary medical school affiliation, (3) to have a multiservice physical therapy practice available for clinical education, and (4) to have a well-established physical therapy clinical education program. Three teaching hospitals in this geographic region met these criteria.

Subjects

From each of the teaching hospitals, six subjects were identified based on their role within the institution: the hospital administrator responsible for the physical therapy service, the physical therapy department director, the CCCE, and three staff members or CIs. Each CI was required to have at least 4 years of experience at that institution and was selected based on availability. Each subject gave informed consent prior to participation in the study.

Data-Collection Instruments

Demographic data were collected from department records during the 4-year period (1984-1988) regarding the following: department organizational structure, staff size, the number of vacant positions, productivity targets, recruitment efforts, new capital equipment (single items costing more than $500) and physical therapy department space acquisitions, new or different responsibilities in the job descriptions, physical therapy case mix, organizational changes in the student program, number of CIs employed, number and level of students accepted, number of contracted schools, student productivity targets, and efforts to recruit students as future employees.

Perceptions about both organizational and professional environments were collected using three survey instruments: the Capacity for Change Index, the Social Climate Scale, and the Standards for Clinical Education in Physical Therapy instrument. The first two assessment instruments were identified from the organizational environment literature and modified for use in this study. The third instrument was selected from the physical therapy practice and education literature. This survey instrument examined perceptions about the physical therapy practice and teaching environment within the organization.

The Capacity for Change Index identifies subjects' perceptions of the following organizational characteristics: occupational specialization, specialized knowledge, the hierarchy of decision making, occupational autonomy, financial rewards, and emphasis on efficiency and effectiveness. Participants indicate the degree to which these characteristics are present in their environment. High scores in these characteristics suggest a complex organizational environment. The creators of this instrument have shown that the complexity of organizations leads to more difficulty in the

change process, with resulting dysfunction when change occurs too rapidly.[22] The instrument was modified slightly by the investigator to reflect appropriate physical therapy terminology. Four questions were added to address the physical therapy student in this environment, using the same question format.

The Social Climate Scale was developed by Moos[23] to assess the psychosocial climate in hospitals. Moos and colleagues have developed several instruments, all with the same framework, relationship dimensions, personal development dimensions, and system maintenance and change dimensions. The Social Climate Scale used in this study was adapted from Moos's Ward Atmosphere Scale, which has descriptors most relevant to the hospital setting.[23] Social climate is defined as the fit between organizational tenets and individuals' needs, as has been developed from early work on the effects of environmental pressures on human behavior.[24] This instrument provides 50 descriptors of interaction between individuals and the organization, allowing the participants to indicate their agreement with each. Social climate assessment is useful when environmental change is taking place, as the impact of the change may be reflected early in the climate of the environment.[23] This instrument provides perceptual data from those in the setting about how individuals within different roles interact with one another, how the service helps individuals grow professionally, and how the service sustains itself during times of change. This instrument was modified slightly by the investigator to reflect appropriate physical therapy terminology.

The Standards for Clinical Education in Physical Therapy instrument was adapted from work done by Barr et al.[25] The instrument provides participants' perceptions about the practice environment as those perceptions relate to standards for student education in these clinical settings. These standards include both organizational and educational expectations for physical therapy practice.

Subject interviews expanded on perceptions identified by the survey instruments. These semistructured interviews consisted of four major questions with several specific follow-up questions. Interview questions are listed in the Appendix.

Procedure

Prior to implementation, the demographic data-collection tools, survey instruments, and interview guidelines were reviewed by a panel of five experts addressing study design and content area. Several changes in the demographic data-collection tool and the interview questions were made following this review. A physical therapy educator with expertise in descriptive analysis independently reviewed the data-collection instruments in relation to the research questions to provide content validation of the data obtained with these tools. Again, minor modifications were made in the interview questions. This procedure established face validity of the data. No effort was made to test the criterion-based validity or reliability of data obtained with the modified instruments.

Data were collected by a single investigator in the following order: demographic data from department records and statistics, three environmental assessment survey instruments completed by the subjects, and a 1-hour semi-structured interview with each subject. All data were collected during a 1-week period at each of the three sites.

Department records and statistics were reviewed, and data were extracted using a data-collection form and then discussed with the department manager or CCCE to confirm their accuracy. For each of the three surveys, subjects were asked to respond twice to each item—once to indicate their response to the item in the present environment and a second time to indicate their response to the item as they perceived it to be prior to the introduction of DRGs in their institution. All survey responses were collected on optical scanning sheets for data-reduction purposes. Interviews were conducted individually with each subject after completion of the surveys. Each interview was tape-recorded for later transcription.

Data Analysis

Demographic data were reviewed for changes over a 4-year interval (1984-1988). Where appropriate, means and ranges were calculated to describe changes in variables. The nature of changes noted was further elucidated through description of each change.

Each of the survey instruments used a five-point Likert scale to elicit responses for each item, which produced ordinal data. Data were entered from optical scanning sheets for computer-assisted data reduction. Each set of item pairs (responses for past and present on each item from all subjects) was analyzed for mean score, frequency count, sign test (two-tailed) result, Spearman rank-order correlation coefficient, and the number of subjects who expressed no change in item score from past to present.

Differences between scores for past and present within each set of item pairs were calculated using a sign test. Sets of item pairs that did not demonstrate significant differences were analyzed for agreement between responses for past and present. Two tests were applied sequentially: the Spearman rank-order correlation coefficient to determine a relationship between responses for past and present within the item pair ($P<.05$) and a comparison of actual item scores for each subject within each item pair. In the latter, a minimum of 66% (2/3) of the subjects demonstrating no difference between scores for past and present within the item was considered clinically significant. These statistical and clinical measures allowed individual items on each of the survey instruments to be placed in one of

three categories: changed from past to present, unchanged from past to present, or unable to meet criteria for the first two categories.

Transcribed interview data were read by the investigator. A qualitative research software package,* was used to assist in the labeling and sorting of interview data.[26] The investigator organized recurrent comments into coded categories called "themes." A *theme* is defined as a common belief, assumption, or meaning stated through comments by subjects.[27] Themes were developed if common statements were found at all three sites and by at least one third of the participants. Verbatim statements were selected from the transcripts to amplify and clarify the subjects' meaning and to demonstrate how the themes were abstracted from the interviews. No efforts were made to compare institutions or categories of subjects with one another in this study.

Results

Demographic Data

Changes were noted over the 4-year period in six demographic characteristics—four involving practice and two involving clinical education. Three demographic characteristics did not change during the 4-year period. Table 1 summarizes the demographic data.

Survey Data

A survey response rate of 100% was achieved, although some subjects left individual items blank if they felt they were unable to respond. This was noted particularly in the Standards for Clinical Education in Physical Therapy instrument and did not exceed two missing values for any one survey item (ie, $n\geq16$).

In the Capacity for Change Index, none of the 13 items were found to be unchanged when the previously

described criteria were applied. Five items demonstrated a statistically significant difference from past to present. Mean scores for past and present, sign test results, and probability values are presented in Table 2. All scores indicated stronger subject agreement with the statement at present than in the past or that the statement had become more accurate from past to present. In the Social Climate Scale, 11 of the 50 descriptive statements were found to be unchanged. For these unchanged items, mean scores for past and present, the number of subjects with scores unchanged from past to present, and the correlation coefficients are shown in Table 3. Significant differences were found in 7 descriptive statements. Mean scores for past and present, sign test results, and probability values of these items are listed in Table 4. In each of the 7 items, sign test results indicate a positive shift from past to present, indicating a favorable change in the environment.

The Standards for Clinical Education in Physical Therapy scale demonstrated generally low mean scores, which suggests that subjects felt standards were met in large part. Fourteen of the 20 standards were unchanged from past to present. Mean scores for past and present, number of subjects with unchanged scores from past to present, and correlation coefficients are given in Table 5. A significant difference was noted in only 1 standard, as shown in Table 6.

Interview Data

Interview data produced 13 themes— 8 in the area of practice and 5 in the area of clinical education. In many cases, these themes were found to be far more prevalent in the interview data than the criteria demanded. The practice themes addressed the practice environment and issues created by the interaction between environment and practitioner. Clinical education themes addressed the learning environment and instructional issues. Practice and clinical education themes are outlined in Table 7.

---

*Ethnograph software package, distributed by Qualitative Research Management, PO Box 30070, Santa Barbara, CA 93130.

Table 1. *Demographic Data*

Characteristic	Change Noted
Physical therapy staff size	PT[a]: increased; mean=27%, range=5%-50%
	PTA[b]: unchanged
	Support staff: variable
Recruitment efforts	Proactive; ongoing activities
	Expanded; new efforts initiated
	Organized; use of recruiters
	Collaborative; working with other institutions
Space/capital equipment[c]	Three or more pieces of capital equipment acquired by each site
	Expansion of 3,000-5,000 sq ft at each site
Job descriptions	Two of three sites noted increased senior staff supervisory responsibilities
CI[d] training	Two of three sites noted formalization of training program and development of new resource materials
Student preparation	All sites changed expectations by preferring or requiring senior students only
	No Change Noted
Physical therapy productivity targets	70%-75% of work devoted to "billable" activities
Student program organization	Single person responsible for CI training and program management
Clinical practice areas	Five or six areas available to students at each site; some recent reorganization

[a]PT=physical therapist.

[b]PTA=physical therapist assistant.

[c]Capital equipment is operationally defined as a single item costing more than $500.

[d]CI=Clinical Instructor.

Practice

Increased illness acuteness.
When questioned about increased severity of illness, interviewees identified two factors that yield a more acutely ill patient population: technology to sustain life under more critical circumstances and earlier discharge of subacutely ill patients, yielding a sicker population in the teaching hospitals. Interviewees commented

> Patients are more acute when they come in, they are more acute when they leave, and we have a shorter time to work with them.

> These are people who should have been dead or would have been dead 4 years ago.

Earlier discharge planning. All
interviewees acknowledged the role of physical therapy in discharge planning to be earlier and more influential from past to present. The CIs and administrators commented

> I feel that we have gotten an increased volume [of patients] since prospective payment went into place because I think physicians and nursing are recognizing that we are instrumental in expediting a discharge.

> Sometimes it means that [the patient's] anesthesia hasn't [even] worn off yet, and you are already in there.

> The emphasis in our practice now is on evaluation and discharge planning from the very first day, with a varying amount of time between those two

[points]: the evaluation and the discharge date.

Streamlined hospital mission.
Hospital administrators and department managers commented particularly on the changing hospital mission. They described this changing mission as a very conscious effort to increase the efficiency of the hospital in the face of scarce financial resources.

> It's not just efficiency, ... but efficiency and effectiveness need to be components of what it is that [we] do.

> I think it's team members working together with ... clearer role responsibilities, but hopefully a more cooperative spirit to get patient care first.

Concerns over quality of care.
More than two thirds of the interviewees commented specifically on quality-of-care issues. Comments addressed not only perceptions of quality of care but the shortcomings in measuring quality of care. Although comments were in agreement that practice was different, there were varied feelings about whether the quality of care had improved or diminished.

> The worst consequence [of PPS] is that we are just not having as much time as we'd like to be able to perform quality treatments, or maybe we need to redefine what quality is.

> I am no less comfortable with the practice of physical therapy here. I think we have increased challenges in terms of acuity of the patient, length of stay, and so forth, but ... I've got a good staff and the coordination among therapists assisting each other and communicating [is good].

> The other [benefit of PPS] might be a greater formal attention to quality of care, and that relates to the development of those standards and certain measured expectations. So we are asking our departments that in the past might not necessarily have had such formal programs for the measurement of quality ... to now have such [a program].

Greater professional
development opportunities. Two thirds of the interviewees, primarily

Table 2. *Capacity for Change Index Items Demonstrating Change from Past to Present*

Survey Item	Mean Score[a]		Sign Test[b]	P
	Past	Present		
Occupational specialization in the acute care physical therapy environment	2.67	4.17	+	.0003
Volume of specialized knowledge needed by physical therapists to function in the acute care environment	2.78	3.89	+	.0001
Relative emphasis placed on the quality of services rendered by the physical therapy department	4.11	4.72	+	.0039
Relative emphasis placed on the efficiency of operations within the physical therapy department	3.11	4.39	+	.0003
Degree of stress the physical therapy department creates for students in clinical education	3.17	3.67	+	.0391

[a]Scale: 1=very low, 5=very high.

[b]+=statistically significant change toward higher score.

CIs and department managers, commented on the opportunity that acute care creates for the right individual. The opportunity includes clinical specialization and experiential learning in a dynamic, fast-moving environment. Two CIs commented

> I think the growth of specialization ... and also just the growth of the individuals within the department.

> The best [part of this environment] is that it is extremely dynamic and challenging. You can direct a lot of your [own] learning.

Who is the *right* individual for this environment? One department manager said

> Their skills, their knowledge base, and practical application of physiology has to be, I think, keener than it was before. Intellectually more capable. Physically more capable ....

New ethical dilemmas. Time constraints, technology, and large numbers of patients have combined to create uneasiness and ethical questions for a majority of the CIs and department managers interviewed. Most CIs and department managers addressed earlier discharge and the lack of sufficient follow-up services in the community and the existence of waiting lists for physical therapy services in the teaching hospital. Comments included

> I have concerns that the moving of a patient out of the hospital too early is not matched by the support in the community to take that kind of patient. That makes me uneasy.

> I think it is awful that physicians can identify that a patient needs a service, and because we don't have sufficient staff to provide the service, then people go without [because of early hospital discharge].

Increased accountability. Increases in accountability were expressed by every interviewee and described in regard to patients, the institution, and other professionals. Such increases were viewed as a positive consequence of PPS, although being accountable was not always easy and created stress for physical therapists.

I frequently feel that physical therapists take on a tremendous amount of responsibility as patient advocates, more than they should, and frequently alone.

> I was always concerned with patients' lack of initiative in ... taking charge of their own condition, and I think maybe DRGs have helped that a little bit. More emphasis on patient education, early discharge, getting them ready right from day 1.

> I think we can't take things for granted as much. We have to really examine closely what we are doing. We have to try to be more efficient with our time, be really clear as to what our goals are.

The need for PPS fine-tuning. Although interviewees recognized the need for cost-containment and the benefits of greater efficiency, all expressed some concern for the patient in the transition to PPS and feared that individual situations of inadequate service had occurred. The CIs commented

> The downside for the patient is, frankly, I get to you when I get to you. I can't guarantee anything.

> I worry a lot about [PPS pressures] clouding the judgment of the people who make surgical decisions, medical decisions, discharge decisions.

Clinical Education

Clinical education themes addressed both the learning environment and the instructional process.

Acute care a valued learning environment. Acute care as a learning experience for students is still viewed by practitioners as valuable and unique. Growing strain on this relationship between student education and acute care, however, is noted. Two CIs commented

> I think it is important for students to be able to experience this setting because they may work in this setting. They have to have a taste for it, but what they need is the guidance to understand how to cope with this setting and how to find favorable things in it.

> What is difficult is when [the students] are ... beginning, if they are not quick

Table 3. *Social Climate Scale Items Unchanged from Past to Present*

Survey Item	Mean Score[a]		Frequency Count[b]	Spearman r^c
	Past	Present		
Staff put much energy into what they do around here	1.44	1.28	15	.79
Few people ever volunteer around here	3.61	3.72	12	.83
The more experienced physical therapy staff offer assistance to the younger physical therapy staff	1.50	1.39	14	.67
Physical therapy staff welcomes and helps new staff get acquainted	1.55	1.50	15	.77
Disagreements among staff are made apparent to others	3.25	3.19	12	.82
Physical therapy students are encouraged to ask questions	1.41	1.35	16	.99
The department is good at taking advantage of unexpected opportunities	2.50	2.39	12	.87
The department emphasizes continuing education and professional development	1.67	1.56	14	.67
Physical therapy staff are encouraged to identify and suggest solutions for problems	2.00	1.56	12	.73
Physical therapy staff set an example of neatness and orderliness for students	2.16	2.16	16	.92
Physical therapy staff participate in planning for student assignments and activities	2.35	2.24	14	.58

[a]Scale: 1=strongly agree, 5=strongly disagree.

[b]No. of respondents with score unchanged from past to present.

[c]$P<.05$.

learners, because they [cause a] drag in the system. [This is] especially [true when] there is very little backup for patient care if you don't get it done yourself.

Recruitment of students seen as a benefit. Another reality of this learning environment is that clinical education has been increasingly recognized as an effective recruitment strategy. Primarily hospital administrators and department managers commented that part of the real value of clinical education is to create a source of potential employees. Although interviewees did not feel that students were used inappropriately as staff, they acknowledged that chances of employing these students and other new graduates were enhanced by a student program. One department manager summarized it this way:

I think that [the hospital administrator] fully recognizes the value of a student program ... in terms of recruiting. Word gets out if you have a good program and a good department. Word gets out via the students to their peers that [this hospital] might be a good place to consider [for a job].

More is expected of students. All interviewees addressed the changing student performance expectations. New student expectations were cited in terms of precision and readiness in performance and the ability to be more independent in their learning. Students must adapt to their environment more quickly, apply clinical skills more readily, and demonstrate

decision making more aptly. The CIs commented

We kind of expect them to adapt ... and be quite clear in their goals and their plans for the patient. They are also more involved in the team meetings and team interactions.

It is very demanding, in terms of being able to integrate the different complexities of each patient into what [each patient] needs.

Asked about the characteristics of a successful student in this setting, CIs commented

To ... use the teaching/learning process for themselves and also with their patients.

... good communications, both verbal and written, organized, assertive, [good] listening skills. A sense of humor would help.

Student learning experiences constrained. More than two thirds of the interviewees commented on the changing nature of student supervision in the acute care setting. Clinical instructors and department managers agreed that students receive more direct supervision, less opportunity for exploration and trial-and-error learning, and greater emphasis on efficiency of treatment and patient outcome. A department manager and a hospital administrator commented

I suspect that the amount of time in direct supervision is probably longer than it has been because the patients are so much sicker.

There is much more reluctance in letting [the students] just sort of try things several times until they get it right.

Rewards of clinical instruction remain intrinsic. Given this increasingly austere backdrop, motivation to teach students in the clinical setting comes mostly from within. Department managers and CIs agreed that a primary motive for clinical education in acute care is personal—the satisfaction in seeing students learn under their direction, the obligation to their profession, and the learning they derive from the clinical instruction process. Although other benefits such

Table 4. *Social Climate Scale Items Demonstrating Change from Past to Present*

Survey Item	Mean Score[a]		Sign Test[b]	P
	Past	Present		
Department administration encourages physical therapy staff to express concerns and frustrations	2.50	1.94	+	.04
Physical therapy staff have some control over their work hours (scheduling)	3.28	2.39	+	.001
Physical therapy staff are encouraged to identify and suggest solutions for problems	2.00	1.56	+	.03
The department approaches problems in an organized fashion	2.78	2.00	+	.04
The department places a high degree of emphasis on budgetary planning	2.61	1.89	+	.02
The department has clearly defined policies and procedures	2.56	1.61	+	.002
Physical therapy staff have regular input in department planning	2.50	2.06	+	.04

[a]Scale: 1=strongly agree, 5=strongly disagree.

[b]+=statistically significant change toward a lower score.

as recruitment were noted by department managers and administrators, CIs see it this way, and a department manager commented on the growth of his staff:

> One of the big rewards is having the person become independent and function as a peer. I like [the person] to achieve the [level] of peer relationships.

> When I see somebody's light go on, ... that learning experience is what makes it all worthwhile.

> My perspective ... has always been [that] you need to put something back into the profession, so I am willing to take [the students] and work with their skills to the point where we hope they can be clinically competent.

> I think the greatest reward is seeing the growth and development of CIs, in terms of both their clinical teaching ability and the ripple effect that it has on their professional life.

Discussion

These results can be considered in two categories: changes in acute care physical therapy practice in these teaching hospitals and changes in clinical education within these environments.

Physical Therapy Practice Changes

Physical therapy in the acute care environment requires an increasing amount of specialized knowledge and, according to the subjects of this study, places growing emphasis on the quality and the efficiency of practice, as evidenced by the data obtained with the Capacity for Change Index. Interview data confirm that more critically ill patients are in the acute care environment and that physical therapists are more involved with these patients. Practitioners are more sensitive to the tension between quality of care and productivity. The widening gap between student preparation and clinical performance expectation noted by subjects is likely the result of this changing aspect of practice as well.

Physical therapists in these acute care settings describe a more central and independent role in patient management for which they feel more accountable. Accountability is a recurring theme in the interview data, emphasizing the need to justify recommendations for treatment intervention, length of hospital stay, and disposition. Physical therapists describe themselves as more eminently involved in such health care decisions. The intensity of work and interdependence of the professional staff noted in the Social Climate Scale support the conclusion that responsibility is believed to have increased in this professional role. Literature cited and demographic data in this study support the growing utilization of physical therapy in an acute care atmosphere otherwise focused on constraint.[12,13,17]

Physical therapists are increasingly challenged by the ethical dilemmas involving financial constraints, distribution of resources, and quality of care for patients. Interview data support the common belief that acute care hospitals are under pressure to contain health care costs in the face of more sophisticated technology, increasingly acute patient case mix, and growing health care personnel shortages. Results of the Capacity for Change Index indicate a perceived increased emphasis on quality and efficiency of operations. These findings combine to support the notion that such pressures have increased the struggle with ethical dilemmas perceived by those in the environment. Subjects have noted that these ethical dilemmas are very real, with some patients' needs remaining unmet. These physical therapists have also indicated that they are uncomfortable with their ability to manage these conflicts. Greater supervisory responsibilities for senior staff, noted in the demographic data, and greater involvement of staff in department problem solving, as seen in the Social Climate Scale data, exemplify efforts to support practitioners facing difficult decision-making responsibilities.

Physical therapists in this study agreed that their role with patients has changed, focusing more on evaluation, treatment planning, and discharge and less on provision of pa-

Table 5. *Standards for Clinical Education in Physical Therapy Instrument Items Unchanged from Past to Present*

Survey Item	Mean Score[a]		Frequency Count[b]	Spearman r[c]
	Past	Present		
The physical therapy service provides an active, stimulating environment appropriate for the learning needs of the student	1.47	1.41	13	.68
Clinical education programs for students are planned to meet specific objectives of the education program, the physical therapy service, and the individual student	1.64	1.52	12	.74
The clinical center has a variety of learning experiences available to the student	1.23	1.23	17	1.00
The physical therapy staff practices ethically and legally	1.06	1.12	16	.68
The clinical center is committed to the principle of equal opportunity and affirmative action, as required by federal legislation	1.41	1.35	16	.99
The clinical center's philosophy and its objectives for patient care and clinical education are compatible with those of the educational institution	1.56	1.50	15	.98
The clinical center demonstrates administrative interest in and support of physical therapy clinical education	1.76	1.94	12	.74
The physical therapy staff is adequate in number to provide a good education program for students	2.23	2.05	12	.65
One physical therapist with specific qualifications is responsible for coordinating the assignments and activities of the students at the clinical center	1.20	1.33	12	.61
Clinical Instructors are selected based on specific criteria	2.33	2.20	11	.76
Clinical Instructors apply the basic principles of education (teaching and learning) to clinical education	2.25	1.87	12	.91
Special expertise of the various center staff is shared with students	1.76	1.52	14	.86
The physical therapy staff is interested and active in professional associations related to physical therapy	2.82	2.70	15	.91
Selected support services are available for students (eg, emergency medical care, health services, library, room, board)	1.94	2.12	14	.85

[a]Scale: 1=strongly agree, 5=strongly disagree.

[b]No. of respondents with score unchanged from past to present.

[c]P<.05.

tient treatment. Interview data confirm earlier discharge planning and a more focused mission of the institution. These changes in acute care affect those providers who serve the patient later in the medical course of care (eg, rehabilitation hospitals, skilled nursing facilities, outpatient services, and home health care). Subjects interviewed share the concern expressed by various authors[7,15,16] about whether these post–acute care providers respond to the changing locus of care.

Subjects in this study described an increasing attention paid to the interpersonal and professional development needs of physical therapists in the acute care setting. Data from the Social Climate Scale support the idea that these acute care physical therapy environments are more sensitive and caring for the human resource needs of its staff. Interview data clearly identify the perception that opportunity exists in terms of professional growth for those in the acute care teaching hospital. It is the belief of these physical therapists that this opportunity

increased over the 4-year period of this study.

Clinical Education Changes

Student clinical performance expectations appear to have increased in accordance with the changing acute care physical therapy environment, yet interview data suggest that student preparation is unchanged. Changes in the nature of physical therapy practice in acute care settings have previously been discussed. These changes should necessitate adjustments in student

Table 6. *Standards for Clinical Education in Physical Therapy Instrument Items Perceived as Demonstrating Change from Past to Present*

Survey Item	Mean Score[a]		Sign Test[b]	P
	Past	Present		
The physical therapy service has an active and viable process of internal evaluation of its own affairs and is receptive to procedures of review and audit approved by appropriate external agencies	1.76	1.41	+	.0313

[a]Scale: 1=strongly agree, 5=strongly disagree.

[b]+ =statistically significant change toward a lower score.

performance for greater clinical readiness and independence in learning. This may explain the findings of closer supervision and less flexibility in learning experiences for students, greater perceived stress on students in this environment, and the recent limitation of affiliations to seniors only in these environments. Ironically, the Capacity for Change Index results indicate that these acute care settings are less flexible to adjust to individual student needs.

Resources for clinical education are unchanged. In the midst of significant environmental change in acute care, the structure, size, and resources of the clinical education program in each of these settings are unchanged according to interview and demographic data. Although the need to support clinical education is recognized by these hospital administrators and department directors, little has been done to change the student education program, as evidenced by the demographic data. Given the previous observation regarding the increased expectations in student clinical practice performance, this lack of additional resources or assistance is seen as a concern by CIs and CCCEs.

Students in the acute care environment must be active in directing and assessing their own learning experience. Characteristics of acute care noted in the survey and interview data, such as shortened patient length

of stay, emphasis on efficiency, and increasing patient complexity, cause the acute care setting to be both a rich and stressful learning environment for students. Activities that take the physical therapist away from direct patient care, such as teaching, are increasingly difficult to justify and have been challenged by hospital administrators and insurers. Continued heavy utilization of physical therapy and emphasis on efficiency cause physical therapy work loads to remain high. Clinical Instructors defined through their interview comments those students who are most likely to succeed in this environment as peo-

Table 7. *Themes Identified from the Interview Data*

Area	Theme
Practice	
Practice environment	The acute care patient population is changing; patients are more critically ill; less critically ill patients are discharged more quickly
	Discharge planning is initiated earlier and with more physical therapy involvement
	The teaching hospital mission has been more clearly delineated and streamlined
Interaction between environment and practitioner	Quality of patient care is a concern but does not appear to have diminished
	Greater professional development opportunities exist for those who choose to stay in the acute care environment
	Ethical questions are increasingly unresolved and are troublesome to practitioners in the acute care setting
	Increases in accountability are acknowledged and viewed as a positive occurrence by practitioners
	Prospective payment systems need fine-tuning at this time as patients continue to "fall through the cracks"
Clinical education	
Learning environment	Student education in acute care is valued and interdependent, yet this relationship has become increasingly strained
	Staff shortages have given clinical education programs a new and powerful benefit as a recruitment instrument
Student instruction characteristics	Student readiness is unchanged, whereas clinical practice expectations in this environment have increased
	Students are now more closely supervised, experience less trial-and-error learning, and have greater emphasis placed on efficiency and patient outcomes
	Professional obligation, generativity, and inherent value of clinical education are still the motivators for Clinical Instructors

ple who are mature, self-motivated, and assertive in their communication style.

Participation in clinical education remains highly valued by those in the acute care environment. Clinical Instructors and CCCEs have described through the interviews their motives for participation in clinical education as largely intrinsic. They express this as part of their own development and professional obligation. Department managers and hospital administrators commented candidly about the positive impact that clinical education has had on new staff recruitment. The Social Climate Scale data also indicated a supportive environment for students and new staff. Clinical education in these acute care environments appears to be in no immediate danger of discontinuation. All participants in the study acknowledge that this clinical learning experience will continue to occur in the acute care setting, whether as a part of the educational program or through early job experiences. It is the belief of these subjects that the specificity of an acute care clinical education experience is essential to the preparation of physical therapists.

There are limitations of this study that should be acknowledged:

1. The study was based on individual perceptions and was retrospective. To the extent that perceptions have been affected by time or personal bias, these data may be flawed.

2. Generalizing of the findings is limited to the participating institutions; however, the themes and conclusions identified serve as a basis for comparison with other institutions and as a framework for future study.

3. The methodology has considered the three sites as one group without efforts to compare the individual institutions with one another. The data may be confounded where differences exist among these institutions.

Appendix. *Subject Interview Questions*[a]

1. In what ways has the provision of physical therapy in this department changed over the past 4 years?
   A. What do (you/the individual physical therapists) do differently in the provision of care to (your/their) patients?

2. How have these changes in the provision of care made you more or less comfortable in (your/the) practice of physical therapy in this hospital?
   A. In what ways have these changes been good or bad for patients?

3. How have these changes in practice that we have been talking about influenced the teaching of physical therapy students in this hospital?
   A. In what ways have the goals of the student program and the goals of the patient care service become more or less compatible?

4. How have these changes in the clinical teaching of physical therapy students made you feel more or less comfortable about clinical education?
   A. In what ways has (your/the) management of the student in the physical therapy department changed, and are these changes beneficial?

[a]Note: Each of the major interview questions and one example of a follow-up question are presented. During the interview, all subjects answered four or five follow-up questions after each major question. All subjects were asked the same major and follow-up questions.

4. The survey instruments from the organizational environment literature were adapted for this study. Although face validity exists for their use, caution should be exercised. Environmental assessment instruments more applicable for physical therapy settings need to be identified.

5. Introduction of PPS policy was a significant environmental factor during the period of time studied. It was not, however, the only source of change. The changes cited in this study cannot be solely attributed to PPS.

Conclusions

Using demographic, survey, and interview data collected from CIs, CCCEs, department managers, and hospital administrators in three New England teaching hospitals, the changing nature of physical therapy practice and clinical education in these environments has been described. These changes are noted at a time during which dramatic modification of the acute care environment is under way, necessitated by spiraling health care costs. These results indicate significant change in the role of the physical therapist within these settings and suggest how these changes influence the clinical education of physical therapy students in these teaching hospitals.

References

1 Rolph E, Lindsey P. *Medicare's Prospective Payment System: The Health Care Community's Reaction and Perception.* Santa Monica, Calif: Rand Corp; 1986.

2 Greenberg W, Southby RM. *Health Care Institutions in Flux: Changing Reimbursement Patterns in the 1980s.* Arlington, Va: Information Resources Press; 1984.

3 Lohr KN, Brook RH, Goldberg GA, et al. *Impact of Medicare Prospective Payment on the Quality of Medical Care: A Research Agenda.* Santa Monica, Calif: Rand Corp; 1985.

4 DesHarnais S, Kobrinski E, Chesney J, et al. The early effects of the prospective payment on inpatient utilization and the quality of care. *Inquiry.* 1987;24:7-16.

5 Morrissey MA, Sloan FA, Valvona J. Medicare prospective payment and post-hospital transfers to subacute care. *Med Care.* 1988;26:685-698.

6 Berman RA, Greene J, Kwo D, et al. Severity of illness and the teaching hospital. *J Med Educ.* 1986;61:1-9.

7 Kosecoff J, Kahn KL, Rogers WH, et al. Prospective payment system and impairment at discharge. *JAMA.* 1990;264:1980-1983.

8 Ruberstein LV, Kahn KL, Reinisch EJ, et al. Changes in quality of care for five diseases measured by implicit review: 1981 to 1986. *JAMA.* 1990;264:1974-1979.

9 Schwartz WB, Newhouse JP, Williams AP. Is the teaching hospital an endangered species? *N Engl J Med.* 1985;313:157-162.

10 Thorpe KE. Why are urban hospitals so high? The relative importance of patient source of admission, teaching, competition, and case mix. *Health Serv Res.* 1988;22:821-836.

11 Vanselow NA. The financial status of U.S. teaching hospitals. *Acad Med.* 1990;65:560-561.

12 Dore D. Effect of the Medicare prospective payment and the utilization of physical therapy. *Phys Ther.* 1987;67:964-966.

13 Davis KD, Gwyer J. *The Impact of the Prospective Payment System on the Delivery of Physical Therapy Services.* Alexandria, Va: American Physical Therapy Association; April 1986.

14 Holt P, Winograd CH. Prospective payment and the utilization of physical therapy service in the hospitalized elderly. *Am J Public Health.* 1990;80:1491-1494.

15 Fitzgerald JF, Fagan LF, Tierney WM, et al. Changing patterns of hip fracture care before and after implementation of the prospective payment system. *JAMA.* 1987;258:218-221.

16 Fitzgerald JF, Moore PS, Dittus RS. The care of elderly patients with hip fracture:

changes since implementation of the prospective payment system. *N Engl J Med.* 1988;319:1392-1397.

17 Rapoport J, Judd-Van Eerd M. Impact of physical therapy weekend coverage on length of stay in an acute care community hospital. *Phys Ther.* 1989;69:32-37.

18 Brown GD. Changing health care environments: implications for physical therapy research, education, and practice. *Phys Ther.* 1986;66:1242-1245.

19 Purtilo RB. Saying "no" to patients for cost-related reasons. *Phys Ther.* 1988;68:1243-1247.

20 Kautzmann LN. An assessment of the impact of the Medicare prospective payment system on level II fieldwork. *Am J Occup Ther.* 1986;40:470-473.

21 Conyne RK, Clack RJ. *Environmental Assessment and Design.* New York, NY: Praeger Publishers; 1981.

22 Hage J, Aiken M. *Social Change in Complex Organizations.* New York, NY: Random House Inc; 1970.

23 Moos R. *Evaluating Treatment Environments.* New York, NY: John Wiley & Sons Inc; 1974.

24 Moos R. Conceptualizations of human environments. *Am Psychol.* August 1973:652-665.

25 Barr JS, Gwyer J, Talmor Z. Evaluation of clinical education centers in physical therapy. *Phys Ther.* 1982;62:850-861.

26 Seidel J. *Ethnograph Manual, Version 3.* Littleton, Colo: Qualis Research Associates; 1988.

27 Bogdan RC, Biklen SK. *Qualitative Research in Education: An Introduction to Theory and Methods.* Boston, Mass: Allyn & Bacon Inc; 1982.

Commentary

The author of this report has provided extensive data with which the reader can evaluate the status of clinical education in three teaching hospitals, prior to and subsequent to the implementation of the prospective payment system of hospital reimbursement of patients receiving Medicare. This topic is of considerable interest to academic and clinical educators in physical therapy, as hospital-based clinical education continues to comprise a large portion of our clinical education programs nationwide.[1] Emery's study provides us the opportunity to examine the effects of a major change in health care reimbursement for a component of the health care industry and to predict the future of educational activities in these institutions. I appreciate the opportunity to comment on the method of inquiry used in this study and on the interpretation of the data and to reflect on further implications of these data for physical therapy education.

The theoretical framework used to guide this research appears to be a positivistic one, utilizing a descriptive research design and both direct and indirect methods of data collection (ie, survey and interview). I point this

out because the interview data are summarized into conceptual themes and supported by narrative data taken from the interview transcripts, which would appear to suggest a phenomenological approach to the development of this segment of the study. The methods the author describes for development of the conceptual framework of the study, for development of the research instruments, and for data collection, however, do not reflect a true qualitative approach to the investigation of this research question. Although conducted in the natural setting, this research does not reflect the appropriate efforts to utilize the investigator as the primary data-gathering tool, the rich description of the environment reflective of long-term participation in the environment, or the interdependence of data collection and data analysis that would characterize a qualitative approach to the question.[2] Although a quantitative approach was appropriately used in this study, I wish to clarify this distinction only as it may contribute to understanding the lack of agreement I found in some of the interview data and proposed themes.

I would agree that the information generated from the personal inter-

views provided the most interesting data in this study. As the author mentions, the introduction of the prospective payment system is not the only source of change to which the results of this study can be attributed. This is especially true of the interview data, given that none of the interview questions appear to have reinforced the concept of identifying change attributable specifically to the initiation of the prospective payment system. This does not represent a significant limitation to my understanding of these data; however, the title of the article might more appropriately refer to the changes in teaching hospital practice and clinical education over a 5-year period, attributable to a wide range of causes. The potential determinants of these changes would have been an interesting additional research question for this study.

I had difficulty interpreting three of the themes of the interview data in the area of practice, based on the narrative data that were provided. Mr Emery states that the teaching hospital mission has been more clearly delineated and streamlined, but the data provided illustrate neither concept. There is no clear understanding from these data regarding the current missions of the teaching hospitals in this study, and particularly whether or not their missions include the education of anyone in health care. The data indicate that the administrators in this study appreciate the recruitment value of their clinical education programs, but will this suffice to maintain a strong commitment to the teaching mission in periods of decreasing health care reimbursement?

I did not find a sufficient amount of data reported to allow the reader to conclude, as the author did, that the quality of patient care does not appear to have diminished. The data reported as supporting the themes of ethical dilemmas and the need for fine-tuning the prospective payment system seem to me to be strong indicators of the decreased quality of health care offered to these subjects' patients, both within the setting and throughout an episode of care.

The practice theme related to fine-tuning the prospective payment system does not communicate a clear construct as written in the article. Perhaps the data available to the author do suggest a specific concept of change needed in the reimbursement system, but the examples of data provided here do not help to clarify or support this confusing theme.

Of the clinical education themes, I had difficulty with two important concepts purported to be findings by the author: the complementary themes of an existing strain in the relationship between the acute care practice setting and the student education program, and the student readiness for practice in this environment. The data reported to support these themes do not seem to adequately describe the strained relationship discussed by the author. Although

data are clearly identified that describe increasing expectations of students in the acute care setting, what data indicate that students are coming into these clinical settings by and large unprepared to meet these expectations? Though the remainder of the interview data may be replete with this sentiment, I did not find the data reported to be convincing of the author's conclusion that there exists a widening gap in what is expected of students in this setting and the students' ability to perform during these affiliations.

If these themes emanating from the interview data provide an accurate description of the status of physical therapy clinical education in teaching hospitals, the implications for education programs are significant. How can students best be prepared in the academic setting to succeed in such affiliations? For example, should students be able to perform efficient and appropriate evaluations and be competent in discharge planning prior to their first acute care affiliation? When should teaching hospital affiliations be sequenced in the rotation of full-time or part-time clinical affiliations? How should academic and clinical educators adjust clinical education objectives for student performance, given the increasingly specialized knowledge utilized in this practice setting? A thorough understanding of some of these implications may allow better use of the teaching hospital as a clinical education resource than currently exists.

One additional idea warrants further discussion. A Clinical Instructor in this study commented that students must have a taste for the acute care setting, "… but what they need is the guidance to understand how to cope with this setting and how to find favorable

things in it." This comment reminds us that we must integrate into this analysis the students' perception of their ability to learn in teaching hospitals. When reflecting on my personal evaluation of clinical education in acute care settings, I have a perplexing dilemma correlating conflicting feedback. Although the data reported here, describing the acute care setting as an increasingly challenging and intellectually stimulating practice setting for physical therapists, are consistent with my feedback from practitioners in acute care hospitals of varying sizes, students with whom I come into contact often have a different perspective. As the Clinical Instructor in this study tells us, it is often hard for the student to find "favorable things" about acute care physical therapy practice. My observations indicate that that student's perceptions are disproportionally weighted with instances of routine and cursory patient evaluations and protocol-driven, technically based treatments. Perhaps the author has other data from this study that would confirm or disconfirm the existence of this conflict between the Clinical Instructor's and the student's perceptions of the level of practice in acute care settings.

Janet Guyer, PhD, PT
Assistant Professor
Graduate Program in Physical
Therapy
Duke University
Durham, NC 27710

References

1 *Current Patterns for Providing Clinical Education in Physical Therapy Education.* Alexandria, VA, American Physical Therapy Association, 1985.
2 Jensen G. Qualitative methods in physical therapy research: a form of disciplined inquiry. *Phys Ther.* 1989;69:492–500.

Author Response

I would like to thank Dr Gwyer for her thoughtful comments on this report. She has raised several important points related to this research to which I would like to respond. Perhaps more importantly, she has identified additional research needs in this area and has suggested several additional research questions. I find her comments both instructive and supportive as we look to future research efforts in this area.

Dr Gwyer's observations regarding the theoretical framework of this study are correct. The study was descriptive, relying on three sources of data: demographic, survey, and interview. The latter two sources express the participants' perceptions of the environment. An interview format was selected as one data source because it offered a greater depth of information and expression than the survey instruments alone. This study did not use a true ethnographic approach. Indeed, I spent only 1 week at each site, with some follow-up, and only as an observer of the system. This does not represent an opportunity to become immersed in the environment and therefore make interpretations as an "insider." The identification of themes from the interview data seems a practical approach to describing commonalities in the interview comments. Of necessity, only a very few examples of interview data were provided in this report to support the themes I identified.

I would like to offer some clarification for the questions that Dr Gwyer raised regarding specific themes. I will resist the urge here to present more interview data, but instead will summarize participants' perceptions in these areas to further elucidate these themes.

The theme of streamlined hospital mission was developed primarily from department manager and hospital administrator comments that centered on efficiency and effectiveness. Hospital administrators talked about greater efficiency through organizational changes such as flattening the organizational structure of the institution, reducing patient amenities such as shuttle bus services and number of reception staff, and increasing the coordinated effort of discharge planning. Department managers spoke more of cooperative efforts between departments and staffs to focus the institutions' efforts more precisely. These efforts included greater centralization of decision making, interdepartmental team building, and related activities. In several instances, department managers described this push toward efficiency and effectiveness in a positive way.

The theme of concerns over quality of care was generated from an interesting and complex set of interview data. I would agree with Dr Gwyer that the data supporting this theme do not appear consistent with some other comments by participants related to growing ethical dilemmas and potential shortcomings of the prospective payment system (PPS). I would also note, however, that participants indicated greater efforts and activities in quality assurance through the demographic and survey data presented in the report. Interview data suggested truly mixed opinions about the preservation of quality, however one might attempt to quantify that. In my view, there are two additional observations to make. Participants agreed that there was greater challenge in maintaining quality of care for patients, but also that greater efforts and attention were being paid in this area. It seemed that participants as a whole were therefore unwilling to say there

was either a net loss or gain in quality. The other point is conceptual and relates to how we define quality. It seems that participants previously viewed high-quality care as an ultimate goal, always something to be striven for, always with room for improvement. As they were pressed in this PPS system, participants seemed more willing to talk about quality as a threshold, a minimal acceptable standard. This change in the conceptual framework that practitioners have of quality may be important to explore further as we continue to assess how we define and measure quality.

The clinical education themes should be carefully considered by clinical educators and researchers. Dr Gwyer raises a question about the purported "gap" between student readiness and acute care teaching hospital expectations. The data support examples of increased clinical educator expectations in terms of independence, efficiency, and self-directedness on the part of the student. There is no evidence that suggests that students are less well-prepared. Rather, available evidence suggests that the gap between expectations and preparation may be widening as expectations have increased. Participants in the study described the "gap" as expanding, commensurate with the increasing demands of PPS. What has changed is the clinical educator's resources of time and attention to assist the student in the full transition to the practice setting. Students are therefore expected to be more independent more quickly, and to develop efficiency in their patient care sooner. Can students be prepared for this prior to arriving in the clinical setting? This question can be debated. One thing is clear from the data: The clinical educator has less time to assist in this transition. Several participants also commented on the increased risk that this presents in the situation in which students need remedial or modified clinical education learning experiences.

Finally, Dr Gwyer raises the important point of the students' perspective on this changing clinical education environment. The students' perspective is outside the scope of this study, but a most important area of future research. Understanding these environments through the perceptions of those in the setting is incomplete without consideration of the students' perspective. If, from the students' perspective, the value of these environments as settings for clinical learning has changed, we need to understand this. I would also suggest that how acute care teaching hospitals contribute to a comprehensive clinical education may be changing, from the students' perspective, based on changes that may be occurring in the students' definition of comprehensive clinical education. As an anecdotal comment, I have observed that students' perceptions of the teaching hospital setting may have more to do with the specific rotation or service the student is assigned to and may have less to do with the institution as a whole. As teaching hospitals have become more streamlined, the broad student exposure has given way to a more specific rotation experience to reflect the organizational structure of these physical therapy departments. Perhaps this means that greater attention must be paid to the context of clinical learning in the future, and not just the institution that houses the clinical education program.

Dr Gwyer has expanded the discussion of this report and offered additional considerations for future inquiry on this topic through her comments. It is my hope that the commentary and my comments in this response will be helpful to readers and will offer clarity and challenge to the research yet to be done in this area.

Michael J Emery, EdD, PT

Research Report

Enhancing Service Productivity in Acute Care Inpatient Settings Using a Collaborative Clinical Education Model

Richard K Ladyshewsky

Background and Purpose. *Exposure of physical therapy students to acute inpatient settings is difficult to achieve because of staff shortages and 1:1 supervision. The purpose of this study was to examine the productivity effects of the 2:1 teaching model in the acute inpatient clinical setting. Changes in patient throughput and the amount of care provided were the measures used to define productivity.* **Subjects.** *The work load measurement statistics of 8 Clinical Instructors (CIs) and 16 physical therapy students were examined.* **Methods.** *The productivity of each CI during a control period was compared with the productivity of the CI-student team.* **Results.** *Each CI-student team's mean productivity was greater during the clinical placement than during the control period when the CI worked independently. Even when the students' productivity measures were prorated by 0.6, the productivity was greater during the student placement than during the control period.* **Conclusion and Discussion.** *The study demonstrates that students make positive contributions to clinical service units that can exceed normal productivity levels of the CI. The 2:1 model has the potential to increase productivity while increasing the numbers of placements for academic programs in limited specialty areas. [Ladyshewsky RK. Enhancing service productivity in acute inpatient settings using a collaborative clinical education model. Phys Ther. 1995;75:503–510.]*

Key Words: *Clinical education, Collaborative, Cooperative, Productivity.*

The exposure of physical therapy students to acute inpatient settings (eg, general medicine, general surgery) is often difficult to achieve. These service areas are also plagued by frequent and chronic staff shortages. It is not surprising, therefore, that it is difficult to find enough clinical placements for students in these areas. When staff shortages exist, shortages of clinical placements may increase due to re-

fusal to accept students because of concerns about institutional productivity. Such shortages create enormous difficulties for academic programs trying to plan clinical learning experiences. Creative methods of maximizing teaching resources are needed if students are to receive a well-rounded education prior to licensure.

The teaching model frequently used in physical therapy clinical education is the one student to one Clinical Instructor (CI) ratio (1:1 model). This model may limit the maximization of teaching resources and has not been shown to provide the most effective strategy for the development of clinical competence. This teaching model typically requires a CI to balance his or her caseload and administrative responsibilities with those of student supervision, evaluation, and teaching. This responsibility creates much anxiety on the part of the both the CI and the student. For the CI, anxiety comes in part from administrative pressure to maintain productivity and quality of

RK Ladyshewsky, MHSc, BMR(PT), is Lecturer, School of Physiotherapy, Curtin University of Technology, Perth, Western Australia, Australia. He was Academic Coordinator of Clinical Education, Division of Physical Therapy, University of Toronto, Toronto, Ontario, Canada, at the time of this study. Address all correspondence to Mr Ladyshewsky at School of Physiotherapy, Curtin University of Technology, Selby St, Shenton Park, Western Australia 6008, Australia.

This article was submitted May 18, 1994, and was accepted February 2, 1995.

patient care.[1] Maintaining this productivity and quality of care often comes at the expense of the student's learning experience.[2] For the student, anxiety comes in part from not having adequate opportunities for supervised practice, feedback, and reflection. Excessive reliance on the 1:1 teaching model may also create major limitations for academic programs trying to place students in a variety of clinical settings.

One model that has been demonstrated to maintain productivity, provide high-quality learning experiences, and increase the number of placements in the clinical setting is the collaborative or cooperative teaching model.[2,3] In this model, two (or more) students are assigned to one CI. The students manage the care of the CI's caseload under the CI's direct supervision. Collaborative teaching refers to situations in which the interactions among students are not based on fixed teacher/learner roles.[4] The participants are viewed as equal partners in the learning process, with the responsibility for learning placed on the students.[4] Ladyshewsky and Healey[5] have described this model in detail. In their experience, they have found that this model encourages peer-based teaching and mutual problem solving. The CI functions as a facilitator, supervisor, and coach, with the students providing the bulk of patient care.[5] This model of teaching also decreases the reliance of students on the CI.[2–5]

This collaborative teaching strategy has been demonstrated to be effective in promoting learning in the clinical setting.[2,3,6–11] As students develop their ability to work together, they are better able to contribute and to use the contributions of their peer(s) to enhance their learning.[12] Further, as individual team members begin to learn collaboratively, they become empowered to promote additional learning among their peer group.[12] This peer-based learning strategy can lead to higher levels of clinical competence.[8] As Neufeld and Barrows[9] have stated, collaborative teaching provides a forum for students to identify their own emotional reactions and skills in

listening, providing criticism, and pooling the collective experiences of the group in finding answers to a problem.

The impact of the collaborative teaching model on institutional productivity has yet to be fully studied. Disadvantages of this model such as increased time for evaluation, setting of objectives, managing different learning styles, differences in rapport between the CI and the students, and the need to share scarce resources can potentially increase the work load for the CI and influence the overall productivity of the supervisor-student team. Unfortunately, there are few evaluations of productivity when using multiple-student–single-instructor models.

Most evaluations looking at the impact of students on clinical agency output have used 1:1 models of student supervision and have focused on "costs to facilities" and not "measures of productivity."[13–21] There have, however, been a handful of studies examining the productivity side of clinical education. Lopopolo[22] found that students produced a net financial benefit per day by increasing the number of patient visits per day. Leiken et al[23] examined productivity using occupational therapy, physical therapy, and radiology technology students in one large metropolitan hospital. The number of treatments provided was used as the productivity measure.[23] In two studies,[23,24] Leiken and colleagues found that the students contributed to the facility's capacity to provide patient care. Kaplow[25] concluded in her review of a physical therapy internship program in Quebec, Ontario, Canada, that the service provided by students outweighed the cost, in time spent, by CIs to supervise and coordinate the program. Ladyshewsky et al[26] also found that physical therapy students did not produce negative effects on overall departmental productivity in an outpatient orthopedic setting. Instead, actual staffing levels, case mix, amount of meeting time, and length of waiting lists were the factors more likely to influence patient throughput.[26] Coulson et al[27] found that senior physical therapy

students in an outpatient setting increased the clinic's net earnings by $216.77 per day and throughput by 3.25 patients per day. Graham et al[28] also demonstrated that longer placements (eg, 5 weeks) produced greater productivity and efficiency than did shorter placements. The student-CI team's productivity (as measured by mean number of patients treated per day, mean revenue generated per day, and mean number of treatment units provided per day) in longer placements (5 weeks) was also substantially higher than when the therapist worked alone.[28]

The basis for this study was to evaluate the patient care productivity of the collaborative teaching model in acute care inpatient settings. A 2:1 model (two students to one CI) was utilized. Differences in patient care productivity between the CI alone and the CI with two students were investigated.

Method

Subjects

Eight CIs employed in six different hospital-based acute inpatient settings and 16 physical therapy students were involved in the study. Five of the CIs had previously supervised students in a 2:1 placement and had received training in managing this type of supervisory arrangement from a workshop program regularly offered by the University of Toronto (Toronto, Ontario, Canada). Five CIs had supervised 7 or more students during the course of their career. The remaining three CIs had supervised 0, 1, and 3 students, respectively. All CIs involved in this study volunteered to supervise 2 students at the same time. The CIs were advised to turn over the majority of their patients to the 2 students and to spend their time in student supervision.

The 16 students who were involved in the study had completed their third year of academic study at the University of Toronto. The University of Toronto Program in Physical Therapy is a 4-year program leading to the Bachelor of Science (Physical Therapy) degree. By the end of the third year, students in this program have completed all studies in cardiorespiratory, neurology, and orthopedic sciences. They have also completed 4 weeks of full-time clinical practice, which occurred at the end of their second year of study. Of the 16 students, only 1 student had a previous 2:1 placement experience. The student pairs were randomly assigned to their placements by the Academic Coordinator of Clinical Education (ACCE) using the university's computerized placement matching system. The paired assignments were then reviewed by the ACCE, and changes were made if there were discrepancies in academic performance (eg, one student with an average grade of 60% and the other student with an average grade of 85%) and previous academic preparation (eg, one student holding a higher degree and the other student possessing only a high-school diploma). The students' cumulative grade point average was used as an academic performance measure. The number of years of pre–physical therapy higher education was used as a measure of previous academic preparation. In all cases, an equitable match was attained. For all of the students, this was their first acute inpatient experience in cardiorespiratory therapy.

Procedure

Workload Measurement System (WMS) data were collected and compared at two different points in time: once during the student placement and once during the control period. The WMS captures time spent in patient care, student supervision/teaching, and administration. Detailed descriptions of the various measures used in the system are presented in Table 1. The student placement was a 5-week full-time placement. The control period was a 1-week full-time period during which the CI worked independently. The data from this week were then multiplied by 5 so that a comparison could be made with the SP data. In Kaplow's study of physical therapy intern productivity, she outlined several considerations for

ensuring reliable and valid data.[25] Data should come from the same institution with and without students, and the case mix across sampling intervals should be approximately the same.[25] This study met the first requirement by using data from the same institutions with and without students. The same CIs were also involved in both components of the study (control period and student placement).

The strategy that I used to ensure case-mix consistency across the control period and the student placement was to capture only 1 week of CI data during the control period. The data were collected from 2 to 4 weeks before or after the actual student placement. A sufficient interval between the control period and the student placement was necessary to ensure that there were no influencing effects on the CI's productivity (eg, preparing for the student before or refamiliarizing oneself with the caseload after the students' departure). The control period had to be close enough to the student placement, however, to ensure that case mix had not changed substantially. I assumed that capturing 5 full weeks of CI data for the control period (with the 2- to 4-week grace period before or after the student placement) could increase the chance that the work unit characteristics would differ from the actual student placement, thus affecting the nature of the comparison. Ladyshewsky et al[26] have described several of these cofactors (eg, changes in staffing, case mix, meeting time, patient volume) that can have an impact on productivity measures.

Neither the students nor the CIs were aware of this study. This blinding was done to ensure that their reporting would be honest and typical of their regular activity rather than being influenced by their knowledge of being in an experiment. The 2:1 teaching model is part of the normal clinical education program at the University of Toronto, and the students and CIs believed they were engaged in a standard clinical placement. The students and CIs did complete an evaluation form asking them for qualitative infor-

mation about the placement experience. The director of each physical therapy service, however, was sent a letter inviting him or her to participate in the study. If the director agreed to participate in the study, I met with the director to discuss the scope and objectives of the study and the methods for ensuring confidentiality. Following each student placement and control period, I met with the director and collected the appropriate data.

Instrumentation

Standardized WMS data were used to measure productivity in these acute inpatient settings. These data are already available in usable format through the Canadian Management Information Systems group created through the merger of the Canadian Management Information Systems (MIS) Project and the Canadian National Hospital Productivity Improvement Program.[29] The WMS data that were utilized in this study are described in Table 1. One weighted unit of time is equivalent to approximately 1 minute of staff time.[29] These data were then manipulated to create five specific productivity indicators. These productivity indicators are also described in Table 1.

Data Analysis

Once all the WMS data were collected, I calculated the productivity indicators. Each productivity indicator for the student placement included the WMS data for the CI and the students. The productivity indicators for each of the eight teams were then grouped together by period (control period and student placement) and averaged. By averaging each of the productivity indicators across the eight groups, one is able to make comparisons between the control period and the student placement.

The data collected during the student placement were analyzed in two different ways: (1) in their pure form and (2) with the student component reduced by a cofactor of 0.6. It was important to factor down the students' WMS data contributions because it

Table 1. *Workload Measurement System (WMS) Data and Productivity Indicators*[a]

Term	Definition
Workload Measurement System (WMS) data	
Direct care weighted units (DCWU)	Direct patient care activities are those activities that are diagnostic, evaluative, and therapeutic activities of the service and that require the presence of the patient
Patient care weighted units (PCWU)	Encompasses both direct patient care activities and indirect patient care activities; the latter are those patient care activities that support or supplement diagnosis, evaluation, and treatment for which the presence of the patient is not required
Attendance days (ADAY)	A 24-hour period during which physical therapy direct care has been provided to a patient; only one attendance may be recorded for the same person in a 24-hour period
Paid worked hours of the Clinical Instructor (WH)	Total paid hours of the employee only; benefit hours are not included (worked hours of the student are not part of this measurement because they are not paid by the agency; any service contribution they provide is therefore considered a benefit)
Productivity indicators (dependent variables)	
Direct care weighted units per worked hour (DCWU/WH)	The number of recorded time units in the direct care category divided by the number of worked hours; DCWU/WH measures the amount of direct care in minutes per hour provided to patients
Patient care weighted units per worked hour (PCWU/WH)	The number of recorded time units in the direct and indirect patient care category divided by the number of worked hours; PCWU/WH measures the amount of direct and indirect care in minutes per hour provided to patients
Attendance days per worked hour (ADAY/WH)	The number of attendances for the sampling interval divided by the number of worked hours; ADAY/WH measures how many patients are seen or treated per hour
Direct care weighted units per attendance day (DCWU/ADAY)	The number of recorded time units in the direct patient care category divided by the number of attendance days; DCWU/ADAY measures the average amount of direct care in minutes spent on each patient
Patient care weighted units per attendance day (PCWU/ADAY)	The number of recorded time units in the direct and indirect care category divided by the number of attendance days; PCWU/ADAY measures the average amount of direct and indirect care in minutes spent on each patient
Non-patient care activity (NPCA)	The amount of actual time in hours spent in activities such as administration, staff development, and didactic teaching

[a]Adapted from *Physiotherapy Workload Measurement System-National Hospital Productivity Improvement Program, Health and Welfare Canada-Statistics Canada Health Division, 1987–1988 Edition.* Ottawa, Ontario, Canada: Minister of Supply and Services; 1988.

would be incorrect to assume that 1 minute of student time was equivalent to 1 minute of CI time. I selected a reduction factor of 0.6 because these students were expected to manage a two-thirds caseload by the end of the placement, as per guidelines established by the University of Toronto clinical education program. This factoring had the net effect of reducing the students' patient care productivity contributions by 40% and served as an efficiency/effectiveness adjustment to the productivity indicator.

Results

Amount of Care Provided per Worked Hour

Table 2 illustrates the mean difference in patient care productivity during the control period and the student placement. The range across the eight facilities for the control period and the student placement is also provided. The total amount of direct care weighted units per worked hour (DCWU/WH) and patient care

weighted units per worked hour (PCWU/WH) provided increased by 106% and 99% from the control period to the student placement. When the students' contribution to DCWU/WH and PCWU/WH was reduced by a factor of 0.6, there was still a net increase in the teams' productivity of 47% and 43%.

Table 2. *Differences in Productivity Indicators From Control Period to Student Placement*[a]

Producivity Indicator	Control Period			Student Placement			% Change	Factor 0.6	% Change
	X̄	SD	Range	X̄	SD	Range			
DCWU/WH	25.57	10.57	17.33–39.73	52.57	17.34	34.35–81.72	+106	56.50	+47
PCWU/WH	39.56	10.49	29.86–49.33	78.56	18.24	48.92–98.63	+99	56.50	+43
DCWU/ ADAY	17.30	6.56	14.33–25.14	27.82	4.14	23.35–35.26	+60	19.39	+12
PCWU/ ADAY	31.11	11.95	17.05–56.58	43.38	12.16	26.33–65.08	+39	30.70.	−1
ADAY/WH	1.48	0.74	0.53–2.67	1.98	0.84	1.16–2.79	+34	NA	NA

[a]See Table 1 for definitions of productivity indicators. NA=not applicable.

Number of Patients Treated per Worked Hour

Table 2 also illustrates the mean difference in the numbers of patients treated during the control period and the student placement. The range across the eight facilities for the control period and the student placement is also provided. The attendance days per worked hour (ADAY/WH) increased by 34% from the control period to the student placement. That is, the two student-CI teams were able to treat 34% more patients as compared with what the CIs normally managed. This particular calculation did not include a factoring component of 0.6, given that it is measuring actual numbers of patients treated per worked hour.

Amount of Care Provided per Patient

Table 2 further illustrates the mean difference in the amount of care provided to each patient during the control period and the student placement. The range across the eight facilities for the control period and the student placement is also provided. The amount of direct care weighted units per attendance day (DCWU/ADAY) and patient care weighted units per attendance day (PCWU/ADAY) increased by 60% and 39% from the control period to the student placement. When the students' contribution was reduced by a factor of 0.6, there was still a net increase in the amount

of DCWU/ADAY of 12%. With respect to PCWU/ADAY, there was a net decrease of 1%.

Amount of Clinical Instructor Time Spent in Non–Patient Care Activities

Clinical Instructors spent approximately the same amount of time managing their administrative responsibilities during the course of the student placement as they did during the control period. During the 5-week control period, CIs spent, on average, 27.04 hours on administrative duties. During the 5-week student placement, CIs spent, on average, 25.26 hours on administrative duties. In addition to this administrative time, the CIs were also able to spend, on average, 27.58 hours on didactic teaching activities during the student placement. During the student placement, therefore, the CIs spent, on average, a total of 52.84 hours on administration and didactic teaching.

Discussion

This study demonstrates that students placed in an acute inpatient setting are able to make a positive service contribution and that this contribution can exceed the unit standard when two students are assigned to one CI. One of the main reasons these productivity results were obtained was that the CI was able to delegate most of his or her direct responsibility for "hands-on" care to the two students. This delega-

tion provides time for the CI to supervise the two students while minimizing any detrimental effects on productivity. Expert treatment can be provided by the CI when necessary.

It is true that if the CI also managed a large caseload in conjunction with the caseload of the two students, the productivity of the unit could theoretically increase even further (providing there were enough patients). This increased productivity, however, could have a detrimental effect on the quality of learning and supervision. This outcome was evidenced in an earlier study by Ladyshewsky,[2] which demonstrated that the quality of supervision and learning decreased (as reported by students) when their CI's personal caseload increased.

Even though this particular study utilized Canadian work-load measurement data, the results are generalizable to most health care institutions at which the physical therapy salary component of the departmental budget is relatively constant (eg, the physical therapists are paid their salary whether students are present or not). What was measured in this particular study was the activity of the CI and the students when providing patient care.

Although this work-load measurement system does not attempt to measure every minute of a physical therapist's time. it does give a good measure of the amount of care provided. The

WMS is part of standard hospital recording in Canada, so most physical therapists are well versed in the reporting method. This method enhances the reliability of their reporting. Because students are learning how to report their WMS data, there is a greater possibility of incorrect reporting. Fortunately, CIs are expected to review these data, and all students receive a 2-hour training session on the Canadian WMS as part of their administrative education in the second year of their program. Both of these safeguards served as important reliability checks. As mentioned earlier, CIs and students were not aware that these data were being collected. Hence, any reporting bias should have been minimized.

The fact that the amount of DCWU/WH and PCWU/WH increased is not surprising, given that there were more "bodies" available to provide patient care. The increase in these values is a function of the mathematics involved in deriving these productivity measures. Only the paid worked hours of the CI were included in the denominator. The numerator, however, included the DCWU and PCWU of all three team members. The reason for calculating the measures in this way is that the students' service contributions to the agency are a benefit. The agency does not pay for them. It is, therefore, only appropriate to consider the cost of the CI's time. What was important to determine was whether the students' contributions to productivity during the student placement were sufficient to equal or outweigh the normal productivity of the CI during the control period.

The increase in ADAY/WH demonstrated that the team was able to manage their caseload responsibilities as well as treat additional patients. For those agencies that bill their patients on a per-attendance basis, the potential for increased revenue is evident. One of the reasons productivity increased in this case was not because there was an unlimited supply of patients for the students to treat. Most acute inpatient units have fixed bed complements and therefore a fixed

number of patients for treatment. Students were able to treat patients from other physical therapists as the students' skill and competence increased. This factor accounted for the increase in the number of attendances per worked hour.

The amount of direct and overall patient care provided per attendance (DCWU/ADAY and PCWU/ADAY) was also found to increase and is a direct measure of the amount of time, on average, spent with each patient. In many ways, these work-load statistics offer a measure of quality, if one assumes more time with a patient is better. Because the single caseload of the CI was divided between two students, each student was able to spend a proportionately greater amount of time with each patient. This is why an increase in the amount of care per patient was seen. With factoring, however, PCWU/ADAY decreased by 1%. By itself, this decrease is insignificant because it is an average measure and reflects the variance in performance among the eight 2:1 teams. This decrease does, however, demonstrate the effect of incorporating the students' efficiency on productivity.

Although beyond the scope of this study, it would have been interesting to measure the impact of students on overall work unit productivity. One would expect to see, at least, a break-even outcome, with students offsetting the decrease in the number of patients seen by other physical therapy staff. In addition, one would expect to see either an increase in administrative time by the other physical therapists (using the time made available by students treating their patients) or an increase in the amount of time these physical therapists spent treating their remaining patients. Both findings have been reported in earlier work undertaken by Kaplow[25] and by Ladyshewsky et al,[26] who found that the influence of students did not have a detrimental effect on overall work unit productivity.

The absorption of the CI's caseload by the two students provided the CI with time to plan and engage in clinical

teaching as well as time to maintain his or her administrative responsibilities. This teaching time is important if the benefits of a cooperative learning strategy, which were described earlier, are going to be realized. The CI needs time to structure the learning environment such that students can learn cooperatively. The fact that the amount of CI administrative time remained relatively consistent between the control period and the student placement period suggests that students utilized the expertise of one another to solve problems. This possibility further reinforces the concept that this model has the potential to decrease the reliance of students on CIs.[2–5]

From a cost-accounting perspective, the additional time that was made available for teaching should not be interpreted as a cost to the agency. Although this "teaching time" costs the agency in the sense that this professional physical therapist could be engaging in some other activity, it ignores the fact that the only reason this time has become available is because the students are providing a free service to the hospital. I believe that this student service contribution should be interpreted as a payback or benefit to the facility. The principle that the investigator is trying to elucidate is that one cannot isolate clinical teaching costs from productivity. Both must be considered as part of the full cost-benefit equation.

One of the critical elements behind the success of this placement model is that the students had completed their clinical studies and had already completed a full-time 4-week placement during their second-year program. Hence, they were able to make a useful contribution to the service. These same results might not have occurred in a clinical teaching situation using junior students.

The data reported in this article are mean data. There were definite differences in the data among the CI-student teams, the ranges of which are shown in Table 2. Not every team demonstrated the same changes in productivity. This finding reflects the difficulty in implementing controls in this type of study, in which there may be different student performance capabilities, different case mixes among acute inpatient settings, different patient acuity levels, different institutional systems in operation, and differences in how the CIs spend their time teaching and supervising. For example, in one particular group in this study, a thoracic surgeon went on holiday in the middle of the placement, which had a dramatic effect on the productivity of the team.

Another important limitation of this study is that it did not measure the quality of patient care provided by the students. This is not an issue exclusive to 2:1 models of clinical supervision. It is an issue for any model of clinical teaching. What is interesting about this particular model of clinical supervision is that it has the potential for improving the quality of care provided by students during a placement. If the CI properly delegates the majority of his or her clients to the students, the CI is in a much better position to oversee the quality of care provided by the students, a finding reinforced in the study by Emery and Nallette.[3] This finding is in direct contrast to the 1:1 situation, in which the CI is constantly struggling to meet the demands of his or her personal caseload of 65% to 75%, for example, with the 25% to 40% caseload of the student. Another important factor to consider about this teaching model, outside of productivity, is that it has the potential to increase the number of acute inpatient placements for university programs.

There was a net positive influence in productivity across the eight facilities. There will always be instances in which a placement may result in a decrease in productivity because of problems related to patient availability, supervision, or student performance. These same issues are not exclusive to 2:1 models of clinical teaching and can be extended to the 1:1 model. Over the course of time, however, one would hope that the facility benefits overall from its student program.

Ideally, further investigations with larger samples would add to the research. It was difficult to find enough CIs who were willing to supervise two students at the same time. The general shortage of acute inpatient cardiorespiratory placements in itself also led to a less-than-ideal sample size.

Repeating this type of analysis in different speciality areas would also determine whether these same productivity benefits occur. Investigations using this type of data analysis on placements of different durations should also be undertaken, as Coulson et al[27] demonstrated that this factor also has an effect on levels of productivity.

This type of productivity analysis varies somewhat from the type of cost-benefit analyses undertaken in the literature. Most cost-benefit studies in the past have looked at very few multiple measures. The impact of students on institutions was often assessed by counting changes in numbers of patients seen or in numbers of treatments provided. Tracking the amount of time CIs spent teaching students and then calculating the cost of this supervision (without considering the service benefit accrued to the agency by the students) has also been undertaken. Other studies have examined changes in the amount of billed revenue when students are placed in an institution.

With the advent of computerized management information systems, much more accurate work-load and productivity information can be collected and analyzed in tandem. Time spent in patient care interventions, administration, and teaching can be easily collected and tied into cost estimations. This approach provides a much more reliable and valid method of cost-benefit analysis. The impact on an individual CI's productivity or the productivity of an entire work unit can also be assessed using these management information systems.

Conclusion

This study has demonstrated that a cooperative model of clinical education using two students assigned to one CI can positively influence a service unit's productivity. In this study, acute inpatient services were examined. The implications of these results should interest ACCEs, CIs, and administrators because all are concerned about the impact of students on institutional productivity. There is clearly much more room for other investigations of this sort. For example, does one get similar results using a different model of work-load measurement? How does placement length influence productivity, and do you get similar types of results with more senior or junior students? What are some of the effects on patient care quality when you have multiple students and one CI? Finally, do you get the same type of effects in different specialty areas?

In spite of these additional research questions, the physical therapy profession can use the current information gleaned from this study to reexamine the way in which it delivers its clinical education programming. Current resource constraints, institutional staff shortages, deficiencies in the number of clinical placements, and the changing nature of our profession require that we reexamine the way we prepare our students.

References

1 Bohannon RW. Statistical analysis of productivity in one physical therapy department. *Phys Ther.* 1987;21:1553–1557.

2 Ladyshewsky R. Clinical teaching and the 2:1 student-to-clinical instructor ratio. *Journal of Physical Therapy Education.* 1993;7:31–35.

3 Emery M, Nallette E. Student staffed clinics and creative clinical education during the times of constraint. *Clinical Management in Physical Therapy.* 1986;6(2):9–10.

4 McDonald BA, Larson CO, Dansereau DF, et al. Cooperative dyads: impact on text learning and transfer. *Contemporary Educational Psychology.* 1985;10:369–377.

5 Ladyshewsky RK, Healey E. *The 2:1 Teaching Model in Clinical Education: A Manual for Clinical Instructors.* Toronto, Ontario, Canada: Department of Rehabilitation Medicine, Division of Physical Therapy, University of Toronto; 1990.

6 Tiberius R, Gaiptman B. The supervisor-student ratio: 1:1 versus 1:2. *Canadian Jour-*

nal of Occupational Therapy. 1985;52:179–183.

7 Abercrombie MLJ. *Anatomy of Judgement.* Hàrmondsworth, England: Penguin Publishing Co Ltd; 1969.

8 DeClute J, Ladyshewsky RK. Enhancing clinical competence using a collaborative clinical education model. *Phys Ther.* 1993;73:683–689.

9 Neufeld VR, Barrows HS. The McMaster philosophy: an approach to medical education. *Journal of Medical Education.* 1974;49:1040–1050.

10 Glendon K, Ulrich D. Using cooperative learning strategies. *Nurse Educator.* 1992;17:37–40.

11 Barrows HS. The scope of clinical education. *Journal of Medical Education.* 1986;61:23–33.

.12 Irby D. Clinical teaching and the clinical teacher. *Journal of Medical Education.* 1986;61:35–45.

13 Ramsden EL, Fischer WT. Cost allocation for physical therapy in a teaching hospital. *Phys Ther.* 1970;50:660–664.

14 Rabkin MT. Reducing the costs of medical education. *Health Affairs.* 1986;5:97–104.

15 Hammersberg SS. A cost/benefit study of clinical education in selected allied health programs. *J Allied Health.* 1982;1:35–41.

16 Chung YI, Spelbring LM, Boisonneau R. A cost benefit analysis of fieldwork education in occupational therapy. *Inquiry.* 1980;17:187–191.

17 Mackinnon JR, Page GG. An analysis and comparison of the educational costs of clinical placements for occupational therapy, physical therapy, speech pathology and audiology students. *J Allied Health.* 1986;15:225–237.

18 Page GG, Mackinnon JR. Cost of clinical instructors time in clinical education-physical therapy students. *Phys Ther.* 1987;67:238–243.

19 Porter RE, Kincaid CB. Financial aspects of clinical education to facilities. *Phys Ther.* 1977;57:905–909.

20 Kling DR, Bulgrin JA. Clinical education costs and benefits: application of a fiscal analysis model. *J Allied Health.* 1987;16:135–147.

21 Pobojewski TR. Case study: cost/benefit analysis of clinical education. *J Allied Health.* Summer 1978:192–198.

22 Lopopolo RB. Financial model to determine the effect of clinical education on physical therapy departments. *Phys Ther.* 1984;64:1396–1402.

23 Leiken AM, Stern S, Baines RE. The effect of clinical education programs on hospital production. *Inquiry.* 1983;20:88–92.

24 Leiken AM. Method to determine the effect of clinical education on production in a health care facility. *Phys Ther.* 1983;63:56–59.

25 Kaplow M. *Cost Benefit of Physiotherapy Internship in Quebec.* Montreal, Quebec, Canada: McGill University; 1980. Thesis.

26 Ladyshewsky RK, Bird N, Finney J. The impact on departmental productivity during physical therapy student placements: an investigation of outpatient physical therapy services. *Physiotherapy Canada.* 1994;45;94–98.

27 Coulson E, Woeckel D, Copenhaver R, et al. Effects of clinical education on the productivity of private practice facilities. *Journal of Physical Therapy Education.* 1991;5:29–32.

28 Graham CL, Catlin PA, Morgan J, Martin E. Comparison of 1-day-per-week, 1-week, and 5-week clinical education experiences. *Journal of Physical Therapy Education.* 1991;5:18–23.

29 Government of Canada. *Physiotherapy Workload Measurement System National Hospital Productivity Improvement Program, Health and Welfare Canada Statistics Canada Health Division, 1987–1988 Edition.* Ottawa, Ontario, Canada: Minister of Supply and Services; 1988.

Performance Issues in Clinical Education

Brief Report

Addressing Problem Areas of First-year Students

Instructors at Stockton State College in Pomona, New Jersey, identified five problems typical of students in the early stage of the entry-level physical therapy program: 1) an inability to view patients holistically, 2) a hesitancy to touch patients, 3) a hesitancy to ask questions of instructors, 4) inaccuracy in evaluation and treatment, and 5) a tendency to take too much time for evaluation and treatment. A laboratory experience was designed to address these problems.

METHOD

Students in the first semester of the entry-level physical therapy program participated in the laboratory experience as a part of the introductory class session in their kinesiology course. Eighteen students completed a brief questionnaire about the five problem areas identified by the instructors before the laboratory experience. The same 18 students completed a similar questionnaire and an evaluation of the experience at the conclusion of the class session. The laboratory consisted of three components that addressed the five problem areas identified.

The first component, designed to address the problem of not viewing patients holistically, was entitled "Five-Minute Mingle." Students were instructed to introduce themselves to three students with whom they were unfamiliar and to obtain the following information: name, place of birth, and recent work or volunteer experience. After the time allotted for mingling had ended, the students were asked to identify the following information about the three students they had introduced themselves to: eye color, type of handshake, and height.

The second component, designed to address students' hesitancy to touch others, was entitled "Human Motion Machine." An initial student was instructed to assume any position and to produce some type of motion. The second student connected to the first student and produced another motion. This continued until all 18 students were connected. After the exercise, the instructor led the students in a group discussion of their feelings about touching and being touched.

The third component of the laboratory, designed to address the problems of questioning, speed, and accuracy, was entitled "Tunnel of Touch." Four tunnels were constructed from

gym mats and treatment tables. The four tunnels were arranged around a central exchange area. Labels identified each tunnel according to a particular color. Students were divided into four teams and were given a starting tunnel color for the team. Each member of the team was also assigned a second tunnel color. Each team member went through the team tunnel and then had to proceed through their second tunnel and then move around the periphery of the tunnels to get back to the original tunnel. Each team was judged on the time needed for completion of the activity and on the accuracy of exchanges by team members. Discussion after the exercise focused on the importance of asking questions that clarified the task, speed, and accuracy to task accomplishment.

RESULTS

Comparison of the students' pre-experience and post-experience questionnaires showed that 28% of the students showed a higher regard for the role of speed in task completion after the exercise, 5% showed a higher regard for accuracy, 5% showed a higher regard for the

importance of observational skills, 5% thought that they were better observers, 50% reported higher comfort levels when being touched, 44% reported higher comfort levels with touching, and 39% were more willing to ask questions as needed following the laboratory experience. The results shown in the Table indicate that students had positive opinions about the laboratory experience.

DISCUSSION

The questionnaire responses indicate that the problem areas identified by the instructors were addressed by the laboratory. In particular, students' levels of comfort with touching and being touched increased, as did their willingness to ask questions when necessary. Whether these initial learning experiences will lead to improved early clinical performance is not known.

Elaine Bukowski, MS, PT

The author is Assistant Professor, Physical Therapy Department, Stockton State College, Pomona, NJ 08240-9988.

Table
Students' Responses to Post-introductory Laboratory Questionnaire (N=18)

Question	%
1. As a whole, the introductory lab was:	
extremely helpful	22
very helpful	56
helpful	22
not really needed	0
worthless	0
2. In terms of your own educational needs, the lab was:	
extremely relevant	17
very relevant	33
relevant	33
somewhat relevant	0
not relevant	0
no response given	17
3. Did you enjoy this lab?	
enormously	11
very much	44
a lot	28
a little	0
not at all	0
no response given	17
4. How would you rate the overall quality of this lab?	
excellent	11
very good	67
good	5
fair	0
poor	0
no response given	17

Reprinted with permission from the *Journal of Physical Therapy Education*, Vol 5, No 2, p 83, 1991.

DESIGN OF CLINICAL EDUCATION

Collaborative Clinical Learning Designs

THROUGH A NEW LENS

Collaboration &

by Jody S Gandy, PhD, PT

MARK BOLSTER

Among the changes that have taken place in clinical education: multiple students supervised by one CI, such as in the 2:1 model discussed on pages 46-54.

History is a kind of telescope. We can use it both to look back on our profession's progress and to look ahead to our profession's future. To be the masters of our own fate, we must continually adjust the focus–and sometimes replace the lens.

Consider clinical education. Approximately half of all PTs are serving as clinical instructors (CIs) right now. The days of working one-to-one with a student in the clinic seem to be numbered, and some of us are feeling anxious or resentful about it. Why should we change a formula that we're so comfortable with, a formula that's worked for so many years?

The answer is simple: It isn't working anymore. Clinical education takes place in the practice setting and by its nature must reflect the context of practice. And during the past 12 years, the context of practice has changed...

...From Service to Service Delivery

In the 1980s, physical therapy services—and health care services in general—were provided primarily in hospitals. In 1983, 41.9% of physical therapy services were provided in the hospital setting. Today, those services are provided primarily in private offices (29.2%), with 25.4% in hospital settings. Other settings include rehabilitation centers (13.1%), home health agencies

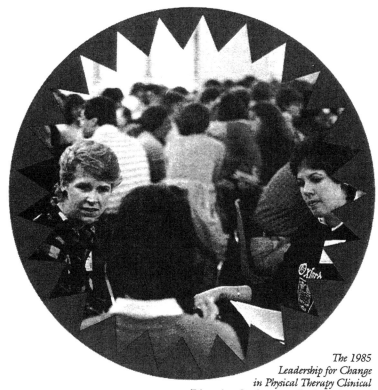

The 1985 Leadership for Change in Physical Therapy Clinical Education Conference at Eagle Rock served as a catalyst for many of the changes taking place in clinical education today.

Interdependence

Whether you're a CI, a CCCE, an ACCE, or a student on affiliation, your role in clinical education is changing. Understanding why can help make the change work for you.

(7.7%), and extended-care facilities (7.4%), with a majority of physical therapists practicing in multiple settings.[1]

In 1985, the focus of health care was on *services* and on documenting changes in patient status through utilization review. Health care looked favorably on physical therapy, and third-party payers usually reimbursed for physical therapy services at a rate commensurate with the charges generated. These services were examined according to quality assurance measures and generally were considered

by administrators to be revenue generators for facilities. Recently established: the prospective payment system (PPS) and Medicare's system based on diagnostic related groups (DRGs), in which services were reimbursed according to average length of stay for patients in the specific DRGs.

As a result of skyrocketing costs, the focus of health care in 1995 is on service *delivery*, which is driven by cost-containment measures, accountability through outcomes effectiveness, accessi-

bility, and controlled or managed care. Dramatic health care reform has taken place at the state level, with managed care at the forefront. Universal access has been discussed—but for now has been tabled—at the national level. Among the issues under debate in the 1990s: rationing of care, diagnostic and treatment codes setting reimbursement rates for all types of services, practice guidelines developed according to diagnosis to provide protocols for the delivery of care, networks for health care providers, "corporatization" of health care, and a system that would rate physician competence.

...From PT Recruitment to PT "Redesign"

In 1985, many facilities reported increasing numbers of physical therapist (PT) and physical therapist assistant (PTA) vacancies and implemented highly competitive marketing strategies.

By 1995, facilities in some regions that have had ongoing difficulty recruiting PTs and PTAs have begun to explore the development and use of "alternative service providers" to meet the demand for physical therapy services.[2] As recent articles in *PT* have indicated,[3-7] in the reengineering of hospitals and the provision of services through provider networks, some PT and PTA positions have been "redesigned" or eliminated. Demand for physical therapy in certain underserved geographical regions and in geriatric and pediatric populations, meanwhile, continues to grow.[8] The American Physical Therapy Association's (APTA) Government Affairs Department reports that consumers now can legally access physical therapy services in 30 states without a physician's referral; however, regardless of direct access, Medicare regulations and managed care plans typically mandate physician referral.

...From Generalization to Specialization to...

In 1985, physical therapy services already had begun an era of expansion in such settings as private practice, industry, long-term and extended care, sports medicine, home health, and schools.[9] Advances in health care technology, the aging of the US population, and changes in exercise patterns were reflected in the roles assumed by PTs and in the growth of physical therapy specialties in such areas as geriatrics, pediatrics, orthopedics, neurology, and sports. Physical therapists were developing knowledge and expertise in specific areas through postprofessional education programs, continuing education, and research. Through the American Board of Physical Therapy

Specialties (ABPTS), the profession launched efforts to evaluate and recognize individual clinical competency in specialized practice areas.[10] In the late 1980s, then, physical therapy was becoming both more expansive and more specialized, offering opportunities in a wide variety of settings with patients throughout the life span.

In 1995, with continued advances in technology and research, the continued aging of America, and the federal legislation providing for individuals with disabilities (ADA), physical therapy remains vested in specialization. More than 1,000 clinical specialists were recognized last year by the profession in seven specialty areas.[10] However, as physical therapy makes strides in the area of specialization, other professions such as medicine are making efforts to increase the number of generalists to meet the needs of populations in underserved geographical regions and to fill the need for primary care providers under managed care.[11] In physical therapy, the role of physical therapists as primary care providers and the need to shift in emphasis from specialization to generalization are topics of debate.[12]

Impact on Clinical Education

In 1985, increased publicity about and demand for physical therapy spurred the development of new PT and PTA education programs with ever-growing applicant pools. A majority of PT programs worked collaboratively through clinical education consortia to develop strategies that would share resources and reduce administrative workload for the academic coordinator of clinical education (ACCE). The trend in clinical education paralleled that in practice and education: expansion. More sites were developed to accommodate individual student and program needs.

By 1995, many physical therapist education programs have transitioned to the postbaccalaureate professional level, in part to meet the demands of the new health care environment[13]; one professional doctoral program is in development. Competition for slots in education programs has increased, with opportunities for physical therapy education expanding international-

ly.[14,15] But higher education itself, like health care, has limited resources and is implementing its own cost-containment measures. The "driver" is the demand—made both by government and by consumers—for institutional accountability regarding resource management, more flexibility to accommodate adult learners, and education programs that increase opportunities for graduates to be employed. In 1995, many academic institutions view physical therapy as one of the professions that can meet these demands—but physical therapist faculty recruitment and the availability of high-quality clinical education sites are problematic.[16]

Since 1985, clinical education consortia have increased in number to help therapists learn how to become effective clinical educators.[17] Clinical education research and publications have provided more information about how to provide and manage effective clinical education programs.[18,19] APTA's voluntary *Guidelines for Clinical Education* have assisted in clinical site and CI development. And, in 1994, APTA provided additional support to reduce some of the administrative tasks associated with clinical education: a standard data-gathering tool called the Clinical Center Information Form, which provides information about clinical sites to academic programs.

Despite these efforts, and despite the fact that the number of clinical education sites has risen approximately 49% since 1985, sites and instructors are even more scarce than they were 10 years ago. Why? The number of PT and PTA graduates requiring clinical learning experiences has almost doubled (Table[9,20-36]), and clinical rotations generally are longer and often coincide with each other. Financial resources are limited, as is the number of qualified CIs; demands for greater patient-care productivity and accountability, meanwhile, have increased. As of 1992, only 53.4% of all CIs attended CI training programs prior to taking their first student.[36]

In addition to the logistical problems of clinical education today, there are challenges to content. Our new graduates increasingly are expected to routinely practice using collaborative and interdisciplinary

Table. Clinical Education—Then and Now

10 YEARS AGO

Professional Programs

- Predominately baccalaureate degree level.
- 106 accredited physical therapist (PT) professional programs—3,434 graduates (mean class size=32).[20,21]
- 68 accredited physical therapist assistant (PTA) programs—995 graduates.[20,21]
- Average number of weeks in length, PT programs: 80, with full-time clinical education comprising 25% of the curriculum; PTA programs: 66, with full-time clinical education comprising 19% of the curriculum.[20,21]
- Mean number of clinical education sites per PT program: 83 (range=21-180 centers).[22]
- PT and PTA programs in aggregate placed 4,636 students in 3,490 clinical education sites for typically two to four full-time clinical education rotations.[9]

Curricula

Based on the 1978 *Standards and Criteria for Accreditation of Physical Therapy and Physical Therapist Assistant Education Programs,* curricula were evaluated in terms of how well they met curricular competencies. Clinical education was broadly defined in the standards as an "organized sequence of learning experiences designed to enhance learning that were adequate in number, accessible to students, and appropriate in scope to meet the clinical education objectives and mission of the academic program."[23,24]

Clinical Education Consortia...

were organized by region and were comprised primarily of academic coordinators of clinical education (ACCEs) and, secondarily, clinical educators, who collaborated in administrative activities, promoted networking and support between ACCEs and clinical educators, provided continuing education programs for clini-

cal faculty, and conducted limited clinical education research. The 16 different consortia represented a total of 72 PT programs.[25]

CIs...

on average had practiced 6.6 years and supervised a total of five students per year. Most CIs had 2 or fewer years of clinical experience before teaching their first student in the clinic and practiced in a variety of settings, with university teaching and community hospitals serving as more than half of the clinical education sites. To become clinical sites, facilities typically initiated contact with academic programs and attempted to accommodate, on request, as many students as feasible from all regions of the country while using a clinical supervision pattern of one CI to one student.[9]

TODAY

Professional Programs

- Predominately at the postbaccalaureate professional level.
- 141 accredited PT programs—5,267 graduates (mean class size=40).[26]
- 165 accredited PTA programs—2,793 graduates.[26,27]
- Average number of weeks in length, PT programs: 83.5, with full-time clinical education comprising 33% (27.6 weeks) of the curriculum[27]; PTA programs: 69.5, with clinical education comprising 27% (18.7 weeks) of the curriculum.[28]
- Mean number of clinical education sites per PT program: 184 (mode=200; range=20-791 clinical sites).[27]
- PT and PTA programs in aggregate placed 8,060 students in more than 5,300 clinical education sites for an average of three or four full-time clinical education experiences.[29]

Curricula

Based on the 1992 *Evaluative Criteria for Accreditation of Physical Therapist Education Programs* and the 1994 *Evaluative Criteria for Accreditation of Physical Therapist Assistant*

Programs, curricula were evaluated in terms of how well graduates met the academic program's established education and student performance outcomes. Clinical education was described in terms of its organization; integration within the curriculum; provision in a variety of practice/health care settings, with delineation of specific learning experiences; and establishment of formal and informal communication procedures between clinical and academic faculty.[30,31] In 1993, the profession endorsed the voluntary *Guidelines for Clinical Education* that provided a structure for assessing the quality of clinical education sites and delineated the roles and responsibilities for providing high-quality clinical instruction by the center coordinator of clinical education (CCCE) and clinical instructor (CI).[32]

Clinical Education Consortia...

were organized by region and state or both and frequently included clinical faculty and, in some instances, academic faculty and program directors. The 31 different consortia represented a total of 206 professional PT and PTA programs[33-35] and collaborated on many initiatives, including 1) administrative activities such as obtaining clinical slot commitments, using consistent evaluation instruments, and conducting joint site visits; 2) networking and communicating between academic and clinical faculty; 3)

providing for a regular clinical faculty development program; 4) conducting clinical education research; and 5) developing strategies for resolving clinical education issues according to region.

CIs...

on average had 5.9 years of clinical teaching experience, of which 3.94 years were spent at their current facility, and supervised a mean of 1.8 students (range 1-21) per year. Clinical sites affiliated with an average of 6.6 PT programs and 2.4 PTA programs. A vast majority of CIs had only 1 year of practice experience before taking their first student and practiced in varied and multiple settings. The most typical supervisory pattern was 1:1 (84.2%), followed by 2:1, 1:2 or more, and 1 PT/PTA CI team to 1 PT/PTA student team. In general, academic programs contacted clinical sites to provide clinical education. In many cases, not only were sites unable to accommodate additional students, but they were developing criteria for selecting programs or finding themselves in situations in which clinical commitments had to be broken. The two most frequent reasons cited by clinical sites for cancellation of affiliations: staffing shortages and patterns (66.4%) and staff inexperience (17.5%).[36]

team approaches, regardless of setting. They need to know how to problem solve, make sound clinical decisions within a variety of facility "pathways" or practice "algorithms," consult with and make referrals to other health professionals, seek information on their own, and accurately assess their own strengths and limitations.

Compelling Realities

All of these realities compel us to "adjust our focus"—even replace that lens—and explore alternatives that more effectively use available limited resources and provide an environment for learning that more closely approximates current and future practice.

An emerging trend in clinical education involves alternative supervisory patterns that encourage collaboration and interdependence; provide for mentoring and role modeling; empower learners; and demonstrate and model effective methods of supervision, delegation, and interpersonal communication.[37,38] These new patterns are flexible in design to accommodate different settings, different learning experiences, and the varying number of qualified CIs. (The computer technology is even available to match clinical sites with students from multiple academic programs, both interinstitutionally and intrainstitutionally.[39-41]) Not all of the new supervisory patterns may be appropriate for every setting; however, the act of exploring them could lead any setting to greater innovation in providing clinical education.

To determine the effectiveness of the new models, clinical educators need to conduct research and publish their findings in the peer-reviewed literature. In the meantime, this issue and future issues of *PT* will provide a forum for PT and PTA clinical educators who have responded to the environment. They will share how they planned, designed, and implemented these patterns and reflect on their experiences. Patterns to be discussed include one CI to two or more students (collaborative/interdependence pattern) (see pages 46-54), one PT/PTA CI team to one PT/PTA student team (supervisory/delegation pattern), and one CI to one first-year student and one last-year student team (mentor

pattern). (A version of this mentor pattern is discussed on pages 51-53.)

Clinical education is essential to the success of physical therapy professional education—and to the success of the profession. Clinical educators have worked hard to develop and refine the way they transmit knowledge, skills, and behaviors that PT and PTA graduates will need. The profession must continue to develop more collaborative and interdependent methods for providing high-quality student learning experiences in varied practice settings that accommodate both the increased number of PT and PTA students and the practice environments these students enter on graduation. *PT*

Jody S Gandy, PhD, PT, is APTA Director of Clinical Education.

References

1 *1993 Active Membership Profile Report.* Alexandria, Va: American Physical Therapy Association; 1994.
2 *Health Professions Education for the Future: Schools in Service to the Nation. Report of the PEW Health Professions Commission.* San Francisco, Calif: UCSF Center for the Health Professions; 1993.
3 Woods EN. Restructuring of America's hospitals: what does it mean for physical therapy? *PT—Magazine of Physical Therapy.* 1994;2(6):34-41.
4 Arthur PR. Patient focused care: acute orthopedic services. *PT—Magazine of Physical Therapy.* 1994;2(7):34-47.
5 Brumfield J. Patient focused care: PT and neuroscience. *PT—Magazine of Physical Therapy.* 1994;2(9):76-85,89.
6 Bullock K. Patient focused care: hospital wide. *PT—Magazine of Physical Therapy.* 1994;2(11):51-60.
7 Sinnott MC. Critical pathways to success. *PT—Magazine of Physical Therapy.* 1994;2(12):55-61.
8 *Human Resources: Facts & Figures.* Alexandria, Va: American Physical Therapy Association; 1993.
9 Clinical Education Database. Alexandria, Va: American Physical Therapy Association; 1985.
10 American Board of Physical Therapy Specialties. *Directory of Certified Clinical Specialists in Physical Therapy 1985-1993.* Alexandria, Va: American Physical Therapy Association; 1994.
11 Littlemeyer MH, Martin D, eds. Rural health: a challenge for medical education. Proceedings of the 1990 Invitational Symposium. *Acad Med.* 65(12S):1990.
12 Woods EN. What's so special about specialist certification? *PT—Magazine of Physical Therapy.* 1994;2(2):46-51.
13 Reynolds JP. Ah-hahs & ambiguities: toward the 21st century in PT education. *PT—Magazine of Physical Therapy.* 1993;1(11):54-62, 117-118.
14 *1993 APTA Applicant Report.* Alexandria, Va: American Physical Therapy Association; 1993.
15 Ellis J. PT program in Scotland offers unique opportunity for US students. *PT Bulletin.* 1994;9(37):5.
16 El-Khawas E. Campus trends 1993. *Higher Education Panel Report.* 1993;8(July):3-27.
17 May BJ, Smith HG, Dennis JK. Combined clinical visits and regional continuing education for clinical instructors. *Journal of Physical Therapy Education.* 1992;6(2):52-56.
18 *Clinical Education: An Anthology.* Alexandria, Va: American Physical Therapy Association; 1992.
19 Deusinger S, Gwyer J, Foord L, DeMont M, Gandy

J, Sanders B. A challenge to clinical educators: compendium for effective clinical education. *Journal of Physical Therapy Education.* 1990;4(2):55-75.
20 *List of Accredited and Developing Professional Physical Therapist and Physical Therapist Assistant Education Programs.* Alexandria, Va: American Physical Therapy Association; 1984.
21 *Physical Therapy Education Program Fact Sheet.* Alexandria, Va: American Physical Therapy Association; 1986.
22 *Report on Clinical Education Faculty in Physical Therapy—1985.* Alexandria, Va: American Physical Therapy Association; 1986.
23 *Commission on Accreditation in Physical Therapy Education. Standards and Criteria for Accreditation of Physical Therapist Education Programs.* Alexandria, Va: American Physical Therapy Association; 1978.
24 Commission on Accreditation in Physical Therapy Education. *Standards and Criteria for Accreditation of Physical Therapist Assistant Education Programs.* Alexandria, VA: American Physical Therapy Association; 1978.
25 *Report on Clinical Education for the Entry-level Physical Therapist: Consortia, Clinical Education Conferences, and Students' Early Patient Contacts.* Alexandria, Va: American Physical Therapy Association; 1986.
26 *List of Accredited and Developing Professional Physical Therapist and Physical Therapist Assistant Education Programs.* Alexandria, Va: American Physical Therapy Association; 1994.
27 *Physical Therapist Education Program Fact Sheet.* Alexandria, Va: American Physical Therapy Association; 1994.
28 *Physical Therapist Assistant Education Program Fact Sheet.* Alexandria, Va: American Physical Therapy Association; 1994.
29 Clinical Education Database. Alexandria, Va: American Physical Therapy Association; 1992.
30 Commission on Accreditation in Physical Therapy Education. *Evaluative Criteria for Accreditation of Education Programs for the Preparation of Physical Therapists.* Alexandria, Va: American Physical Therapy Association; 1992.
31 Commission on Accreditation in Physical Therapy Education. *Evaluative Criteria for Accreditation of Education Programs for the Preparation of Physical Therapist Assistants.* Alexandria, Va: American Physical Therapy Association; 1994.
32 Clinical Education Guidelines and Self-Assessments. Alexandria, Va: American Physical Therapy Association; 1993.
33 *Clinical Education Resource Guide.* Alexandria, Va: American Physical Therapy Association; 1994.
34 Teschendorf B, Gramet P, Heubusch L. Group development of a clinical education instrument. *Journal of Physical Therapy Education.* 1988;2(1):10-12.
35 *1992 Clinical Faculty Survey.* Alexandria, Va: American Physical Therapy Association; 1992.
36 May BJ, Smith HG, Dennis JK. Combined clinical visits and regional continuing education for clinical instructors. *Journal of Physical Therapy Education.* 1992;6(2):52-56.
37 DeClute J, Ladyshewsky R. Enhancing clinical competence using a collaborative clinical education model. *Phys Ther.* 1993;73:683-696.
38 Solomon P, Sanford J. Innovative models of student supervision in a home care setting: a pilot project. *Journal of Physical Therapy Education.* 1993;7(2):49-52.
39 Hughes C. *Final Report to the APTA Board of Directors on a Project to Design, Implement, and Evaluate a Multischool/Student Computer Site Matching Program.* Slippery Rock, Pa: Slippery Rock University; 1993.
40 Ladyshewsky R. Review of computerized matching program to assign physical therapy students to clinical placements. *Journal of Physical Therapy Education.* 1993;7(2):67-71.
41 Dennis JK, May BJ. Computer assisted student clinical placements. *Journal of Physical Therapy Education.* 1990;4(2):87-92.

Clinical Teaching and the 2:1 Student-to-Clinical-Instructor Ratio

Richard Ladyshewsky, MHSc, BMR (PT)

ABSTRACT: The clinical education of physical therapists has traditionally used teaching ratios of one student to one clinical instructor (1:1 model). This pilot study examined a clinical supervision approach in which one clinical instructor supervised two students concurrently (2:1 model). Nineteen 2:1 placements were investigated. Questionnaires were completed by third-year physical therapy students (n=38) and their clinical instructors (n=19) after the placement. The results suggested that most clinical instructors and students were pleased with their teaching and learning experiences, respectively. Specific advantages unique to the 2:1 learning experience were identified.

INTRODUCTION

To foster the application of knowledge, skills, and attitudes learned by students in didactic educational sessions, clinical experience is a routine component of physical therapy curricula. It is in the clinical setting that students are expected to demonstrate competence in practice. One means of enhancing the learning experience is to encourage active student participation in the clinical placement.

Students will benefit from the clinical experience if they can contribute actively to the learning process.[1,2] The multiple-student–single-instructor model is one means of achieving more active learning. In this model, students develop their abilities to work cooperatively and to promote learning among their student team members because of the requirement to work in groups. This is achieved by delegating the case load of the clinical instructor (CI) to the two or more students and establishing parameters for joint practice. Not only does this require the students to work collaboratively in planning the appropriate method(s) of care for their patient(s), it also reinforces the team concept.

A cooperative learning style is not naturally adopted by all students in the clinical setting. Students may be dependent, competitive, or cooperative in their learning style.[3,4] A *dependent* learner requires a significant amount of guidance and support from the CI. This style may be appropriate for beginning students, but it is inappropriate for students further along in their education. *Competitive* learners, on the other hand, try to outperform other students. This type of behavior interferes with learning and prevents development of a team-centered style of practice. Changing this type of learning behavior involves giving students opportunities to work in groups with clearly defined objectives for goal accomplishment.

Cooperative learners possess an adaptable learning strategy. They can engage in joint problem-solving sessions and share previous experiences. This learning strength allows cooperative learners to replicate the concept of the team approach so commonly referred to in patient care.

Cooperative learning is often referred to as *collaborative* learning and can be defined as a form of indirect teaching in which students work collaboratively in solving problems (either academic or clinical) that have been organized by their instructor.[5] This learning strategy is quite different from traditional teacher and learner roles, because students are partnered in the learning process and work through clinical problems as a team that may or may not include the CI. Students in this learning milieu are viewed as equal partners in the learning process and are responsible for achieving their own learning objectives.[6]

Johnson and Johnson stated that the collaborative learning model is desirable in situations requiring problem solving or complex task analysis and in scenarios where a standard of performance is expected.[3] Such situations are common to the physical therapy clinical setting. Learning models that reinforce the concept of collaboration, therefore, must be encouraged to facilitate acquisition of these clinical skills.

Most studies on collaborative learning have focused on academic or classroom-based

learning.[3,7,8] The results of these studies strongly support the collaborative teaching model. The results of other studies also have demonstrated that students achieved much higher levels of achievement and productivity when learning was done on a collaborative basis.[6,9] Collaborative learning studies in clinical health education, however, are fewer in number than studies completed in the classroom. Of the few studies that have been undertaken, there is some evidence to support the concept of a collaborative learning strategy.[10-14] This concept involves organizing students into small groups (two or more) and structuring problems or learning situations for them to work through. The method of supervision and the structuring of the learning experiences are the most important features of a collaborative model, because students may continue to work independently in multiple-student–single-instructor models and not obtain the benefits of a collaborative learning approach.

Abercrombie was one of the first individuals to support the collaborative learning approach in medical education.[10] Her research demonstrated that positive medical judgment was enhanced at a much faster rate when small groups of students worked on formulating a clinical diagnosis together. The rationale behind this finding was that the group members could share their knowledge and collectively utilize their previous clinical experiences. This minimized any unshared biases or incorrect presuppositions.[10]

Other investigators examined the multiple-student–single-instructor model (3:1, 2:1) from a more operational perspective.[11-13] Their descriptive analyses indicated that multiple-student–single-instructor models are effective in meeting clinical education objectives, maintaining departmental standards for productivity, patient care, quality assurance, documentation, and patient satisfaction. Students who experienced this learning model had a much more positive attitude towards this type of instruction than students who remained in traditional 1:1 models.[13] The CIs who participated in the 2:1 ratio also presented a much more positive attitude

Mr Ladyshewsky is University Coordinator of Clinical Education, Department of Rehabilitation Medicine, University of Toronto, 256 McCaul St, Toronto, Ontario M5T 1W5.

towards collaborative teaching than those who continued to engage in traditional 1:1 supervision.[13]

Several advantages result from a multiple–single-instructor (2:1) teaching ratio: stronger students support weaker students, the frequency of superficial questions presented to the CI decreases, students provide mutual companionship, and dependency on the CI decreases.[12] Specific disadvantages also were identified, such as additional paperwork, different learning styles among the students, and differences in rapport among the group, but these were minimized when specific strategies were implemented by the CIs.[12] These strategies included structuring feedback, ensuring cooperative and individual work time, establishing clear learning contracts, clarifying student roles for patient care, and outlining basic ground rules for the learning experience.[12]

Declute and Ladyshewsky demonstrated that physical therapy students who undertook clinical experience in collaborative learning models scored significantly higher in all measured areas of clinical competence (patient evaluation, program planning, implementation of treatment, communication, documentation, and professional behavior) compared with their counterparts in more traditional 1:1 instructional models.[14]

The hypothesis of this study was that learning is enhanced when collaborative or cooperative learning methods are implemented. The support in the literature prompted the University of Toronto Division of Physical Therapy to apply this method of learning in the clinical setting. A principle impetus for the initiation of this teaching model in the clinical environment was a decreasing supply of placements for students in the metropolitan Toronto area and the need to seek more efficient placement and supervision models. The purpose of this investigation was to assess the effectiveness of the multiple-student–single-clinical instructor ratio (2:1) as a means of supervising students.

METHOD

Clinical instructors at University of Toronto-affiliated health care facilities were asked to submit 2:1 placements for the period of May 1990 to August 1990 on a volunteer basis. All clinical experiences were full-time and 4 weeks in duration. Nineteen facilities offered to pilot the 2:1 placement model. This resulted in 19 pairs of students and 19 CIs for the study. The type of placements offered are described more fully in Table 1.

The physical therapy students involved in this study were third-year students in a four-year undergraduate bachelor of science (physical therapy) program. Forty-seven percent (n=17) of the students were admitted directly into the program from high school. Nineteen percent (n=7) of the students had 1 or 2 years of previous university preparation when admitted into the program. Thirty-three percent (n=12) of the students had 3 or more years of previous university preparation when admitted to the program. Students at this level have completed studies in basic sciences, pathophysiology, and clinical management of patients in cardiorespirology, neurology, and orthopedics and have completed 4 weeks of full-time clinical practice.

PROCEDURE

Students selected their placement choices for the May 1990 to August 1990 clinical placement period from a list of available placement options. They were not informed which placements were 2:1 in nature. The actual assignments then were distributed among the students using a computerized random matching process. After these initial assignments were made, the list of students assigned to 2:1 placements was reviewed by the investigator. When unequal matches existed between students in the 2:1 placements, the investigator substituted another student to create a better match. Criteria used for the matching process were students' academic background prior to admission to the physical therapy program (eg, direct entry from high school, 1 year of university, previous degree) and cumulative grade point average.

A workshop was provided for the CIs before the commencement of the 2:1 placements. This workshop was available to CIs involved in the study and to other interested CIs. Fifty-two percent of the CIs involved in the study (n=10) attended the workshop. The workshop discussed strategies for implementing the 2:1 model and provided an overview of the principles of collaborative teaching.

At the end of each placement period, the CIs and students involved in the pilot project completed a questionnaire about the 2:1

placement. The questionnaire items developed by the investigator in collaboration with a senior physical therapy student as part of an independent research project. The rationale for item generation was based on issues raised in the literature and concerns voiced by CIs during the workshop sessions. The items were pretested by the Division of Physical Therapy's Clinical Education Committee. This committee is composed of 10 center coordinators of clinical education, each based in a different teaching facility. These individuals are responsible for the development and implementation of the student program in their agency. The questionnaires differed for the student group and the CI group to obtain specific information relevant to their respective roles. The questionnaire format included both closed- and open-ended responses.

The student questionnaire requested information about the type of placement, method of assigning patients, case load volume, and variety. Questions about the learning relationship with the other student and with the CI also were included. Some of the questions asked included, "How did the instructor spent his/her time with you?", "Were there any incidents involving a personality conflict with the other student?", "Describe the amount and method of supervision received by the CI." "Do you feel your evaluation was influenced by the performance of the other student," and "Describe how you received feedback." Students also rated the overall placement learning experience and could make additional comments.

The CI questionnaire requested information about the instructor's level of previous clinical teaching experience. Information about teaching role also was solicited, along with a breakdown of clinical teaching, administrative, and patient-care responsibilities. The CI was asked to rate the placement model in terms of learning opportunities available for students and ease of implementation. An opportunity to make additional comments was provided at the end of the questionnaire.

DATA ANALYSIS

Summaries of the questionnaire responses were organized into frequency distributions by CI and student groups. Cross tabulations were computed using selected variables to ascertain whether any significant interactions existed within a group. The Chi-square test was used to test for significance ($P \leq .05$).

RESULTS

Clinical Instructors

Nineteen CIs responded to the survey. The characteristics of this group of CIs are

Table 1
Clinical Placement Assignments (n=19)

Type of Placement	n
Specialty	
Orthopaedics	6
Neurology	6
Cardiorespirology	7
Facility	
Acute care hospital	16
Rehabilitation center	3

described in Table 2. A large proportion of the CIs who volunteered to participate in this pilot project had considerable clinical and supervisory experience.

The CIs also carried a rather large clinical or administrative case load during the implementation of the 2:1 placement. The breakdown of their duties is described in Table 3. The amount of patient care and administrative activity that continued to be provided specifically by the CI during the placement was considered high, given that CIs were advised to assign the majority of their case load to the two students. Despite the CIs' tendency to be actively involved in patient care or administrative activity, the students commented that the CIs were actively involved in the learning experience.

In inpatient orthopedic settings, 2:1 placements were easier to implement than 1:1 placements. In outpatient orthopedic settings, 2:1 placements were as easy to implement as 1:1 placements. At orthopedic settings, CIs assigned most of their patients to the students and engaged in more supervisory activities. Sixty-six percent (n=4) of CIs in orthopedics carried a personal case load less than 25% of normal.

In neurology settings, CIs indicated that 2:1 placements required more time and effort to implement. In cardiorespirology settings, CIs were split into two groups regarding the ease of implementation. Some felt that 2:1 placements required more time and effort to implement, whereas others felt that there was no difference between the 2:1 and 1:1 models. In cardiorespirology and neurology settings, CIs carried higher personal patient case loads than their orthopedic counterparts. Sixty-six percent (n=4) of the CIs in neurology carried personal patient case loads 25% to 50% of normal. All of the CIs (n=7) in cardiorespirology spent 25% to 50% of the time in patient care or departmental administrative activity.

Instructors for the most part preferred to assign patients directly to the students or involve them, to a certain extent, in the selection process. The CIs also reported that feedback on a student's performance was provided both on an individual and group basis. This appears appropriate because part of the patient load carried by the students was shared.

One concern raised by CIs during the 2:1 workshop was the possibility of pairing students with different levels of clinical competency. Three fourths of the CIs (n=14) stated that the students in the student group performed at similar levels. This may have resulted from the preplacement matching performed by the investigator or some other

factor(s). When CIs were asked to comment on the appropriateness of matching students by academic background and grade-point average, 90% of the CIs (n=17) supported this concept.

Twenty-six percent of the CIs (n=15) reported that their students performed at different levels. Correspondingly, these same CIs spent more time with the weaker student. Despite these performance differences, the CIs indicated that the team continued to work well.

Table 4 provides additional comments of the CIs about the 2:1 placement compared with previous 1:1 experiences. When learning objectives were only partially fulfilled by the students, this was often related to a weaker student's inability or to a lack of patient variety. The majority of CIs in orthopedic, neurology, or cardiorespirology settings felt that the 2:1 experience was an appropriate learning model for their specialty.

Table 2
Characteristics of Clinical Instructors (n=19)

Characteristic	n (%)
Number of years of clinical experience	
<2 years	2 (10)
2–5 years	6 (32)
>5 years	11 (58)
Number of students supervised in the past	
0–2	4 (21)
3–6	7 (37)
7–10	4 (21)
10+	4 (21)
Previous experience with 2:1 supervision	
Yes	11 (58)
No	8 (42)

Table 3
Clinical Instructor Activity During 2:1 Placement (n=19)

Activity	n (%)
Supervision and teaching time	
0–25%	1 (5)
25%–50%	6 (32)
50%–75%	8 (42)
+75%	4 (21)
Patient care time	
0–25%	8 (42)
25%–50%	11 (58)
Administration time	
0–25%	14 (74)
25%–50%	4 (21)

Table 4
Outcomes of 2:1 Placements as Reported by Clinical Instructors (n=19)

Outcome	n (%)
Fulfillment of student learning objectives	
Yes	13 (68)
Partially	6 (32)
2:1 model implementation difficulty for clinical instructor	
Substantially more difficult than 1:1 model	3 (16)
More difficult than 1:1 model	9 (47)
Same to manage as 1:1 model	2 (11)
Easier to manage than 1:1 model	5 (26)
Overall impression of 2:1 model as a learning experience for students	
2:1 model is better than 1:1 model	13 (68)
2:1 model is the same as 1:1 model	3 (16)
2:1 model is worse than 1:1 model	3 (16)

Of particular interest was the lack of a relationship between clinical and student supervisory experience and reported ease of 2:1 placement implementation. Clinical instructors with a good foundation of clinical and supervisory experience often reported that 2:1 placements required more time and effort than traditional 1:1 models. This impression represented nearly 60% of the total CI group (n=11). In contrast, some CIs with minimal clinical and supervisory experience reported that the implementation of 2:1 placements was the same as, or easier than, traditional 1:1 models. These comments represented the remaining 40% of the group (n=8). This 60%–40% split persisted even when previous experience in a 2:1 placement was considered.

More than three fourths of the CIs (n=14) identified various additional factors that influenced the 2:1 experience. In situations where there were insufficient numbers of patients available for two students, the willingness of other clinical units to provide patients and to assist in supervision was beneficial. Practice settings in which students can work closely together (eg, gym settings or single/adjacent units) also lighten the work of the CI, because both students can be readily observed. Environments with a large variety of patients for students to assess and treat were viewed as suitable areas for 2:1 learning experiences. Several CIs reported that a high level of administrative activity or a large personal case load had a negative impact on the learning experience.

Students

Thirty-six students responded to the questionnaire, resulting in a 95% response rate. In 66% of the student pairs (n=13 pairs), students occasionally shared patients. Fifty-eight percent of the students who were part of this shared-patient group (n=15) reported that their roles in the management of the patient were quite clear. The remaining 42% of this group (n=11) commented that their roles were occasionally unclear, particularly when they were responsible for planning and coordinating their patient's care.

Eighty-nine percent (n=32) of the students stated that they had an adequate number of patients for their case load. Seventy-seven percent (n=28) reported that there was sufficient variety of patients. Ninety-seven percent (n=35) of the students reported no incidence of personality conflict with the other student. In the one case where a student reported a conflict, the student commented that the quality of learning in this placement was still outstanding.

When students gave their impressions of the extent to which their CI was involved in patient care, almost 50% of students (n=17) reported that their CI spent a significant portion of the day treating his or her private case load. The varying degree of patient care responsibility undertaken by the CI was found by the students to affect the quality of supervision and quality of learning. When the CI was not heavily involved in patient care, 91% of the students considered the quality of supervision to range from "good" to "outstanding." There was a demonstrable reduction in the students' perception of the quality of supervision when a CI's patient care responsibility increased. Seventy-five percent of the students who felt that their CI was heavily involved in patient care stated that the quality of supervision was only "satisfactory" to "good." This rating difference between the two groups was significant (χ^2=11.2; df=3; P=.01).

This rating difference was apparent in the students' evaluation of quality of learning. When the CI's availability decreased because of patient care commitments, the student's rating of the learning experience was lower. This finding also was significant (χ^2=24.12; df=6, P=.0005).

A major concern expressed by students entering a 2:1 placement was the possibility that their performance might be compared with the other student. Eighty-six percent of the students (n=31) felt that their evaluation was not influenced by the performance of the other student. Fourteen percent of the students (n=14) felt that their evaluation was influenced by the performance of the other student.

Overall, students in the 2:1 supervision model were favorably impressed (Table 5). Eighty percent of the students (n=29) stated that they would not oppose another 2:1 placement if such an assignment was given. The remaining 20% (n=7) would not choose another 2:1 placement.

Many of the proposed benefits of collaborative learning models not discussed previously also were reported individually in the questionnaire by the students. Students indicated that they practiced their skills on each other and engaged in joint problem-solving activities without interrupting the CI. Students also were able to help each other by correcting each other's mistakes; this led to a more effective consolidation of ideas. The presence of a colleague also reduced the stress associated with entering a new and unfamiliar environment.

Sixty-four percent (n=23) of the students indicated that specific characteristics of the facility positively influenced their 2:1 learning experience. The availability of other staff for supervision when the principal CI was occupied was extremely useful, as were environments that allowed students to work in close proximity with each other and with the CI. Settings with a large variety of patients with differing functional levels provided enough interesting cases to be shared between two students. One student commented that the scheduling practice of the outpatient department (ie, 20-minute block bookings) allowed the CI to balance her time more effectively between the two students. One negative influence mentioned was the acute nature of patients in an intensive-care setting. This made independent decision making and treatment implementation difficult, because the student had to wait for the CI to finish with the other student before she could implement specific "high-risk" treatments.

DISCUSSION

The comments provided by the CIs and students in this exploratory survey suggest

Table 5
Students Impressions of 2:1 Learning Experience (n=36)

Aspect	n (%)
Quality of supervision	
Outstanding	17 (47)
Good	13 (36)
Satisfactory	4 (11)
Poor	2 (6)
Quality of learning environment	
Outstanding	16 (45)
Good	12 (33)
Satisfactory	7 (19)
Poor	1 (3)
Overall impression	
Outstanding	12 (33)
Good	16 (45)
Satisfactory	5 (14)
Poor	3 (8)

that 2:1 placements are a viable alternative to traditional 1:1 placements in specific clinical environments. These comments. however. should be considered in the context of other factors that may have affected the opinions solicited from the CIs and students in the questionnaires.

Finding enough CIs willing to supervise two students simultaneously was difficult. although several attempts were made to solicit volunteers. The CIs who volunteered to participate in the project may have biased the investigation towards a positive outcome. because more than half of the instructors had previous experience with 2:1 teaching. The positive results solicited in the questionnaire may reflect this volunteer bias.

The success of the 2:1 model may be related to the type of practice setting. Orthopedics was the clinical specialty in which 2:1 placements were easiest to implement. Clinical instructors in cardiorespirology and neurology stated that more effort was required on their part to successfully implement the 2:1 placement. This finding should be interpreted with some caution. Most CIs. particularly in neurology and cardiorespirology settings. did not delegate the majority of their case load to students and continued to carry between 25% and 50% of a normal case load. This would have increased the implementation effort.

The investigator did not explore reasons why some of the CIs in these two specialty areas carried a 25% to 50% of normal case load throughout the 2:1 learning experience. Staff shortages and growing patient waiting lists may increase the administration's reluctance to free up staff for student supervision. Other plausible explanations might be that CIs are reluctant to release "their" patients to students or that clinical education is not viewed as important. What was observed. however. was that the more a CI was involved in direct patient care. the lower the student's rating of quality of supervision and learning.

Given that the CIs in neurology and cardiorespirology were carrying 25% to 50% of a normal case load in conjunction with supervising two students. one strategy that these CIs may have utilized was to give the students more independence for patient care. These students had very little clinical experience to date. and this delegation of patient care responsibility may explain why some students found their patient management roles to be unclear.

Clinical instructors. for the most part. stated that their student pairs were well matched and performed at equivalent levels. Five CIs. however. felt that one of their two students

performed at a lower level. Despite this performance difference. the CIs commented that it did not pose any problems for the learning team. One of the cited advantages of collaborative learning arrangements is that stronger students will support weaker students during the placement.[12] This may explain the continued success of the learning experience and is worthy of further study.

Five students felt that their evaluations were influenced by the performance of the other student. It is not known whether these same five students were rated as performing at a lower level by their CI. Clinical instructors. therefore. must always be aware of the natural tendency to make comparisons and must ensure that they base evaluative judgments on observable. definable criteria.

The need to match students appeared to be an important concern for CIs. Ninety percent of the CIs (n=17) felt that the matching process used by the investigator should continue. Matching students with similar academic backgrounds is no guarantee that they will demonstrate similar clinical performance. but it probably is the only method that academic coordinators of clinical education (ACCEs) have for matching students. Further investigation should examine learning experience outcomes when students are assigned to their placements randomly. without any intervention from the ACCE. An increase in problematic performance differences between students or an increase in personality conflicts would support the need for a matching strategy.

The amount of the CI's experience did not have any predictive value on his or her ability to successfully manage a 2:1 ratio. The CI's sense of whether the 2:1 placement model required more or less effort than the 1:1 model was more dependent on the CI's understanding and use of specific collaborative teaching strategies than on experience alone. This finding is supported by an earlier investigation by Tiberius and Gaiptman.[12]

A small proportion of students (n=8) would choose the 1:1 approach over the collaborative model. This is interesting. because only 8% (n=3) of the students rated their placement experience as "poor." This suggests a preference on the part of some students for more individualistic. one-on-one teaching. Some students also may have preferred the traditional 1:1 teaching model because of concerns that their performance may have been compared with that of the other student.

CONCLUSION

Shortages of clinical placements and the need to educate therapists capable of work-

ing alongside other health professionals prompted the Division of Physical Therapy at the University of Toronto to develop and evaluate an alternative model of clinical education. Evaluation of new clinical placement models is imperative to identify factors necessary for successful learning while optimizing clinical teaching resources. More investigation of collaborative teaching models in different clinical specialty and practice environments is needed to enhance the generalizability of these results.

Better controls to ensure that case-load delegation is maintained throughout the learning experience would address some of the implementation issues raised in this study. Investigation of possible matching strategies to ensure optimal performance of the learning team would be extremely useful. as would identifying formal training criteria for CIs.

ACKNOWLEDGMENTS

This study was supported by a grant from the Ministry of Health. Government of Ontario. Canada. The author gratefully acknowledges the assistance of Kim Kushida. BSc. PT: the Division of Physical Therapy's Clinical Education Committee: and the clinical instructor community that participated in this study.

REFERENCES

1. Irby D. Clinical teaching and the clinical teacher. *Med Educ.* 1986:61(9):35-45.
2. Stritter FT. Hain JD. Grimes DA. Clinical teaching re-examined. *J Med Educ.* 1975:50(12):876-882.
3. Johnson DW. Johnson RT. *Co-operation. Competition and Individualization.* Englewood Cliffs. New Jersey: Prentice Hall: 1975.
4. Pratt D. Magill. MK. Educational contracts: a basis for effective clinical teaching. *J Med Educ.* 1983:58:462-467.
5. Bruffee KA. Collaborative learning and the "conversation of mankind." *College English.* 1984:46:635-652.
6. McDonald BA. Larson CO. Dansereau DF. et al. Cooperative dyads: impact on text learning and transfer. *Contemporary Educational Psychology.* 1985:10:369-377.
7. Slavin R. Cooperative learning: can students help students to learn? *Instructor.* March 1987:74-76.78.
8. Smith R. A teacher's view on cooperative learning. *Phi Delta Kappan.* May 1987:663-666.
9. Johnson DW. Maruyama G. Johnson R. et al. Effects of cooperative competitive and individualistic goal structures on achievement: a meta-analysis. *Psychol Bull.* 1981:89:47-62.
10. Abercrombie MLJ. *Anatomy of Judgment.* Harmondsworth: Penguin: 1964.
11. Emery M. Nalette E. Student staffed clinics and creative clinical education during the times of constraint. *Clinical Management in Physical Therapy.* 1986:2:6.9-10.
12. Tiberius R. Gaiptman B. The supervisor-student ratio: 1:1 vs. 1:2. *Can J Occup Ther.* 1985:32(4):179-183.
13. Healey E. Wells PA. Collaborative learning in the clinical setting: effect on attitudes and performance. Unpublished manuscript: 1988.
14. Declute J. Ladyshewsky R. A retrospective analysis of performance outcome in collaborative versus individual clinical placement models. Unpublished manuscript: 1991.

Research Report

Enhancing Clinical Competence Using a Collaborative Clinical Education Model

Background and Purpose. The purpose of this study was to determine whether students in collaborative (two students to one Clinical Instructor [2:1]) learning placements differed on measures of clinical competence as compared with their peers in traditional (1:1) clinical placements. **Subjects.** The population examined consisted of intermediate-level students in the physical therapy program at the University of Toronto. **Methods.** The outcome measure of clinical competence in this study was a weighted score acquired from the university's Evaluation of Clinical Competence (ECC) form. Seven subgroup clinical competence scores as well as the total clinical competence score were analyzed. **Results.** The collaborative learning group demonstrated significantly higher scores on all aspects of the ECC instrument. **Conclusion and Discussion.** This result suggests that achievement of clinical competence in patient evaluation, program planning, implementation of treatment, communication, management skills, professional behavior, and documentation were enhanced through collaborative learning. [DeClute J, Ladyshewsky R. Enhancing clinical competence using a collaborative clinical education model. Phys Ther. 1993;73:683–697.]

Key Words: Clinical competence; Cooperative learning; Education: physical therapist, clinical education.

Jennifer DeClute
Richard Ladyshewsky

Historically, the education for professional occupations has been founded in apprenticeship, in which the student learns alongside a mentor or skilled professional.[1] Most allied health programs continue to maintain this focus by including clinical placements in their curriculum. During these placements, students work with a practicing clinician to develop the knowledge, skills, and attitudes necessary for entry into their selected profession. During this clinical training period, the students are expected to transfer their theoretical knowledge into real-world professional skills and behaviors.[2–4]

There is overwhelming agreement in the literature regarding the value and importance of clinical education in physical therapy and other allied health programs.[2–11] Well-developed clinical education programs are essential components of a professional training program, as they are an important determinant of the quality of health care to be received in the future. *Clinical education* has been defined as "learning by doing in the presence of a clinical model."[7(p1079)] This definition emphasizes the concept that enhanced learning results from the active participation of the learner.[12,13] Some feel that this characteristic is the most influential factor in

J DeClute, BSc(PT), is Staff Physical Therapist, Sunnybrook Health Sciences Centre, 2075 Bayview Ave, North York, Ontario, Canada M4N 3M5. She was an undergraduate student in the physical therapy program at the University of Toronto, Toronto, Ontario, Canada, when this study was completed in partial fulfillment of her degree requirements.

R Ladyshewsky, MHSc, BMR(PT), was Academic Coordinator of Clinical Education, Division of Physical Therapy, University of Toronto, 256 McCaul St, Toronto, Ontario, Canada M5R 3C7, at the time of this study. Address all correspondence to Mr Ladyshewsky c/o 403 Riverton Ave, Winnipeg, Manitoba, Canada R2L 0N6.

This study was part of an earlier investigation on collaborative learning by Mr Ladyshewsky that was supported in part by a grant from the Ministry of Health of Ontario.

This study was approved by the University of Toronto Department of Rehabilitation Medicine's Ethics Review Board.

This article was submitted November 21, 1991, and was accepted May 25, 1993.

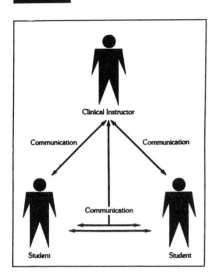

Figure 1. *Collaborative/cooperative model in clinical education.*

clinical learning, whereas others believe that the learner's present level of ability and knowledge is the major determinant of learning.[10,13,14]

There are many factors in the clinical environment that influence the learning process and subsequently the outcome of a given learning experience. For example, each facility is unique in the patient population it serves, its physical space, equipment, policies and procedures, and special programs.[15] Learning environments, however, must first fulfill the "safety needs" of the learner in order to facilitate the learner's intellectual needs.[13] In clinical practice, this translates into a nonthreatening environment in which students are free to practice unfamiliar or recently acquired techniques without the fear of embarrassment when making mistakes.[13]

Clinical education has also been defined as the transfer of abilities, ideas, and beliefs from instructor to student through the direct interaction with patients.[3,16] This definition emphasizes the importance of the role of the Clinical Instructor (CI). There is a relatively large amount of literature outlining effective and ineffective characteristics of the CI.[3–7,10,15,17] The amount of literature that is available

on the subject would suggest some degree of "face validity" to the notion that the CI is a major determinant of the quality of clinical learning that results. Essentially, the CI is responsible for the construction of an environment in which the learner applies and integrates previously acquired information.[13] The CI thereby adopts the role of a facilitator and directs the natural process of learning.[13] It is this role, that of facilitator, that must be emphasized among instructors if self-directed learning and problem-solving skills are to be developed by students.

Clinical education in physical therapy programs typically uses a ratio of one student to one CI (1:1 ratio). Even though this is the most commonly used approach, it has not been validated to any great extent. The 1:1 ratio is also a major limiting factor for universities as they begin to expand their enrollments in order to respond to an increasing public demand for physical therapy services. Program expansions in physical therapy require a larger base of clinical training sites and instructors to supervise the students in a 1:1 teaching model. With most facilities already experiencing staff shortages, more creative means of educating physical therapy professionals need to be examined. One such approach is a collaborative or cooperative model of clinical teaching in which two or more students are assigned to one CI (2:1 ratio).

Figure 1 displays the general communication flow within the collaborative or cooperative model.[18] Ladyshewsky and Healey,[18] in their experience in working with this teaching model, have found several interesting things. First, the cooperative model has been found to encourage collaboration and cooperation among students and has promoted more open communication among all members of the learning team. Second, although the students still maintain the responsibility for their own patients and caseload, they have been encouraged to consult with one another when questions arise about patient care. This type of collab-

oration or consultation among students has decreased their reliance on the CI.[18–20]

Based on their work in evaluating this model, Ladyshewsky and Healey[18] believe that 2:1 approaches encourage more collaboration among peers. This collaboration, however, does not occur naturally, and those who have examined cooperative learning models report that instructors must express the expectation that the students will work together.[21–24] For example, the instructor may also need to arrange joint teaching sessions with the students or have the students prepare a project together to enhance their cooperative skills.

To provide adequate supervision for more than one student, Ladyshewsky and Healey[18] believe that the CI needs to delegate part, if not all, of his or her caseload to the students. The students assume responsibility for patient care usually equal to or greater than the caseload normally carried by the CI. Ladyshewsky and Healey[18] believe that caseload delegation is imperative if the CI is to have the time to appropriately facilitate the learning experience.

The use of collaborative or cooperative learning techniques is well documented in the educational, psychological, and medical education literature.[11,19–28] Cooperative learning organizes students into small groups in which they assist each other to integrate skills, knowledge, and problem-solving abilities, thereby increasing self-esteem and acquiring a more positive attitude toward learning (E Healey, PA Wells; unpublished manuscript; 1988).[22,23,26,27,29] Collaboration is not a new concept. It permeates many aspects of everyday life and appears to be a natural tendency for humans who often seek help and who divide work loads to make work easier.[24,25] Bruffee[25] has argued that what distinguished collaborative learning from traditional classroom practice was that it changed the social context in which students learn. He comments that students' work tended to improve when they got help from peers. Furthermore, the students learned from each other and from the activity of helping itself. Collaborative learning, therefore, appeared to harness the powerful educative force of peer influence, which had been, and largely still is, ignored and wasted by traditional forms of education.[25]

If one accepts this premise for learning, it makes sense to facilitate models of learning that integrate social interaction, preferably at the peer level. This format of learning provides a forum for students to identify their own emotional reactions and skills in listening and providing criticism and to pool the collective experiences of the group in finding answers to a problem.[22] This approach to learning has shown that learning from one's peers in a group format enhances learning and comprehension.[22,23,26,27,29]

With respect to enhancing clinical judgment, strategies that enable students to be well versed in the theory behind disease or pathology is a necessity. Abercrombie[29] found that clinical judgment was augmented in medical students when they collectively solved problems. She involved groups of 12 medical students in a series of eight 1½-hour discussions concerned with seeing, language, classification, evaluation of evidence, and causation. Those students who took the course did significantly better in activities requiring clinical judgment than the students who did not take the course. Specifically, when the students who took the course were observed, they tended to discriminate better between facts and conclusions, to draw fewer false conclusions, to consider more than one solution to a problem, and to be less adversely influenced in their approach to a problem by their experience of a preceding one.[29] Neufeld and Barrows[22] have also illustrated how one can enhance learning by pooling the collective expertise and experience of medical students in biomedical problem-solving activities.

There appear to be disadvantages to the collaborative model such as increased time for evaluation and objec-

tive setting, managing different learning styles, unproductive competition, differences in rapport, and the need to share potentially scarce resources.[20] These disadvantages can be minimized, however, if effective supervision strategies are put into place before the placement.[20] Ladyshewsky and Healey,[18] in their experience in developing 2:1 models of clinical education, also point out that many of these disadvantages or challenges can be minimized by ensuring that the students receive adequate supervision and feedback and that the placement is planned well in advance.

The purpose of our study was to determine whether students who experienced a collaborative (2:1) learning placement differed on measures of clinical competence as compared with their peers in traditional (1:1) clinical placements. The purpose and expected outcome of clinical education in physical therapy and other clinically based allied health disciplines is the production of competent practitioners.[4,5,30,31] Hence, it is important to measure the educational experience of this new model against a valid and reliable measure of clinical competence.

Method

Measurement Instrument

The outcome measure used in this retrospective study was a weighted score acquired from the Evaluation of Clinical Competence (ECC) form utilized by the University of Toronto (Ontario, Canada) program in physical therapy. The ECC form is a behaviorally anchored rating scale composed of 33 items ranked on a progressive ordinal scale. The 33 items are grouped into seven different subcategories of clinical competence: patient evaluation, program planning, implementation of treatment, communication with patient/family, communication/management skills, documentation, and professional behavior. Each of the 33 competency standards delineated in the ECC form is weighted by a factor of 1 to 3, depending on its importance to overall clinical compe-

tence. These competency standards are also broken down into four statements, each describing a higher level or ranking of competence. The higher the ranking received, the higher the competency level achieved. Figure 2 outlines one of these behaviorally anchored competency measures used in the ECC instrument. The weighted scores in each of the seven subcategories as well as the total clinical competence scores were used to compare group means for the 2:1 and 1:1 placement groups.

The ECC form demonstrated reliability factors of .591 and .624 when used on senior (fourth-year) and intermediate (third-year) physical therapy students, respectively.[32,33] These were very strong measures in support of the ECC form, given that it has been suggested that the maximum reliability coefficient generally achieved is .30 for clinical evaluations.[32,33] Loomis[32,33] was also able to demonstrate that the ECC form possessed adequate measures of content, concurrent, and construct validity.

Sample

Both the CIs and students involved in this retrospective analysis of performance were part of an earlier study at the University of Toronto that examined implementation issues related to the 2:1 teaching model in cardiorespiratory, orthopedic, and neurology settings.[19] A questionnaire format was used to obtain this information and involved 19 CIs and 38 third-year physical therapy students. The results of this study demonstrated that the placement model was effective in achieving a positive educational outcome.[19]

Students in the University of Toronto undergraduate physical therapy program are required to complete eight 4-week blocks of full-time clinical practice. Students complete 4 weeks of clinical practice at the end of their second year, 16 weeks at the end of their third year, and 12 weeks at the end of their fourth year of study.

The third-year students in this study completed their four clinical place-

21. To ***assist the patient/family/others to assume responsibility for implementing treatment,*** the student:

MID	FINAL	
____	____	does not teach the patient/family/others the ward or home therapy.
____	____	needs reminding to teach patient/family/others the ward or home therapy.
____	____	teaches patient/family/others the ward or home therapy.
____	____	In addition, teaches the patient/family/others to monitor their own therapy, and conveys the importance of compliance.

Comments:

Figure 2. *Example of Evaluation of Clinical Competence item. The Clinical Instructor selects the behavior (both at midterm and final) that most typically describes the student's average performance. The behaviors are ranked progressively, culminating in a level that is representative of a newly graduating physical therapist. The item is scored by multiplying the value of the behavior (1=lowest competency-4=highest competency) by a weighting factor of 1 to 3. The weighting factor that is applied is a function of the item's importance in overall clinical competency. (Reprinted courtesy of Joan Loomis, Department of Physical Therapy, Faculty of Rehabilitation Medicine, University of Alberta, Edmonton, Alberta, Canada.)*

ments during the months of May through August of 1990. Each student was required to complete one placement (4 weeks) in each practice setting (cardiorespiratory, orthopedics, and neurology). The remaining placement was a repeat of one of these three placements, but in a different subspecialty area. As a result, no one student repeated the same type of clinical rotation during his or her summer placements. Sixty-four students in the third year of the program consented to participate in the study. This meant that there was a possible total of 256 evaluations available for analysis. Of this total, 38 evaluations were the result of 2:1 placements. The remainder were evaluations from placements of a 1:1 ratio.

The 38 students in the 2:1 group were fairly similar in age. Sixty-seven percent of the students were between 20 and 24 years of age, 27% were between 25 and 29 years of age, and the remaining 6% were between 30 and 34 years of age. There were, however, differences in the level of previous academic preparation within the 2:1 group. Forty-seven percent of the students had only high-school qualifications prior to starting their physical therapy studies. Thirty-four percent of the students had 3 or more years of university education prior to starting their physical therapy studies. The remaining 19% of the students had either 1 or 2 years of university education prior to entering the program. The characteristics of the 1:1 group were not investigated.

Students were assigned to all placements by the Academic Coordinator of Clinical Education (ACCE) using a computerized matching system. Students ballot for five placement options per period within a specific area of clinical practice. The computer system then uses a lottery method to assign the students to a specific placement, based on their five placement selections. The resulting student-pair assignments were then reviewed by the ACCE. Student pairs with a large difference in preadmission academic background and/or grade point average were separated, and a student with more similar qualifications was assigned to one of the students in the pair. Given that the ACCE had access to all student records, appropriate matches (based on academic standing and preadmission status) could be found. For example, students with high academic standing and previous university preparation would form a matched pair. Students admitted to the program directly from high school with average marks would form another pair. This matching process was carried out in an effort to minimize potential differences in student performance.

The CIs who were part of this earlier study were not randomly selected, as it was difficult to elicit support from the CI community for the project. Hence, those who were interested in undertaking this teaching model volunteered to participate in the project. Of the 19 instructors, 58% had 5 or more years of clinical experience, 32% had 2 to 5 years of clinical experience, and 10% had less than 2 years of clinical experience. Seventy-nine percent of the instructors had previously supervised three or more students, and 58% of the instructors also had previous experience supervising two students at the same time. This same group of instructors were responsible for completing the ECC forms for each of the students in the 2:1 pairs. Again, characteristics of the CIs who evaluated the 1:1 group were not investigated.

Control for Learning Effects

To control for the possible learning effects a collaborative placement might have had on subsequent clinical performance, all student evaluations that occurred after the completion of a 2:1 placement were disqualified from the study. For example, a student who completed a 2:1 placement in May would have his or her remaining three 1:1 placement scores removed from the data analysis. In those few instances in which a student had more than one 2:1 placement, only the evaluation scores from the first 2:1 placement were included in the analysis. The disqualified clinical placement scores were not analyzed further to determine whether the competency levels attained by students in their 2:1 placement persisted in later placements. Given that all students were placed in different facilities and clinical specialities each month, it would be difficult to conclude whether their collaborative

Table. *Clinical Competence Scores for Collaborative (2:1) Group (n=28) Versus Individual (1:1) Group (n=80)*

Clinical Competence	1:1 Group		2:1 Group		
	X̄	%	X̄	%	t
Patient evaluation	3.36	84	3.60	90	2.61[a]
Program planning	3.22	80	3.48	87	2.67[a]
Implementation of treatment	3.52	88	3.73	93	2.98[a]
Communication with patient/family	3.48	87	3.68	92	2.29[b]
Communication and management skills	3.56	89	3.74	94	2.05[b]
Documentation	3.36	84	3.61	90	2.16[b]
Professional behavior	3.58	90	3.79	95	2.82[a]
Total clinical competence score	3.42	85	3.66	92	3.34[c]

[a] Significant at $P=.02$.

[b] Significant at $P=.05$.

[c] Significant at $P=.01$.

learning performance in 1 month had an impact on their performance in a different subspecialty area in a later month.

The criteria previously described resulted in 28 collaborative (2:1) placements (May, n=5; June, n=11; July, n=7; August, n=5) and 183 traditional (1:1) placements for study. All 28 collaborative (2:1) placement scores were utilized in this study. To determine whether there were any cumulative learning or competence effects in the 2:1 group, a one-way analysis of variance (ANOVA) of the 2:1 scores across the 4 months was carried out. The possibility existed, for example, that students in a 2:1 placement in August would perform better than those who had their placement in May because the former would have already had 3 months of clinical experience. The ANOVA, however, revealed no significant difference in the 2:1 scores on a month-by-month basis ($F=.345$, $df=3$, $P>.05$). Again, this lack of a cumulative learning or competence effect was likely due to the fact that students change their clinical subspecialty area every month. This monthly changing of placements requires the students to master new and often different clinical skills and behaviors.

Because there was no appreciable cumulative learning or competence effect across the 4 months in the 2:1 group, we randomly selected 20 subjects from the 1:1 group for each placement month to form the comparison group. This selection process resulted in a 1:1 sample group of 80 subjects. A one-way ANOVA was also carried out across these four subgroups to determine whether there were any significant differences in the 1:1 scores across the 4 months. The subjects' scores were found not to be significant ($F=.49$, $df=3$, $P>.05$), and these subjects were therefore believed to comprise an equivalent comparison group.

The students in the collaborative (n=28) and individual (n=80) learning groups also had similar academic grade point percentages at the time of their placement assignments. The average grade point percentages were 77% (B+) and 74% (B), respectively (on a four-point scale, these percentages would be 3.3 and 3.0, respectively). A *post hoc* examination of these grades revealed no statistically significant difference at the .05 level. It would appear, therefore, that there were no gross differences in knowledge level between the groups on entry into their clinical placements. Had there been a large difference in

academic grade points between the two groups (eg, a significantly higher grade point average for the 2:1 group), the results achieved might have been due to knowledge level alone and not collaboration.

Data Analysis

The purpose of this study was to determine whether there were any differences in performance scores between the 2:1 and 1:1 placement groups. A two-tailed *t* test for independent samples at a predefined significance level of .05 was utilized to measure the ECC score differences between the 2:1 and 1:1 groups. This same test was undertaken for each of the seven subscore items that comprise the ECC form (ie, patient evaluation, program planning, implementation of treatment, communication with patient/family, communication and management skills, documentation, and professional behavior).

Results

The Table presents the mean overall ECC scores and mean subscores for the 2:1 and 1:1 groups. The percentage column describes these same mean scores as a percentage value. The percentage score is derived by taking the mean score and dividing by 4.00. A score of 4.00 is the highest score one can achieve.

All seven clinical competence subcategory scores/percentages and the total clinical competence score/percentage of the 2:1 placements were found to be statistically significant at the .05 level. On *post hoc* examination, four categories (ie, patient evaluation, program planning, implementation of treatment, and professional behavior) were significant at the .02 level. The total clinical competence scores were significant at .01. It is interesting to note that these four subscores were significantly lower than the .05 level, suggesting a fairly strong relationship between the 2:1 model and these measures. Moreover, the overall ECC score for the 2:1 group was significantly higher than that for the 1:1 group at .01. Even if one were to dismiss the .05 level of significance for a lower probability indicator, these three items still suggest some effect as the result of the collaborative model.

Discussion

The results of this study support the argument that clinical competence, as measured by the ECC form, is enhanced through a process of collaborative learning. On closer examination, it can be seen that the four areas of clinical competence most enhanced by collaborative learning (ie, patient evaluation, program planning, implementation of treatment, and professional behavior) involved a higher degree of clinical judgment. A secondary finding of the study was the lack of a significant difference in competency scores in the collaborative placements from May to August. Intuitively, one would expect that scores toward the end of the summer placement period would have risen as the students acquired more experience. This was not the case and was likely due to the students having to change their clinical rotation every 4 weeks, thus reducing the potential for a cumulative learning or competence effect.

There are some limitations to the results of this study that are noteworthy. Although the results are very favorable, this study only examined differences between group means. Second, as this study was retrospective, we had little control over the characteristics of the students in each group or the characteristics of the specific placement, including the environmental variables and the characteristics of the CIs. The CIs in this study, for example, frequently did not assign the majority of their caseload to their students.[19] This was due to a variety of reasons. Delegating the CI's entire caseload to the students is a central tenet inherent in the 2:1 model. In our study, the CIs' independent patient loads ranged from 25% to 50% of normal.[19] This resulted in the CIs being overloaded with the responsibility of a partial caseload as well as the increased administrative

duties required to oversee two students. These responsibilities may have interfered with the ability of the CIs to observe the students' performance on sufficient occasions and might have influenced the students' final evaluation scores. One could argue that in the 1:1 model, the caseload demands of the CI in conjunction with the need to supervise a student produces a similar type of pressure. This may produce similar influences with respect to evaluation scoring.

As described earlier, the CIs who supervised the students were found to have "considerable clinical and supervisory experience."[19] Specifically, 79% of the CIs had supervised at least three students in the past, and 58% had previous experience in the management of a collaborative learning placement.[19] The remaining CIs in the 2:1 group all had supervised students previously but had supervised fewer than three students.[19] It is possible that the favorable outcome of the collaborative learning experiences might be due to the fact that the majority of the CIs in the 2:1 group were more experienced and more familiar with teaching techniques than were the CIs in the 1:1 group. This is difficult to surmise, however, given that the experience base of the CIs in the 1:1 group was not examined. All instructors who undertake student supervision have the opportunity for gaining experience through university-sponsored workshops and are given guidelines and assistance through extensive written documentation concerning their role as an instructor. Hence, large differences in teaching experience would be minimized by the university's instructor development program and requirement that each CI have at least 1 year of full-time clinical experience. A review of the students' evaluations of their placements for both the 1:1 and 2:1 groups also indicated no overt differences in quality of instructor skill.

Another explanation for the positive results may be that the CIs who volunteered to participate in the 2:1 group prefer this type of clinical teaching

experience. Their scoring, as a result, may have been biased positively in order to support their preference for this type of clinical teaching model. This scoring effect, however, is controlled to a certain extent by using an objective evaluation form (ie, the ECC instrument). The instructions that accompany this instrument are quite clear in describing the expected competency levels the students must exhibit in order to receive a certain score. The CIs and students were also unaware at the time of this study that these scores would be used in a study. Hence, any experimental effects or scoring bias was kept to a minimum.

These results do suggest, however, that there is an increasing need for further research into this important area of health professional education using both qualitative (student diaries, observation, student/CI interviews) and qualitative methods of analysis similar to that undertaken in this study. A study that evaluates 2:1 placements whereby CIs completely delegate their caseload would be beneficial, as would replication of this study within other university programs and other levels of student training (eg, senior students). The effect of matching students using academic background and grade point average also deserves further exploration. For example, are the same outcomes achieved when students are matched without consideration of any other variables. Two influences this study did not examine were the potential effects of age differences among the groups and the impact of previous academic training on performance. Examination of the effects of collaborative learning on individual performance (rather than groups) would also be very informative and useful to clinical educators.

Conclusions

The results of this study appear to support the growing body of literature in favor of collaborative learning in the health care professions. The achievement of clinical competence in the areas of patient evaluation, program planning, implementation of treatment, communication with patient/family, communication and management skills, professional behavior, and documentation during third-year physical therapy clinical fieldwork placements all appeared to be enhanced through collaborative learning. This finding implies that clinical placement ratios of two students per CI may be a viable alternative to the traditional 1:1 ratio.

A more widespread use of collaborative learning placements would serve several purposes. First, it appears to support the enhancement of overall clinical competence. Second, it should increase the total number of available placements in the clinical setting. This greater availability would allow increased enrollment in physical therapy programs and allow universities to meet the growing demand for rehabilitative services. Third, it reinforces the concept of a team approach to problem solving and the delivery of health care.

References

1 Tompson MA, Tompson C. The evolution of standards for the fieldwork component of the curriculum. *Canadian Journal of Occupational Therapy*. 1987;54:237–241.

2 Edwards M, Baptiste S. The occupational therapist as a clinical teacher. *Canadian Journal of Occupational Therapy*. 1987;54:249–255.

3 Tompson MA, Tompson C. The Canadian approach to fieldwork. *Canadian Journal of Occupational Therapy*. 1987;54:243–248.

4 Dinham SM, Stritter FT. Research on professional education. In: Wittrock MC, ed. *Handbook of Research on Teaching*. 3rd ed. New York, NY: Macmillan Publishing Co; 1986:952–970.

5 Jarski RW, Kulig K, Olson RE. Clinical teaching in physical therapy: student and teacher perceptions. *Phys Ther*. 1990;70:173–178.

6 Peat M. Enid Graham Memorial Lecture: Clinical education of health professionals. *Physiotherapy Canada*. 1985;37:301–307.

7 Emery MJ. Effectiveness of the clinical instructor: students' perspective. *Phys Ther*. 1984; 64:1079–1083.

8 Gartland GJ. Teaching the therapeutic relationship. *Physiotherapy Canada*. 1984;36:24–28.

9 *Undergraduate Medical Education Bulletin (Center for Studies in Medical Education, Faculty of Medicine, University of Toronto)*. September 1989:1.

10 Stritter FT, Hain JD, Grimes DA. Clinical teaching reexamined. *Journal of Medical Education*. 1975;50:876–882.

11 Johnson DW, Maruyama G, Johnson R, et al. Effects of cooperative, competitive and individualistic goal structures on achievement: a meta-analysis. *Psychol Bull*. 1981;89:47–62.

12 Tiberius R, Magnon J. Ten beliefs about teaching and learning. *Undergraduate Medical Education Bulletin (Center for Studies in Medical Education, Faculty of Medicine, University of Toronto)*. September 1989:2.

13 Griffiths P. Creating a learning environment. *Physiotherapy*. 1987;73:328–331.

14 Ausubel D, Novak J, Hanesian H. *Educational Psychology: A Cognitive View*. 2nd ed. London, England: Holt, Rinehart & Winston; 1978.

15 Scully RM, Sheppard KF. Clinical teaching in physical therapy education: an ethnographic study. *Phys Ther*. 1983;63:349–358.

16 Daggett CJ, Cassie JM, Collins GF. Research on clinical teaching. *The Review of Educational Research*. 1979;49:151–169.

17 O'Shea HS, Parsons MK. Clinical instruction: effective and ineffective teacher behaviors. *Nursing Outlook*. 1979;27:411–415.

18 Ladyshewsky R, Healey E. *The 2:1 Teaching Model in Clinical Education: A Manual for Clinical Instructors*. Toronto, Ontario, Canada: Department of Rehabilitation Medicine, Division of Physical Therapy, University of Toronto; 1990.

19 Ladyshewsky R. Clinical teaching and the 2:1 student to clinical instructor ratio. *Journal of Physical Therapy Education*. 1993;7:31–35.

20 Tiberius R, Gaiptman B. The supervisor-student ratio: 1:1 versus 1:2. *Canadian Journal of Occupational Therapy*. 1985;52:179–183.

21 Glendon K, Ulrich D. Using cooperative learning strategies. *Nurse Educator*. 1992;17: 37–40.

22 Neufeld VR, Barrows HS. The McMaster philosophy: an approach to medical education. *Journal of Medical Education*. 1974;49:1040–1050.

23 Slavin RE. *Cooperative Learning*. New York, NY: Longman Inc; 1983.

24 Bruffee KA. The art of collaborative learning: making the most of knowledgeable peers. *Change*. 1987;19:42–47.

25 Bruffee KA. Collaborative learning and the conversation of mankind. *College English*. 1984;46:635–652.

26 McDonald BA, Larson CO, Dansereau DF. Cooperative dyads: impact on text learning and transfer. *Contemporary Educational Psychology*. 1985;10:369–377.

27 Slavin RE. When does cooperative learning increase student achievement? *Psychol Bull*. 1983;94:429–445.

28 Pennebaker DF. Teaching nursing research through collaboration: costs and benefits. *J Nurs Educ*. 1991;30:102–108.

29 Abercrombie MLJ. *Anatomy of Judgement*. Harmondsworth, Middlesex, England: Penguin Publishing Co Inc; 1969.

30 Aston-McCrimmon E. Trends in clinical practice: an analysis of competencies. *Physiotherapy Canada*. 1984;36:184–188.

31 Barrows HS. The scope of clinical education. *Journal of Medical Education*. 1986;61: 23–33.

32 Loomis J. Evaluating clinical competence of physical therapy students, part 1: the development of an instrument. *Physiotherapy Canada*. 1985;37:83–88.

33 Loomis J. Evaluating clinical competence of physical therapy students, part 2: assessing the reliability, validity and usability of a new instrument. *Physiotherapy Canada*. 1985;37:91–98.

Commentaries

Following are three commentaries on "Enhancing Clinical Competence Using a Collaborative Clinical Education Model."

The authors of this article distinguish themselves by their courageous challenge of an old and traditional model of teaching and evaluation in clinical education. The effectiveness of our typical 1:1 apprenticeship model has neither been adequately documented nor empirically validated, yet its ubiquitous use persists. These authors have introduced and studied a model of clinical education that could directly benefit both our students' learning and our Clinical Instructors' productivity in practice. These outcomes are critical in this time of personnel shortage, rising need for clinical education placements, and redefinition of the physical therapist as an autonomous professional who must seek and use collaborative methods to enhance patient care.

The authors should also be complimented on selecting as a measurement tool one of the only evaluation systems that has been demonstrated in physical therapy—at least in some clinical contexts—to be psychometrically sound.[1,2] In addition, their effort to recognize some of the variables that might affect the validity of the evaluation (eg, rater bias, student and instructor characteristics) is also an important facet of this article. Clinical educators must be vigilant in identifying aspects of the evaluation process, the clinical setting, or the learning experience that may compromise the decisions they make about students' readiness to progress in school, graduate, and enter practice.[3]

The intent of the collaborative model is to facilitate cooperation among members of the health care team, encourage individual accountability for learning, and maximize personnel resources in the clinical training phase of physical therapy education. The collaborative model clearly emphasizes interaction between the student members of the learning triangle.[4] Although I would agree that interaction among peers is an important aspect of being a professional, I am concerned that the model overemphasizes collaboration between students and underemphasizes the importance of collaborating with experts who provide the primary sources of role modeling so important in shaping the behavior of our future colleagues.[5] Our efforts to reduce intimidation and provide support for the learner in clinical education should not be overshadowed by our obligation to have students regularly interact with and respond to direction from experts who are themselves providing direct patient care. Specific guidance for Clinical Instructors adopting the collaborative model is needed to balance these factors.

I am also concerned that the collaborative model may tend prematurely to promote independence of the learner. Stritter[6] has described a developmental approach to clinical instruction in which the learner deliberately, systematically, and gradually assumes independence from the instructor. Critical in this approach is believing that students can and should be responsible for learning and that the goal of education is for each student to become independent of the instructor. Users of the collaborative model must be sensitive to each student's readiness to accept responsibility for the facets of this paradigm. Specific training of both students and Clinical Instructors is essential to enable accurate assessment of such readiness.

Having a well-defined domain of professional practice is an essential feature of any competence system.[3] The conclusions made from this study rest on two important assumptions. First, the authors appear confident that the seven categories of performance are independent and mutually exclusive. This assumption allows them to treat the scores derived from using the Evaluation of Clinical Competence (ECC) as meaningful in their own right. Considerable overlap, however, may be occurring between and among categories. For example, communication with patients and family members inevitably occurs during patient evaluation and program planning. With no assurance that the categories are mutually exclusive, comparison of scores in different categories may be suspect. In addition, association between total scores of the two groups may be inflated if the individual categories lack independence. Use of either the categories as independent entities or the total score as reflective of the contributions of categories would be preferable.

The second assumption made by the authors concerns an expressed relationship between a problem-solving ability and four of the seven performance categories (patient evaluation, program planning, treatment implementation, and professional behavior). This conclusion is not well supported by the study results or addressed comprehensively in the discussion. We have much to learn about the process of problem solving in clinical practice, including the possibility that "much of what has been termed problem solving is really pattern matching and requires only recognition of specific sets of information."[7(p57)] Clinical educators must not only seek a more thorough understanding of problem solving as a component of clinical competence, but also must be trained specifically to construct specific learning experiences to facilitate this ability.

For raters to assess performance accurately and to infer competence from that performance, each component of the domain must be clearly defined and regularly updated to reflect the requirements of practice.[3] The authors express considerable confidence in the ECC as an instrument for measuring clinical competence. Before making any overall conclusions about whether competence has indeed been measured, I would caution the authors to consider whether this instrument has been adequately updated to include performance characteristics required of the physical therapist today. In addition, because "the validity of any assessment of clinical competence will depend on the nature, number and variety of problems and the range of settings in which performance is sampled,"[7(p57)] I ask whether use of the ECC fostered an adequate sampling of clinical encounters and whether the instrument was established to be equally useful in a variety of clinical settings.[8] Questions also remain about the nature of training and consistency of using the instrument by the multiple raters. Evidence that these issues have been addressed is needed to justify the conclusions of the authors regarding competence of the students in either study group.

Patient characteristics, caseload mix, characteristics of the social and organizational setting, and other moderating variables of the teaching and learning setting can, at times, compromise conclusions made via clinical competence assessment.[8] The lack of information about students in the 1:1 comparison group raised the possibility that differences in ECC scores may have been due to learning style, attitudes, or other personal characteristics that could affect learning and performance.[5] Further information about the characteristics of both groups of students is essential to determining whether group differences occurred as a result of teaching variables or individual subject differences (or both).

Dinham and Stritter note that "a complex environment and multiple instructors can make it difficult to isolate the impact of specific instructors and teaching behaviors."[5] Not only is more information about the characteristics of participating instructors needed to justify the conclusions about group differences, but examination of the behaviors actually exhibited by each group of instructors is essential. Information about whether the teaching behaviors expected in the collaborative model[4] actually occurred in the 2:1 group is essential if conclusions about competence differences are to be ascribed to use of this model. Observation, logs, and interviews may have substantiated the extent to which different teaching strategies were used and can be attributed to the outcome(s) of this study.

The topic, research design, and study outcome presented in this article raise several issues critical to the growth and development of physical therapy clinical education. Issues related to teaching and learning, the instrumentation and process of assessing clinical competence, and variables affecting the context of clinical education require further study to enhance the effectiveness of this phase of the entry-level curriculum. I hope that these comments will facilitate further dialogue among physical therapists interested in clinical education.

Susan S Deusinger, PhD, PT
Director and Assistant Professor
Program in Physical Therapy
Washington University School of
  Medicine
Campus Box 8083, 660 S Euclid Ave
St Louis, MO 63110

References

1 Loomis J. Evaluating clinical competence of physical therapy students, part 1: the development of an instrument. *Physiotherapy Canada.* 1985;37:83–88.

2 Loomis J. Evaluating clinical competence of physical therapy students, part 2: assessing the reliability, validity and usability of a new instrument. *Physiotherapy Canada.* 1985;37:91–98.

3 McGaghie WC. The evaluation of competence. *Evaluation and the Health Professions.* 1980;3:289–320.

4 Ladyshewsky R, Healey E. *The 2:1 Teaching Model in Clinical Education: A Manual for Clinical Instructors.* Toronto, Ontario, Canada: Department of Rehabilitation Medicine, Division of Physical Therapy, University of Toronto; 1990.

5 Dinham SM, Stritter FT. Research on professional education. In: Wittrock MC, ed. *Handbook of Research on Teaching.* 3rd ed. New York, NY: Macmillan Publishing Co; 1986:952–970.

6 Stritter FT. *The Learning Vector: A Developmental Approach to Clinical Instruction.* Chapel Hill, NC: The University of North Carolina Press; 1983.

7 McGuire C. Perspectives in assessment. *Acad Med.* 1993;68:S3–S8.

8 Kane MT. The assessment of professional competence. *Evaluation and the Health Professions.* 1992;15:163–182.

I appreciate the opportunity to review and comment on this most interesting manuscript. I find the topic and methodology used by the authors to be very timely in our clinical education literature, in light of the recent changes in the practice environment. I particularly value the examination of a clinical education model, which builds on the availability of a valid and reliable clinical performance instrument. Further, exploration of this model in the context of current constraints on clinical practice make this model of great interest to clinical educators in both the clinical or academic settings. The suggestion that this model can both enhance the learning experience of the student and assist in alleviating the pressure on clinical educators to provide this valuable professional learning experience is very exciting and should be of interest to a wide audience of health professional educators and practitioners.

I agree with the authors' premise that the role of the Clinical Instructor is to serve as the facilitator of learning, perhaps the most significant ingredient of a successful learning experience. This puts responsibility on the student for the learning experience, a responsibility that is highly consistent with the student's future professional role. This premise appears to be supported by the finding that student scores between collaborative and traditional instructional ratios were different regardless of the clinical education block, suggesting that the instructional experience, including the Clinical Instructor's role, is paramount in the clinical learning experience.

I appreciate the authors' careful explanation of the collaborative-learning model and the detail with which they have linked this model to the needs of physical therapy clinical education. The authors appropriately point out that this model of learning enhances collaboration and cooperation among students, and it therefore increases the resource that students can be to one another, decreasing their reliance on a clinical mentor. I agree with the authors' explanation, which is well supported in the cited literature.

Several limitations of the study have been pointed out. Some are significant and deserve careful consideration when interpreting and generalizing these results. Of these limitations, I am particularly concerned about two: (1) the lack of information about the Clinical Instructor and student characteristics in the 1:1-ratio instructional group and (2) the apparent "senior" nature of the Clinical Instructors (both as instructors and as practitioners) for the 2:1-ratio instructional group. Although it is difficult to criticize missing information in the 1:1-ratio instructional group, it is equally difficult to ascertain that the cause for difference between these groups is certainly related to the different instructional methodology. Certainly, future studies will need to examine through a controlled, prospective comparison other sources of difference between these instructional methods, to include but not be limited to (1) previous student learning experiences,

(2) self-selection into a preferred learning style group (eg, 2:1 ratio), and (3) other factors that bias the results toward the experimental group.

Related to this lack of information about the 1:1-ratio Clinical Instructor groups is the apparent "senior" nature of the Clinical Instructors in the 2:1-ratio instructional group. Although it is difficult to suggest that the Clinical Instructors for the 2:1-ratio instructional group are more senior than the Clinical Instructors for the 1:1-ratio instructional group without the characteristics of both Clinical Instructor groups being available, one must suspect that such a difference exists. A majority of the 2:1-ratio group Clinical Instructors had supervised three or more students previously and had more than 5 years of clinical practice experience. This represents a significantly greater than average level of experience for Clinical Instructors both in terms of their teaching and their practice. The degree to which this level of experience may have favorably influenced these results is potentially significant. Future work should include sufficient information about the characteristics of each of the Clinical Instructor groups.

I also agree with the authors that methodological issues such as matching the student pairs to be more similar and sampling only intermediate (third-year) clinical education experiences may limit the degree to which these data can be generalized. The effects of a more diverse student sample and matching options will be useful to ascertain. Future research in these areas would augment and clarify this initial report.

Finally, I would like to raise a conceptual issue in the design of this study for consideration. The use of the Evaluation of Clinical Competence (EEC) developed by Loomis in this study raises an interesting dilemma. This instrument has well-documented validity and reliability data available for physical therapy student groups similar to the sample used in this study. These reliability data are ac-

ceptable, making this tool a valuable resource for clinical education research. Actual experience with the tool by Clinical Instructors participating in the study further enhances its application here. On closer examination of the tool, and as described by the authors, it is apparent that student scores using the instrument are hierarchical within each category, with higher scores given for increasing independent performance within each category. I question whether the 2:1-ratio instructional method is one that promotes more rapid assumption of responsibility and therefore independence. With a single instructor working with two students, one of the students is always functioning more independently and with indirect supervision from the instructor. This may promote greater, earlier independence or at least the appearance of greater independence. If one instructional method yields a higher score when using the EEC instrument, it is possible that the differences noted in this study are more a function of the measurement instrument than the actual differences among the student groups in their performance. I suggest that future studies also include the use of other evaluation instruments, which may not use level of independence as a measure of competence in clinical practice. Use of other clinical performance evaluation instruments may provide further insight in this area.

I commend the authors on their contribution to the clinical education literature with this research report. Explanation of this innovative clinical instruction model and its effectiveness comes at a very challenging time in clinical education. The education community will find this report most helpful. I hope that my comments here serve to further strengthen this initial work and will contribute to future research in this area.

Michael J Emery EdD, PT
Associate Professor
Academic Coordinator of Clinical
* Education*
Department of Physical Therapy
University of Vermont
305 Rowell Bldg
Burlington, VT 05405

The United States is influenced and driven by intricately linked forces that shape the nature of professional education. Some of the contemporary forces that are propelling change in professional higher education include the exorbitant national debt, limited opportunities for individuals to benefit from higher education, scrutiny of fundamental values and beliefs of what constitutes "quality education" by addressing the outcomes of the educational process, and health care reform as it relates to education in health professions such as physical therapy. These forces have spurred educators and practitioners alike to closely examine more innovative and cost-effective methods of providing high-quality physical therapy education that are linked to stated outcome measures for its graduates. Thus, as demonstrated by this article, one of the burgeoning and promising areas for scholarly inquiry in physical therapy education is clinical education.

DeClute and Ladyshewsky are to be commended for their scholarly inquiry into a collaborative clinical educational model using clinical competence as an outcome measure. Collaborative clinical education has frequently been discussed and encouraged by educators, but little empirical evidence has been noted in the physical therapy literature on the subject.[1-3] Based on the authors' review of the literature, enhancing the effectiveness of students' learning during clinical education is of equal concern to both Canadian and US physical therapy programs. Even though clinical education is important and valued in both nations, without the provision of a contextual framework for this study, the reader might assume that one could easily implement the collaborative clinical education model in the United States similarly as in Canada without possible modifications. Thus, it would have been beneficial for the authors to provide the reader with a clear contextual framework to examine the nature of clinical education in relation to higher education and health care in Canada. This would ensure that appropriate comparisons and adaptations might be considered if electing to adopt this model of clinical education in the United States.

In this study, the authors compared the success of using the collaborative 2:1 learning placement with that of using the 1:1 learning placement, based on student clinical competency measures on an instrument determined to yield valid and reliable results. The authors also provided anecdotal information that this model promoted three areas of clinical education: (1) more open communication among all members of the learning team, (2) increased consultation between students when questions arose about patient care, and (3) decreased reliance on the Clinical Instructor (CI).

On *post hoc* examination of the seven significant clinical competence subcategories, the areas for which collaborative learning in the 2:1 placement model were most enhanced were patient evaluation, program planning, implementation of treatment, and professional behavior. These four areas were interpreted to involve a high degree of clinical judgment. These findings seem to contradict the authors' experience with the collaborative model, which should correlate more highly with the remaining clinical competence categories, described by the authors as communication with patient/family, communication/management skills, and documentation. The authors do not adequately reconcile this difference for the reader. Possible reasons are not offered as to why the 2:1 placement model as compared with the 1:1 placement model resulted in a higher degree of clinical judgment rather than communication and cooperation. In a related issue, reference was not made as to whether the term "clinical judgment" was determined based on factor analysis, prior research by Loomis, or a term selected by the authors. How "clinical judgment" was interpreted

remains unclear, and this confusion may misrepresent the outcome of the study.

Although DeClute and Ladyshewsky clearly acknowledged significant limitations of this study, some necessitate further discussion. One of the critical flaws of the study is the absence of any information on the backgrounds of the CIs participating in the 1:1 clinical placement model. Conclusions drawn about the 2:1 placement model as compared with the 1:1 placement model based on the lack of comparable data are suspect, at best. One could speculate that the CIs participating in the 1:1 placement model may have been inexperienced clinical educators with limited exposure to students, had limited clinical experience, represented a different age spectrum, and differed in their previous academic preparation. All of these factors would contribute to outcome differences in the study. Likewise, the authors did not address whether any of the CIs participating in the study had previously been involved in a 2:1 clinical placement model as a student. A compelling argument can be made for the role of pedagogy in teaching and the impact this may have when the learner becomes a CI. If the student participating in the 2:1 collaborative learning model experiences positive outcomes, then this may have a direct impact on the success of that individual's ability to provide collaborative learning experience in the future.[4]

The study's basic premise was to compare the competence of the learners in two different clinical placement groups. Yet, the characteristics of the students participating in the 2:1 clinical placement group were investigated, whereas students assigned to the 1:1 group were not addressed. This represents a second major flaw in the study that affects the validity of the study. In addition, the authors make some basic assumptions about the student as a learner in the design by pairing students of like academic performance based on preadmission background and/or grade point average (GPA) after completing a comput-

erized matching. Justification for this decision should have been grounded in the literature, which presents mixed reviews as to whether preadmission background and GPA are good predictors for success in clinical education.[5-7] Likewise, given that the results indicated no significant differences between the GPAs of both groups, an argument could be made for not pairing the student learners in the collaborative model.

Another interesting finding in the study was the lack of a significant difference in competency scores in the collaborative placements from May to August. The authors speculate that this is a result of "students having to change their clinical rotation every 4 weeks, thus reducing the potential for a cumulative learning or competence effect." Some evidence exists to support the notion that student learning is specific to the clinical environment and that competence is reached only on those core skills that are frequently encountered and experienced by the student across a number of placements.[8] If this is true, then education may have to reassess the concept of "variety" and "competence" as perhaps paradoxical terms. Exposure to a variety of clinical settings and patients may provide a different kind of learning experience than learning that occurs in the same clinical environment over an extended period of time. Grossman's theoretical model of teaching addresses the notion of expertise in content knowledge, pedagogical knowledge or the "how" of what we do, and an understanding of the context in which learning is placed.[9] Hence, the variables of length of time and variety of settings in clinical education may both be critical to students' ability to develop entry-level competence, but in different ways. One can speculate that content knowledge may allow for the development of knowledge and skill in clinical competence. Pedagogical knowledge and an awareness of the dynamic context in which clinical practice exists may help the student to better understand the "how" of what physical therapists do, which frequently changes depending on the clinical environment.

Certainly, further studies that investigate the 2:1 clinical placement model by comparing length and variety of clinical placements would assist in clarifying how these variables affect student performance outcomes. Another twist would be to examine how the intervention of student instruction about this model of clinical education prior to attending a 2:1 clinical placement model affects outcome performance.

Lastly, the authors chose to examine two clinical placement models using quantitative outcome measures. Yet, by their own admission, historically the effectiveness of this model can be found in qualitative processes that transform the CI's role from teacher to facilitator by encouraging self-directed learning, problem-solving skills, cooperative and collaborative learning, and open communication between and among students and the CI. Comparing the process of how student learning occurs in both models may provide insight as to how to more adequately prepare students to enter physical therapy practice.

These criticisms aside, the authors are to be commended for taking the initiative and risk to provide the education community with one of the few empirical studies that examines an alternative model of providing clinical education other than the traditional 1:1 clinical placement model. Hopefully, they will consider this to be a beginning area of focused research investigations with the potential to examine many implications and variations on the theme of the 2:1 clinical placement model such as its cost-effectiveness, personnel effectiveness, impact on the availability of clinical sites, and examination of the learning process as reported by the CI and the student(s). Given the results of this study, the authors should be encouraged that alternative models of providing clinical education warrant further investigations and that their effort has generated information by which other clinical education models will be examined.

Jody Shapiro Gandy, PhD, PT
Director of Clinical
 Education/Education Systems
American Physical Therapy
 Association

1111 N Fairfax St
Alexandria, VA 22314

References

1 Emery MJ, Nalette E. Student-staffed clinics: creative clinical education during times of constraint. *Clinical Management in Physical Therapy.* 1986;6(2):6–10.

2 Versteeg M, Strein J, Fitch D, Darnell R. Utilization of rotatory clinical faculty members in physical therapy education. *Journal of Physical Therapy Education.* 1987;1:21–26.

3 Graham C, Catlin P, Morgan J, Martin E. Comparison of 1-day-per-week, 1-week, and 5-week clinical education experiences. *Journal of Physical Therapy Education.* 1991;5:18–23.

4 Kirkpatrick H, Byrne C, Martin M, Roth M. A collaborative model for the clinical education of baccalaureate nursing students. *J Adv Nurs.* 1991;16:101–107.

5 Dettman M, Linder M. Significance of prior experience on students' clinical performance. *Journal of Physical Therapy Education.* 1988;1: 7–9.

6 Balogun J. Predictors of academic and clinical performance in a baccalaureate physical therapy program. *Phys Ther.* 1988;68:238–242.

7 Rheault W, Shafernich-Coulson E. Relationship between academic achievement and clinical performance in a physical therapy education program. *Phys Ther.* 1988;68:378–380.

8 Missiuna C, Polatajko H, Ernest-Conibear M. Skill acquisition during fieldwork placements in occupational therapy. *Clinical Journal of Occupational Therapy.* 1992;59:28–39.

9 Grossman P. *The Making of a Teacher: Teacher Knowledge and Teacher Education.* New York, NY: Teachers College Press; 1990.

Author Response

We wish to thank Dr Deusinger, Dr Emery, and Dr Gandy for sharing their views on our work. The kind remarks they have made about our study are appreciated. The more critical issues that they have brought forward concerning our work certainly bring to light some interesting issues, and we offer the following thoughts in response.

One specific concern that Dr Deusinger raises is that the 2:1 model overemphasizes collaboration between students at the expense of collaborating with experts who provide the primary source of role modeling for students. This argument assumes that only the Clinical Instructor (CI) or the expert can teach the student. Although we do not disagree with the point that the expert plays a major role in clinical education, the literature suggests that students can be a powerful influence on each other in terms of acquiring new knowledge and skill.[1]

Dr Deusinger is also concerned that the model may promote premature independence of the learner. We would argue that the increased collaboration and joint problem solving that occurs in a 2:1 model (between all parties) actually enhances competence and therefore enables the students to be more independent at an earlier stage. Deusinger's comment, however, about the need for specific training of students and CIs in cooperative models of education is very insightful. Successful implementation of this model is grounded in the application of appropriate teaching strategies.[2] For this model to be successful, there must be a balance of peer-based learning, paced independence, and professional role modeling.

Our statement that suggests a relationship between problem-solving ability and four of the seven performance categories (patient evaluation, program planning, treatment implementation, and professional behavior) has been challenged by Dr Deusinger. She points out that much of what has been termed "problem solving" is actually pattern matching and requires only recognition of specific sets of information. If one accepts this definition as a component of problem solving, then it can be argued that the 2:1 model may be a powerful means of enhancing performance because of the visual learning strategies that occur throughout the placement.[3] Observing how the other student behaves professionally, how he or she approaches an evaluation, and how he or she implements treatment can be a strong means of modifying and improving one's own performance.

We believe quite strongly, however, that beyond pattern recognition, other elements of problem solving such as working through difficult clinical cases and problems is facilitated using a collaborative approach. This is because students bring previous experiences and knowledge to a situation and can share this information with their peers. This student-centered learning has been demonstrated to promote higher levels of academic achievement and performance.[4–10] In the end, it is probably irrelevant whether competence is achieved through pattern recognition, through discussion and analysis of problems, or through a combination of both. If a higher degree of competence in the student(s) is achieved, and this is accomplished through a cooperative learning strategy, then this model of learning should be encouraged.

Another issue that Dr Deusinger raises is the possibility that the Evaluation of Clinical Competence (ECC) instrument has not been adequately updated. As a result, it may not reflect today's requirements for competent practice. We only partially agree with this statement because it is quite true that physical therapy has changed since the development of the ECC tool. One of the benefits of this evaluation tool, however, is that it is behaviorally based and looks more at "how" tasks are performed. Hence, changes within physical therapy prac-

tice can be readily accommodated using the tool's existing format. The ECC tool focuses more on global physical therapy attributes (eg, how well one manages time, documents results, interprets results, communicates, plans interventions, and collects information). Furthermore, the students involved in this study were placed in traditional practice environments. It was for these environmental contexts in which the ECC was developed.

Deusinger, Emery, and Gandy all express concern over the lack of information describing the 1:1 group (both students and CIs). Their points are well taken about whether it was variation in teaching style, individual subject differences, or a combination of both that had an effect on the results. A prospective design would have enabled us to collect this information and would have added more strength to our discussion. Analysis of the actual behaviors exhibited by instructors in both the 2:1 and 1:1 groups would also have been useful. Again, a prospective study design would have captured this information.

Dr Emery raises the point that the 2:1 model may or may not promote more rapid assumption of responsibility and therefore independence. This more rapid assumption of responsibility and independence may be the direct result of the instructor working with one of the students, thereby forcing the other student to function more independently. Dr Emery argues that if this is the case, then an evaluation instrument that uses a hierarchical approach (such as the ECC) may favor those students who are forced to function more independently. This assumption is correct if, in fact, students in the 2:1 model are required to assume independence earlier than students in the 1:1 model. We would argue that the assumption of responsibility and independence in the 2:1 model does not differ much from the assumption of these characteristics that occurs in the 1:1 model. Instructors in the 1:1 model typically carry an independent caseload separate from that of the student. In this capac-

ity, the student in the 1:1 model is still left to act and think independently because the CI is occupied with his or her own direct patient care responsibilities. In this situation, the student must still acquire a level of independence within a given time frame. Because of this, we do not believe that the hierarchical nature of the ECC tool was biased in favor of the 2:1 group. We would agree, however, that validation of our results using other instruments, as suggested by Emery, would be a useful means of establishing more certainty around this issue.

Dr Gandy raises an interesting point about the lack of a contextual framework for this study, given that it occurred within the Canadian health care system, which is fundamentally different from that in the United States. The payment structures and medicolegal differences that exist between the two nations certainly would require that anyone interested in implementing this model take these differences into consideration.

Prior to implementing the 2:1 model, it is important that its impact on one's working environment be fully assessed.[3] From here, strategies to ensure that the model will be successful can be developed. Fortunately, there is experience with the multiple-student–single-instructor model in the United States.[11] Emery and Nalette[11] have demonstrated quite successfully how this teaching model can work within the American health care context.

One specific difference that sets the two nations apart is the manner in which clinical education programs are administered. In Canada, there are 13 physical therapy programs. Each program has a specified geographic region in which to place its students. Students from other programs wanting to undertake a placement in that region must arrange this placement through the appropriate university. In addition, the National Association of Clinical Educators in Physiotherapy, which consists of all physical therapy program Academic Coordinators of

Clinical Education (ACCEs), has well-established time frames and policies for organizing placements during summer placement periods. These procedures centralize much of the placement planning, facilitate the matching of students into 2:1 relationships, and help to minimize many of the overlaps and competition for affiliation sites seen in the United States.

Dr Gandy expresses some concern about our interpretation of clinical judgment. We selected the term "clinical judgment" to describe those skills that require a high degree of problem solving with respect to patient care (ie, collection of client data, interpretation of the data, and establishment and implementation of an appropriate intervention).

Our anectodal statement that communication skills are enhanced in a collaborative model is challenged by Dr Gandy in light of the fact that the study illustrated that skills involving clinical judgment actually improved the most. Although we do state, anecdotally, that communication skills are enhanced in a 2:1 model, our purpose in undertaking this study was not to identify which competencies might improve more than others. Given that communication skills are very much shaped by one's own personality, sense of comfort within an environment, and previous experience, they are perhaps less influenced by collaboration. Although the communication skills of the 2:1 group improved over those of the 1:1 group, other skills such as patient evaluation, program planning, treatment implementation, and professional behavior appeared to fare better. These latter four competencies or behaviors are not as well established in students (unlike communication style) and may, therefore, be more amenable to modification and change when challenged in a collaborative model.

Dr Gandy criticizes our approach about pairing students according to grade point average (GPA) and preadmission academic background. We would agree with Dr Gandy that the decision to pair students according to GPA and preadmission background has mixed reviews in the literature.[12,13] There is evidence in the literature, however, to suggest that there is a positive linkage between academic achievement and clinical performance.[14-16] Usage of GPA and preadmission academic background is also something that ACCEs can readily put into place and hence our decision to use these criteria as matching variables. Psychological tests or personality inventories are more difficult to implement, require specific training, and have not been shown to have satisfactory levels of predictive ability on performance.[17]

It would be interesting to randomly assign students to their 2:1 placements without considering any other variables. Dr Gandy suggests this as a future approach to study whether similar results are achieved. It would be difficult, however, to draw any conclusions about performance if the GPA scores of the two groups under study were found to be significantly different. For example, if the 2:1 group performed at a higher level and possessed significantly higher GPAs than the 1:1 group, which also happened to perform poorly, these positive results may have been the result of better academic preparation in the 2:1 group, and not the result of collaboration. At least having the confidence that the two groups have roughly equivalent GPAs serves as a control and provides some assurance to the investigators that some other factor, outside of academic GPA, led to the enhanced performance in the collaborative group.

Lastly, Dr Gandy criticizes us for taking a purely qualitative approach to this problem. The purpose of this particular study was not to investigate the qualitative aspects of a collaborative clinical education model but to look at competency in a 2:1 model of clinical education using a measuring instrument as our outcome measure. Issues relating to the role of the instructor, communication, problem-solving styles, and methods of teaching are, of course, important and valuable aspects worthy of study. These qualitative perspectives have been examined in part by Ladyshewsky.[18,19] Other studies[2,11,20,21] have also begun to examine some of the qualitative aspects of collaborative models, and the reader is encouraged to review these studies for more information.

Again, we would like to thank Dr Deusinger, Dr Emery, and Dr Gandy for their insightful criticisms and praises. Our work was quite exploratory in nature and appears to have raised many more questions about this teaching model. We hope that our study and the dialogue stemming from the commentaries will inspire further research and discussion into how we might best educate and prepare our future practitioners in physical therapy.

Richard Ladyshewsky, MHSc, BMR(PT)
Jennifer Declute, BSc(PT)

References

1 Bruffee KA. The art of collaborative learning: making the most of knowledgeable peers. *Change.* 1987;19:42–47.

2 Tiberius R, Gaiptman B. The supervisor-student ratio: 1:1 vs. 2:1. *Canadian Journal of Occupational Therapy.* 1985;52:179–183.

3 Ladyshewsky R, Healey E. *The 2:1 Teaching Model in Clinical Education: A Manual for Clinical Instructors.* Toronto, Ontario, Canada: Department of Rehabilitation Medicine, Division of Physical Therapy, University of Toronto; 1990.

4 Johnson DW, Maruyama G, Johnson R, et al. Effects of cooperative, competitive and individualistic goal structures on achievement: a meta-analysis. *Psychol Bull.* 1981;89:47–62.

5 McDonald BA, Larson CO, Dansereau DF. Cooperative dyads: impact on text learning and transfer. *Contemporary Educational Psychology.* 1985;10:369–377.

6 Johnson DW, Johnson RT. *Cooperation, Competition and Individualization.* Englewood Cliffs, NJ: Prentice Hall; 1975.

7 Abercrombie MLJ. *Anatomy of Judgement.* Harmondsworth, Middlesex, England: Penguin Publishing Co Inc; 1969.

8 Slavin RE. *Cooperative Learning.* New York, NY: Longman Inc; 1983.

9 Slavin RE. When does cooperative learning increase student achievement? *Psychol Bull.* 1983;94:429–445.

10 Neufeld VR, Barrows HS. The McMaster philosophy: an approach to medical education. *Journal of Medical Education.* 1974;49:1040–1050.

11 Emery MJ, Nalette E. Student-staffed clinics: creative clinical education during times of constraint. *Clinical Management in Physical Therapy*. 1986;6(2):6–10.

12 Gough HG, Hall WB. The prediction of academic and clinical performance in medical school. *Research in Higher Education*. 1975;3: 301–313.

13 Pickles B. Correlations between matriculation entry requirements and performance in the diploma program of physiotherapy at University of Alberta. *Physiotherapy Canada*. 1977; 29:249–253.

14 Tidd GS, Conine TA. Do better students perform better in the clinic? *Phys Ther*. 1974; 54:500–505.

15 Peat M, Woodbury MG, Donner A. Admission average as a predictor of undergraduate academic and clinical performance. *Physiotherapy Canada*. 1982;34:211–214.

16 Colliver J, Verhulst S, Williams R. Using a standardized patient examination to establish the predictive validity of the MCAT and undergraduate GPA as admission criteria. *Acad Med*. 1989;64:482–484.

17 Nayer M. Admission criteria of entrance to physiotherapy schools: how to choose among many applicants. *Physiotherapy Canada*. 1992; 44:41–46.

18 Ladyshewsky R. Clinical teaching and the 2:1 student to clinical instructor ratio. *Journal of Physical Therapy Education*. 1993;7:31–35.

19 Ladyshewsky R. Enhancing learning and productivity in cardiorespirology using a collaborative model of clinical education. *Physiotherapy Canada*. 1993;45:4. Abstract.

20 Pennebaker DF. Teaching nursing research through collaboration: costs and benefits. *J Nurs Educ*. 1991;30:102–108.

21 Glendon K, Ulrich D. Using cooperative learning strategies. *Nurse Educator*. 1992;17: 37–40.

CLINICAL
Education Series

by Kathryn Haffner Zavadak, PT,

Christine Konecky Dolnack, MS, PT,

Susan Polich, PT, and

Mark Van Volkenburg, PT

Colla

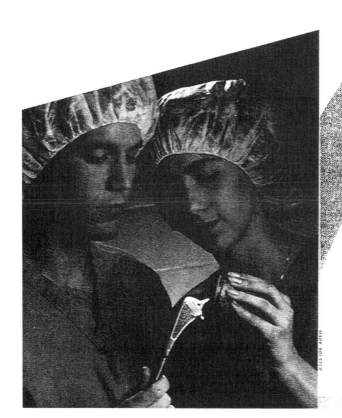

Reprinted from *PT—Magazine of Physical Therapy.* Zavadak KH, Donack CK, Polich S, Van Volkenburg M.
Collaborative models. 1995;3(2):46-54. With the permission of APTA.

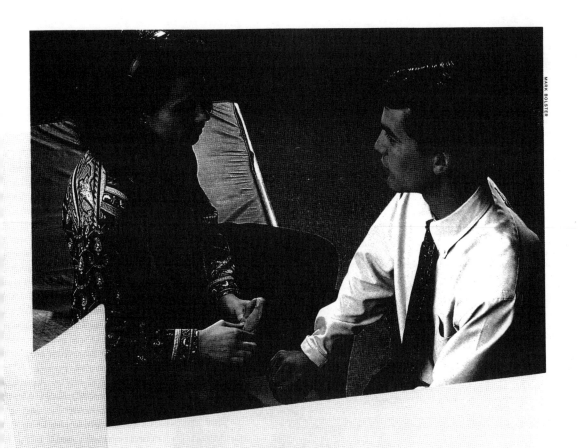

ative Models

Two facilities adapted the 2:1 collaborative model of clinical education—and not only met the demand for more placements but boosted their own productivity

Clinical education is changing. As Gandy (page 40) says, "The days of working one-to-one with a student in the clinic seem to be numbered." Innovative clinical education models are being explored to meet new needs. In the "2:1" model, one clinical instructor (CI) manages two students who learn as a student team.

Recent literature on the 2:1 collaborative learning model has addressed philosophy, advantages and disadvantages, and strategies for success.[1-3] However, although

Ladyshewsky and Healey[1] discussed how CIs can prepare for two students, the literature has not described how to structure the clinical education experience day by day and week by week. Each facility in effect must create its own "model."

This article focuses on how St Margaret Memorial Hospital (SMMH) and the University of Pittsburgh Medical Center (UPMC), Pittsburgh, Pa, planned and carried out 2:1 collaborative learning experiences, handling pitfalls and devising solu-

Are you a CCCE, CI, or student participating in an innovative clinical education model? Contact Jan Reynolds, PT Magazine, 1111 N Fairfax St, Alexandria, VA 22314-1488; 800/999-2782, ext 3182.

Figure 1. The SMMH Experience

WEEK 1

Day 1: Both students are introduced to the staff, oriented to the facility, and familiarized with SMMH's basic policies and procedures by the CCCE, who also talks with the students about the philosophy, goals, and advantages and disadvantages of the 2:1 model. At this meeting, expectations are clearly defined, and the two students acknowledge their understanding of both the model and the expectations (eg, emphasize collaboration, not competition; tell the CI how they feel the experience is going; bring up problems). The students spend the rest of the day observing different PT clinicians.

Day 2: The CI meets with the students individually to review background information and goals for the experience. Neither student expresses concerns about the model at this time. Both state they are willing to try it.

The CI meets with both students to discuss collaborative learning, taking this opportunity to emphasize the expectations previously reviewed by the CCCE. "Collaborative goals" are established by allowing the students to identify areas in which they each feel particularly strong and other areas in which they believe they need work. The students agree that because they attend different schools, they have different academic backgrounds they can draw upon to help each other. They then devise a concrete plan to meet their goals, including such team projects as creating a log for students in the clinical education program and team-teaching patient education classes on rheumatologic disease management.

The students spend the remainder of the day participating in orientation activities or assisting the CI with selected components of patient treatment.

Day 3: This is the first full day that the students treat patients. The CI divides her caseload of seven patients (seen twice daily) between the two students. She now is freed to work with the students both individually and collaboratively, and the students begin to take more responsibility for patient treatment programs.

Day 4: After observing several patient evaluations, the students decide to collaborate on performing an evaluation. Prior to the evaluation, they develop a list of questions to ask when completing a patient's history and agree on areas to examine during the evaluation. The CI notes that their combined list is more complete than their individual lists would have been. One student evaluates the patient's upper extremities, and the other student evaluates the patient's lower extremities. The CI assists with joint-deformity inspection and laxity testing. After the evaluation, the students collaborate with each other and with the patient to form and document goals and treatment plans.

WEEK 2

The students each carry a caseload of two or three patients, each treated twice daily. Each student performs two or three new evaluations this week.

Most collaboration takes place prior to and during evaluations, but some collaboration also occurs during treatment, especially when the treatment requires two people (eg, with a patient who requires the assistance of two people to do a transfer). As they increase their own caseloads, the students begin to work more independently.

At the end of this week, the CI meets with the students individually to discuss their satisfaction so far. They voice no complaints; however, in a subsequent team meeting, one student expresses discomfort when the CI asks a question of both

students. She explains that she does not want to answer the question first because that might make her seem "competitive"; however, she also does not want to hesitate because that might give the appearance of not knowing the answer. The other student replies, "If you're concerned, just say so, and we'll work it out." This situation demonstrates that the students do have some issues to address in forming a working relationship. In the opinion of the CI, this expression of discomfort will pave the way for other concerns to be brought forth and discussed; without this frank discussion, the relationship between the students may have been completely different.

WEEK 3

This is the busiest week in the clinic. The students are assigned to treat four patients who had been evaluated over the weekend and to evaluate two new patients. Because caseloads are high in the physical therapy department, the CI also evaluates two new patients and then transfers them to the students for treatment. The team thus adds a total of eight patients to their caseloads, which is more than would have been seen by the CI individually. This removes some of the pressure from other staff members.

At this point, the CI's role begins to evolve into one of giving confirmation and guidance rather than assistance. The students are beginning to rely on each other for hands-on help.

WEEK 4

During this week, each student carries a caseload of three to five patients, each treated twice daily. Collaboration becomes increasingly difficult because of these higher individual caseloads. To ensure that the students have time to collaborate, the CI does some careful planning. For instance, "mini-rounds" are instituted, in which the students and the CI discuss each patient's status, areas in which further evaluation is needed, and options for treatment. The students are encouraged to problem solve through exchanging ideas, evaluating those ideas for effectiveness, and developing backup plans. Discharge planning also is initiated during these meetings, exposing the students to more patients and ideas than typically exist in the 1:1 model. Both students report that this is enriching their learning experience.

As the students seek guidance from each other, the CI's presence is needed less than it might be needed in the traditional 1:1 model. The CI has more free time for projects, paperwork, and reading. The students are encouraged to seek the guidance of the CI any time they feel the need.

The students' midterm evaluations are done separately. Because adequate one-to-one time has been spent with each student, the CI does not find it difficult to evaluate the students as individuals.

WEEKS 5 TO 8

New individual and team goals are derived from the midterm evaluations. At this point, the students feel comfortable discussing individual areas of strengths and weaknesses with each other. They plan ways in which they can help each other achieve their individual goals.

Each student carries a caseload of five or six patients, each treated twice daily.

During weeks 7 and 8, a final evaluation is completed before each student departs. The students then provide the CI and the CCCE with feedback about the 2:1 experience.

The CI resumes her caseload without difficulty as each student departs.

---

tions. It is important to emphasize that there are many ways to adapt the 2:1 model; this article discusses only two of them.

The SMMH Experience

A 267-bed, acute care, community-based teaching hospital with a 30-bed rehabilitation unit, SMMH specializes in rheumatology, orthopedics, family practice, and gerontology. The physical therapy department consists of both inpatient and outpatient services in rheumatology, orthopedics, gerontology, neurology, occupational health, and sports medicine. Care is provided by 24 physical therapists (PTs), 6 physical therapist assistants (PTAs), and 8 physical therapy aides. The department currently affiliates with 18 schools and provides clinical education for approximately 20 to 22 PT and PTA students per year.

The physical therapy department at SMMH has provided traditional 1:1 clinical education experiences ever since it came into being, experimenting briefly in 1986 with an alternative model. In the 1990s, three factors led the clinical education staff at SMMH to explore alternatives in more depth:

1. As new schools were being established in the region, more clinical education sites were needed to accommodate the greater number of students, and the overall number of affiliations provided by St Margaret were increasing.
2. Changes within the health care system had resulted in shorter lengths of stay for inpatients and an increase in the number of persons treated as outpatients, which meant that staff were shifting from inpatient to outpatient care and fewer inpatient therapists were available to serve as CIs.
3. It was time to try something new!

Because a commitment to take students on the inpatient rotation had been made a year before the impact of the first two factors was understood, there were not enough CIs for all of the incoming students—that is, under the traditional 1:1 approach to clinical education. The physical therapy department therefore decided to pilot a 2:1 model that would offer both a solution to the shortage of CIs and a potential for increased productivity.

Step 1. Learn more about 2:1. A version of the 2:1 model was implemented at SMMH in 1993. Because the students had not been encouraged to collaborate with each other, the experience was similar to the "individualistic" model defined by Ladyshewsky and Healey,[1] in which two students work independently while sharing the same CI.

Although the students reported that the experience was "adequate," the CI believed it was less than optimal for several reasons. Staffing patterns and case volume, for example, had required that the CI carry her own caseload in addition to the students' two separate caseloads. Because of the demands of her own caseload, it was difficult for the CI to find adequate time to spend with each student. The CI believed that this factor had the greatest impact on the quality of the experience for both the students and the CI. As a result of this first experience, the center coordinator of clinical education (CCCE) determined that more information about 2:1 models was needed.

After attending a 1-day seminar on collaborative learning—during which guidelines were shared for planning the 2:1 experience, discussing the model with administration, and soliciting support for the model from staff—the CCCE decided that the entire physical therapy department needed to be better educated about the model.

Step 2: Educate administration about the advantages and disadvantages of 2:1. The CCCE met with the director of the physical therapy department to explain the theory of collaborative learning as described by Ladyshewski.[1,2] Based on what had been learned from the previous 2:1 experience and from a review of the literature, the CCCE and the director agreed that the CI would need to carry either no caseload or a very low caseload (no more than 20% of a normal caseload) so that the CI could be free to teach, observe performance, and facilitate discussion and learning situations.

Potential benefits to the productivity of the department were identified: Under a 2:1 model, two students under the supervision of one CI would be able to carry a caseload exceeding that of a typical staff member. Because it was projected that some staff would need to "cover" the CI (ie, carry a slightly higher caseload than the CI would carry during the first 1 or 2 weeks of the experience until the students' caseloads increased), the director suggested that these aspects of the 2:1 model be discussed with staff.

Step 3: Educate staff. With the support of the director, the CCCE and senior PT in

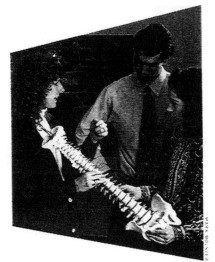

clinical education held two in-service meetings for the physical therapy department's clinical education study group. (All other staff were informed about 2:1 models during administrative meeings and departmental in-service programs.)

The first meeting explained the theory of collaborative learning (versus that of individualistic learning) and the concepts central to student team learning. Both the students' responsibilities and the role of the CI—and how they would differ from those of the 1:1 model—were discussed, including caseload distribution, method of supervision, and how students would utilize each

other as resources in problem solving. The study group was informed that the CI's caseload would need to remain at a reduced level until the orientation process was completed and the students' caseloads were increased. The CCCE then sought feedback to determine interest in trying the model and willingness to support the CI.

Most study group members expressed support; however, some said they were concerned because they felt that exceptional organization skills would be needed to carry out this model and that there could be personality conflicts and competition between the students. Using a problem-solving format, the second meeting addressed potential problems with the 2:1 model, including the temporary increase in staff caseloads. Strategies suggested to overcome these problems included 1) organizing and planning for the experience, 2) discussing competition versus collaboration with the students before they began the experience and giving them a plan for what to do if they began feeling "competitive" or encountered other problems, and 3) planning how to manage the increased caseload.

Step 4. Solicit support from administration, academic coordinators of clinical education (ACCEs), and staff. Administration and staff agreed to launch a second, collaborative version of the 2:1

Staff were shifting from inpatient to outpatient care, and fewer inpatient therapists were available to serve as CIs.

model. Because of time constraints, the model was not discussed with the ACCEs until midterm; however, no drawbacks were noted as a result of this delay.

Step 5: Choose the "right" CI. The CCCE identified proper selection of the CI as essential to success. The director, the CCCE, and the senior PT in clinical education agreed that the CI would need solid organizational skills, flexibility, and a willingness to try something new. Because this trial of the 2:1 model would rely on collaboration between the students, the CI also would need to have a solid understanding of adult learning theory (ie, the learner is self-directed, communicates expectations and needs, and participates in planning and evaluating the learning experience). As it happened, the same CI who had taken part in the previous 2:1 experience was identified as having these qualities and was willing to try a 2:1 model again.

Step 6. Plan the experience. The CCCE met with the CI 2 weeks before beginning the 2:1 experience to discuss the specific steps in implementation. The CI read the CCCE's notes and a manual on the 2:1 model.[1] The CCCE and the CI then developed student schedules that allowed time for a lecture-format orientation to the 2:1 model, including time to discuss collaborative learning goals and plans. Both the CCCE and the CI believed that the orientation process and the first 2 weeks would be critical because they would set the tone for the entire clinical education experience.

Step 7: Initiate! The CCCE identified two students who were scheduled for affiliation at the same time. They were at the same academic/clinical level (second year), and each had had a 1:1 clinical education experience, but they attended different schools. They began the 2:1 experience on the same day and ended 1 week apart (because of differences in length of affiliation between the schools). As a result of time constraints, the 2:1 collaborative learning model was discussed with only one of the students prior to the clinical affiliation. Both students were encouraged—both individually and as a team—to express any concerns they might have about the 2:1 model.

Figure 1 contains a week-by-week, day-by-day description of these students' 2:1 experience.

Perceived advantages. Students reported that under the 2:1 model:

1. They found the environment to be less threatening (especially early in the affiliation) because they were able to support each another when fielding questions and trying new skills and because they were able to practice techniques on each other before treating a patient.

2. They had the opportunity to learn both from their own experiences and from each other's experiences.

3. They were exposed to each other's caseloads and therefore to a greater variety of patients, diagnoses, and potential treatment solutions, and they had more discussion about patient care than had been available in the 1:1 model.

4. They received more individual attention from the CI than they had received under the 1:1 model, and it was easier to

---

Figure 2. The UPMC 2:1 Student Learning Contract[a]

I **Objective:** Completion of a minimum of six comprehensive patient evaluations.

Criteria:
A Completion within 48 hours of patient arrival unit.
B 90% accuracy, using current quality improvement (QI) standards,[b] with guidance from the clinical instructor (CI) and peer.
C As evaluated using the University of Pittsburgh performance evaluation.

II **Objective:** The student will have designed six comprehensive plans of care.

Criteria: As in I-A, I-B, and I-C.

III **Objective:** The student will have attended all Physical Therapy Department meetings and educational opportunities, as directed by the Coordinator of Education.

Criteria: Attendance rolls.

IV **Objective:** The student will have attended all weekly patient staffings, reporting on patient status and writing all progress and summary notes in 7 of 8 weeks.

Criteria: As in I-B and I-C; on the chart within 24 hours.

V **Objective:** The student will demonstrate good interpersonal relationships and communication skills with CI, peers, and health professionals. This includes participating in problem-solving discussions and joint treatments with peer.

Criteria: As in I-C.

All other objectives as listed in the affiliating school's student clinical performance evaluation and discussed with the Center Coordinator of Clinical Education.

[a]Objectives to be met by completion of the affiliation.
[b]These standards are the minimum performance standards required of any physical therapist at UPMC.

approach the CI because she was not treating patients.

The CI reported a positive 2:1 experience. She said she had more time to observe student performance, give instruction, facilitate discussion, and emphasize problem solving, which she believed resulted in better insight into and appreciation of each student's strengths and weaknesses and more time to design individual experiences to fit individual student needs. The CI felt that because she had no caseload of her own, she was able to give more immediate feedback and was able to provide more hands-on experience to the students. The CI also reported learning from the students and developing and using more personnel management, time management, interpersonal, and administrative skills than she had been able to use in traditional 1:1 clinical education. As the students became more independent, even more of the CI's time was freed for student evaluation, projects, and research.

The combined student-CI caseload usually exceeded the typical caseload carried by an individual staff member. With no students, the CI's average number of patient visits per day was 9% higher than the staff average; with one student, 39% higher; with two students, 49% higher, at approximately five more patient visits per day.

Did patients benefit from the 2:1 model? Because the students did not have to wait for the CI to finish treating a patient before she could give assistance, patients did not have to wait as long for treatment sessions to proceed. Research is needed, however, to determine whether the increased sharing of ideas under the 2:1 model results in increased treatment effectiveness.

Perceived disadvantages. The students identified what they thought might prove to be disadvantages of the 2:1 model. They were uncertain, for example, how to interact with each other—when to lead and when to follow—and they were worried that the CI would compare them with each other or that an air of competitiveness would develop between them. However, once expectations were made clear and the students saw how the experience was struc-

tured and got to know each other, these concerns disappeared.

A disadvantage surfaced when one of the students had several patients in the clinic at once. Rather than struggle (and thus learn) to manage a number of patients simultaneously, this student requested help from the other student. Likewise, when one student did not know what to do in a given situation, she would go to the other student for suggestions rather than think through potential solutions. The CI believed this tendency compromised the students' independence. She brought it to

their attention. After discussion, the students agreed not to assist each other so readily and to consider possible solutions on their own and present the options to each other only for discussion or confirmation.

It also must be noted that—occasionally—one student would give the other student incorrect instruction.

The staff and facility noted no disadvantages to the 2:1 model.

The UPMC Experience

A 1,200-bed, multifacility teaching hospital specializing in trauma, transplantation medicine, and oncology, The University of Pittsburgh Medical Center (UPMC) is a university-based alliance of hospitals, institutes, and health science schools. The physical therapy department consists of 30 PTs and 8 PTAs who provide inpatient and outpatient services at Presbyterian University Hospital and Montefiore University Hospital and specialized services in the Balance and Vestibular Laboratory at the Eye and Ear Institute, all in Pittsburgh. PTs

and PTAs can rotate through nine teams: two acute medicine teams; neurotrauma, cardiopulmonary, transplantation, orthopedic, outpatient, and neurosurgery teams; and a 20-bed rehabilitation unit. The physical therapy department currently affiliates with 20 schools and provides clinical education for 35 full-time students per year. The circumstances that precipitated the decision to try the 2:1 collaborative teaching model at UPMC were similar to those that precipitated the decision at SMMH.

Step 1. Learn more about 2:1. The CCCE's initial opinion about the 2:1

> **[The CI] said she had more time to observe student performance, give instruction, facilitate discussion, and emphasize problem solving, which she believed resulted in better insight into...each student's strengths and weaknesses.**

model was negative because of incomplete information. After attending a seminar that thoroughly explained the 2:1 principles, the CCCE said he would give serious consideration to implementing the model—but only under the right circumstances. The right circumstances arose when a sudden, rapid turnover of staff resulted in the limited availability of experienced CIs for scheduled students.

Step 2: Educate administration. As in the process at SMMH, the CCCE educated the director of physical therapy about the basic tenets of collaborative learning and convinced the director that the 2:1 model would not have a negative impact on productivity.

Step 3: Educate CIs. All CIs attended an in-service program to introduce them to the idea of the 2:1 model.

Step 4: Choose the "right" CI. As did the CCCE at St Margaret, this CCCE identified the selection of the CI as one of the key elements for the success of this model. When the decision to implement the 2:1 model was made, the CCCE already had been considering a CI whose characteristics included competence as a clinician, solid organizational skills, a strong interest in adult learning—and a desire to explore a new challenge.

To alleviate stress, ease transitions, and outline expectations, the chosen CI reviewed all the available literature and discussed the logistics with the CCCE. This not only reduced anxiety about the experience but initiated the preparation of staff, including the orientation of the entire rehabilitation team and the creation of learning goals.

Step 5: Educate the "team." The rehabilitation unit was selected as the clinical education site because it was a more "controllable" unit from an organizational standpoint, was smaller in size, and the CI of choice was located there. The rehabilitation team received a special in-service training on specific plans and goals for the 2:1 experience, with emphasis placed on the fact that caseloads would shift the CI's responsibilities and timetables would be altered. Staff were made aware that temporary increases in their own caseloads prior to and after the experience might occur.

Step 6: Plan the experience. Circumstances at UPMC did not allow staff much time to prepare for the students' arrival. The CI recognized that planning therefore would be even more critical to success.

In contrast to the lecture orientation given to the students at SMMH, students at UPMC would be presented with an initial learning contract (Fig 2), an outline of a general plan, and guidelines for the 2:1 model (Fig 3). (The CI later identified these documents as critical to providing structure and setting clear expectations.) The students would be asked to sign the documents as proof that they understood the expectations, and each student would be asked to keep a diary of his or her experience. It was decided that to avoid influencing the students in recording their thoughts, the CI would see the diaries only after the students had completed the experience. The CI also would keep a diary.

Step 7: Inform the schools. Both ACCEs of the affiliating schools were advised of the plan to implement the 2:1 model.

Step 8: Initiate! The students at UPMC were at different academic levels (one student was a first-year student; the other was a second-year student). They also began and ended their affiliations 1 week apart. The student who arrived first was advised of the plan for the experience on her first day; the other student was notified via a letter in a welcome packet prior to her arrival.

It was decided purely out of interest that the students would take the Myers-Briggs Type Indicator[4]—a Jungian-based assessment tool that describes such personality traits as degree of introversion or extroversion, intuitiveness, and judgment and decision-making styles—before they began the 2:1 experience. The test indicated that they had very different personality types.

Figure 4 contains a week-by-week, day-by-day description of these students' 2:1 experience.

Figure 3 UPMC Student Guidelines for 2:1 Model[a]

The students and clinical instructor (CI) will work as a team. To foster this relationship, the students will work as equal peers. Although each will be assigned his or her own caseload, the fellow student, or peer, will serve as immediate backup or support service. The CI will serve as mentor, helping to guide decisions, monitoring progress of the team and of each member of the team, and counseling whenever necessary.

Your peer should be your first line of defense. All questions should first be taken to your peer. After discussion, the CI should be informed of your decision. The CI then has the responsibility to correct, modify, or concur with your decision. When assistance is needed during a treatment session (standby for safety, for example), you should ask your peer first for help. If your peer cannot be of assistance, consider rearranging your treatment plan to allow time for your peer to assist you. If that cannot be accomplished, consult with the CI. If you need to leave the department, your peer should cover for you. Again, this may make the rearranging of treatments or other preplanning necessary.

Your CI may request that you interrupt your patient's treatment to participate in a collaborative learning activity. This may take place when your peer or another therapist has an interesting treatment or patient. Please be ready at any time to join in one of these "collaborative teaching moments."[b]

Feel free to try out a new treatment or skill of which you are unsure on your peer. Freely communicate and critique each other's work, with a professional demeanor.

Keep a diary of your feelings or anything else you feel is important. I will ask you for this diary when you leave, but I will not ask to look at the diary before then. Your CI will also keep a diary.

The team will hold meetings at least once per week. At these meetings, we will discuss our patients, your treatment plans, patient goals, and progress toward these goals. We may modify your plan based on these discussions. Your CI also will ask about your comfort level with the 2:1 model. I ask that you express yourself in that meeting, but if you need to talk privately, I am always available.

You will be given a midterm and a final evaluation, using your school's guidelines. Your progress will be judged individually, not as a team. That is, you will be judged for *you*, not for your peer.

As this is a new venture for all of us, these guidelines may be modified at any time.

Student _____ Date _____

CI _____ Date _____

[b]*This has been modified to account for patient safety, busy schedules, and other conditions that make leaving difficult.*

Perceived advantages. Some of the same advantages of the 2:1 collaboration model identified by the students at SMMH also were identified by the students at UPMC, such as feeling less hesitant about asking each other questions and being able to share different ideas and views. Other benefits cited by the students: increased motivation through constructive, team-oriented competition; increased willingness to be self-reliant; and increased teamwork.

The CI at UPMC reported many of the advantages reported by the CI at SMMH. She also reported that the different arrival times, different departure times, and different academic levels—which the literature indicated may be disadvantageous[1]—actually were advantageous. Staggered starts prevented the CI from being overwhelmed by two new students at once. Because the

second-year student had an earlier start, the CI was able to give the first-year student the additional attention she needed, and the second-year student was able to boost her own confidence by helping to orient the other student. (This may not have been the case had the first-year student started first.) The CI found that the students' different education levels complemented each other: Weaknesses were addressed and the knowledge base of both students was increased through their interaction.

Perceived disadvantages. Potential drawbacks identified by the students were similar to those identified at SMMH and included the potential for increased competitiveness between the students and favoritism on the part of the CI. Less reliance on the CI's professional expertise also was cited as a potential disadvantage.

Because of the carefully structured atmosphere and involvement of the CI, however, these potential disadvantages did not materialize in practice.

One disadvantage of 2:1 models—a disadvantage that was described by Ladyshewsky and Healey[1]—did emerge at UPMC: One student "overpowered" the other. This tendency became evident during the second week of the collaborative experience. Management techniques were used to help the stronger, more assertive student soften her approach in professional communication. Simultaneously, and without coaching, the less assertive student rose to the challenge created by her peer: She became more assertive and confident and was able to suggest techniques to her peer that would help with communication. According to the CI, the first-year student

---

Figure 4. The UPMC Experience

WEEK 1

Day 1: The second-year student (Student A) is oriented to the facility and its policies by the CCCE and to the rehabilitation team and its policies by the CI. The learning contract and expectation documents are reviewed and modified to include the student's goals.

Student A observes patient treatment with the CI. Rehabilitation team members assist with the CI's caseload to allow orientation time for the CI and student.

Day 2: The CI treats her entire caseload (eight patients, treated twice daily) while A observes.

Day 3: The student begins to perform partial treatments as the CI directs.

Day 4: Partial-to-complete treatment programs are performed by Student A with patients selected by the CI, who chooses uncomplicated cases to allow Student A some early confidence-building independence.

Day 5: Student A performs complete treatments on selected patients. Student A and the CI each have four patients, treated twice daily.

Week 1 resembles a classic 1:1 clinical education experience.

WEEK 2

Day 1: The first-year student (Student B) is oriented to the facility and its policies by the CCCE. Student A orients Student B to the rehabilitation team and its policies as the CI observes. The learning contract and expectation documents are reviewed and modified to include Student B's goals, and both students review their contracts together and begin to plan collaborative experiences. Rehabilitation team members are requested to assist with the CI's and Student B's caseloads to allow time for orientation.

Day 2: Student A performs her first evaluation while the CI observes. This student carries a caseload of four patients (who originally belonged to the CI's caseload), treated twice daily. Student B observes the CI treating the remainder of the patients in the CI's caseload.

Days 3 and 4: Student A treats the patients in her caseload while the CI observes from a distance and intervenes as needed. When intervention is necessary, both students observe. Student B provides partial treatment for uncomplicated patients.

The CI observes the students discussing problems and solutions. The students occasionally consult with the CI before discussing problems with each other, as they originally were instructed.

Day 5: Student A continues to evaluate and treat patients as the CI observes from a distance. Student B provides partial treatments for the patients remaining in the CI's caseload, with guidance from the CI. The CI meets with both students to discuss patient progress and problem solve for patients who have more difficult conditions or who are not making progress.

Both students are encouraged to discuss concerns about the 2:1 model with the CI; neither voices complaints at this time.

WEEK 3

Day 1: Student B performs full treatments on the patients remaining in the CI's original caseload, with the CI's guidance. Student A evaluates patients and provides treatment, with occasional guidance from the CI. Each student carries a caseload of five patients, treated twice daily.

Days 2 and 3: The students collaborate on a patient evaluation. Because this evaluation is the first for Student B, she performs only part of the evaluation, and Student A completes it. The students collaborate on treatment plans and goals.

Day 4: Student B performs a complete evaluation with a patient who has no complications. The students confer first with each other and then with the CI when problems arise (eg, when the students are uncertain of a patient's family and social situation and therefore are unable to write appropriate goals for discharge).

Day 5: Midterm evaluations are performed separately, and the the CI and both students hold their weekly progress meeting.

WEEKS 4 TO 6

Each student carries a caseload of five patients treated twice daily. The students continue to perform all patient evaluations and treatments and participate in rounds and discharge-planning meetings. They attend other learning experiences individually, including observation of surgery and of other health professionals. When one student is absent from the clinic, her peer treats both the patients in both caseloads.

The CI's duties during this time include monitoring of students, teaching interactions with both students simultaneously, and limited management duties.

Weekly progress meetings are held.

WEEK 7

Student B receives her final evaluation, and the CI resumes Student B's portion of the caseload when Student B departs.

WEEK 8

Student A receives final evaluation and departs. The CI resumes the full caseload, which numbers eight patients treated twice daily.

would not have progressed in assertiveness and professional communication if she had not been challenged by this interaction with a peer.

Another disadvantage mentioned in the literature is the tendency of CIs to compare the students.[1] The CI's diary—in which she logged numbers and types of patients treated, evaluations performed, and student responses—was useful in helping her keep the students' identities separate and avoid comparing them.

The staff and facility reported no disadvantages to the 2:1 model.

Collaborating for the "Real World"

Although the experiences of SMMH and UPMC were different, both facilities considered the collaborative learning model to be a "success." Preliminary indications are that, in both facilities, the combined productivity of the students and CI exceeded the productivity of an individual PT carrying a typical caseload. Both facilities found that the constraints of the 2:1 model as described in current literature do not have to be impediments. In fact, learning to work under unfamiliar conditions with persons who have different levels of education and different personality traits may help prepare students to assume their professional roles in the "real world."

Both facilities found the following elements to be essential to the success of the collaborative 2:1 model: thorough education and orientation of staff, administration, and students to the philosophy of collaborative learning; selection of the "right" CI; a manageable caseload for the CI; and clear expectations.

Plans for the future at SMMH and UPMC include piloting the model on different rotations and with different CIs. As the demand for placements continues to grow, consideration may be given to other collaborative models, such as the 3:1, 4:1, and 5:2 models, some of which will be discussed by PTs and PTAs in future issues. *PT*

Kathryn Haffner Zavadak, PT, is Senior Staff Physical Therapist in Clinical Education/Rheumatology, Department of Physical Therapy, St Margaret Memorial Hospital, Pittsburgh, Pa. She served as CI for the 2:1 experience at SMMH. Christine Konecky Dolnack, MS, PT, is CCCE, St Margaret Memorial Hospital. Susan Polich, PT, is Instructor and ACCE, Duquesne University, John G Rangos, Sr, School of Health Sciences, Department of Physical Therapy, Pittsburgh, Pa. At the time this article was written, she was a PT III at the University of Pittsburgh Medical Center, where she served as CI for the 2:1 experience. Mark Van Volkenburg, PT, is Director, Harmarville Rehabilitation Center, Pittsburgh, Pa. At the time this article was written, he was CCCE, Department of Physical Therapy, University of Pittsburgh Medical Center. The authors thank Karl R Gibson, MS, PT, for his support and feedback.

References

1 Ladyshewsky R, Healey E. *The 2:1 Teaching Model in Clinical Education: A Manual for Clinical Instructors.* Toronto, Ontario, Canada: Department of Rehabilitation Medicine, Division of Physical Therapy, University of Toronto; 1990.

2 Ladyshewsky R. Clinical teaching and the 2:1 student-to-clinical-instructor ratio. *Journal of Physical Therapy Education.* 1993;7(1):31-35.

3 DeClute J, Ladyshewsky R. Enhancing clinical competence using a collaborative clinical education model. *Phys Ther.* 1993;73:42-56.

4 *Myers-Briggs Type Indicator: What's Your Type?* Pittsburgh, Pa: Training and Development Department, University of Pittsburgh Medical Center; 1993.

Collaborative Learning— 4:1 MODEL

A CI, an ACCE, a physical therapy manager, and

a student share insights about a 4:1 model of supervision implemented by

Northwestern University.

In the first installment of an ongoing series on innovative models in clinical education, *PT* interviews Babette Sanders, MS, PT, Instructor in Physical Therapy, Northwestern University Medical School, Chicago, Ill, and Staff Physical Therapist and Clinical Instructor (CI), Evanston Hospital, Evanston, Ill; Jean Rogers, MA, PT, Academic Coordinator of Clinical Education (ACCE), Programs in Physical Therapy, Northwestern University; Diane Merkt, PT, Physical Therapy Manager, Evanston Hospital; and physical therapy student Julie Bliven.

The 4:1 clinical education experience implemented by Sanders and her colleagues in July 1995 was one of the first in the country.

The CI's Perspective: Babette Sanders

PT: Your situation may be somewhat unique. You're a full-time faculty member *and* a CI for one of the university's clinical sites. What types of clinical education models have you participated in?

Sanders: We've used almost every type of model, including the 1:1. The 2:1 model is the one most commonly used in the Chicago area. Most clinical educators in our region emphasize creativity, regardless of the model, and they try to be open to any kind of collaborative arrangement.

PT: How would you describe the physical therapy program's philosophy about clinical education prior to implementing the 4:1 model?

Sanders: We were committed to exposing a majority of students to collaborative learning before they graduated. In a way, a university *has* to believe in collaborative learning. After all, it is—or should be—a logical extension of the classroom learning experience.

PT: The implementation of the 4:1 model with Northwestern students was part of a pilot study that you're conducting with Jean Rogers. Why did you choose the 4:1 for this pilot?

Sanders: Like all programs, we were having trouble finding clinical education slots—specifically, acute care slots. I happen to practice part-time at Evanston Hospital, a 550-bed teaching hospital that has outpatient and rehabilitation services. Its acute care team provides all care at the patient's bedside, including physical therapy—there's no central gym. I believed Evanston had the caseload volume and variety required to provide four students with high-quality learning experiences. The students would be able to work with a wide range of patients—from those needing crutch-walker training to those with heart transplants. They'd have exposure to general/medical/surgical care, orthopedics, neurology, intensive care, and critical care.

PT: Is intimate knowledge of the clinical site on the part of the education program essential for implementing the 4:1?

Sanders: Yes—but no more so than for implementing any other type of model, including the 1:1. In a collaborative model, however, it may be even more important to know your *students* well. Can they handle the independence? Can they be supportive of each other? It was a big advantage for me to be both a faculty member and a CI. Another big advantage was that, in our academic calendar, students are gone for the month of July. That meant that I could serve as a CI full-time for those 4 weeks, with the school paying my salary.

PT: Was it a struggle to get people to "buy in" to the 4:1 model?

Sanders: I approached Jean Rogers, the ACCE, with the pilot idea. She was 100% supportive. Our only concern was liability, because I would be paid by the university, not the hospital. We determined that the university would indeed cover me and the students. The physical therapy manager at

"The most important skill for the CI...is the ability to accurately and quickly assess a student's abilities— and to let go immediately when you sense the student is ready."

—Babette Sanders

Evanston Hospital, Diane Merkt, was enthusiastic about trying something new. The hospital had its own concerns about liability; once those were clarified, there were no obstacles. The hospital liked the idea of being involved in something that was so timely and important.

PT: How did you educate hospital staff about the model?

Sanders: We met with the acute care team and the entire physical therapy staff in April to explain the model. There was only one hitch. Between the time of this meeting and the start of the experience, the CCCE left. That meant that the new CCCE was coming into the 4:1 experience cold. But she did a great job, even though she had no previous experience with the model.

PT: Did you rely on any literature to help you explain or plan the experience?

Sanders: The work of Richard Ladyshewsky and his colleagues[1-3] was helpful. Although they didn't write specifically about the 4:1 model, the issues of collaborative learning that they explored are the same regardless of model.... As a student at Temple University, Philadelphia, Pa, Maureen Triggs Nemshick[4] wrote her master's

thesis on setting up a 2:1 collaborative experience. She outlined the different components that make a collaborative experience work—such as the match of facility needs to program needs and the quality of student-to-student interaction and student-to-CI interaction. That also was helpful. Although I didn't use these sources for the day-to-day operations of the 4:1, I am using them now to build the framework of our study.

PT: We'll talk later about that study. How did you adapt the 4:1 model?

Sanders: We decided to involve two different levels of students. We created a "hybrid" model: For 2 weeks, two second-year students participated in a 2:1 experience with another CI. In weeks 3 through 6, they were joined by two first-year students in the 4:1 experience, for which I served as CI. In weeks 7 through 9, the second-year students resumed the 2:1 experience with the other CI.

PT: Did you choose the students based on whether they were ready for the 4:1?

Sanders: No. The students selected themselves. They based their decision on some written information we gave them about the model and about the facility. The strong reputation of the hospital was a big attractor, and all of the students knew me because I was a faculty member. One of them said she was choosing the 4:1 model because she thought it would be a great experience.

PT: What's different about designing a 4:1 experience?

Sanders: In the 4:1 model, the CI has to trust that students will function independently and that they will know when they're in over their heads and need to get help. For this experience, I ensured that I had time alone with every student every day, whether it was for troubleshooting or for evaluating a patient. Sometimes I would accompany the student as an "aide" during a treatment session. It's also important to set up formal, weekly meetings, both with each individual and with the "student team." During team meetings, we discussed how we were doing as five people in a clinical education program. We handled procedural matters at that time, such as scheduling to ensure that the students weren't getting only orthopedic experiences.

PT: **What else is different about designing a 4:1 experience?**

Sanders: You have to design a caseload that allows the appropriate level of independence for each student. In our case, we had to work around the academic experiences that the first-year students hadn't had yet. Those students, for example, hadn't received formal training in MMT [manual muscle testing]. Working with the general/medical/surgical population, then, was appropriate, because that population typically doesn't require formal MMT. We also didn't schedule first-year students to evaluate patients with neurological dysfunction, for obvious reasons; but we did schedule them to be the "aides" to the second-year students, who *were* able to perform these evaluations. In that way, the first-year students could have the exposure, but not the primary responsibility.

PT: **What's the most important skill for the CI in a 4:1 experience?**

Sanders: The ability to accurately and quickly assess a student's abilities—and to let go immediately when you sense the student is ready for a given responsibility.

PT: **What was your biggest challenge?**

Sanders: As the CI for the 4:1, I had a number of concerns. Would I really be able to meet four people's needs? To be in four places at the same time? To ensure that patient care was not compromised in any way? The CI has those types of questions going into any new experience. You have to be aware of both the upside and the downside. As many butterflies as I had, however, I believed I could do it. That's the key to anything.

PT: **What are the advantages and disadvantages of the 4:1 for the patient?**

Sanders: Some patients may not like being treated by a team of students. Period. So that's obviously a disadvantage. But the

advantages can be substantial. In the 1:1 model, students don't necessarily go to the CI with questions, because they're worried that they'll be judged. In the 4:1 model, however, a student can go to his or her peers for confirmation and additional information. That kind of collaboration is bound to result in better care for the patient. And because the basic sciences are still fresh in the minds of the first-year students, they can actually help the second-year students keep in touch with that knowledge base.

PT: **What does a 4:1 experience mean for the clinical site?**

Sanders: For one thing, it means greater productivity. More patients can be treated; patients can have quicker access to services. The CI cannot carry a full caseload; for example, I was able to treat only two patients during those 4 weeks. But even if, at a minimum, two students each carry half a caseload and the other two treat only a few patients, the total number of patients treated is greater than that treated by the therapist under normal conditions. For the university, of course, the 4:1 model means there are three additional slots opened up! And these days, that's the bottom line.

PT: **What does a 4:1 experience do for staff?**

Sanders: Having four students in a department can make staff feel as though their clinic is a place of learning. It's a psychological benefit. Plus, depending on the volume, the students' extra caseload coverage may allow a department to identify new projects. That does require some planning up-front, however.

PT: **What was the most rewarding aspect of this experience for you as a CI?**

Sanders: The way the students responded to it. So many times in other types of clinical education experiences, the CI has to ask the student, "Well, *what do you think?*" Not in the 4:1. By the time a student made the decision to page me, for example, the student had already gone through a lengthy decision-making process, gathering as much information as possible from the

---

Tips for Implementing the 4:1 Model

1. **For the CCCE and CI:** Evaluate your staff and their willingness—and your own willingness—to "give up" the 1:1 model. For the collaborative learning experience to be successful, everyone involved should recognize that there is a shortage of high-quality clinical education experiences and believe that the 4:1 model is a viable solution.

2. **For the ACCE:** Is the caseload volume of the facility large enough to accommodate four students? Most facilities can handle two students; not all can handle four. Know how the physical therapy service works. And if the facility believes that it can do a good job with the 4:1 model, be encouraging!

3. **For the education program:** Ensure that students learn how to collaborate in the classroom before they enter the clinical site. Show them how team problem solving relates to the clinical education experience.

4. **For the CI, ACCE, and CCCE:** Work together to evaluate the potential benefits for the academic and clinical staff, the facility, and the students.

5. **For the CCCE:** Ensure that the CI is able to "let go" and allow students to live up to their own abilities.

nurse or the social worker and conferring with his or her peers. The students basically made their own decisions and came to me only for confirmation, rather than asking me early on, "What should I do?" Even the first-year students were independent with their selective caseload. And all of the students were supportive of each other.

PT: **In what way?**

Sanders: I periodically scheduled a second-year student to function as an "aide" to a first-year student. It was gratifying to see the second-year students move into the "CI" mode. One said to me, "It's really interesting to watch a first-year student. I have to make sure I'm organized in my own thought process before I can give guidance." The 4:1 model helped the students develop their teaching and supervision skills.

PT: **It sounds as though this was a positive experience for everyone. Was there anything you would do differently?**

Sanders: Nothing substantial. The only thing I would do differently is make sure that every student had a pager!

PT: **Across all settings, the focus today is on "outcomes effectiveness." The education community needs to know which collaborative models are most effective. What outcomes did you decide to measure for your study?**

Sanders: The effects of the 4:1 model on student performance and facility productivity.

PT: **How did you collect these data?**

Sanders: First, we developed a list of critical questions and did pre- and post-experience interviews with each of the principal players—the entire acute care team, including non-physical therapists; the CI for the 2:1 experience; myself for the 4:1 experience; and all of the students individually.

PT: **What types of questions did you ask?**

Sanders: Questions such as "What do you think a typical day will be/was like?" and "What will be/were the benefits of having

"It's a two-way street. The physical therapy profession has been guilty of thinking only about how clinical sites can meet students' needs. We need to think about how students can meet clinics' needs."

—Jean Rogers

students at multiple levels?" All of the students and the CIs kept daily journals; we're looking at those for themes. The hospital maintained productivity numbers and collected patient satisfaction information. Although we won't be able to correlate patient satisfaction directly to the 4:1 experience, we will be able to see whether patient satisfaction was lower or higher than usual during the month of July 1995.

PT: **Does the 4:1 model prepare students for managed care?**

Sanders: The collaborative learning model is an important part of the changing health care system. It helps students, practitioners, and the profession as a whole move away from the feeling that PTs are the center of the universe. Students may be especially susceptible to that feeling. Team models such as the 4:1 can help prepare new graduates for critical paths, increased collaboration with other health care professionals, increased delegation, and the changing nature of health care itself.

The ACCE's Perspective: Jean Rogers

PT: When Babette Sanders first approached you about the 4:1 model, did you have any reservations?

Rogers: I thought it was a wonderful idea. I was familiar with the 4:1 model implemented by the physical therapy program at the University of Michigan, which to my knowledge is the only other program to implement this model. I liked the idea of combining first-year and second-year students. In my opinion, *that's* what made this experience really special.

PT: **Why did the idea of combining different levels of students appeal so much to you?**

Rogers: For one thing, it was particularly appropriate for an acute care site. In the acute care setting, physical therapists have to assess patients and help them become functional enough for discharge to another setting. Assessment and discharge-planning skills are especially important. With their more highly developed assessment skills, the second-year students can help mentor the first-year students.

PT: **Another reason why the 4:1 model appealed to the university must have had to do with the shortage of clinical sites.**

Rogers: Of course. Here as elsewhere, the number of slots aren't rising with the number of students that need to be accommodated. The demand is far greater than it was even 5 years ago. But the even bigger attraction was the promise of developing better decision-making and team-building skills in the students.

PT: **From the university's point of view, were there special liability concerns?**

Rogers: With collaborative learning models, there is the fear that students will see patients alone when they are not ready to do so, potentially increasing the risk of malpractice exposure for the supervising CI, the facility, and the university. But the irony is that unprepared students may be *more* likely to see patients alone in a 1:1 model!

PT: Why is that?

Rogers: In the 1:1 model, the CI often has his or her own caseload to manage. The intent with a 4:1 model is that the CI will be a full-time CI with no caseload. The CI therefore can better observe the students in the initial weeks of the experience to determine who has the ability to be independent—and to what degree of independence.

PT: Why is it difficult for many physical therapists to "give up" the 1:1 model?

Rogers: I've been an ACCE for 11 years. When I was a student—that was a long time ago!—I went on "clinical affiliations" with at least one or two peers, and at the time I thought that it would have been better to have a 1:1 situation. It's only natural to think that a student will get more attention and feedback that way. Many of us "grew up" with the 1:1 model and prefer what's familiar. But if we cling to that model, we're denying everyone a great opportunity! Again, if there is only one student, that CI has to divide his or her attention between the student and a caseload. But if there's one full-time CI with multiple students, the CI can concentrate solely on the students and the way they are managing patients.

PT: Is it fair to say that collaborative models require more work on the part of clinical sites?

Rogers: Only in the sense that these models require a lot of advance planning. It used to be that you could plan experiences a week before the students arrived. Not with the 4:1! To organize an experience that meets everybody's needs, the caseload has to be carefully designed, and students have to be carefully assessed. Babette was physically and mentally exhausted after the first week. But that passes. In general, education programs ask facilities to commit to taking students a year or two in advance, when many facilities are in such flux today that they don't know whether they'll be in existence next year! The collaborative model becomes just one more change that clinicians have to deal with, and, for some clinics, it's one change too many.

> "With a shorter LOS, students have to learn to set short-term goals, and they can't always use all of those detailed evaluation skills they're learning in school. "
>
> —Diane Merkt

PT: How can education programs help clinics deal with the change?

Rogers: These days, clinics want to be in control of at least *something* in their environment. Especially when clinical education experiences involve multiple students of different levels or from different programs with different schedules, the education program should explain the process in detail. For example, the first wave of students can actually help orient the second wave to facility procedures and equipment ordering. These are discreet tasks that are easy to follow up, so they work from an educational standpoint and also can help the clinic maintain some sense of control over the experience.

PT: What is the education program's role in preparing *students* for collaborative models?

Rogers: We need to teach them how to communicate their thought processes so that they can maximize their consultations with the CI. We need to model collaboration in the classroom as much as possible, through clinician visits and field trips. We expect our students to be members of problem-solving teams in the classroom, and we need to make it clear how that relates to the practice environment in general and the

clinical education experience specifically.

PT: What advice would you give to people interested in finding out more about collaborative models?

Rogers: Do what we did—we read Ladyshewsky's work, and when we had questions, we called him directly! Or call us! [See contact information below.] People *are* available to help.

PT: What do you believe is the future of clinical education under managed care, given the increased caseload volume and fewer visits?

Rogers: We all have to find creative ways to provide high-quality health care services and clinical education. Facilities will be looking more critically at the economic impact of clinical education, and, for some of them, clinical education may become a lower priority. Some therapists believe that students should pay tuition to the clinic instead of the university for the period of the affiliation.

PT: As an educator, how would you respond to that argument?

Rogers: We all should be concerned about the cost of education. Universities and health care facilities alike are experiencing cutbacks in funding. Most universities distribute the cost of the student's education across all terms of enrollment, including terms when students are in clinical facilities. If we expect students to pay tuition to universities *and* facilities, we will further increase the students' financial burden. We all need to sit down together to assess how the resources of clinical facilities and education programs—including those of students—can be used more effectively.

PT: Is the sense of professional duty to student education diminishing?

Rogers: Many PTs don't view educating others as our responsibility—unless the "others" are patients or patient families. In the medical profession, there's an established tradition, an expectation that you will teach: Advanced residents are expected to teach new residents, new residents are expected to teach medical students, et cetera. But it's a two-way street. The physical therapy profession has been guilty of thinking only about how clinical sites can fulfill students' needs. Programs need to think about how students can help meet clinics' needs—how students can be included in treating patients, conducting research, and providing community outreach in a way that enhances the clinic's practice. That's what students want, too. As one recently said to me, "I want to know what it's really like out there. I *want* to know the bad stuff."

The PT Manager's Perspective: Diane Merkt

PT: **What was your reaction when you were approached about the 4:1?**

Merkt: I was ready for it. Other teaching hospitals in our area had participated in the 2:1. I thought the 4:1 would be a good opportunity for Evanston Hospital.

PT: **Why?**

Merkt: We have a good relationship with Northwestern; two of their faculty members are on our staff; our staff participate in lab practical exams at Northwestern; and I hire one or two Northwestern graduates every year. The 4:1 was another way of maintaining that rapport. I knew I'd have support from administration because of the research project involved and—especially in these times—because Northwestern was paying one of the CI's salaries.

PT: **Were staff enthusiastic about taking part in a 4:1 experience?**

Merkt: They were hesitant. They hadn't had enough exposure to it. I network a great deal, so I was less skeptical. Even though this experience went well, some would still hesitate—the 2:1 model is more "comfortable" for many PTs.

PT: **What were the positives of the 4:1 for your staff?**

Merkt: The staff liked having the students around and the questions that they asked. The CI and the students identified a need—for gait-training handouts—and

> ✑
>
> "I eventually want to be able to handle whatever patient comes my way, so I didn't want to just 'follow someone around.' I wanted to develop independence."
>
> —Julie Bliven
>
> ✑

answered it, and the staff appreciated that: one less thing they had to do. The 4:1 also allowed staff to take vacations at the same time. It theoretically would have allowed us to take on more special projects; however, it's hard to plan for special projects in the acute care setting, where the caseload volume fluctuates so much.

PT: **Were there any negatives?**

Merkt: On a couple of occasions, we had to "flex" our full-time employees' regularly scheduled hours to accommodate fluctuations in caseload so that students would have an optimal experience. Now and then, working with students was difficult for some of our younger staff, particularly those who rotated through other sites and services and had a more variable schedule.

PT: **How did patients respond?**

Merkt: We had no appreciable increase in patient complaints. Collaborative models may work best in acute and inpatient settings—especially when care is provided bedside—because patients are used to having multiple care providers. Two years ago we had a 2:1 experience in Evanston Hospital's outpatient department. The patients

were not as accepting, and the CI ended up having to take on some of the students' caseload.... Of course, acute care poses its own challenges. With the shorter length of stay, students have to learn to set short-term rather than long-term goals, and they can't always use all of the detailed evaluation skills they're taught in school. They have to develop a sense of what's important to test and what to let go.

PT: **Is there anything you would do differently?**

Merkt: I'd have the students fill out time cards, with productivity deductions made for their meetings, just as "real" staff do. And I'd make better use of the opportunity to do special projects, primarily by assigning teams of PTs to projects rather than just one individual who may not be able to take advantage of the time because of a sudden influx of patients.

PT: **In general, how did the 4:1 experience affect productivity?**

Merkt: Our target productivity rate for a staff PT is 78% to 80%. The study being done by Babette Sanders and Jean Rogers will provide specific data. From the facility's point of view, the students' productivity levels were high enough to justify a full-time CI—and that's important.

A First-Year Student's Perspective: Julie Bliven

PT: **What did you expect to get out of the 4:1 experience?**

Bliven: The CI and the ACCE talked with us about the model, but I didn't have many preconceived notions. I didn't know I'd be working so closely with the second-year students, for example.

PT: **What did you *want* to get out of the experience?**

Bliven: I eventually want to be able to handle whatever type of patient comes my way, so I didn't want to just "follow someone around." I wanted to develop some independence.

PT: **When did you first realize that you**

were in the "real world" of the clinic?

Bliven: Right away. I saw my first patient less than 2 hours into my first day.

PT: **What happened with that first patient?**

Bliven: After reviewing the chart, the CI [Sanders] and I discussed my initial game plan. The patient was a woman with diabetes who had a femoral bypass. She already had an amputation; she knew that if she didn't exercise, she would risk losing another limb. But she was resistant. She ended up being my patient—a very challenging first patient! I eventually became independent in her treatment sessions.

PT: **Describe a typical day in your 4:1 experience.**

Bliven: We first-year students would look at a chart after the CI had reviewed it. One of us would write notes. The CI would ask us what we "got out of it," then, "Do you think you can start this session alone?" She'd usually come into the treatment room 10 or 15 minutes after we started.

PT: **How did you decide on who would do what?**

Bliven: The CI screened the patients. If the patient required a basic evaluation, a first-year student would do it and a second-year student would act as the "aide." If the patient required a more in-depth evaluation, a second-year student would do it, and a first-year student would act as the "aide." I liked that system. If I missed something, one of the others would catch it! When we disagreed, we'd discuss it later and give each other feedback: "I really liked it when you...."

PT: **Were there any difficult moments?**

Bliven: Sure. One patient did not want to do *anything*. He had a total hip replacement and bowel problems, and he was miserable. All he did was complain. I was the "aide," but when I became frustrated with the patient, I "took charge." It wasn't that I thought my approach was better; it was that my instinct to get control of the situation took over. I learned that this is something I

need to work on as a team player.

PT: **How did you finally deal with that patient?**

Bliven: All of a sudden, we figured out what made him tick! He just needed encouragement—a lot of it. "That's great!" "Way to go!"

PT: **Were you involved in any non–patient-care activities?**

Bliven: We all worked on an in-service program for the clinical staff, and we created handouts on gait training for staff to give patients. It felt good to do something that needed to be done.

PT: **What else did you like?**

Bliven: The one-to-one meetings with the CI and learning whether the strengths and weaknesses I thought I had were the same ones that she saw.

PT: **What did you learn about those strengths and weaknesses?**

Bliven: My strength is in developing rapport with patients, but I need to learn more about how to get information from them. And I need to improve my note-writing skills... The 4:1 experience reinforces the fact that everyone is different—coworkers, patients. Rapport with other professionals—physicians, nurses, occupational therapists—is just as important as good rapport with patients. As "aides," we needed to act the part and follow the other student's lead. It made me think about what it would be like to communicate with and delegate to physical therapist assistants and physical therapy aides.

PT: **Ultimately, why do you think the 4:1 worked for you?**

Bliven: Because I knew I wanted to work both independently and as a team member. If a student isn't ready to do that, it's not going to work. You need to take initiative, such as randomly selecting some patient charts to read. What also made the experience work was that I already knew the CI. I didn't have to spend a lot of time getting to know someone. I felt comfortable telling her when I needed assistance.

PT: **You have more clinical education experiences ahead of you. Would you like them all to be 4:1?**

Bliven: The 4:1 was a great first experience. I was able to develop my style by picking and choosing from four different ideas and opinions! But now I'm ready for the 1:1, to further develop my own style and independence.

PT: **You had the opportunity to witness managed care firsthand. What most impressed you?**

Bliven: The reduced length of stay. So many patients just didn't seem ready to go home. For one of the patients I treated, for instance, safety was a big issue; he wasn't ready to be discharged to the home. The CI and I explained this to the physician, but the insurer wouldn't cover any additional days, and the patient was discharged.... As a student, I'm still learning what I need to know about pathology and treatment. I can't say that I've seen the impact of managed care yet. *PT*

This article was based on interviews conducted by Jan Reynolds, Contributing Editor.

Babette Sanders will be giving a platform presentation on the 4:1 model at APTA's Physical Therapy '96 Conference in Minneapolis, Minn, June 14-18, 1996. Sanders and Jean Rogers also will be presenting a short course, "Collaborative Learning in Acute Care: An Exciting Way to Meet Today's Health Care Challenges." They welcome reader questions. Sanders can be reached at 312/908-9405 or b-sanders2@nwu.edu; Jean Rogers, at 312/908-6787 or jro343@nwu.edu.

References
1   Ladyshewsky R, Healey E. *The 2:1 Teaching Model in Clinical Education: A Manual for Clinical Instructors.* Toronto, Ontario, Canada: Department of Rehabilitation Medicine, Division of Physical Therapy, University of Toronto; 1990.
2   Ladyshewsky R. Clinical teaching and the 2:1 student-to-clinical-instructor ratio. *Journal of Physical Therapy Education.* 1993;7(1):31-35.
3   McClure J, Ladyshewsky R. Enhancing clinical competence using a collaborative clinical education model. *Phys Ther.* 1993;73:42-56.
4   Nemshick M. *Physical Therapy Clinical Education in a 2:1 Student-Instructor Ratio Education Model.* Philadelphia, Pa: Temple University; 1994. Master's thesis.

Planned Small-Group Experience: Model for Part-time Clinical Education

Gail C Grisetti, EdD, PT

ABSTRACT: The planned small-group experience is an alternative part-time clinical education model designed around seven sessions. Three sessions occur at the academic institution, and four sessions take place at clinical sites. Students are sent into the clinic in small groups with a packet of specific objectives to accomplish. Objectives relate directly to classroom material. Each session is a separate module, allowing clinics to participate in a single session or in several sessions. Students rotate each clinical session through different facilities with different group members. The experience constitutes one semester of part-time clinical education. The subsequent semester, students complete an 8-week, individual, part-time clinical affiliation. This model addresses problems associated with part-time clinical education and the lack of uniformity in student experience. During the four years it has been used at Old Dominion University, the model has been evaluated favorably by clinicians and students.

INTRODUCTION

Part-time clinical affiliations traditionally have been a component of physical therapy education. These affiliations provide students with on-site clinical instruction by a licensed physical therapist for several hours per week and occur during the semester while classroom instruction continues. Walish, Olson, and Schuit[1] suggested that part-time clinical education builds students' self-confidence in the affective and psychomotor domains. Part-time clinical education allows students to practice in a limited context. Movement between the clinic and the classroom allows students to build skills and to integrate into the professional role gradually. Experiences gathered during part-time affiliation stimulate interest in mastering classroom material and demonstrate application of this material.

Dr Grisetti is Associate Professor and a Coordinator of Part-time Clinical Education, School of Community Health Professions and Physical Therapy, Old Dominion University, Norfolk, VA 23529-0288.

Historically, physical therapy students were assigned to part-time clinical affiliations on an individual basis early in their professional education. The academic institution provided students and clinical coordinators with a list of various goals and objectives for students to meet while accompanying the therapist on rounds.

Kondela and Darnell[2] identified several problems with part-time clinical education: a limited number of clinics located within a reasonable driving distance of the academic institution; demands experienced by clinical faculty involved in year-round clinical education; and conflicts exhibited by students struggling to complete course work while participating in a 14-week part-time affiliation.[2] Recent trends in staffing patterns at clinical sites, competition among schools for individual clinical placements, and the introduction of the entry-level master's-degree student have created new challenges. These challenges illustrate the need to develop creative ways to provide part-time clinical education.

In 1989, the School of Community Health Professions and Physical Therapy at Old Dominion University in Norfolk, Va, adopted a new format for part-time clinical education in response to these challenges. The new model is called the planned small-group experience (PSGE), and it has been introduced into the entry-level master's-degree curriculum.

MODEL DESIGN

The format for the PSGE is a 7-week series of sessions that begins 7 weeks into the first semester of the first year. The seven sessions are divided between the clinical sites and the academic institution. The initial session is held at the academic institution and orients students to the geographical area, provides an overview of the types of facilities available, and discusses the behaviors desired in the clinic. The instructor gives an in-depth presentation to students on the rationale of the PSGE model and answers questions regarding the content of the packet. This session is led by the academic coordinator of part-time clinical education (ACCE) and may include presentations by area clinical coordinators regarding expectations of student performance.

The sequence of sessions is displayed in the Figure. Sessions 1, 3, and 7 occur at the academic institution, and sessions 2, 4, 5, and 6 occur at clinical sites. Session titles reflect the content of the module. The PSGE model is designed specifically to allow facilities to accept students for one to four sessions. The PSGE is followed in the spring semester by 8-week individual clinical assignments.

MODEL CONCEPT

The PSGE model integrates specific content areas of the curriculum into the part-time clinical affiliation. It provides a structured format for clinical instructors so that material is covered uniformly in all facilities. On-site participation occurs in small groups of three or four students assigned to a facility for a particular session. Students receive instruction and practice skills based on a sequence of topics predetermined by the academic faculty. The clinical instructor provides activities and directs experiences related to that topic during the half-day experience.

Specific information is provided by the ACCE regarding tasks that must be completed during the session. This structure encourages planning and analysis by the clinical instructor in preparation for the visit and closely relates the time spent in the clinic to course work. Material beyond the level of the student at that time is not covered. Perry[3] suggested that determining and developing clinical objectives closely related to the curriculum adds to the effectiveness of clinical education.

Clinical Activities

Activities performed during the on-site sessions are based on curriculum contained in the first semester and are progressive in their development and integration of skills. The activities involve an increasingly difficult sequence of tasks and problem-solving strategies.[2] The format also introduces students

Reprinted with permission from the *Journal of Physical Therapy Education*, Vol 7, No 2, pp 60-62, 1993.

to the process of clinical decision making used by the clinical instructor.[4,5]

It is important, therefore, for the academic faculty to review the first-semester curriculum. Course content which will become objectives for the clinical sessions must be identified. These objectives are translated into activities to be completed during the various sessions. Because completion of these activities is mandatory, clinical coordinators must carefully review the list of activities to determine whether their facility can provide the student group with these activities.

The initial letter of request to the clinical coordinators mailed by the ACCE contains a list of activities to be completed during each session. The clinical coordinator can agree to participate in from one to four sessions, depending on the ability of that facility to provide the activities. Coordinating activities between the academic and clinical faculty has helped PSGE to be one in a series of clinical experiences leading to the first full-time affiliation at the end of the first year of course work.

Students rotate to four different facilities during each of the four on-site sessions. Group members also rotate so that students can work with different class members during each session. The rotation of sites and student group members helps familiarize students with local clinical sites available for the 8-week part-time affiliation and subsequent full-time affiliations.

During sessions two and four, student small groups share in the completion of the objectives; the information gathered will be synthesized and presented in both oral and written formats. The second session (at the academic institution) allows students to share information gathered during their first week at the clinics. In this session, files are created by the various groups of students; the files feature a description of the type and size of the facility, types of patients treated, number and type of personnel, and methods of documentation. Students use these files as references to prepare for upcoming sessions, when they will rotate into a different clinic, and to assist in determining their 8-week individual part-time affiliation during the spring semester.

During sessions five and six, each student is responsible for completing the packet of objectives. The activities performed in sessions five and six depend on mastery and recall of material from sessions two and four.

Evaluation of Student Performance

Student performance is evaluated by the ACCE and the clinical instructor. The ACCE bases the student's grade on responses to questions in the packet. This method of evaluation applies particularly to weeks two and four, when information is gathered, questions are answered, and interviews conducted. The ACCE reviews the packets after the first two on-site sessions.

After the last two sessions (when specific skills are performed), the packets are signed and reviewed by the clinical instructor who has evaluated the student's ability to perform the transfer technique, gait-training, or modality during that session. The ACCE assigns a grade of "Pass" or "Fail" to the student's performance. At Old Dominion University, the Pass/Fail grade becomes a letter grade when the student completes the 8-week individual part-time affiliation during the spring semester.

PROBLEMS IN PART-TIME CLINICAL EDUCATION

The PSGE model addresses several new concerns in providing part-time clinical education. These include the diversity in the background of graduate students admitted into the entry-level program, the fluctuation in staffing patterns in facilities, and comments from clinical instructors concerning the skill level of students during the first semester.

Volunteer/Employment Experience

The entry-level master's-degree program was instituted at Old Dominion University in 1987. Students entering the program have a wide and varied background in physical therapy. Their experience may include one or two years of paid employment as a physical therapy aide or several months of observation as a volunteer with virtually no hands-on experience. Students may never have experienced the acute care environment and may have worked only with an outpatient orthopedic population.

Presently there is no way to evaluate the quality or content of students' previous experience. The initial part-time clinical experience is an important first step in equalizing some of these background differences. It is an opportunity for the academic institution to ensure that entry-level master's-degree students receive an equal foundation in basic skills regardless of their backgrounds.

To implement the model, the ACCE must review the volunteer or work experience of each student to determine the type and nature of prior exposure to physical therapy. Incoming students provide information on the length of their experience in the clinic, the type of facility in which they volunteered or worked, and the tasks they performed.

This allows the ACCE to identify areas where students may have acquired knowledge prior to entering the program. This information will be used in making the initial assignments.

To equalize their experiences, students are placed in clinics where they can gain the greatest amount of new information—rather than placing them in clinical areas that may reinforce skills associated with their volunteer or work experience. The skills learned by students during volunteer or work experience may not represent what the students have been taught and tested on in the classroom. Students' previous training in volunteer or work settings cannot be assumed to represent classroom content. The initial part-time affiliation is an important time for the academic institution to direct students to areas that will contribute to the general knowledge base established during the first year.

Clinical Site Staffing

Reduced and variable staffing patterns have made finding part-time clinical sites difficult. Unexpected changes in staff may cause facilities to cancel part-time affiliations or to decline the initial request for a placement made by the ACCE. Part-time students in the first semester cannot assume a patient load, and, in the understaffed department, the part-time affiliate may be viewed as less desirable than a full-time affiliate who can take an expanded role in patient care.

The first-semester student requires the most individual attention and the closest supervision from the clinical instructor during the half-day session. This level of supervision may be viewed as reducing time spent with patients when staffing is reduced. The flexibility of the PSGE model means that even understaffed or contracted departments can accept students. Accepting a part-time student for 14 weeks may be impossible for the understaffed clinic, but accepting three students for a single 4-hour session with a specified format has proved manageable.

Concerns of Clinical Coordinators

During the initial part-time affiliation, students are in the very early phases of skill acquisition. Clinical coordinators have reported that the benefits of part-time affiliation are diminished if the student has had limited exposure to patient care during volunteer training and has only started to learn skills in the classroom. The PSGE model addresses this problem through the packet of specific objectives and the scheduling of clinical sessions during the semester.

Students develop their repertoire of skills before they reach sessions five and six. The students' gradual introduction into the clinical setting eases students' performance anxiety. They can demonstrate more skills to the clinical instructor by sessions five and six because they are in the final six weeks of the first semester.

BENEFITS OF THE MODEL

Since the implementation of the PSGE model at Old Dominion University, the problem of finding part-time affiliations has reduced dramatically. The success in finding sites applies to both the planned small-group sessions and to the subsequent 8-week individual affiliation. The option of accepting students for one to four sessions has eased pressure on clinical instructors. They can accept students when it is most convenient or most appropriate for them in light of the objectives for that session.

The structure of the model reduces the total number of individual assignments needed and eases competition for sites in areas where fluctuating staffing patterns may make finding part-time affiliations difficult. The planning required makes the students' visit more of an event than the traditional part-time affiliation. The workload of having students in the clinic is distributed among more staff members.

Clinical instructors have reported that the structured format clarifies the tasks to be accomplished during each session. This seems to be especially important during the first semester, when clinical instructors are trying to evaluate students' knowledge and skill levels. The PSGE packet of objectives eliminates much of the guesswork from their decisions. The structured format allows clinical instructors to serve in a more clearly defined teaching role. The structure also provides direction for physical therapists who may have been newly designated as clinical instructors.

CONCLUSION

Part-time clinical education appears to directly benefit students, but the problems associated with finding sites make the task difficult and time consuming. Rather than abandoning part-time clinical education, ACCEs should explore other ways to provide students with this opportunity. The PSGE model provides structure and guides development of students' first clinical contact. In addition, the PSGE model reduces the number of clinical slots needed per year. The overall benefit of the PSGE model suggests that this format addresses the significant problems and concerns experienced by academic institutions facing the challenge of part-time clinical education.

ACKNOWLEDGMENT

Appreciation is extended to Ms. Patricia Windom-Sachon for her contribution to the conception of the PSGE model. Ms. Sachon was a full-time faculty member at Old Dominion University when the model was developed.

REFERENCES

1. Walish J, Olson R, Schuit D. Effects of a concurrent clinical education assignment on student concerns. *Phys Ther.* 1986;66:233–236.
2. Kondela P, Darnell R. Receptivity to full-time early clinical education experience. *Phys Ther.* 1981;61:1168–1172.
3. Perry J. A model for designing clinical education. *Phys Ther.* 1981;61:1427–1432.
4. Payton O. Clinical reasoning process in physical therapy. *Phys Ther.* 1985;65:924–928.
5. Echternach J, Rothstein J. Hypothesis-oriented algorithm for clinicans: a method for evaluation and treatment planning. *Phys Ther.* 1989;66:1388–1394.

Figure
Sequence of sessions for planned small-group experience model.

   I.   Introduction (Academic Institution)
      Orientation to PSGE model. Review of packet of objectives. Discussion of professional behaviors. Orientation to geography of area.

   II.   Clinical Site Investigations (Clinical Sites)
      Investigation of facilities by type of setting. Identify the type of facility and patient population served. Describe the philosophy of the institution and review the table of organization for the department. Review the system of documentation, types of records, and referral sources. Identify the number and type of personnel. Tour the facility and describe the size and layout of the physical therapy department. Interview a physical therapist.

   III.   Presentation and Discussion of Findings from Session II (Academic Institution)
      Information gathered by student groups is presented in oral and written format. Reference files are created.

   IV.   Introduction to Clinical Decision Making (Clinical Site)
      Chart review: disease process investigation and interviews. Review charts provided by the clinical instructor. Retrieve essential data. Discuss the condition of the patient or the disease process affecting the patient. Interview the physical therapist and the patient in relation to the condition or disease process.

   V/VI.   Transfer/Gait Training or Modalities (Clinical Site)
      During session, half of the students practice transfers and gait activity while the other half practice modalities. During the next session, the groups reverse activities. Review charts and the disease or condition affecting the patient. Understand why the disease or condition requires that transfer or gait activity or modality. Perform the activities and record them in the chart. Repeat with other patients as time allows.

   VII.   Discussion and Review of Experiences (Academic Institution)
      A wrap-up session. Students complete evaluation forms, add to the reference files on clinics, and discuss experiences.

PEER COACHING IN CLINICAL TEACHING
Formative Assessment of a Case

FRANCINE P. HEKELMAN
STEPHEN P. FLYNN
PAMELA B. GLOVER
SIM S. GALAZKA
Case Western Reserve University
School of Medicine

J. ARCH PHILLIPS, Jr.
University of Georgia

Increasingly, medical education, and family medicine in particular, is focusing on improving clinical teaching. Peer coaching represents one alternative for improving and enhancing instruction. It enhances clinicians' understanding and use of new skills by demonstration, practice, and nonevaluative feedback from their colleagues. This article introduces the idea of peer coaching as an approach to faculty development. It uses a 1½-year formative assessment of one family physician's teaching practices and beliefs to describe the process.

EVALUATION & THE HEALTH PROFESSIONS, Vol. 17 No. 3, September 1994 366-381
© 1994 Sage Publications, Inc.

C linical teaching is one of the most complex and multifaceted tasks facing clinicians in an academic medical setting. Because of the complex nature of the medical education process, medical education, and family medicine in particular, is increasing the emphasis on improved clinical teaching and learning (Daggett, Cassie, & Collins, 1979). In addition, teaching in family medicine is further complicated by factors such as working within an ambulatory setting, frequent rotations, and unpredictable and random clinical cases, thus obviating any reasonable efforts for preplanned clinical teaching. Within this context, sensitive medical educators acknowledge the significance of the preceptorship model in which critical teaching and learning occurs for most students and resident physicians in a series of one-on-one encounters.

In the fall of 1991, the Department of Family Medicine at Case Western Reserve University embarked on a peer coaching project designed to improve the clinical teaching skills of faculty. This project appears to break new ground in medical education as a thorough literature search produced no evidence that peer coaching has been previously adapted to medical education in the clinical setting. The goal of this project is to help clinician teachers recognize current teaching behaviors and teaching practices and then to improve those teaching styles and behaviors. A further goal is to help clinician teachers develop the ability to adapt teaching strategies to fit the needs of the individual student. As clinician teachers learn to recognize their own teaching behaviors and practices, they should also become more sensitive to the strategies employed by their colleagues. This, in turn, will allow clinician teachers to evolve into a community of peer coaches who work together to enhance medical education. The need for such a program is made clear by evidence gathered by the faculty development educator through interviews and observations of the clinician teachers in the ambulatory settings. This includes a range of counterproductive teaching behaviors among physician faculty (Daggett et al., 1979; Hekelman, 1990; Hekelman, Vanek, Kelly, & Alemagno, 1993). These included:

1. With few exceptions, faculty did not view teaching as a central function of precepting.

2. Faculty tended to *do* for learners versus facilitating *doing* by the learner.
3. Faculty demonstrated limited sensitivity to learner differences, and, when differences were recognized, teachers had difficulty adjusting patterns of interaction accordingly.
4. Faculty acknowledged a very narrow repertoire of basic teaching strategies—their teaching tended toward single pattern responses in teaching encounters regardless of the situation at hand.

The purpose of this article is to assess the formative development of the peer coaching program to date as a faculty development mechanism for improving and enhancing the physicians' repertoire of clinical teaching skills. Implementation of peer coaching is described in conjunction with a formative analysis of the teaching practices and beliefs of one family physician to illustrate the process. The assessment and educational activities in the case reported span a 1½-year time frame.

Peer coaching, a deliberate systematic intervention to bring about instructional improvement, evolved as one alternative to failed efforts to bring about more effective teaching behaviors through traditional in-service programs (Joyce & Showers, 1980, 1982; Joyce, Weil, & Showers, 1992; Schon, 1987). As described earlier, peer coaching is a process that engages clinicians in an agreement to help one another become better instructors. The peer coaching model develops a shared language and set of common understandings essential for collegial study to gain new knowledge and skills. It is a cyclical process in which clinicians' understanding and use of new skills is enhanced by demonstration, practice, and through feedback from colleagues.

PEER COACHING PROJECT

Six physician faculty from the department of family medicine were invited to participate as peer coaches and were paired in dyads to observe, interact with, and, ultimately in the course of this project, to coach each other.

To the best of our knowledge, no research has been conducted that examines reflective teaching skills through peer coaching to improve clinical teaching in medical education. Textual formats and qualitative studies have only recently begun to be used for research in teaching in medical education. This format was found particularly useful in describing the richness of the peer coaching process and allows educational researchers to represent the dialogic and evolving character of collaborative efforts that occurred between the physician teacher and the coach. Experience to date with this project suggests that changes in teaching behaviors and routines is a long-term proposition.

The peer coaching project described in this report was designed to span a 3-year period. The three stages of the clinical supervision process—pre-observation, observation, and post-observation—served as a framework for periodic feedback to the six participants regarding their teaching proficiency (Berliner, 1988; Goldhammer & Cogan, 1969).

Stage One: Pre-Observation

The faculty development educator described teaching within the context of the ambulatory setting, and an initial profile of the six participants was developed. The purpose of the initial assessment was two-fold: (a) to match the tasks of the physician teachers to the goals of the peer coaching program; and (b) to determine the efficiency of the proposed dyads. The assessment profile included the Learning Styles Inventory, Myers-Briggs Type Indicator, and a self-assessment of pedagogical expertise (See Appendix). Assessment of pedagogical expertise was based upon the 14 assumptions of an expert pedagogue and the developmental level of the teacher (Berliner, 1988). Next, selected readings from both general education and medical education on clinical teaching were sent to each participant. This was followed by 2 half-day videotaped observation sessions to obtain a baseline data of the instructional behaviors used by the physician teacher. A half-day workshop was then held that focused on heightening awareness of the use of teaching routines and practices, enhancing sensitivity to cues in the environment that change or alter teachers' decision-making processes, as well as to cues that alter the outcome of the clinical teaching encounter. Participants viewed and critiqued their baseline videotapes in small groups and in their dyad.

Stage Two: Observation

Clinician teachers were observed a minimum of three times and a maximum of four times during the first year of the project, while they were teaching residents, medical students, and nurse practitioners. After each observation, the teacher and faculty development educator met and analyzed the teaching behaviors used during the encounter. Clinician teachers also observed their colleagues teaching in the clinical sites twice during this period of time and analyzed the teaching behaviors used. They then participated in two workshops that used videotapes of teaching as an instructional method for reflecting on teaching behaviors and teaching practices. Through these processes, the clinician teachers described their teaching behaviors and participated in reviewing, critiquing, and analyzing videotapes of their own teaching and that of their colleagues. These activities were designed to facilitate the clinical teachers' development into effective peer coaches working collaboratively to improve medical education.

Stage Three: Post-Observation

In the third stage of this project, clinician teachers select one or more teaching behaviors used personally or by a colleague and develop proficiency in using one or more new teaching strategies. This process includes observation, practice, and nonevaluative feedback. At this stage, the peers will become proficient at self-monitoring and set directions for further development, practice, and collaboration.

THE CASE REPORT

This case report reflects the perspectives of the physician as teacher and the faculty development educator/coach. Given that the project focuses on both teacher change and the collaborative process between the clinician teacher and the coach, an effort has been made to capture the richness of the interaction occurring between the two faculty members.

The clinician teacher and the coach met for the first time in 1986 while working on a faculty development training grant. The two were somewhat different. The clinician teacher was a physician and a fellow trained in research in family medicine. The coach was a nurse with a Ph.D. in curriculum and instruction with years of experience in education and nursing. The clinician teacher was an assistant professor who had been teaching in a residency program for 3 years. His interests included residency curricula, faculty development, and clinical instruction. For 5 years, the clinician teacher and the coach cotaught the monthly faculty development program at the community-based residency site and collaborated on a number of other educational and research activities. Through the years, they came to trust and respect each other. Both were dedicated to the improvement of teaching.

The clinician teacher and the coach had different areas of expertise and different expectations of the peer coaching process. The clinician teacher's interest rested with what was happening to his medical students and residents and the need to attend to his other duties as a practitioner and administrator. The coach's focus was on successfully implementing the peer coaching program. The coach adapted the peer coaching process from the general education setting to the clinical teaching context. She defined peer coaching as a systematic and deliberate approach to improving clinical instruction through studying the theoretical basis of instruction. Peer coaching involves observing multiple demonstrations of clinical teaching, practice with feedback, and coaching to provide companionship, analysis, and adaptation. Peer coaching requires parity in addressing the interests and expertise of both the coach and the clinician teacher. The coach encouraged the clinician teacher and the other peer coaches to participate in defining the goals, objectives, methods, and outcomes of the project.

The clinician teacher was interested in changing his teaching behavior and chose to focus on two microskills of clinical teaching— eliciting student questions and using and providing feedback. He read articles forwarded by the coach that included information and studies on the developmental levels of teachers, teaching routines, and the microskills of teaching that he selected for improvement. Videotape served as a mechanism for reviewing, both independently and with colleagues, the teaching behaviors the clinician teacher selected for improvement. The clinician teacher talked about his observations of himself on videotape as a part of a planned educational intervention with the coach. He also shared the tapes with other peer coaches in an effort to obtain their feedback. The coach focused on the clinician teacher's change in teaching behaviors and teaching practices. Her aim was to understand how the clinician teacher interpreted what he was doing when he was teaching, or the mental scripts he used related to teaching. This was accomplished by observing the cues received from the student, the environment, and/or the patient that either altered his routine response to the student, delayed it, or let it stay the same.

STAGES OF THE CLINICIAN TEACHER'S PROGRESS

STAGE ONE: A PROFILE OF THE CLINICIAN TEACHER

During the project's first year, a profile of the clinician teacher was obtained and included a Learning Style Inventory, the Myers-Briggs Type Indicator instrument, and a self-assessment of pedagogical expertise.

The Learning Style Inventory, which evaluates using a combination of a variety of learning behaviors, revealed that the clinician teacher's preferred style of learning was to learn abstractly and through hands-on experience. The Myers-Briggs Type Indicator instrument revealed that the clinician teacher was an extrovert who was intuitive; he employed feeling and perception in his day-to-day activities. Using the 14 assumptions of an expert pedagogue and the developmental levels (greenhorn, advanced beginner, proficient, expert) described by Berliner (1988), the clinician teacher rated his level of development in teaching as proficient. The clinician teacher's teaching practices, as he entered the peer coaching program, reflected a certain level of pedagogical expertise. He possessed significant subject matter knowledge in family medicine and significant years of experience in practice and teaching. He was comfortable with the clinical setting and seemed to have a rich fund of personal knowledge to draw upon.

Initially, the coach also observed the clinician teacher for 2 half-days and identified those behaviors that the physician teacher seemed to use most often and those behaviors that were used infrequently. For example, he rarely offered feedback to residents during the 2 half-days of observation.

STAGE TWO: CLINICIAN TEACHER'S
AWARENESS AND REFLECTIONS ON TEACHING

During the second stage of his teacher development, the clinician teacher participated in 3 half-day peer coaching workshops. Workshops focused on presenting the theoretical underpinnings of teaching, observation of teaching in the clinical setting, practice, and feedback. These workshops were followed by videotaped observations of the clinician teacher while teaching. Debriefing occurred after each clinical teaching encounter, during which the clinician teacher acknowledged sensitivity to certain teaching routines and behaviors and verbalized about his teaching practice in interface with the coach. The clinician teacher also viewed his videotapes with the coach and reflected on the behaviors he was trying to enhance. The coach focused on the clinical skills the clinician teacher chose to improve and the impact of those skills in producing the desired outcome of the teaching encounter.

The coach focused on the language and routines of teaching in a clinical setting using a process similar to that of practitioners in diagnosing and managing patients. It seemed comfortable to both parties. The clinician teacher began to work on the microskill of eliciting information from students. As he did, positive things began to happen. He described this in a conversation with the coach.

> We had a situation occur yesterday when I was being taped where the resident wanted to prescribe a certain antibiotic and I would have used a different one. I had to force myself to let the resident proceed with her treatment plan, which was okay, rather than imposing my preference in this situation. It is much easier to take control and direct the student to select the medication I prefer than it is to elicit information from the resident about her choice of antibiotic, especially when I would not choose the medication she selected. (Interview, June 9, 1992).

In the medical world, teacher-centered control is important. However, in teaching students and residents to become practitioners, it is important to note when to give up control or transfer control gradually until the resident as learner is independently capable of managing the patient safely. The more information clinician teachers can elicit from the student, the more comfortable they can be in transferring control.

One possible interpretation of changes in the clinician teacher's practice of teaching is that his ability to be critically reflective about his teaching behaviors and routines developed concurrently with the educational interventions introduced and practiced in the workshops. Structured questions related to the clinician teacher's selected microskills in relation to the outcomes of the encounter provided for reflection on what he was doing. Other contributing factors include the repeated videotaping sessions with debriefings, as well as the observations of peers.

The clinician teacher began sharing his experiences frequently with his coach. This text presents excerpts of his understanding of the changes he made in clinical teaching.

> As a student, I learned mostly from observation and reflection. I always searched for underlying concepts and principles. I was never very good at remembering isolated or unrelated bits of information. Over time, I developed a more active, hands-on learning style to compliment my abilities with observation and reflection. Now I like to observe, try things out, reflect, and get feedback. This learning style is very compatible with the peer coaching process which I have enjoyed and benefited from.
>
> My clinical teaching style had evolved from primarily facilitative in my early years to a more authoritative and expert style as I gained confidence in my clinical and teaching roles. I am naturally restless and cannot sit still for any length of time. I have an active, "busy," interventionist teaching style. I sometimes found myself talking too much and intervening too quickly. I was quick to give answers and often did not allow the learner adequate time to think or problem solve. While this may have been efficient and appropriate for some situations (and easier for me), I knew this style was not the most effective for promoting autonomy and responsibility in most learners. Furthermore, I was not happy with my ability to give and receive feedback. Finally, I did not feel adept at surfacing some of the emotional issues underlying many physician-patient and teacher-learner encounters.
>
> Coaching has helped me to redevelop a more facilitative teaching style by focusing on the micro-skills of eliciting questions, the use of "wait time," and providing time for learners to problem solve. I am continu-

ing to work on giving better feedback. I am becoming more comfortable with receiving feedback from my colleagues and want to learn to elicit more feedback from medical students and residents. I still need to work on becoming more comfortable with emotionally charged precepting encounters.

Sharing experiences with the coach and other clinician teachers represents an attempt to heighten awareness and sensitivity on the part of the physician teachers to the nature of teaching in the clinical setting. The focus is on teacher reflection and changes in teaching practice and teaching behaviors. The result provided for an oral dialogue between the clinician teacher and the coach. The following conversation is an example of how nonevaluative feedback can guide change in teaching behaviors and routines.

The clinician teacher and the coach met in the precepting room. The coach set the stage for the session by asking the clinician teacher, "what area of teaching do you wish to work on improving?" "I think I'd like to focus on 'wait time' and eliciting information from the resident as to what he/she learns." In past encounters, the clinician teacher has used questions to seek information from residents and then proceeded to answer his own questions without providing sufficient wait time. He is observing a second year resident on a videotape monitor as she works with a mother and her baby. After the resident leaves, the coach offers nonevaluative technical feedback. She notes the number of times the clinician teacher paused and waited for responses rather than offering information. The coach asks the clinician teacher for his perceptions regarding the wrap-up with the resident. The clinician teacher perceives that he did not jump in immediately and that he did provide wait time. He notes that the student seems more comfortable and that by waiting for the resident to give him the information, he was taking himself out of the expert role.

As the clinician teacher noted at the end of the first Project year:

This is a whole new way to get to know someone. And it is a humbling experience—you see yourself on tape and think, ["I could have done that better"]. We don't get many opportunities at such a personal level to engage in activities that will improve teaching. The peer coaching program has provided a new avenue for professional growth. This is one of the most exciting things that I am involved in. I am beginning to see some changes in the way I do things, and I recognize that this is a natural extension of what we do all the time—teaching patients and precepting residents one-on-one—only this program involves teaching the teacher one-on-one (i.e., precepting the preceptor). (Interview, June 14, 1992)

The physician teacher has begun to develop reflective teaching practice within a community of colleagues. As his repertoire of clinical teaching skills develops, both teacher and coach will begin to identify different models of teaching that can best be used in the ambulatory setting. Working with his peers, the clinician teacher hopes to facilitate the integration of peer coaching into his residency site.

DISCUSSION

The project described in this report breaks new ground in medical education and, halfway through the 3 years, has yielded some very interesting preliminary findings and work in progress:

1. All clinician teachers who have participated in the full complement of activities have affirmed the value of peer coaching as a viable tool for professional development. Due to problems of scheduling and professional demands, one dyad withdrew from the project.

2. Each clinician teacher has identified improvement in some aspect of his/her teaching and attributed gains to the project.

3. Uniformly, the participants report a heightened awareness of the importance of teaching. Several now view precepting as a teaching function rather than a supervisory activity.

4. Where peer coaching relationships were initially anxiety laden and distant, they have now become comfortable collegial interactions, which are both anticipated and welcomed.

5. Clinician teachers are demonstrating markedly greater willingness to guide students and residents through the decision-making process rather than making clinical decisions for them. There is notably greater tolerance for ambiguity on the part of the teacher, especially if patient safety is not in jeopardy.

6. Self-analysis of clinical teaching is becoming a routine, leading to shifts in individual teaching behavior to fit the situation of the moment.

7. Clinician teachers desire and seek feedback from students and residents regarding their teaching and its appropriateness and effectiveness.

8. Peer coaching is labor-intensive and time-consuming. The participants in this project feel that it is well worth the time and effort. They perceive long-term outcomes which are not generally apparent in short-term, quick-fix activities.

Several emerging outcomes need to be highlighted. Given that precepting is often viewed by physicians in practice as necessary and time consuming, all peer coaching participants have taken a different view as a result of participation in the project. They have reported that heretofore they would have viewed the preceptor role as that of supervisor to make sure that effective clinical practice was delivered, rather than viewing that role as a critical field-site teaching function for physicians in training.

It is also important to comment on the observed development of colleagueship around teaching roles and functions. Professionals outside the field of education per se more often than not tend to view the teaching function as something that they do because they are content experts transmitting knowledge. These six peer coaches see teaching as a developing, interacting process and, hence, are seeking ways for enhancement. In particular, they are experimenting with strategies to cause learners to take more active roles and greater responsibility for their own learning, to test assumptions if you will. These physician teachers are thus reflecting quite a different pattern from that normally observed in similar settings.

Unquestionably, approaches such as peer coaching are labor-intensive and time-consuming on the part of both trainers and trainees. Our experience to date suggests that the time commitment is worth the investment. Project peer teachers see teacher development as a continuous and on-going process of their professional life. They talk about continuity and longitudinal development as a part of their commitment to teaching. Implementing and managing a peer coaching (or any other teaching improvement) project is not without its problems. Demands on physician teachers are many and varied and their time is often not their own. Preceptor schedules and assignments make continuity with a particular resident or student difficult to achieve and maintain. Neither can one lose site of the fact that, in clinical teaching settings, patients drive the curriculum. Case presentations tend to include problems of diagnosis and treatment occurring in an unpredictable order or pattern. For these same reasons, mastery and refinement of a particular teaching skill is extraordinarily difficult. In spite of the many limitations, the intervention appears to work and those participating physicians report enthusiastically about their opportunities to focus on teaching.

At this point of analysis of the progress of the project, two of the three dyads remain intact and engaged. Of the two dyads, one is much more motivated and active. The second dyad paired a novice teacher, with less than 2 years of clinical teaching experience, with a more experienced teacher. This dyad took longer in its evolution to develop an effective working relationship. The third dyad consisted of a community practitioner and a senior faculty member who were not consistent and committed. Although this dyad attended workshops and participated in observation, the demands of a busy practice and administrative responsibilities precluded effective participation.

REFERENCES

Berliner, B. (1988, February). *The development of expertise in pedagogy.* Charles Hunt Memorial Lecture, presented at the meeting of the American Association of Colleges for Teacher Education, New Orleans, LA.

Daggett, C., Cassie, J. M., & Collins, G. F. (1979). Research on clinical teaching. *Review of Educational Research, 49,* 151-169.

Goldhammer, R., & Cogan, M. (1969). *Clinical supervision.* New York: Holt, Rinehart & Winston.

Hekelman, F. (1990). *An analysis of physicians' instructional behaviors in the family practice setting.* Unpublished doctoral dissertation, Kent State University, Ohio.

Hekelman, F., Vanek, G., Kelly, K., & Alemagno, S. (1993). Characteristics of family physicians' clinical teaching behaviors in the ambulatory setting. *Teaching and Learning in Medicine, 5,* 18-23.

Joyce, B., & Showers, B. (1980, February). Improving in-service training: The message of research. *Educational Leadership*, pp. 380-385.

Joyce, B., & Showers, B. (1982, October). The coaching of teaching. *Educational Leadership*, pp. 4-10.

Joyce, B., Weil, M., & Showers, B. (1992). *Models of teaching*. Needham Heights, MA: Allyn & Bacon.

Schon, E. (1987). *Educating the reflective practitioner*. San Francisco, CA: Jossey-Bass.

APPENDIX
Peer Coaching Self-Assessment Profile

Instructions: Based on David Berliner's five stages of development of pedagogical expertise, rate yourself on the 14 propositions of pedagogical-content knowledge expertise. Place a check in the appropriate box.

1. Novice—deliberate
2. Advanced Beginner—insightful
3. Competent Performer—rational
4. Proficient—intuitive
5. Expert—a-rational

Propositions regarding expertise in pedagogical-content knowledge	1 Novice	2 Advanced Beginner	3 Competent	4 Proficient	5 Expert	Comments (continue on back, if necessary)
I excel in the domain of teaching Family Medicine in the clinical setting						
I have well-practiced routines which I use when teaching in the clinical setting						
I am sensitive to social and contextual situations when teaching in the clinical setting						
I have a general plan when teaching in the clinical setting, but I am flexible and react to what the student is doing						

When teaching in the clinical setting, I analyze the problems and know where students are likely to go wrong in their thinking								
When teaching in the clinical setting, I focus on the important aspects of instruction in a given situation								
When teaching in the clinical setting, I am able to discern meaningful patterns in the teaching/learning encounter								
When solving teaching problems in the clinical setting, I feel I have a rich fund of personal knowledge and experience to draw upon								
When analyzing a teaching problem in the clinical setting, I find it easy to make predictions, assumptions, and hypotheses about the situation								
When teaching in the clinical setting, I pay attention to things that are about to go wrong for the student								
When teaching in the clinical setting, I find it easy to zero in on the critical aspects of an encounter								
When teaching in the clinical setting, I am comfortable trying a variety of different instructional strategies								
I am confident in my abilities as a teacher in the clinical setting and am comfortable with that role								

Interdisciplinary/
Multidisciplinary
Clinical Learning
Designs

Making Interdisciplinary Education Effective for Rehabilitation Students

Jan Perkins
Joyce Tryssenaar

ABSTRACT: Interdisciplinary education has been recommended as a way of preparing students for team practice after graduation. There is debate in the literature over the best way to implement interdisciplinary education sessions, and many factors can influence their effectiveness. This paper is a case description report of a pilot project developed to promote interdisciplinary learning. The Northern Studies Stream of McMaster University's School of Occupational Therapy and Physiotherapy in Ontario, Canada developed a project that combined students from the occupational therapy and physiotherapy programs for small group tutorials held during clinical placements. The project incorporated suggestions from the literature in order to encourage cooperation and interdisciplinary learning. Participants were mature, second-degree students with similar levels of clinical experience. The sessions were a required part of the academic course, but were ungraded. Tutorials focused on issues relevant to clinical practice for both groups and were facilitated by faculty from both professions. Evaluation was positive, suggesting student characteristics (eg, level of experience and maturity) and session design features that may be helpful in planning future interdisciplinary education experiences.

The presence of interdisciplinary teams in health care practice today is prevalent, and often required. This has evolved in part because no one person or discipline can have expertise in all the areas of specialty knowledge needed for high quality care of clients with complex disorders.[1,2] An interdisciplinary approach is particularly recommended when dealing with specific client populations with chronic and complex conditions, and with clients who traditionally have difficulty dealing with the health care system (eg, the elderly, and persons with mental illness or developmental disorders).[3-6] In addition to the possible positive effects on quality of care, a team approach has been proposed as a

Reprinted with permission from the *Journal of Allied Health*. Perkins J, Tryssenaar J. 1994;23:133-141.

means of improving treatment efficiency[7] and optimally meeting the health needs of the community.[8]

Although the theoretical rationale for interdisciplinary teams is generally accepted, the results in many cases do not live up to expectations.[9] There is considerable potential for dysfunction in a treatment team. Role conflicts often develop among different professional groups.[10-12] Laatsch, Milson, and Zimmer suggest that, in many cases, health professionals still do not function as cooperative members of a health care team and know surprisingly little about each other's professional roles.[13] These findings are not difficult to understand in light of the inherent conflict between the recognition that tasks must be shared, and the desire to protect a professional "turf."[14]

As practitioners and educators struggle with how to improve team functioning, a logical starting point has been to examine interdisciplinary education. Based on the hypothesis that students demonstrate in practice what they learn in the classroom, it seems reasonable to assume that interdisciplinary education would be one of the best ways to encourage interdisciplinary practice. The writings of Sommer, Silagy, and Rose support the belief that multidisciplinary education is a worthwhile means of improving the quality of interaction and level of cooperation between health professionals.[8]

The World Health Organization defines interdisciplinary education in the health sciences as:

> The process by which a group of students (or workers) from the health-related occupations with different educational backgrounds learn together during certain periods of their education, with interaction as an important goal, to collaborate in providing promotive, preventative, curative, rehabilitative, and other health-related services.[15]

It has been suggested that for successful interaction after graduation, health professionals should be educated in a manner that fosters such interdisciplinary collaboration.[16,17] Unfortunately, interdisciplinary education has often encountered problems that limit its acceptance and effectiveness.[9,14,18]

Considerable thought has gone into designing interdisciplinary educational encounters, and many suggestions have been made. Sommer, Silagy, and Rose have outlined the broad aims of interdisciplinary education as follows: to engender mutual respect among members of different professions; to improve the understanding of the need for teamwork and the methods to achieve teamwork; and to introduce the roles of different health care practitioners.[8] To meet the desired goals for team practice, educational experiences should be specifically designed to help students learn to work interdependently, while incorporating their feelings and knowledge about one another.[13] Content, timing, and group mix are also important factors to consider.

McKeil et al and Norman suggest that, in order to allow students the opportunity to first develop a professional identity, the best time to promote the team approach is in the senior portion of a professional program, or in continuing education after graduation.[17,19] A contrasting view is expressed by Kindig, who suggests interdisciplinary education occur early in a professional program in order to encourage interaction before professional identity becomes too rigid to allow shared territory. This can then be reinforced after clinical experience.[20] Blockstein argues for a clinical focus for interdisciplinary education, in continuing rather than basic education, so as to provide material relevant to practice. He also feels that in continuing education, students will be adult learners whose maturity and sense of security in their role will help make the education a success.[14] For interaction during basic education, Connelly suggests giving some academic credit, an opinion shared by Lynch, who indicates that using "add on" sessions can diminish the apparent importance of interdisciplinary education,[21,22] and send the message that interdisciplinary education is not important enough to be included in the regular curriculum.

PROJECT

Background

The School of Occupational Therapy and Physiotherapy is a program within the larger Faculty of Health Sciences at McMaster University, Hamilton, Ontario. As evidenced by their mission statement, the Faculty of Health Sciences places considerable emphasis on interdisciplinary collaboration:

> We are a Faculty of Health Sciences characterized by interdisciplinary, interprofessional, interfaculty, and interinstitutional cooperation, working to achieve our goals of excellence in education, research, and service. . . . We value and will actively encourage collaboration among individuals and groups within the Faculty and beyond to achieve common goals.

Also included is a component directed towards education:

> Central to our mission is the preparation of health professionals and scientists who can contribute to humane and cost-efficient health care, continue independent and efficient learning, adapt to change and initiate change, and collaborate within interdisciplinary teams.

One can see that these philosophical tenets direct and support interdisciplinary education. Satin identifies such support as a key factor for success, and suggests making interdisciplinary education a primary program goal on a par with other major educational goals.[23]

Within the Faculty of Health Sciences, academic events are planned to facilitate interdisciplinary education. These include half-day to two-day workshops on gender issues, sexuality, and palliative care; a shared orientation for students; and a community health day. These involve all health sciences schools and departments and, whenever possible, follow principles of problem-based learning within small groups made up of students from several disciplines. While attendance is required, it should be noted that these are added to the regular course of study for each discipline, rather than an integral part of the academic course. As indicated in the literature, these "add on" efforts may not be the most effective way of promoting interaction.

The School of Occupational Therapy and Physiotherapy has additional opportunities for shared education in the regular curricula, as both programs follow the same academic schedule. Courses are organized in a block (or unit) system, with each unit containing a problem-based tutorial course, a seminar course, and a clinical skills laboratory course. After the second unit of the program, students start clinical practice at the end of each unit, with the problem-based tutorials continued, though less freqently, during clinical practice. Interdisciplinary learning occurs in an inquiry seminar course offered in the introductory unit of the programs, and in all courses in the final academic unit required for completion of the occupational therapy and physiotherapy programs, which includes material on management and professional issues relevant to both groups.

This paper describes a case study of a pilot project specifically designed to promote interdisciplinary contact for occupational therapy and physiotherapy students. Students completing clinical practicums typically meet in small-group tutorials to discuss cases and concerns related to their clinical work. Those students who participated in a satellite Northern Studies Stream (NSS) of the main program were placed in interdisciplinary groups for these tutorials, with tutoring shared by faculty from both professions.

Assumptions

Tutorials were developed using information from the literature, and previous experience of the faculty. Several assumptions were inherent in structuring and setting goals for the tutorials. It was assumed that combining professionals from several disciplines results in more highly integrated client care,[12,17] that chronic and complex health care problems benefit from coordinated interdisciplinary team care,[5] and that learning together will prepare health professions students for successful future interdisciplinary team practice.[8,11,16,24]

One of the goals of the interdisciplinary tutorials was to facilitate future professional interaction, and another was to provide the opportunity for students to translate knowledge regarding interdisciplinary care into action through practice in a safe environment. The timing was an important consideration. Faculty felt that the educational experience would be more effective if students first had some understanding of their own professional role and discipline, and in particular would be improved by students having had some experience working with clients. On the other hand, it was assumed that delaying interdisciplinary interaction until after graduation might compromise the health professional's initial effectiveness as a member of a health care team.

Sitting together in a lecture class or discussing a philosophical issue in a classroom setting was felt to be less effective than discussing a case presentation or real life health care problems.[17,25] Additional support for this approach comes from Shepard et al who emphasize that real or simulated clinical and nonclinical experiences are necessary to develop students' understanding of both the consumer's identification of his or her own health care needs, and the roles and responsibilities of other team members.[26] In addition, the authors share Lynch's contention that learning that is integrated into the core curriculum of a program will more effectively model and encourage interdisciplinary education than supplementary sessions.[22]

A final assumption, also supported by Shepard, is the belief that faculty from all professions represented by the students need to be active role models in the learning environment. For this reason, contrary to the usual tutorial group practice in which one tutor is responsible for the group, tutoring of each group was shared by faculty from each of the professions.[26]

MODEL

For this interaction, tutors used the practice model of Ivey et al which describes an increase in shared expertise, and a decrease in professional autonomy along a continuum from parallel practice to a full interdisciplinary team approach.[5] Their model allows flexibility, because for any given situation, a different point on the continuum may represent optimal practice. Physiotherapy and occupational therapy have areas of practice which overlap, and, thus, a model emphasizing the sharing of knowledge became a logical choice.

METHOD

The NSS physiotherapy and occupational therapy students involved were all second-year students doing a six-week clinical practicum in northwestern Ontario. The students have regular tutorials with a faculty member during their clinical practice. These tutorials may be held weekly or, at the discretion of faculty and students, longer tutorials may be held biweekly. At the time of writing, the interdisciplinary tutorials had been completed with one tutorial group of students each year for the past two years.

Usual tutorial group size in the program is six students and one tutor. Because the number of students participating in the NSS program varied, the tutorial group size each year also varied. In the first year, the tutorial group involved three occupational therapy and two physiotherapy students, and in the second year, the group included six occupational therapy and three physiotherapy students. The tutoring was shared both years by faculty members from each profession. The occupational therapy students were working with adult clients, primarily in the areas of gerontology and neurology. The physiotherapy students were seeing clients with neurological conditions. Some clients were seen by students from both professions, either in the same facility, or as clients were transferred between facilities.

The NSS has a specific objective to expose all participating students to issues relevant to rural or remote practice. In departments that are small or located in rural settings, practicing therapists must be generalists in their own discipline, have flexibility in their practice role, and appreciate the value of contributions from other health care team members. The NSS faculty felt that an interdisciplinary approach to the clinical tutorials could enhance student preparedness for rural practice. They therefore expected the NSS students to share experiences that reflected the unique features of practice in each of the very different settings of northwestern Ontario.

In addition to the general NSS objectives, each tutorial group generated their own learning objectives. The first year group developed the specific objective to learn more about the other profession's role. They elected to use time to discuss specific case management strategies with a view to improving their own treatment of clients, and of learning how to harmonize overall client care within a team. Additional, more specific objectives dealt with such matters as improving abilities to write medical charting, and assessment and treatment techniques of use to both groups.

The second year group differed from the first in that it included two students completing practicums in outlying communities. They were linked to the main group by audio teleconferencing. This group also developed their own learning objectives to supplement those provided by the NSS, which included learning about each other's facilities and client profiles, learning to appreciate the other discipline's role, making case presentations involving treatment issues for both professions, and discussing academic assignments that students were completing during their clinical practice.

Evaluation of individual and group performance was done within the tutorial group. Brief feedback on interaction, applicability of the content, group process, and usefulness of the tutorials was encouraged in each session, with more detailed evaluation in a focus discussion, facilitated by the faculty tutor, during the final session. For the participating students, this was the fifth unit in which they had tutorial group learning, and they were experienced and comfortable with the open and frank evaluation process. Particular attention was given during evaluation and additional focus discussion to the interdisciplinary aspects of the tutorials. As stated earlier, the clinical tutorials were an academic requirement without an academic grade, so no formal marks were given.

RESULTS

Both groups of students reacted positively to the tutorials. The students and the faculty tutors were surprised to find that the occupational therapy and physiotherapy students had an incomplete understanding of the other profession's role, even when dealing with similar client populations, despite shared classroom seminars at the beginning of the program. All of the students reported that the interaction helped increase their awareness of the other profession and encouraged collaboration. This was particularly useful for them at a time when they were doing clinical work in interdisciplinary teams.

The case presentations and resultant discussions developed broader pictures of clients' situations than might have occurred in unmixed groups. Students were often surprised and somewhat chagrined to realize the extent to which their treatment focus had left them unaware of the broader picture. Some students were able to coordinate treatments for individual clients as a result of their tutorial discussions.

With regard to the setting for the interdisciplinary interaction, the students felt the clinical tutorials were a useful place to interact with the other discipline, as discussion could be linked to real world situations. They also preferred to have the opportunity to share tutorials without the pressure of grading. This allowed them to become accustomed to the interaction in a relaxed atmosphere, and they thought the experience would be valuable for the final academic unit, which is completely interdisciplinary.

The teleconference tutorials in the second year added another dimension and reinforced the cooperative atmosphere. Teleconferencing requires an organized group structure, thoughtfulness, and awareness of presentation skills. When done well, this encourages the development of a cooperative group structure. On the other hand, while the group has the potential to work efficiently with teleconferencing, the interaction may become less fluid. Tutors approached the experience with the aim of using the medium to enhance student learning of interactive communication skills. With this positive approach, rather than considering the teleconferencing a necessary compromise, the students found the level of interaction could be maintained, and the interdisciplinary aspect of the experience was unchanged.

DISCUSSION

Several factors contributed to the success of the NSS tutorial experiences, which have implications for future interdisciplinary sessions. The students all had a previous undergraduate degree, and were generally mature adult learners. The professions involved had areas of overlap, and students were at the same level of academic and clinical experience. This may have eased the process of developing a cohesive group. It was, of course, also important that the educators involved shared a belief in the value of interdisciplinary education in the educational process.

The interdisciplinary tutorials were used with students at a stage in their learning in which they were comfortable with their own professional roles and able to tolerate discussion and critical appraisal from another discipline, but before their perception of professional roles became rigid. This timing permitted sharing without arousing concerns over professional turf. The tutorials were a part of academic requirements, with the implicit message that they were considered important, but without pressure to compete for academic grades.

The use of real case presentations placed the client at the center of the process, and encouraged integration of academic and clinical knowledge. These clinical discussions imitated the structure of interdisciplinary teams the students will encounter in their professional careers, and open discussion in this setting diluted professional insularity. Management suggestions generated in the tutorials helped streamline the students' service delivery, while reinforcing the main issue of care of the client.

The NSS tutorials have demonstrated the potential for including meaningful interprofessional education in a health professions program. Students appreciated the experience and felt that they had gained valuable insight into another professional area of practice. These shared sessions encouraged occupational therapy and physiotherapy students to develop an interdisciplinary team perspective prior to graduation, and hopefully will assist in the transition from student to professional. Although successful team approaches to health care suggest that professionals educated in traditional discipline-specific programs can and do work well together, expanding undergraduate education to include interdisciplinary experiences may facilitate this method of service delivery.

REFERENCES

1. Halstead LS. Team care in chronic illness: a critical review of the literature of the past 25 years. *Arch Phys Med Rehabil.* 1976;57(11):507-511.
2. Hutt A. Shared learning for shared care. *J Adv Nurs.* 1980;5(4):389-396.
3. Bachrach LL. The legacy of model programs. *Hosp Community Psychiatry.* 1989;40(3):234-235.
4. Helm PA, Kevorkian CG, Lushbaugh M, Pullium C, Head MD, Cromes GF. Burn injury: rehabilitation management in 1982. *Arch Phys Med Rehabil.* 1982; 63(1):6-15.
5. Ivey SL, Brown KS, Teske Y, Silverman D. A model for teaching about interdisciplinary practice in health care settings. *J Allied Health.* 1988;17(3):189-195.
6. Runciman P. Health assessment of the elderly at home: the case for shared learning. *J Adv Nurs.* 1989;14(2):111-119.
7. Infante MS, Speranza KA, Gillespie PW. An interdisciplinary approach to the education of health professional students. *J Allied Health.* 1976;5(4):13-22.
8. Sommer SJ, Silagy CA, Rose AT. The teaching of interdisciplinary education. *Med J Aust.* 1986;157(1):31,34,36-37.
9. Satin DG. The future of geriatric and interdisciplinary education. *Educ Gerontol.* 1986;12(6):549-561.
10. Hannay DR. Problems of role identification and conflict in multidisciplinary teams. In: Barber JH, Kratz CR, eds. *Towards Team Care.* Edinburgh, Scotland: Churchill Livingstone; 1980:3-17.
11. Canadian Association of Occupational Therapists. *Position Paper on Role Overlap Between Occupational Therapists and Other Health Professions.* Toronto, Canada: CAOT Publications; 1989.
12. Welch Cline RJ. Small group communication in health care. In: Ray EB, Donohew

L, eds. *Communication and Health: Systems and Applications.* Hillsdale, NJ: Lawrence Erlbaum Associates; 1990.

13. Laatsch LJ, Milson LM. Zimmer SE. Use of interdisciplinary education to foster familiarization among health professionals. *J Allied Health.* 1986;13(1):33-42.

14. Blockstein WL. Interdisciplinary continuing education. *Mobius.* 1983;3(3):60-75.

15. *Learning Together to Work Together for Health.* Geneva, Switzerland: World Health Organization; 1988. Tech Rep Series 769.

16. Brown M. Interdisciplinary teaching provides allied health students a new look at health information management professionals. *JAHIMA.* 1992;63(11):50-53.

17. McKiel RE, Lockyer J, Pechiulis DD. A model of continuing education for conjoint practice. *J Continuing Educ Nurs.* 1988;19(2):65-67.

18. McPherson C, Wittemann JK, Hasbrouck CS. An interdisciplinary team approach to development of health professions education. *J Allied Health.* 1984;13(2):94-103.

19. Norman G. Interdisciplinary education—rhetoric, reality and research. *Pedagogue.* 1991;3(3):2. (Available from McMaster University, Hamilton, Ontario, Canada.)

20. Kindig DA. Interdisciplinary education development for primary health care team delivery. *J Med Educ.* 1975;50(pt2):97-110.

21. Connelly T Jr. Basic organizational considerations for interdisciplinary education development in the health sciences. *J Allied Health.* 1978;7(4):274-280.

22. Lynch BL. Cooperative learning in interdisciplinary education for the allied health professions. *J Allied Health.* 1984;13(2):83-93.

23. Satin DG. The difficulties of interdisciplinary education: lessons from three failures and a success. *Educ Gerontol.* 1987;13(1):53-69.

24. Madsen MK, Gresch AM, Petterson BJ, Taugher MP. An interdisciplinary clinic for neurogenically impaired adults: a pilot project for educating students. *J Allied Health.* 1988;17(2):135-141.

25. Byrne C. Interdisciplinary education in undergraduate health sciences. *Pedagogue.* 1991;3(3):1,3-8. (Available from McMaster University, Hamilton, Ontario, Canada.)

26. Shepard K, Yeo G, McGann L. Successful components of interdisciplinary education. *J Allied Health.* 1985;14(3):297-303.

Appreciation is expressed to Erica Snippe-Juurakko and Erica Seely for their assistance with this project.

Jan Perkins, MSc, and Joyce Tryssenaar, MEd, BSc, OT, are both assistant professors, School of Occupational Therapy and Physiotherapy, Faculty of Health Sciences, McMaster University, Northern Studies Stream, Lakehead University, Thunder Bay, Ontario, Canada P7B 5E1.

Teaching the Multidisciplinary Team Approach in a Geriatrics Miniresidency

J. EDWARD JACKSON, M.D., WIGBERT WIEDERHOLT, M.D., and
ROBERT KATZMAN, M.D.

Abstract—The miniresidency program in geriatrics begun in 1985 at the University of California, San Diego, School of Medicine acquaints practicing health professionals with a multidisciplinary team approach to the care of geriatric patients. The two-week program features participation in a multidisciplinary outpatient clinic, home visits, social work and nutrition consultations, and conferences with patients and families. Miniresidency members also participate in neurologic and neuropsychological evaluations and attend day care for demented adults. The 71 health professionals who completed the program during its first 20 months showed significant improvement on their scores between the pre- and posttests: the mean of all scores in the pretest was 51 out of a possible 80 (SD 15); the mean of all scores in the posttest was 75 out of a possible 80 (SD 4); $p < .001$. The 77% who returned post-program evaluation questionnaires found the program "useful" or "very useful." *Acad. Med.* 65 (1990):417–419.

The multidisciplinary team approach is increasingly recognized as useful and cost-effective in caring for elderly patients.[1-4] This is particularly true for the frail elderly and for patients with dementing illnesses, who have a disproportionate share of social, economic, and functional problems in addition to the traditional medical problems that physicians are trained to manage.

Although multidisciplinary geriatrics teams are increasingly common, the authors have been unable to find reports of any program specifically designed to teach the multidisciplinary team process to practicing health professionals.

The authors started a miniresidency program in geriatrics at the University of California, San Diego (UCSD), School of Medicine. This article describes the program and reports the authors' observations of its effectiveness.

Dr. Jackson is assistant clinical professor, Division of General Internal Medicine/Geriatrics, Department of Medicine; Dr. Katzman is professor and chair, Department of Neurosciences; and Dr. Wiederholt is professor, Department of Neurosciences; all at the University of California, San Diego, School of Medicine.

Correspondence and requests for reprints should be addressed to Dr. Jackson, UCSD Medical Center, H-811-E, 225 Dickinson Street, San Diego, CA 92103.

Other articles about geriatrics training appear on pages 382, 412, and 414.

Method

The overall objective of the miniresidency is to familiarize health professionals with a multidisciplinary team approach focusing on the patients' functional status. Special attention is given to the diagnosis and care of the demented patient.

To participate effectively in the multidisciplinary team process, the miniresidency participants must have some knowledge of the skills, limitations, and roles of all team members. While this requires that each participant possess certain basic knowledge, it is not expected that an individual will acquire all of the knowledge and skills used by team members from other disciplines. The specific educational objectives for the miniresidency are available from the authors.

The authors believe that interaction with actual patients and their problems will produce more lasting improvements in knowledge, attitudes, and behavior than would simple lecture-centered sessions. Instruction is primarily in the form of clinical preceptorships, directed reading, and tutorial sessions with program faculty. Involvement with a variety of health professionals, in a multidisciplinary team, forms the core educational experience.

The miniresidency is centered around the Seniors Only CARE (SOCARE) multidisciplinary geriatric outpatient clinic. The SOCARE team includes faculty from the departments of internal medicine, psychiatry, neurosciences, nursing, social work, nutrition, and occupational therapy at UCSD. Patients' problems are discussed from many perspectives at weekly team rounds, as well as informally among team members. In evaluating demented patients, the SOCARE team works closely with neurologists and neuropsychologists from the Alzheimer's Disease Research Center (ADRC) at UCSD, functioning as one of six State of California Alzheimer's Disease Diagnostic and Treatment Centers.

The miniresidency is a full-time, two-week-long program. Participants attend team-care rounds, geriatrics, medicine, psychiatry, and neurology clinics, social work sessions, psychometric testing sessions, and occupational therapy sessions; they also accompany a nurse practitioner on home evaluation visits and participate in day care activities for demented patients at the Alzheimer's Family Center. Tutorial sessions with the program director, and with the team member from the participant's own field, help put these diverse experiences into a practical perspective.

For this study, pretests and posttests of the program were used to assess the participants' knowledge of geriatrics. The pretest helped identify areas of weakness and strength for the participants. Statistical comparisons between pretest and posttest scores were performed using Stu-

Table 1

Mean Scores Achieved by 71 Health Professionals on Each Component of Tests Given before and after Completion of a Miniresidency in Geriatrics, University of California, San Diego, School of Medicine, 1985 – 1988*

Test Component	Maximum Possible Score	Pretest Score		Posttest Score		
		Mean	SD	Mean	SD	% Change†
General geriatrics	50	33	6.98	48	2.38	+44
Dementia	25	15	4.59	22	2.65	+49
Drug use	25	14	5.29	23	1.60	+64
Nursing	35	26	4.64	33	2.09	+27
Home evaluation	20	16	2.22	19	0.96	+20
Social work	25	19	3.14	23	1.88	+21
Mean of all scores	80	51	15.2	75	4.03	+48

*The authors established a miniresidency in geriatrics in 1985 to familiarize health professionals with a miniresidency team approach focusing on the patients' functional status. To investigate the effectiveness of the program, the 71 professionals who had completed the miniresidency through June 1988 were given tests before and after the program on a variety of geriatrics topics.

†Comparisons between the pre- and posttest scores were performed using Student's paired t-test with the Boniferroni corrections.

dent's t-test for paired data with the Boniferroni correction.[5]

Six months after completion of the program, a questionnaire was mailed to all participants regarding their current clinical geriatrics activities, as well as their assessments of the miniresidency and its various components.

The health professionals studied in this investigation were all those who completed the miniresidency in geriatrics from the program's beginning in April 1985 through June 1988. The majority of these came from the fields of nursing (35%), medicine (27%), social work (20%), and psychology (13%); some were from more than one field. Across these groups, 39% were educators. The participants came from California (66%), other states (24%), and other nations (10%).

Results

All participants showed improvement in their knowledge of clinical geriatrics (see Table 1).

All participants expressed satisfaction with the program. Postprogram questionnaires were returned by 37 of the 48 participants (77%) to whom they were mailed. Seventy-three % (27 of 37) rated the program "very useful," while 27% (10 of 37) rated the program "useful," on a five-point Likert-type scale ranging from "not useful" to "very useful." All the participants continued to be active in geriatrics, in clinical, educational,

research, and/or administrative activities.

The most consistent benefits perceived were (1) an improvement of specific knowledge both about dementia — its diagnosis and global impacts on patient family and society — and about drug use in older patients; (2) an understanding of the multidisciplinary team process and its importance in caring for elderly patients. All the participants indicated that they would recommend the miniresidency to their colleagues. Home evaluations, SOCARE team rounds, SOCARE clinics, and the research neurology clinics were the most highly appreciated components of the miniresidency. Participants felt uniformly that a two-week program was preferable to a one-week program in allowing them to assimilate and organize the large amount of material covered during the miniresidency. At present, the authors are aware of four comprehensive geriatrics assessment clinics that have been started by miniresidency participants.

Discussion

The UCSD miniresidency in geriatrics has been, and continues to be, effective in its overall goal of familiarizing practicing health professionals with the multidisciplinary team approach to the care of geriatric patients. Pretest scores indicated that the participants had room for substantial improvement in their knowl-

edge of geriatrics, despite prior interest and active involvement in geriatrics.

Substantial, significant increases in all areas of geriatrics knowledge were demonstrated between the pre- and posttests. The largest improvements were seen in the participants' knowledge areas of dementia and drug use, reflecting both the relative weakness of the typical practitioner's knowledge as well as the specific research and clinical interests of program faculty.

This type of intensive, full-time clinical preceptorship is a practical approach to educating practicing health professionals in the multidisciplinary team approach geriatrics care. It is difficult to envision how a series of lectures or workshops could convey nearly as meaningful a sense of the process of the multidisciplinary geriatrics care team. Similarly, there is no substitute for contact with actual patients to bring home to participants the clinical problems in the care of the frail and demented elderly. Active participation in the team process and tutorials with faculty are crucial to developing an understanding of the multidisciplinary geriatrics care team.

The miniresidency is a successful mode for updating and increasing the knowledge and improving the skills of practicing health professionals. This process is particularly important for the care of the elderly, where both basic science and clinical practice are rapidly advancing. In addition, the miniresidency is an excellent way for health professionals who do not have clinical backgrounds (for example, researchers in neurosciences, epidemiologists, program administrators) to learn about the realities of geriatrics care. Because most multidisciplinary geriatrics care teams function in a manner fairly similar to the one described here, the UCSD miniresidency experience should be generalizable to other centers.

This work was supported in part by the University of California, San Diego, Academic Geriatrics Resource Program; the National Institute on Aging Alzheimer's Disease Research Grant AG-05131; and State of California Alzheimer's Disease Diagnostic and Treatment Center Grant.

The authors gratefully acknowledge the many members of the UCSD Seniors Only CARE team, UCSD Alzheimer's Disease Research Center, and Alzheimer's Family Center who made this program possible. They appreciate the special assistance of Ms. Valerie Krikes in the preparation of the manuscript.

References

1. Williams, T. F. Comprehensive Functional Assessment: An Overview. *J. Am. Geriatr. Soc.* **31**(1983):637–641.

2. Calkins, E. OARS Methodology and the "Medical Model." *J. Am. Geriatr. Soc.* **33**(1985):648–649.

3. Ernst, N. S. Interdisciplinary Team Approach to Geriatric Care. In *The Aged Patient, A Sourcebook for the Allied Health Professional*, N. S. Ernst and H. R. Glazer-Waldman, eds., pp. 3–11. Chicago, Illinois: Year Book Medical Publishers, 1983.

4. Charatan, F. B., Foley, C. J., and Libow L. S. The Team Approach to Geriatric Medicine. In *Principles of Geriatric Medicine.* R. Andres, E. L. Bierman, and W. R. Hazzard, eds., pp. 169–175. New York: McGraw-Hill, 1985.

5. Box, G. E. P., Hunter, W. G., and Hunter, J. S. *Statics for Experimenters.* New York: John Wiley & Sons, 1978, pp. 107–123.

Network Cooperative Clinical Learning Designs

Innovative Models of Student Supervision in a Home Care Setting: A Pilot Project

Patricia Solomon, MHSc, PT
Julie Sanford, MSc, PT

ABSTRACT: Physical therapy students require exposure to community and home care clinical placements to prepare them adequately for future practice trends. Alternative models of student supervision can maximize the use of a clinical education site. This pilot project examined the productivity, suitability, and feasibility of two models of student supervision in a home care setting. A collaborative model, where one clinical instructor supervised two students, had some disadvantages when implemented with junior-level students. A sharing model of supervision, where two clinical instructors supervised one student part-time, had organizational and educational advantages in a home care setting.

INTRODUCTION

The transition from institutional to community care remains a challenge to the health care system. Home care, in particular, is one of the most rapidly growing fields within health care.[1] An increasing number of reports suggest that home care is an efficacious model for health care delivery.[1-3]

Home care is "the provision of equipment and services to the patient in the home for the purpose of restoring and maintaining his or her maximal level of comfort, function, and health."[1(p124)] A more complete and accurate identification of patient problems is made by health care professionals in a non-institutionalized setting where patients can be directly observed operating in their own environment.[3] The home setting may be the most appropriate place for teaching health care professionals about the influence of social, psychological, and environmental factors of disease.[2]

Physical therapists gain unique practice skills in a home care setting. Opportunities to use wellness and prevention models of practice may be infrequent in acute care institutions. Common medical problems such as ageism; ethical issues dealing with death and dying; and the social, psychological, epidemiological, and environmental aspects of maintaining health are not as evident in an acute care, disease-oriented setting.[1,2]

Students who treat patients in the home suddenly realize the full impact of patient problems[2] and become aware that a more holistic approach to care is required.[4] Students must be adequately prepared to understand how assessment, treatment, and evaluation skills can be adapted to home care environments.[1,5,6] Given the direction of health care, it seems reasonable to require physical therapy students to have a clinical education experience in the home environment.

One limitation to increasing the number of students exposed to home care is the apprenticeship model of supervision, where one therapist supervises one student. Models with more than one student per therapist have not been popular with clinical instructors. Supervisory models must maximize the use of a facility as a clinical education site.

Supervisory models where students are supervised by more than one therapist also are not widely reported. A requirement of one clinical instructor per student limits the bank of available supervisors, particularly in full-time affiliations, because therapists who are employed part time are not utilized. Because therapists in home care spend a large proportion of their time traveling, organization and communication between multiple supervisors could be complex, making this model impractical.

Little has been written in the physical therapy literature about alternative models of student supervision, although the need for further study has been identified.[7] Use of alternative models of supervision in the home would expose more students to home care. Models where clinical instructors supervise two or more students simultaneously would allow many more students to practice home care than would a traditional apprenticeship model of supervision. Successful adoption of a model that uses more than one clinical instructor per student would allow more part-time staff to be clinical supervisors. The objectives of this pilot project were to assess the suitability, feasibility, and productivity of two models of student supervision in a home care setting.

METHOD

Supervisory Models

Two models of supervision were evaluated concurrently during two 4-week, full-time clinical placements. The Mohawk-McMaster physiotherapy program uses a block system of integrated academic and clinical study within the curriculum. Two months of academic study precede 1 month of clinical study in the same content area. The pilot project occurred during the clinical components of two consecutive blocks of study. In the first block, students gain experience with various simple musculoskeletal problems. In the second block, expectations for student performance are increased, but the caseload of patients with musculoskeletal problems is the same. Students were undergraduates in the second year of a 3-year program. They were considered junior-level students because their previous clinical experience was limited to one part-time, 4-week placement.

Model 1 (the *collaborative* model) consisted of placing two students with one clinical instructor. Model 2 (the *sharing* model) consisted of placing one student with two clinical instructors, so that each therapist supervised the student part time. In the sharing model, the student was with one clinical instructor 2 days per week and with another clinical instructor 3 days per week.

Six therapists volunteered to be clinical instructors during the pilot project. Six students were randomly chosen from a class of 26 and gave consent to participate in the project in the clinical component of the block. In each block, two students were assigned to the collaborative model and one student was assigned to the sharing model. A total of four

Ms Solomon is Assistant Professor, School of Occupational Therapy and Physiotherapy, Faculty of Health Sciences, Mohawk College/Chedoke Campus, McMaster University, Sanatorium Road, Hamilton, Ontario, Canada L8N 3T2. Ms Sanford is Assistant Professor, School of Occupational Therapy and Physiotherapy, McMaster University, and Research Coordinator, Physiotherapy Department, St. Peter's Hospital, Hamilton, Ontario, Canada.

Reprinted with permission from the *Journal of Physical Therapy Education*, Vol 7, No 2, pp 49-52, 1993.

students and two clinical instructors participated in the collaborative model. and two students and four clinical instructors participated in the sharing model.

Outcome Measures

Questionnaires were designed to be completed post-placement by students and clinical instructors. The questionnaires assessed the following dimensions:

1. The effect of the supervisory model on student and therapist satisfaction. A 7-point scale measured the intensity of the therapists' and students' levels of satisfaction. A score of 1 represented "extremely dissatisfied," and a score of 7 represented "extremely satisfied."

2. Advantages and disadvantages of the home care placement from student and supervisor perspectives. To generate criteria that contribute to a satisfying clinical education experience. 26 senior-level students from the Mohawk-McMaster physiotherapy program were asked to list conditions that contributed to a satisfactory or unsatisfactory clinical experience. These conditions were formulated into statements. Students in the pilot project were asked to indicate which, if any, of the statements applied to their home care placement.

A similar process was used to develop criteria for the clinical instructors. Six experienced clinical instructors were asked to generate criteria that contribute to the quality of their experience as an educator. Therapists participating in the study were then asked to indicate which of these they had experienced during the placements.

3. Students' perception of the degree of difficulty required to meet their educational objectives. A 7-point scale ranging from 1 (extremely difficult) to 7 (extremely easy) measured the intensity of the students' perceived difficulty.

4. The effect of supervising students on the productivity of the clinical instructor. Home care managers gathered information on each therapist to determine the mean number of patient treatments per day by month as an index of productivity. This information was gathered for the six therapists participating in the project for three months prior to the start of the placements. The mean number of daily patient visits for the 3-month period during which the therapists did not supervise students was compared with the mean for the month during which the therapists were involved in clinical education.

Both questionnaires were pretested for face validity and comprehension by senior-level students or supervising therapists.

5. Students completed open-ended questions about the learning experiences gained in the home care placement and the positive and negative aspects of their experience.

Further qualitative data were gathered from the clinical instructors after the placements. Each clinical instructor participated in a standardized interview to explore the supervisory strategies used during the placement.

RESULTS
Satisfaction

Students. The mean of all students' ratings of satisfaction with the educational experience was 6.4, indicating a high overall rating of home care as a satisfying learning experience. Three of the four students in the collaborative model ranked the placement as 7 (extremely satisfying). The fourth student in the collaborative model ranked the placement as 5 (slightly satisfying). This student stated that the limited number of patients treated influenced his satisfaction with the placement. Both students participating in the sharing model ranked the placement as 6 (moderately satisfying).

Clinical instructors. The mean global rating of the clinical instructors' satisfaction with the placement was 6.16. slightly less than the students' rating. One of the two clinical instructors participating in the collaborative model ranked the placement as 4 (satisfying). The other clinical instructor ranked the placement as 7 (extremely satisfying). All four clinical instructors participating in the sharing model rated their satisfaction with the placement as 6 or 7, indicating moderate to extreme satisfaction.

Advantages and Disadvantages

Students. All four students in the collaborative model stated that using the other student as a resource and to provide additional feedback was an advantage. Two students used each other to practice techniques and found this to be beneficial. One student stated that observing another student's treatment style was an advantage. None of the potential disadvantages, such as the supervisor comparing the two students or insufficient time for feedback. were experienced by the students.

We examined students' answers to the open-ended question about positive and negative aspects of the placement. Students in the collaborative model identified decreased variety and number of patients in their caseload as disadvantages of the model. These

were the only negative aspects directly attributed to the model of supervision.

The two students in the sharing model stated that it was particularly beneficial having two clinical instructors because this relieved the stress of spending extended time with one individual. Both students in this model felt that it was valuable to experience different therapist styles of patient assessment and treatment.

Clinical instructors. Both clinical instructors in the collaborative model stated that constant supervision of two students was stressful. One clinical instructor divided her caseload into two parts and, subsequently, each student had only three patients per day. She felt that this limitation in caseload number was a major disadvantage of the collaborative model. This limitation was not experienced by the other clinical instructor in the collaborative model. Both instructors in the collaborative model found that the students used each other as resources and that this relieved some supervisory responsibility.

Clinical instructors in the sharing model enjoyed the opportunity to complete some of their daily activities without the student present. Therapists treating patients whose presenting problem was not musculoskeletal in origin or patients with complex conditions could do so when the student was with the other clinical instructor. This model of supervision necessitates additional time for clinical instructors to meet to evaluate the student and for ongoing communication about the student's status. This time, however, was not documented as a disadvantage.

All clinical instructors felt that good academic preparation, the student's ability to self-evaluate. and the fact that being involved in clinical education contributed to their learning, contributed to a positive clinical placement. These criteria are independent of the model of supervision.

Difficulty Achieving Objectives

Students reported difficulty achieving their educational objectives. The mean rating for all students was 3.1 on the 7-point scale. The mean rating of the degree of difficulty for students in the sharing model was 2.5, compared with a mean rating of 3.0 for students in the collaborative model.

Productivity

The therapists mean number of patient visits per day during student placements was compared with their mean number of visits per day for the three months prior to the students arrival. The productivity of therapists involved in the collaborative model increased from a mean of 5.28 patients per day to a mean of 6.8 patients per day. A reverse trend was experienced by the clinical instructors involved in the sharing model.

The mean number of patient visits per day decreased from a mean of 6.18 to 5.46.

DISCUSSION

If implemented correctly, the collaborative model has several educational advantages. Students can problem solve together, use each other as resources, and alleviate some of the responsibilities of the supervisor.[8] Tiberius and Gaiptman[8] found that the single most important benefit of the collaborative model was a decrease in the amount of superficial questions asked by students. If the clinical instructor treats the students as two separate entities and does not promote collaboration, however, then the advantages of this model may not be as apparent. When the specific supervisory strategies used by the clinical instructors were explored, it appeared that the therapist who was not as satisfied with the collaborative model did not promote teamwork between the students. Her students commented on the small number of patients to which they were exposed.

There are other potential disadvantages to the collaborative model. The therapist must evaluate each student and provide feedback independently. This is difficult in an environment where students and therapists are together constantly. Therapists also stated that the continual presence of two students was stressful. In an institutional setting, the student can more easily attend rounds and access the library or other colleagues, giving the clinical instructor time to complete noneducational activities. This is difficult to orchestrate in the home care environment. Specific times could be designated for reflective learning, students could accompany other colleagues to gain an appreciation of the roles of other team members, or students could accompany other therapists treating patients with interesting conditions to use the strategy in home care.

One unanticipated disadvantage was the crowded environment when three individuals (one clinical instructor and two students) visited the patient's home. Some homes and apartments could not accommodate these numbers. Clinical instructors should assess whether there are patients with less complex problems that the student could see independently or with another student without direct supervision. This would provide clinical instructors with some independent time, decrease the number of individuals in the patient's home, and foster student independence.

Clinical instructors in the sharing model did not experience stress from spending extended time with the student. Another advantage of the sharing model was that patients whose conditions were complex could be treated when the student was with the other therapist. This model allows part-time therapists to supervise students, a suggested advantage of the model.[9] For successful implementation, therapists using a sharing model must view themselves as partners in student supervision. Ongoing communication is essential and can be time consuming. Our productivity information verifies this. The clinical instructors in our project, however, perceived that the advantages of supervising a student outweighed any additional time required for ongoing communication.

Both models had unexpected benefits. Students in the collaborative model practiced giving feedback on clinical performance to a colleague. This is a high-level skill required of all clinicians, particularly as clinical instructors. The sharing model of supervision provided students with broader clinical experience, provided opportunities to develop time-management skills, and promoted greater autonomy in students.[9] Students in our study felt it was advantageous to be exposed to two different approaches to patient care. They also appreciated exposure to a greater variety of patient problems.

Concerns have been expressed about accommodating physical therapy students in community settings.[1] These include safety issues of leaving students in the home alone and transportation of students within the community setting by the therapist. This may leave doubt as to whether inexperienced or junior-level students should be exposed to the home care environment. The elimination of junior-level students from clinical practice in home care would limit the overall number of students exposed to this unique aspect of patient care. The students in our study had 4 weeks or less of previous full-time clinical experience, but they did not have difficulty dealing with the complex caseload. Further studies should determine the minimal skill level required before assigning students to a home care placement. For a collaborative model to be most successful, it may need to be restricted to senior-level students who can make visits independently.

Exposing greater numbers of students to home care has benefits other than providing increased numbers of clinical placements and a varied learning experience. Students tend to practice in placement areas that they have experienced in the past.[10] Providing students with a clinical placement in a community setting may encourage recruitment of new graduates in this area. This becomes even more important in view of the trend toward increased demand for development of community health care services. Future studies should examine whether exposure to community health care influences choice of practice after graduation.

Early exposure to community practice is crucial. Many students entering the health care program view their role as curative and hospitals as an exciting technological milieu.[11] Students should be exposed to differing aspects of patient care early, while they are forming their professional identity. This may be related to our students' perception of the difficulty in achieving objectives. The students may have approached their placements with the medical, curative model foremost in their mind. Because the majority of the caseload consisted of elderly patients or patients with chronic conditions, students may have had difficulty understanding how specific assessment and treatment objectives could be adapted to this population.

The need for more health care professionals trained to work with the geriatric population is a common theme in the literature. Most patients seen in home care are over age 65. Students require clinical practice with geriatric patients to integrate the specialized knowledge and skills required to treat the aging population effectively. In a survey of 101 accredited American physical therapy programs, only 4% offered a clinical experience in geriatrics.[10] Students may lack clinically based experience to complement theoretical models introduced in the classroom. Clinical placements are needed where students can develop skills in geriatric care. Home care is an ideal setting for exposure to geriatric care.

When supplied with a list of disadvantages commonly experienced by students in clinical placements, the students in this study did not identify any that occurred during their clinical placement. This may be due to a reluctance to give negative feedback to clinical faculty who may evaluate them on other occasions. When responding to the open-ended question about negative aspects of the placement, students stated that a lack of variety in caseload type and a decrease in caseload number compromised their learning experience. This also could be an advantage, because with decreased patient numbers students can explore cases in depth. The impact of the patient's illness on the quality of life and living conditions can be examined. There is little opportunity for this in an acute care setting, where therapists may be responsible for more than 20 patients per day.

Maintaining productivity while participating in clinical education is a major concern with administrators. The productivity of the clinical instructors in the collaborative model increased during our pilot project. The postplacement interview revealed that this was due largely to an attempt to increase caseload numbers in response to student feedback midway through the placement. Further study is required about the productivity of both senior- and junior-level students in the traditional apprenticeship model as well as in the collaborative and sharing models. Productivity may be increased substantially if senior-level students visit patients independently.

Several limitations apply to this study. The sample was small, and the results are not amenable to statistical analyses. These results cannot be generalized to other physical therapy programs that do not use a block system in their curriculum, although many similar issues may be present when providing placements in the community. The process of clinical education is complex and multidimensional and does not lend itself to easily measured outcomes. Several variables potentially could affect clinical instructor and student performance and satisfaction during the clinical placement. Factors other than the supervisory model may have contributed to the results. Further study is warranted.

CONCLUSION

Physical therapy students require clinical placements in the community to expose them to this growing sector of the health care system. Home care is an excellent setting in which to gain this experience.

The collaborative model of supervision in home care has some potential disadvantages when implemented with inexperienced students. Unless students work together as a team, they may not gain the full benefits of the clinical placement. A sharing model of supervision is an acceptable alternative in home care.

Further study should delineate the most effective alternatives for clinical supervision in a home care setting with both senior- and junior-level students. One model that would integrate the strengths of both models is the assignment of two students to two supervisors.

ACKNOWLEDGMENTS

The authors acknowledge the ongoing support of physical therapists at the Hamilton-Wentworth Homecare Program. This project was supported by a grant from the Ontario Ministry of Health.

REFERENCES

1. Council on Scientific Affairs. Home care in the 1990s. *JAMA.* 1990;263:1241–1244.

2. Sankar A. Stephen LB. The home as a site for teaching gerontology and chronic illness. *J Med Ed.* 1985;60:308–312.

3. Ramsdell JW. Swart JA. Jackson E. Renvall M. The yield of a home visit in the assessment of geriatric patients. *J Am Geriatr Soc.* 1985;33:169–174.

4. Harris R. Graduate training in geriatrics: new dimensions and trends. *Aging.* 1979;295-296:28–34.

5. Van Ort S. Woodtli A. Williams M. Prospective payment and baccalaureate nursing education: projections for the future. *J Prof Nurs.* 1989;5(1):25–30.

6. Gleeson C. Kearney T. Lawless C. Morris H. Domiciliary care with a multidisciplinary emphasis: a South Australian success. *Physiotherapy.* 1989;75(6):351–353.

7. Henry J. Clinical environment and resources for clinical education: panel summation and discussion. In: *Clinical Education: Present Status/Future Needs.* Alexandria, VA: Department of Education, American Physical Therapy Association; 1988;73–79.

8. Tiberius R. Gaiptman B. The supervisor-student ratio 1:1 versus 2:1. *CJOT.* 1985;52(4):179–183.

9. Gaiptman B. Forman L. The split placement model for fieldwork placements. *CJOT.* 1991;58(2):85–88.

10. Granick R. Simson S. Wilson L. Survey of curriculum content related to geriatrics in physical therapy education programs. *Phys Ther.* 1987;67:234–237.

11. Benor D. Hobfoll S. Prywes M. Important issues in community-oriented medical education. In: Schmidt H. et al. eds. *New Directions for Medical Education: Problem-Based Learning and Community-Oriented Medical Education.* New York, NY: Springer-Verlag; 1989.

"What Do I Do Now?"

In many regions, CIs and CCCEs are miles away from the schools with which they are affiliated—and miles away from each other. This group of physical therapists has overcome the distance to improve clinical teaching skills and solve problems.

By Susan Scherer, PT, CCCE

Sooner or later, all of us come into contact with a student in the clinic. Many of us become clinical instructors (CIs) and center coordinators of continuing education (CCCEs). For the physical therapist who is a CI, typical patient-care issues may seem simple in comparison with those issues that must be addressed with students. Our group of CIs and CCCEs, who work at a number of facilities across Colorado, holds monthly meetings to discuss and help solve problems both typical and unique among clinical educators—problems like these.

Case 1: "I Don't Know If I Can Do It Right"

Your student has indicated that she learns best by first observing, then practicing the technique with her instructor (you), and then using the technique with patients. You are a therapist with a busy orthopedic caseload, and you have little time available between patient visits; however, you schedule some extra time in the mornings for a review session with the student.

Today you have several patients who have conditions that call for the same treatment technique. Because the student has observed you perform this technique several times and has practiced it at least once under therapist supervision, you believe the student is ready to use the technique on her own with patients. Just before the first patient arrives, however, the student states she isn't ready and refuses to use the technique with patients. She says she just doesn't know if she can "do it right."

What do you do now? As a result of our group discussions, we have concluded that many problems common to clinical education can be resolved through simple organizational and planning techniques. Plan some learning experiences before the student arrives so that you can observe his or her skill level. Allow the student to observe treatment and ask pertinent questions. You might even give the student an assignment to observe particular situations and report observations back to you. Engage the student in discussion of alternative approaches to treatment *before* you both see the patient.

Clinical Management

Reprinted from *PT—Magazine of Physical Therapy.* Scherer S. "What do I do now?" 1992;12(2):66-69. With the permission of APTA.

If this procedure had been followed with the student in this case example, it is unlikely that her discomfort with patients would have been a surprise. At this stage, however, the CI probably should go ahead and treat the patient and arrange some other learning experiences for the student.

Allowing the student to perform parts of the evaluation or treatment also may be helpful in decreasing student anxiety—and may help you identify problem areas early. You might have the student perform the manual muscle test after you have taken the patient's history, for example, or have the student provide ultrasound and massage therapy to gain some hands-on experience in palpating muscle tone.

A brief discussion after each encounter gives you the chance to give both positive feedback and constructive criticism. "You did a nice job of placing your hands appropriately during the manual muscle test, but the patient had to move from the sitting position to the supine position three times. Is there any other way you could have sequenced the evaluation?" With just a little bit of advance planning, you can help the student add one skill to another and allow her to learn using her preferred method: first observing, then practicing with the instructor, then using the techniques with patients.

Case 2: A Matter of Style

Your student is pleasant and attentive but just isn't "getting the picture" when it comes to setting goals and carrying out treatment plans. You are frustrated with his lack of

progress. Should you just hold your comments for your midterm evaluation of his performance and hope he gets it together in a few weeks?

This case brings up several important issues, including the frustrating role of the clinical instructor and the importance of the performance evaluation. Our group has used the Myers-Briggs Type Indicator to gain insight into own needs and behaviors. The Learning Styles Analysis also has been helpful to us. Both these evaluations allow the clinical instructor to identify his or her own preferred styles of learning and relating, making decisions, and structuring the environment. Perhaps the student in this case recognizes that there are many options but has difficulty narrowing down the choices, whereas you are more practical and can immediately decide on what you think is the best goal and plan. The question in this case is: Can you two work together in a positive way? If you know that your style contradicts that of the student, sometimes a conscious decision to put aside your preference is required. Although this may be difficult, it may be enjoyable and valuable to "try on" a different style.

This case also reminds us that the midterm and final evaluations are important but cannot take the place of regular communication between student and CI. *Nothing stated in your midterm or final evaluations should be totally new information to the student.* The best way to help the student learn to set goals and devise plans is to communicate your expectations clearly and concretely—from day one. Our group has spent many meetings discussing how to use the midterm evaluation to state performance expectations. We have

found that, although they can be tedious, the BLUE MACS (Mastery and Assessment of Clinical Skills) are a valuable tool in defining expected performance.

To make the evaluation process somewhat less threatening to the student, list the BLUE MACS skills (or the skills determined by the school) that the student is working on during the affiliation, and give the student a copy of that list. Before the formal evaluation, have the student check off those skills he or she feels have been accomplished. At the same time—but separately—you should check off the skills *you* feel the student has completed. This allows both parties to assess the situation without being influenced by the other party. At the time of the formal evaluation, these lists can be compared and discussed, and the final evaluation can be made. By structuring the evaluation in this manner, you also may gain valuable information about how accurately the student assesses his or her own strengths and weaknesses.

Our group also has spent a lot of time defining which skills from the BLUE MACS can be completed in our clinics; deciding which skills are most appropriate for the first or final affiliations; and interpreting what the indicators mean. With the assistance of the University of Colorado physical therapy school, each of our clinical affiliation sites has determined the skills that can be accomplished in its clinic. In conjunction with our group, the academic coordinator of clinical education (ACCE) at the school has developed a list of which BLUE MACS skills the student can be expected to complete at which level. This information has been especially helpful for those facilities

Colorado Clinical Educator's Forum

Among all the issues pressuring physical therapists today, one thing remains clear: the necessity of high-quality clinical education. The arguments for and against entry-level doctorates, professional autonomy, and direct access all emphasize the importance of maintaining and improving our clinical affiliation programs and clinical instruction skills. Physical therapy schools have combined resources into "consortia" for clinical education and use academic faculty to teach courses for clinical instructors (CIs) who are affiliated with those schools.

Many areas of the country—especially in the West—have a great need for education and support for CIs, but the physical therapy schools geographically are far apart and have limited available resources. For clinics in these areas, there is a simple alternative to consortia, one that we in Colorado have been using for 10 years: the Clinical Educator's Forum (CEF).

The CEF began with only five or six CIs who met to discuss problems related to student clinical education. Now the CEF is run by elected officers, including a chairman, a vice chairman, a secretary, and a treasurer. Thirty-five facilities belong to the CEF.

Goals are established annually by the officers. Although the CEF is not an official committee of the APTA, specific goals may be determined by the educational affairs committee of APTA's Colorado Chapter. The CEF developed *Standards for Clinical Instructors,* a document that is used as the basis for continuing education for CIs. The CEF has also joined forces with the University of Colorado Curriculum in Physical Therapy to provide an annual clinical faculty institute to CIs.

Monthly meetings are planned by the elected officers of the group. An expert may be invited to speak about a relevant clinical education topic such as burnout or legal issues in clinical education. Meeting time also is used for discussion of current literature or for work on current projects. Time always is set aside for interaction among the CIs. We usually hold the meetings in a consistent place and at a standard time, but we also have rotated host facilities. The CEF year runs from September through June, with no formal meetings held in December or during the summer.

Dues are collected annually. Those facilities that pay dues receive a copy of the minutes of each monthly meeting, complete with handouts or other pertinent information. The money collected from dues is used to cover mailing costs and speakers' fees and to reduce the cost of the clinical faculty institute.

—S.S.

---

that are starting new affiliations with the physical therapy school.

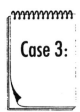

Case 3: A Difference in Perception

You have been out of school for two years now and feel you have gained a tremendous amount of knowledge. Your first student is 10 years older than you are, has had three careers before entering the physical therapy profession, and is resisting your attempts to teach her. She thinks her life experiences will carry her through, but you find her defensive. She doesn't relate well to the patients. What do you do?

This case is typical and very frustrating for the CI. When our group discussed this case, the role of the CCCE was raised. Administratively, the CCCE is responsible for 1) establishing and maintaining contracts with the affiliating schools and 2) training and monitoring the CI's performance. Although it may be difficult for the CCCE to be involved with the clinician and student on a daily basis, the CCCE should be available as needed and should be the mediator or liaison between the student and the clinician. As soon as the problem is identified, the CCCE should spend time with the clinician and the student individually and then with the clinician and student together to find some solutions. The CCCE may be involved throughout the entire affiliation. *The CCCE should not take over the planning and teaching functions of the clinician* but should facilitate the communication between these two individuals.

In this case our group decided that the CCCE definitely should be involved. The student was having difficulty seeing herself as others see her, and we realized that the technique described in Case 2 for use in the formal evaluation would help the clinician and CCCE give informal feedback to the student in a less threatening manner and encourage the student's self-assessment skills. It was a new thought to most of us that these same evaluation forms could be used *throughout* the affiliation and for something other than a formal evaluation! Sometimes it is a helpful exercise for the student to write a subjective, objective, assessment, plan (SOAP) note about his or her day. This allows the student to organize subjective feelings and objective data in a meaningful way and often helps the student develop insights he or she otherwise might not have developed.

Our group has been a forum for discussion of current issues in clinical education. Other pertinent topics have included clinical decision making, legal issues related to clinical education, and the development of standards for clinical educators. Our goals are to provide an avenue for discussion of clinical education issues, to provide an opportunity to meet and talk with other CIs who have varied clinical experiences, and to promote a consistent, high-quality performance among CIs. We hope our experiences will be helpful to others involved in clinical education.

The questionaire to the right was given to clinical instructors before one of our group-sponsored courses. Are you ready to be a CI? **CM**

Susan Scherer, PT, CCCE, is a physical therapist at the National Jewish Center in Denver, CO.

Self-Assessment Quiz

1. Feedback to the student should be focused primarily on areas of weakness that require improvement. **T F**

2. The student's learning style may be a factor in selection of their caseload. **T F**

3. It is not necessary to discuss rationale for different evaluation and treatment techniques with a student because the student has undergone extensive academic work related to this. **T F**

4. When setting specific goals for the student's clinical learning experience, the following persons routinely should be involved (circle all that apply):
   a. Center coordinator of clinical education
   b. Student
   c. Academic faculty
   d. Physical therapy staff
   e. Clinical instructor

5. When should planning for an effective student affiliation occur?
   a. Before the student arrives.
   b. While the student is at the facility.
   c. Both are equally important.

6. When should a clinical instructor begin to prepare for a final student evaluation?
   a. On the first day of affiliation.
   b. At the midterm evaluation.
   c. During the week before final evaluation.
   d. On the day before final evaluation.

7. Effective learning experiences meet which criteria? Circle all that apply.
   a. They are appropriate to the level of experience.
   b. They provide opportunities for the student to succeed.
   c. They can be planned prior to student arrival.
   d. They allow students to practice the desired behaviors.
   e. They are evaluated for effectiveness.

8. Which of the following is not a way to facilitate development of self-assessment skills in a student:
   a. Have student perform frequent verbal self-assessments and discuss them with the clinical instructor.
   b. Inform student of ways to improve.
   c. Have student perform a self-evaluation using his or her school's forms prior to midterm and final evaluations.
   d. Have student write SOAP notes about his or her experiences on a particular day.

Answers: 1.F 2.T 3.F 4.b,e 5.c 6.a 7.all 8.b

Variation in Lengths of Training among Residents Enrolled in Pediatrics and Internal Medicine Training Programs

ROBERT A. HOEKELMAN, M.D., and RUTH M. PARKER, M.D.

Abstract—Data were gathered in 1987 from 180 pediatrics and 302 internal medicine residency training programs about (1) the length of vacation provided their residents, (2) time allowed them for absence from work for reasons other than vacation, (3) how many of them during the previous three years had been required to extend their training to make up absences from work, and (4) whether a system was in place to cover their unexpected absences from work. All these variables affect the duration—but not necessarily the quality—of training that residents actually experience. The data show that these variables demonstrated wide ranges that depended on the postgraduate year of training, the discipline, the program size, and the program type (university, university-affiliated, freestanding, or military). The Accreditation Council for Graduate Medical Education, training program directors, and the American Board of Pediatrics and the American Board of Internal Medicine each need to consider these variables in making their respective decisions about accrediting training programs, verifying the clinical competence of trainees, and certifying program graduates. *Acad. Med.* 65(1990):257–266.

It is assumed that physicians in training within various medical disciplines have similar educational experiences in terms of numbers and types of clinical exposures. To this end, the Accreditation Council for Graduate Medical Education (ACGME) sets and applies minimal educational standards for training through residency review committees established for each discipline. In this way, the ACGME accredits each training program periodically, usually every five to seven years. The educational standards applied relate to the program's institutional affiliation, scope of training, curriculum, learning experiences, staff, facilities, and size, and the evaluation procedures used to measure resident and faculty performances. Accreditation is essential for training programs in order to attract trainees wishing to become certified in their medical disciplines. As one of the criteria for certification, the various specialty boards require completion of a specified number of years of training in accredited programs. Training program directors attest to the specialty board that the training of each resident has or has not been completed satisfactorily.

Despite all this effort to set standards, there are differences in the educational experiences provided to residents. These differences depend on (1) the sizes and locations of training programs, which dictate the numbers and types of patients seen, the frequencies of night and weekend call, and the quantity, variety, and quality of faculty available for teaching; and (2) program policies that relate to the durations of training residents actually experience—that is, policies that govern the length of vacation provided each year and the amount of time allowed for absence from work due to sickness and other reasons that the resident is not required to make up through extended training time.

The purpose of the study reported in this article was to investigate how much variation existed in the lengths of the vacations and allowable leaves of absence without required make-up time provided by pediatrics and internal medicine residency training programs in the United States.

Method

In January 1987, an eight-item, one-page questionnaire was sent to the directors of all 657 accredited pediatrics and internal medicine residency training programs located in the United States and listed in the 1986–1987 Directory of Graduate Medical Education Programs.[1] (The questionnaire was not sent to the directors of the 15 listed programs located in Puerto Rico.) The questionnaire queried the directors on (1) whether the program was a university program, a university-affiliated program, a freestanding program, or a program located in a military hospital; (2) the number of residents currently enrolled in each of the four post-graduate years (PGY-1, PGY-2, PGY-3, and PGY-4); (3) the number of weeks of vacation allowed for each level of trainee; (4) the program's policy concerning making up absences from work (excluding vacation); (5) whether records of days absent from work were kept and, if so, who kept them; (6) the numbers of residents who had completed three years of training by June 1984, June 1985, and June 1986 who had had absences from work (excluding vacations) that exceeded three months; (7) the numbers of residents who had completed three years of training by June 1984, June 1985, and June 1986 who had been required to make up time; and (8) whether a resident was regularly scheduled to provide coverage for unexpected house-officer absences from work (a sick-call resident).

Of the 225 pediatrics residency program directors queried, 180 (80%) responded to the initial mailing; 302 of

Dr. Hoekelman is professor and chairman, Department of Pediatrics, University of Rochester School of Medicine and Dentistry, Rochester, New York. Dr. Parker was a Robert Wood Johnson Clinical Scholar, University of Pennsylvania School of Medicine, when this study was conducted and currently is assistant professor, Department of Internal Medicine, Emory University School of Medicine, Atlanta, Georgia.

Correspondence should be addressed to Dr. Hoekelman, 601 Elmwood Avenue, PO Box 777, Rochester, NY 14642. Reprints will not be available.

Table 1

Numbers and Percentages of 180 Pediatrics and 302 Internal Medicine Residency Programs, by Type and Size, 1987*

| Program Type | Program Size | | | | | | Total, by Type | |
| | Small | | Medium | | Large | | | |
	No.	%	No.	%	No.	%	No.	%
Pediatrics								
University	15	16.3	26	28.3	51	55.4	92	51.1
University-affiliated	8	27.6	16	55.2	5	17.2	29	16.1
Freestanding	26	55.3	18	38.3	3	6.4	47	26.1
Military	8	66.7	4	33.3	0	0.0	12	6.7
Total, by size	57	31.7	64	35.6	59	32.8	180	100.0
Internal medicine								
University	4	5.3	15	19.7	57	75.0	76	25.2
University-affiliated	22	33.3	28	42.4	16	24.2	66	21.8
Freestanding	69	46.9	52	35.4	26	17.7	147	48.7
Military	6	46.2	7	53.8	0	0.0	13	4.3
Total, by size	101	33.4	102	33.8	99	32.8	302	100.0

*In January 1987, the authors sent a questionnaire to the directors of all 657 U.S. pediatrics and internal medicine residency programs in order to determine how much variation existed in the lengths of the residents' vacations and allowable leaves of absence without required make-up time. The data above describe the programs that responded.

the 432 internal medicine residency program directors did so (70%). We did not use a second mailing to increase this response rate because it was considered sufficiently high to satisfy the purposes of the study and the percentages of responses from directors of the four program types — university, university-affiliated, freestanding, and military — were essentially the same as the percentages of distribution of those four program types within the total sample for each of the two disciplines studied (see Table 1).

The data were analyzed according to the variables of discipline, program type, and program size, by use of frequency distributions and cross tabulations.

The authors defined the four program types, for each of the two disciplines, as (1) a *university program* — a residency training program conducted primarily by a university department of pediatrics or internal medicine and located in a general hospital, a children's hospital, or a Veterans Administration hospital; (2) a *university-affiliated program* — a residency training program located in a community hospital, a children's hospital, or a Veterans Administration hospital *not* conducted primarily by a university department of pediatrics or inter-

nal medicine, but whose residents are recruited and enrolled as students in a university's graduate medical education program; (3) a *freestanding program* — a residency training program located in a community hospital, a children's hospital, or a Veterans Administration hospital that has no affiliation with a university with respect to conducting graduate medical education programs for residents; and (4) a *military program* — a residency training program located in a U.S. Army, Air Force, or Navy hospital that has no affiliation with a university with respect to conducting graduate medical education programs for residents. These groupings differ from those used by the Accreditation Council on Graduate Medical Education (ACGME) when classifying participants in residency training programs by their relationship to a medical school.

There were 35 children's hospitals in the sample — 31 were university programs, one was university-affiliated, and three were freestanding. Thirty (86%) of these hospitals responded to the questionnaire. There were 13 Veterans Administration hospitals in the sample — three were university programs, five were university-affiliated, and five were freestanding. Ten (77%) of these hospi-

tals responded to the questionnaire. Data from the children's and Veterans Administration hospital respondents were included with those of each of the categories of training programs they represented, rather than in separate children's and Veterans Administration hospital categories.

Program size for each of the two disciplines was determined by categorizing the programs that responded into three groups (small, medium-sized, and large) according to the number of residents enrolled. Thus, for the 180 pediatrics programs the numbers of residents enrolled ranged from five to 110. Fifty-seven of the programs had 15 or fewer residents enrolled and were designated small programs, 64 had between 16 and 34 residents enrolled and were designated medium-size programs, and 59 had 35 or more residents enrolled and were designated large programs. (Notice that the numbers of programs in the groups are approximately equal.) For the 302 internal medicine programs, the numbers of residents enrolled ranged from four to 159. A total of 101 of the programs had 26 or fewer residents enrolled (small programs), 102 had between 27 and 46 residents (medium-sized programs), and 99 had 47 or more residents (large programs). Here again, the numbers of programs in the groups are about the same. Response rates for the three program sizes within the entire sample could not be determined because the numbers of residents enrolled in the programs that did not respond were not known. Table 1 shows the numbers and percentages of responding programs by program type and size.

Results

The data obtained from the responding programs are presented here in terms of the number of residents enrolled, the length of vacations provided to them, the other absences from work allowed to them and experienced by them, and the use of a sick-call resident system to cover them when they were unexpectedly absent from work.

Number of Residents in Training

The residents enrolled in all the responding pediatrics programs during the 1986–87 academic year were fairly evenly distributed among the first three training years (1,734 in PGY-1, 1,642 in PGY-2, and 1,568 in PGY-3), showing no strong tendency towards the "pyramid" effect—that is, significant losses between PGY-1 and PGY-3. There were 218 PGY-4 residents enrolled; 25% of the 180 pediatrics programs had one PGY-4 resident and 26% had two or more.

On the other hand, the responding internal medicine programs enrolled 23% fewer PGY-2 and PGY-3 residents than PGY-1 residents (3,764 from PGY-2 and 3,745 from PGY-3 versus 4,910 from PGY-1). This reflects the enrollment of "transitional-year" residents who enter other, non-internal-medicine, training programs following their first postgraduate year. There were 436 PGY-4 residents enrolled; 23% of the 302 internal medicine programs had one PGY-4 resident, and 34% had two or more.

Table 2 shows (1) the number of residents enrolled in the responding pediatrics and internal medicine programs at all levels of training, by each program type and size; (2) the per-

Table 2

Numbers and Percentages of Residents Enrolled in 180 Pediatrics and 302 Internal Medicine Programs, by Program Type and Size, 1986–87*

Program Type and Size	No. Programs	No. Residents	% All Residents, by Program Type	% All Residents in All Programs
Pediatrics				
University				
Small	15	177	5.1	3.4
Medium	26	661	19.1	12.8
Large	51	2,616	75.7	50.7
Total	92	3,454	99.9†	66.9
University-affiliated				
Small	8	101	14.0	1.9
Medium	16	387	53.8	7.5
Large	5	231	32.1	4.5
Total	29	719	99.9†	13.9
Freestanding				
Small	26	300	36.3	5.8
Medium	18	380	46.0	7.4
Large	3	146	17.7	2.8
Total	47	826	100.0	16.0
Military				
Small	8	96	58.9	1.9
Medium	4	67	41.1	1.3
Large	0	—	—	—
Total	12	163	100.0	3.2
All programs	180	5,162	—	100.0
Internal medicine				
University				
Small	4	86	1.6	0.7
Medium	15	536	10.2	4.2
Large	57	4,630	88.2	36.0
Total	76	5,252	100.0	40.9
University-affiliated				
Small	22	410	15.7	3.2
Medium	28	1,092	41.8	8.5
Large	16	1,109	42.5	8.6
Total	66	2,611	100.0	20.3
Freestanding				
Small	69	1,261	27.3	9.8
Medium	52	1,818	39.3	14.1
Large	26	1,543	33.4	12.0
Total	147	4,622	100.0	35.9
Military				
Small	6	115	31.1	0.9
Medium	7	255	68.9	2.0
Large	0	—	—	—
Total	13	370	100.0	2.9
All programs	302	12,855	—	100.0

*In January 1987, the authors sent a questionnaire to the directors of all 657 U.S. pediatrics and internal medicine residency programs in order to determine how much variation existed in the lengths of the residents' vacations and allowable leaves of absence without required make-up time. The above data describe the programs that responded.

†This total does not equal 100% because the component percentages were rounded.

Table 3

Numbers and Percentages of 180 Pediatrics and 302 Internal Medicine Residency Programs with Specified Vacation Lengths, by Level of Training and Program Type, 1987*

Program Type for Each Postgraduate Year	No. Programs	Percentage of Programs with Specified Length of Vacation		
		Two Weeks	Three Weeks	Four Weeks
Pediatrics				
PGY-1				
University	92	34.7	32.6	32.6
University-affiliated	29	34.5	34.5	31.0
Freestanding	47	27.8	34.0	38.2†
Military	12	100.0	0.0	0.0
All programs	180	36.7	31.7	31.7
PGY-2				
University	92	7.6	48.9	43.5
University-affiliated	29	3.4	51.7	44.8
Freestanding	47	6.4	48.9	44.6†
Military	12	50.0	16.7	33.3
All programs	180	9.4	47.8	42.8
PGY-3				
University	92	4.3	47.8	47.8
University-affiliated	29	3.4	41.4	55.2
Freestanding	47	6.4	42.6	51.0†
Military	12	33.3	16.7	50.0
All programs	180	6.7	43.9	49.4
Internal medicine				
PGY-1				
University	76	44.7	32.9	22.4
University-affiliated	66	39.4	37.9	22.7
Freestanding	147	40.8	38.1	21.1
Military	13	100.0	0.0	0.0
All programs	302	44.0	35.1	20.9
PGY-2				
University	76	9.2	56.6	34.2
University-affiliated	66	7.6	56.1	36.3
Freestanding	147	12.9	58.5	28.6
Military	13	38.5	38.5	23.0
All programs	302	11.9	56.6	31.5
PGY-3				
University	76	5.3	59.2	35.5
University-affiliated	66	3.0	56.1	40.9
Freestanding	147	10.2	54.4	35.4
Military	13	30.8	23.1	46.1
All programs	302	8.3	54.6	37.1

*In January 1987, the authors sent a questionnaire to the directors of all 657 U.S. pediatrics and internal medicine residency programs in order to determine how much variation existed in the lengths of the residents' vacations and allowable leaves of absence without required make-up time. The above data present the vacation lengths of the programs that responded.

†One medium-sized, freestanding program gave five weeks of vacation in each of the four years of training.

centage of all residents enrolled, by each program type and size; and (3) the percentage of all residents these numbers represent for all the pediatrics and internal medicine residency training programs that responded. Thus, 66.9% of all these pediatrics residents were enrolled in the university programs, while only 40.9% of the internal medicine residents received

their training in such programs. Freestanding programs accounted for 35.9% of the internal medicine trainees and 16% of the pediatrics trainees. The university-affiliated programs were lower on the list, accounting for 20.3% of the internal medicine and 13.9% of the pediatrics trainees. The military hospitals trained relatively few residents—

approximately 3% for each discipline.

Length of Vacation

The length of vacation that residents received during each of the three years of training varied by their levels of training, their disciplines, and the types and sizes of the programs in which they were enrolled. Tables 3

Table 4

Numbers and Percentages of 180 Pediatrics and 302 Internal Medicine Residency Programs with Specified Vacation Lengths, by Level of Training and Program Size, 1987*

Program Size for Each Postgraduate Year	No. Programs	Percentage of Programs with Specified Length of Vacation		
		Two Weeks	Three Weeks	Four Weeks
Pediatrics				
PGY-1				
Small	57	54.4	21.1	24.5
Medium	64	32.8	31.3	35.9†
Large	59	23.7	42.4	33.9
All programs	180	36.7	31.7	31.7
PGY-2				
Small	57	19.3	49.1	31.6
Medium	64	7.8	43.8	48.4†
Large	59	1.7	50.8	47.5
All programs	180	9.4	47.8	42.8
PGY-3				
Small	57	12.3	50.9	36.8
Medium	64	7.8	34.4	57.8†
Large	59	0	47.5	52.5
All programs	180	6.7	43.9	49.4
Internal medicine				
PGY-1				
Small	101	52.5	41.6	5.9
Medium	102	45.1	33.3	21.6
Large	99	34.3	31.3	34.3
All programs	302	44.0	35.1	20.9
PGY-2				
Small	101	16.8	66.3	16.8
Medium	102	10.8	58.8	30.4
Large	99	8.1	45.5	46.5
All programs	302	11.9	56.6	31.5
PGY-3				
Small	101	9.9	68.3	21.8
Medium	102	8.8	52.9	38.2
.Large	99	7.1	42.4	50.5
All programs	302	8.3	56.6	37.1

*In January 1987, the authors sent a questionnaire to the directors of all 657 U.S. pediatrics and internal medicine residency programs in order to determine how much variation existed in the lengths of the residents' vacations and allowable leaves of absence without required make-up time. The above data present the vacation lengths of the programs that responded.

†One medium-sized freestanding program gave five weeks of vacation in each of the four years of training.

and 4 demonstrate these variations. The data presented in the tables show that in general (1) vacation time increased each year; (2) the pediatrics residents got more vacation time at all levels than did the internal medicine residents; (3) the university-affiliated and freestanding pediatrics programs provided more vacation time to their residents than did the university and military pediatrics programs; (4) the university-affiliated internal medicine programs provided more vacation time to their residents

than did the other types of internal medicine programs; and (5) the larger the program size, the longer the vacation time provided to residents in both disciplines, except that among the pediatrics programs, the medium-sized ones provided longer vacations during each year of training than did the large ones.

During the 1986–87 academic year, less than half of all the programs in both disciplines provided four weeks of vacation to their residents at any of the levels of training. Indeed, only

37.1% of the internal medicine programs allowed four weeks of vacation for their residents in PGY-3; those in PGY-2 and PGY-1 fared less well (31.5% and 20.9%, respectively). As noted above and shown in Tables 3 and 4, the pediatrics programs were more generous in this respect. At the PGY-4 level of training (not shown in the tables), 57% of the pediatrics and 44% of the internal medicine programs allowed four weeks of vacation. Eight of the pediatrics and six of the internal medicine programs that provided two to three weeks of vacation for their PGY-2 and PGY-3 residents reported that they allowed them one to two weeks each year to attend medical meetings or for independent study.

Absences from Work

The number of weeks, in addition to vacation time, that the pediatrics and internal medicine training programs allowed their residents to be absent from work because of illness, maternity leave, paternity leave, or family crises (illness, death, or discord) varied considerably by program type and size both within each discipline and between the two disciplines, as shown in Table 5. Only 6.7% of the pediatrics programs and 7.6% of the internal medicine programs allowed no such absences, requiring residents to make up *all* time missed from work. Some programs (17.2% of the pediatrics and 20.5% of the internal medicine programs) had no policy governing these absences. These respondents indicated that absences from work beyond vacation time were allowed without residents' having to make up the time, but that the amount of time allowed depended on (1) the individual circumstances surrounding leaves for sickness, maternity, paternity, or family crisis; (2) the number of consecutive weeks absent from work; (3) the training year during which the absence occurred — that is, absences during the PGY-1 year were more likely to require make-up than those occurring during PGY-2 or PGY-3; (4) the specific service to which the resident was assigned during the absence — that is, absences during intensive care unit assignments were more likely to require make-up than those occurring during other assignments; and (5) the resident's overall performance, with high-performing residents being less likely to be required to make up time away from work than poorly-performing residents.

Of the 180 pediatrics residency programs responding, 127 (70.6%) stated that they kept records of the times

residents were absent from work. The university programs were least likely (58.7%) and the military programs most likely (91.7%) to do so. The university-affiliated and the freestanding programs kept such records at rates of 79.3% and 82.9%, respectively. The small and medium-sized programs were most apt to keep such records (77.2% and 78.1%) and the large programs least apt to (55.9%).

Similar distributions for keeping records of residents' absences were reported by the 302 internal medicine programs — 71.2% of all the programs, 57.3% of the university programs, 80.3% of the university-affiliated programs, and 77.1% of the freestanding programs. However, only 61.5% of the military programs did so. The small internal medicine programs kept records of residents' absences most frequently (84.8%), while the medium-sized and large programs did so less frequently (65.7% and 64.6%, respectively).

The responsibility for keeping absence-from-work records in the 482 pediatrics and internal medicine programs fell to the program chairman's office (77.2% of all programs), to the chief resident (14.7% of all programs), or to the individual resident (8.1% of all programs). There was little variation in assignments of this responsibility among the disciplines or by program type or size within them. Thirteen of the respondents volunteered that while they kept records of residents' absences, they did so only for absences that exceeded one week.

Of the approximately 4,700 pediatrics residents (enrolled in the 180 responding programs) who were scheduled to complete three years of training on June 30 in 1984, 1985, or 1986, 94 (2%) were required to make up time missed from work. For the same period, 136 (1.7%) of the approximately 8,200 internal medicine residents enrolled in the 302 responding programs were required to do so. Neither the lengths of make-up time required in these instances nor whether this time was taken from unused vacation periods or added onto

the end of the three years of training was determined through the questionnaire. There was no tendency in relation to program type or size, or over the three years surveyed, to require make-up time more frequently or less frequently.

There were 57 pediatrics and 63 internal medicine programs that provided 12 weeks of vacation over the three years of training. Of these, 22 pediatrics and 28 internal medicine programs had policies that allowed up to 15 extra weeks of absence from work for other reasons during the three years of training, without requiring make-up. Thus, any illness, maternity, paternity, or family crisis that led to any days away from work in these programs caused their residents to exceed three months of absence from work during the three-year training period. This is the extreme circumstance, but one that must have affected large numbers of residents. Yet only 31 pediatrics and 12 internal medicine residents enrolled in these 50 programs who completed their three years of training at the end of June in 1984, 1985, or 1986 were required to make up time. There surely were many more who were not required to do so, as there must have been among those enrolled in programs that provided less than 12 weeks of vacation, but who were absent from work more than three months overall. They must have numbered many more than the 94 pediatrics and 136 internal medicine residents (of the over 18,000 enrolled annually in all of the responding programs) who were required to make up time either during or following the three years of training that ended on June 30, 1984, 1985, or 1986. Indeed, 28 of the pediatrics and 48 of the internal medicine program directors spontaneously responded that they would allow residents from three weeks to three months of absence from work beyond vacation time during the three years of training without requiring that this time be made up.

The specific issue of the amount of time that each program allowed for

Table 5

Numbers and Percentages of 180 Pediatrics and 302 Internal Medicine Residency Programs with Specified Weeks of Absence Allowed Residents (beyond Vacation Time) during Three Years of Training without Requiring Make-Up Time, by Program Type and Size, 1987*

Program Type and Size	No. Programs	Percentage of Programs with Specified Weeks of Absence Allowed					
		None	1-2	3-4	5-6	7-15	No Policy
Pediatrics							
University							
Small	15	20.0	0.0	6.7	13.3	26.7	33.3
Medium	26	7.7	7.7	15.4	15.4	26.9	26.9
Large	51	7.8	5.9	17.6	13.7	39.2	15.7
All programs	92	9.8	5.4	15.2	14.1	33.7	21.7
University-affiliated							
Small	8	12.5	0.0	12.5	12.5	50.0	12.5
Medium	16	0.0	6.3	31.3	0.0	50.0	12.5
Large	5	0.0	20.0	20.0	0.0	60.0	0.0
All programs	29	3.4	6.9	24.1	3.4	51.7	10.3
Freestanding							
Small	26	0.0	11.5	26.9	15.4	34.6	11.5
Medium	18	5.5	5.5	27.8	16.7	27.8	16.7
Large	3	33.3	0.0	66.7	0.0	0.0	0.0
All programs	47	4.3	8.5	29.8	14.9	29.8	12.8
Military							
Small	8	0.0	25.0	37.5	12.5	12.5	12.5
Medium	4	0.0	0.0	0.0	25.0	50.0	25.0
Large	0	—	—	—	—	—	—
All programs	12	0.0	16.7	25.0	16.7	25.0	16.7
All pediatrics programs	180	6.7	7.2	21.1	12.8	35.0	17.2
Internal medicine							
University							
Small	4	0.0	0.0	25.0	25.0	0.0	50.0
Medium	15	13.3	6.7	13.3	13.3	20.0	33.3
Large	57	12.3	3.5	24.6	8.8	35.1	15.8
All programs	76	11.8	3.9	22.4	10.5	30.3	21.1
University-affiliated							
Small	22	13.6	4.5	18.2	18.2	22.7	22.7
Medium	28	7.1	10.7	21.4	10.7	21.4	28.6
Large	16	0.0	12.5	12.5	12.5	25.0	37.5
All programs	66	7.6	9.1	18.2	13.6	22.7	28.8
Freestanding							
Small	69	13.0	8.7	23.2	8.7	26.1	20.3
Medium	52	0.0	9.6	26.9	17.3	30.8	15.4
Large	26	0.0	0.0	34.6	7.7	42.3	15.4
All programs	147	6.1	7.5	26.5	11.6	30.6	17.7
Military							
Small	6	0.0	33.3	50.0	0.0	16.7	0.0
Medium	7	0.0	14.3	14.3	14.3	42.8	14.3
Large	0	—	—	—	—	—	—
All programs	13	0.0	23.1	30.8	7.7	30.8	7.7
All internal medicine programs	302	7.6	7.6	23.8	11.6	28.8	20.5

*In January 1987, the authors sent a questionnaire to the directors of all 657 U.S. pediatrics and internal medicine residency programs in order to determine how much variation existed in the lengths of the residents' vacations and allowable leaves of absence without required make-up time. The above data present the lengths of the allowable weeks of absence, if any, of the programs that responded.

maternity leave was not addressed in the questionnaire. However, nine program directors commented that they had had one resident over the prior three years who had had to make up time taken away from work because of pregnancy. On the other hand, three program directors commented that their programs allowed between 30 and 60 days (in addition to vacation time) for maternity leave that did not have to be made up. One of these programs also allowed seven days for paternity leave that did not require make-up.

Use of a Sick-Call Resident System

A sick-call resident system provides coverage for residents who are unexpectedly absent from work for any reason.[2] Residents are assigned to this function within the program's schedule, usually while they are on a subspecialty elective. The system ordinarily provides coverage for night and weekend duties, although in some programs week-day assignments are also covered by the sick-call resident. The system is designed to reduce stress among residents who must assume the added work and on-call hours created by a peer's unexpected absence and to reduce stress among the residents who are absent from work — stress caused by the reason for the absence itself and the guilt of adding to their colleagues' already heavy work load.

A sick-call resident system was used in 37 (20.6%) of the 180 responding pediatrics programs. Thirty of the 92 university programs (32.6%), five of the 29 university-affiliated programs (17.2%), two of the 47 freestanding programs (4.3%), and none of the 12 military hospital programs had a sick-call resident system. Large programs were more likely to have such a system (30.5%) than were medium-sized programs (21.9%) or small programs (8.8%).

Of the 302 responding internal medicine programs, 98 (32.5%) had a sick-call resident system. Thirty-two of the 76 university programs (42.7%), 24 of the university-affiliated programs (36.4%), 42 of the 147 freestanding programs (29.2%), and none of the 13 military hospital pro-

grams had a sick call resident system. Again, large programs were more likely to have such a system (45.5%) than were medium-sized (34.3%) or small programs (17.8%).

Those pediatrics and internal medicine programs without a sick-call resident system either used the chief resident of hired part-time physicians to cover for residents who were sick or absent from work for other reasons, or had no backup system at all. In the latter instance, the extra work load was assumed by residents assigned to the same service as the absent resident.

Discussion

The data presented in the previous section are discussed in relation to (1) requirements, promulgated by the pediatrics and internal medicine residency review committees of the Accreditation Council for Graduate Medical Education, for accreditation of training programs; (2) training requirements that applicants to the American Board of Pediatrics and the American Board of Internal Medicine must meet for certification; and (3) recent attempts to reduce the stress experienced by pediatrics and internal medicine residents during training.

The special requirements for residency training in pediatrics[3] and in internal medicine[4] generated by their respective residency review committees make no mention of the length of vacation that should be provided residents or of restrictions on leaves of absence for any reason during training. The residency review committee for internal medicine, however, does make specific recommendations regarding work schedules, which were implemented on October 1, 1989. These include (1) being on call every third or fourth night during inpatient rotations and on call no more than every third night, regardless of the assignment; (2) working no more than 80 hours per week, averaged over four weeks; (3) being free of hospital duties at least one day out of seven; and (4) drawing assignments to the emergency department that do not exceed 12 continuous hours and are followed by at least 8 hours off duty.

Recommendations 2, 3, and 4 are identical to requirements implemented by the New York State Department of Health on July 1, 1989. New York State's limitation that residents can work no more than 24 consecutive hours in direct patient care activities when assigned to inpatient services is not included among the recommendations of the internal medicine residency review committee. The pediatrics residency review committee currently makes no recommendations to limit residents' work schedules, but one of its revised requirements (effective January 1, 1990) is that "resident on-call rotations should occur with an average frequency of every third or fourth night in any year of the program and the schedule should be designed to provide a monthly average of at least one day out of seven without assigned duties in the program."[3] In a 1985 memorandum, the residency review committee stated, that "absenteeism (illness, maternity leave, etc.) which exceeds three months in three years, excluding approved vacation, could adversely affect the attainment of educational objectives, except in very unusual circumstances."[5]

The American Board of Pediatrics, on the other hand, requires at least 33 months of training for residents. In its booklet of information for applicants it states that "absences in excess of three months, whether for vacation, sick leave, maternity leave, etc., must be made up."[6] Further, the board requires residency program directors, in completing its Verification of Clinical Competence Form for each applicant, "describe any periods of absence from the training program that have not been made up by the applicant. This would include any absences, maternity/paternity leaves or sick leave taken in addition to the vacation and sick leave normally allowed each resident. The Board recommends that absences from a program beyond three months during the three years of training be made up by additional periods of training."[7] If the program director believes that an absence of more than three months is justified and that the candidate is qualified to take the board examination, a letter of explanation can be sent by the director to the board's credentials committee for review.[8]

The American Board of Internal Medicine makes no statement in its Policies and Procedures booklet that limits the amount of absence from work that residents may be permitted during their three yeas of training.[9] It explains in a November 19, 1984, memorandum to program directors that this reflects a flexible policy of the board concerning acceptable reductions in its training requirements and leaves to the discretion of program directors the length of absences from work that is permitted residents without requiring make-up. Justification of absences greater than one month per year, exclusive of vacation time and acceptable to the board, is expected from the program director.

The American Board of Pediatrics' posture regarding the length of absences from work permitted residents without requiring make-up presents difficulties for both residents and program directors. The data presented in Tables 3 and 4 show that 31.7% of the responding pediatrics programs allowed 12 weeks of vacation during the three years of training; by board criteria, this would allow no time for absences due to illness or maternity, paternity, or family crises without requiring make-up or getting program-director justification for such absences. The weeks of absence allowed without having to be made up by most of the rest of the programs, shown in Table 5, indicate that large numbers of pediatrics residents were not meeting American Board of Pediatrics length-of-training requirements during the period surveyed in this study. If program directors reported all residents' absences from work to the board on its Verification of Clinical Competence Form, most of these residents would be required to extend the length of their training beyond three calendar years. Program costs for resident stipends, fringe benefits, and malpractice insurance would rise appreciably, and residents would be delayed in starting practice or subspecialty fellowship training. It would also interfere with the timing for spouses' training or job placements in other communities. This could explain why only 2% of the pe-

diatrics residents were required to make up time at the end of their training over the three years surveyed.

The stress caused by worrying about having to make up time, in addition to the already high levels of stress residents experience during training, should be of great concern to program directors. Methods for reducing these high levels of stress in pediatrics and internal medicine programs have been recommended by many individuals and groups involved in directing residency training. The most recently published recommendations emphasize the importance of flexibility in scheduling residents' work hours and in allowing adequate vacation time and absence from work when needed for other reasons.[10,11] It is disappointing that so many programs allow their residents only two or three weeks of vacation each year and require invasion of this time to make up for other absences, and that so few programs have implemented a sick-call resident system.

As noted in the introduction to this report, there are many variables that influence the quality of residency training; the amount of time spent at work over the three years of training may be the least of these. The quality of training programs is the focus of residency review committees, and those for pediatrics and internal medicine have focused on the training program's structure (institution and faculty), process (curriculum and clinical experiences), and outcome (success of its trainees on board-certifying examinations) in judging a program's quality. Other outcomes of training, such as the quality of medical care former trainees deliver, are difficult to measure and are influenced by intervening variables not related to the quality of training received. The residency review committees have chosen not to focus on duration of training, except for the number of years spent at it, perhaps recognizing that even this is arbitrary and that the learning gained during one week of training in one program is equal to that gained during two or three weeks in another. Rather, they have depended heavily on program directors to determine when their

trainees are ready to "come out."

Nevertheless, the problem of wide variations in the length of training experienced by pediatrics and internal medicine residents and its effect upon the quality of their education and their lives needs to be resolved.

There are no easy solutions. Standardizing vacations to allow four weeks during each year of training would reduce some of the variation in length of training and the levels of stress among residents, but this would be difficult for small programs to implement without increasing the work load of residents not on vacation or without reducing the number of patients covered by the residents. Standardizing the length of absence from work allowed for other reasons (for example, to ten, 20, or 30 days during each year of training or, over the three years, to 30, 60, or 90 days) would present the same advantages and disadvantages. In addition, some program directors, residency review committee members, and specialty board members would be concerned that the overall duration of training for substantial numbers of residents would be shortened at a time when the number of residency review committee-required clinical experiences are increasing, and that some residents would take advantage of the system to maximize their time away from work.

It would seem most appropriate for the boards of pediatrics and of internal medicine to adopt flexible policies that transfer to program directors the responsibility to determine within reasonably broad limits how much time each resident should spend at work during each year of training. However, program directors would have to do this diligently and with the greatest of care and wisdom.

The authors thank the 482 pediatrics and internal medicine residency training program directors who provided the information upon which this report is based.

References

1. *1986–1987 Directory of Graduate Medical Education Programs.* Chicago, Illinois: American Medical Association, 1986.

2. Parker, R. M., Hoekelman, R. A., and Napodano, R. J. Illnesses and Other Causes of Unexpected Absences From Work During Residency Training *J. Med. Educ.* **66**(1987):959–968.

3. *Revised Requirements for Residency Training in Pediatrics*. Chicago, Illinois: Accreditation Council for Graduate Medical Education. [Fourteen-page memorandum to directors of pediatrics residency programs] February 18, 1989.

4. *Special Requirements for Residency Training Programs in Internal Medicine*. Chicago, Illinois: Accreditation Council for Graduate Medical Education. [Fifteen page memorandum to directors of internal medicine residency programs] September 27, 1988.

5. *Revised Special Requirements*. Chicago, Illinois: Accreditation Council for Graduate Medical Education. [Ten-page memorandum to directors of pediatrics residency programs] February 19, 1985, p. 9.

6. *Booklet of Information*. Chapel Hill, North Carolina: The American Board of Pediatrics. 1988, p. 16.

7. *Verification of Clinical Competence Forms*. Chapel Hill, North Carolina: The American Board of Pediatrics. [Four-page memorandum to pediatrics program directors] March 21, 1988.

8. Oliver, T. K., Jr., Senior Vice-President, American Board of Pediatrics. Personal communication. August 30, 1989.

9. *Policies and Procedures*. Philadelphia, Pennsylvania: American Board of Internal Medicine, 1988.

10. Hoekelman, R. A. Stress Experienced during Pediatric Residency Training: Its Causes, Consequences, Recognition, and Solutions. *Am. J. Dis. Child.* **143**(1989): 177–180.

11. Resident Services Committee, Association of Program Directors in Internal Medicine. Stress and Impairment during Residency Training: Strategies for Reduction, Identification and Management. *Ann. Intern. Med.* **109**(1988):154–161.

Academic/
Clinical
Faculty
Learning
Designs

Faculty and Clinical Education Models of Entry-Level Preparation in Pediatric Physical Therapy

Wayne Stuberg, and Irene McEwen

Meyer Rehabilitation Institute; Division of Physical Therapy Education; and Department of Anatomy, University of Nebraska Medical Center, Omaha, Neb (W.A.S.); and Department of Physical Therapy (I.M.), University of Oklahoma, Oklahoma City, Okla

The need for pediatric physical therapists has escalated through the growth of physical therapy and the expansion of federally mandated programs for children and youth in the schools. The increased demands in early intervention and educational programs, which are already challenged by growth in student numbers and limited faculty, is a challenge in preparing entry-level practitioners ready to work in pediatrics. This article presents faculty and clinical education models currently being utilized in physical therapy education for pediatrics. The relationship of these models to the development of pediatric practitioners and the current trends in physical therapy education are also discussed.

According to estimates from the American Physical Therapy Association (APTA), approximately 7 to 10% of practicing physical therapists are pediatric practitioners.[1] The need for a greater number of physical therapists qualified to provide services for children and their families has been well-documented throughout *Pediatric Physical Therapy*. Over the past decade, the need for pediatric physical therapists has escalated because high-risk infants have survived and federally mandated programs for children and youth have expanded to cover the age range from birth through high school. The shortage of therapists is also influenced by the intervention methods used by pediatric therapists, which often require the direct skills of a physical therapist, rather than the utilization of modalities, equipment, or paraprofessionals.[2] In support of efforts to alleviate the shortage of pediatric therapists, one of the long-term goals of the Section on Pediatrics of the American Physical Therapy Association is to increase the number of physical therapists from all educational levels who enter pediatrics.[3]

The objective of this article is to discuss the faculty and clinical education models currently being utilized in physical therapy education. The relationship of these models to the development of pediatric practitioners and the current trends in physical therapy education will also be discussed.

0898-5669/93/0503-0123$3.00/0
PEDIATRIC PHYSICAL THERAPY
Copyright © 1993 by Williams & Wilkins

Address correspondence to: Wayne Stuberg, PhD, PT, Director, Department of Physical Therapy, Meyer Rehabilitation Institute, University of Nebraska Medical Center, 600 S. 42nd Street, Omaha, NE 68198-5451.

FACULTY MODELS

The need for increasing the number of physical therapists in pediatrics and other areas of practice is exacerbated by a critical shortage of physical therapy faculty.[4] As a result of the faculty shortage, many physical therapy programs have turned to nontraditional and creative means to provide educational content for entry-level students. This may be especially true for pediatric content, given the shortage of pediatric faculty and pediatric physical therapy's relatively small proportion of the overall practice arena, compared with such specialties as orthopaedics and general acute care.

There are three common faculty models by which physical therapy education programs provide pediatric content: (a) full- or part-time faculty with academic appointments, (b) part-time faculty who are employed by clinical facilities that are affiliated with the college or university, or (c) part-time faculty who work in clinical settings outside of the college or university system.

Within each of these broad categories, there are a number of possible permutations that have been utilized by physical therapy programs across the United States. Each of these faculty models will be described, followed by factors that need to be considered to assure that the faculty model employed satisfies standards of quality for entry-level preparation.

Full- or Part-Time Academic Faculty

The faculty model in which pediatric physical therapy faculty have full-time academic appointments is probably the most common and has traditionally been favored. Some faculty hold part-time academic appointments. This is less common because it may be difficult to meet conventional academic expectations on a part-time basis.[5]

The traditional academic roles of teaching, service, and research, with the amount of time spent on each role varying

Stuberg W, McEwen I. Faculty and clinical education models of entry-level preparation in pediatric physical therapy. *Pediatric Physical Therapy*. Vol 5, pp 123-127. Reprinted with permission.

with the mission or emphasis of the college or university are usually filled by full-time faculty. A 1990 survey of criteria used to evaluate physical therapy faculty found that criteria related to teaching and scholarship were used by more colleges and universities than criteria related to service and clinical activities.[6] This was true of both baccalaureate and entry-level master's degree programs. Faculty research has become increasingly expected and valued in physical therapy programs.[1,7]

Faculty in tenure track positions at major research universities often need to demonstrate excellence in research to become tenured. A probationary period, which is usually 5 or 6 years, is allowed to complete credentials required for tenure, which if granted, allows faculty to remain in the position. This is particularly true for the increasing number of faculty who have doctoral degrees. Faculty who hold nontenure track positions or who work at colleges or universities that do not place an emphasis on research, may be able to focus on the teaching and service faculty roles.

In addition to their teaching and research responsibilities, academic pediatric physical therapy faculty often participate in clinical practice. The settings in which they practice can vary widely. Settings may include faculty practice clinics, college or university physical therapy department facilities, clinics in community programs, contracts with educational programs, or private practice. The amount of time spent in clinical practice and the amount of reimbursement received beyond their base faculty salary, if any, is usually negotiated with the departmental administrators.

Full-time or part-time faculty can be hired with either "hard money," which has been authorized on a continuing basis by the funding source (such as the university), or with "soft money." Soft money usually comes from grants or contracts, so continuous funding of the position is not certain, or funding is for a set time and certain to end. Positions funded through soft money can become available for individual faculty members to assume teaching responsibilities of other faculty who have grants or contracts supporting part or all of their salaries. Research, training, and service programs can be financed by this external funding mechanism.

Soft money positions can provide good opportunities for pediatric faculty although job security is not assured. For example, these arrangements allow new faculty to gain teaching experience without the pressure of the ticking tenure clock. Some positions provide opportunities to work with other pediatric faculty, to be involved in research, to gain experience in writing grants, and to influence policies and programs of state agencies. Soft money positions can also offer an opportunity for clinicians to experience academic life without committing to a hard money position, for which a doctoral degree is increasingly desirable, if not required.[1]

The courses taught by pediatric faculty who hold academic appointments vary considerably. Some faculty teach only pediatric courses or the pediatric components of courses (such as a pediatric unit in an orthopaedics class or the pediatric content of a neurological rehabilitation class). Other pediatric faculty teach both pediatric content and other physical therapy curriculum content.[5] Three factors seem to influence the type of courses that pediatric faculty teach: (a) the size of the faculty; (b) whether or not the program has a postentry-level pediatric program; and (c) the expertise of the pediatric faculty and the program's teaching needs. In a large faculty the chances of having an academician with pediatric background is greater, which allows for greater pediatric focus in the curriculum. In the case of postentry-level programs, there is often greater opportunity for the student to focus on a specialty area such as pediatrics. The third factor that was mentioned, faculty

expertise, relates to the ability of the curriculum to provide entry-level pediatric curriculum content through full- or part-time faculty vs utilization of clinical faculty. Although clinicians are more actively involved in pediatric practice they are not typically aware of pediatric curriculum requirements for accreditation nor do they have the teaching expertise of full-time academicians.

Part-Time University Affiliated Adjunct Faculty

Universities with physical therapy programs are often affiliated with clinical facilities that serve as training sites for students of various disciplines and may provide academic faculty with opportunities for clinical practice. Pediatric rehabilitation centers, child development centers, children's hospitals, and laboratory schools are pediatric facilities that are commonly affiliated with universities. Physical therapists who are employed in these settings may also teach in affiliated academic programs, on a permanent or temporary basis.

The time commitment of affiliated faculty to the academic program will vary with the needs of both the program and the clinical setting. Versteeg et al.[8] described a physical therapy education program that contracted with affiliating hospitals for two physical therapists to serve as half-time adjunct faculty in the academic program. In this example, adjunct faculty assumed many of the roles of full-time academic faculty, including classroom teaching, student advising, research, and faculty and program governance. As a result of their many academic responsibilities and their half-time clinical roles, early program participants were reported to feel as though they had two full-time jobs. To avoid stress associated with excessive amounts of work, the authors recommended ongoing clarification of expectations and responsibilities, and avoidance of scheduling conflicts.

In contrast, affiliated faculty in other physical therapy education programs may not assume all of the traditional faculty responsibilities. For example, affiliated pediatric faculty may teach the pediatric content of a course, or may teach a separate pediatric course, but do not participate in other faculty roles, such as research, publication, student advising, or governance meetings.

Affiliated faculty can teach in either the academic or the clinical setting. Some clinical settings, such as a university child development center, may have classroom space and other facilities that can be used by physical therapy students. When affiliated faculty teach academic content in their clinical settings, they can often combine didactic and clinical experiences for students. Affiliated faculty who teach in academic settings may also be able to provide clinical experiences to support the classroom content.

Part-Time Adjunct Faculty From Outside the University

Part-time pediatric physical therapy faculty can also be recruited from among physical therapists who are not affiliated with the college or university. These faculty may work in clinical settings or other academic settings, and may be from the local area or from virtually anywhere in the world. As with other faculty, they may teach parts of courses or entire courses, but usually assume only the teaching aspects of the faculty role during their part-time assignments. Sometimes these faculty are recruited to help fill gaps left by vacant positions; at other times they are recruited because they have particular expertise in an area of pediatric physical therapy.

Local clinicians might present only one or two sessions of a class, or could participate in classroom and/or laboratory sessions throughout a school term. Creative scheduling is usually necessary when part-time faculty travel from outside the local area. A program with a pediatric faculty vacancy, for example, recruited a therapist from out of state to teach the didactic content of a pediatric elective course during 2 week-long visits. There were 15 contact hours with the students during each visit, which were spaced 6 weeks apart. Before the first visit and between the two visits, the students had laboratory experiences in pediatric sites with local clinical faculty who had been selected specifically for this educational experience and had participated in development of course objectives.

Other options are to bring in visiting faculty for intensive weekend or week-long courses, or to have visiting faculty participate in only a portion of a longer-term course. The ways in which visiting faculty can contribute pediatric physical therapy content are nearly endless, being limited only by the resources of the educational program and the schedules of the faculty and students.

The faculty model used may be based on choice or perhaps the consequence of faculty shortages. If faculty with pediatric experience are not part of the full-time staff, affiliated faculty with pediatric experience or community resources can be utilized to assure adequate exposure of the students to pediatrics.

Quality Considerations

Regardless of the faculty model used, the quality of student's educational experiences is an essential consideration. The quality of faculty has an obvious influence on student's acquisition of pediatric physical therapy knowledge, attitudes, and skills. In addition, the Commission on Accreditation in Physical Therapy (CAPTE) of the American Physical Therapy Association requires that certain faculty standards be met for entry-level program accreditation.[9] Evaluative criteria for accreditation of educational programs include requirements for each faculty member to have documented expertise in teaching; demonstrated effective teaching and evaluation of students; and involvement in scholarly and professional activities, and community service. Each of these are to be consistent with the philosophy of the physical therapy program and the college or university.

The disciplinary expertise and teaching skills of the faculty are important, but do not solely influence the quality of student's educational experiences. The many nonteaching roles and responsibilities of faculty also affect the quality of student's experiences, either directly or indirectly. These roles and responsibilities usually include: student advising and counseling; curriculum review, evaluation, and modification; departmental meetings and committees; college or university governance; research and other scholarly activities; publication; clinical practice; participation in professional organizations; provision of continuing education; other community service; and personal professional development.

The quality of students' experiences with pediatric academic faculty can also significantly influence students' interest in working in pediatric settings when they graduate. It is important that faculty teaching pediatric content not only provide high quality academic and clinical educational experiences for students, but that they are available to advise students, serve as positive role models, and lend support to students as they decide upon and take their first jobs.

CLINICAL EDUCATION MODELS

According to Moore and Perry,[10] clinical education is; "the portion of the student's professional education that involves practice and application of classroom knowledge and skills to on-the-job responsibilities. This occurs at a variety of sites and includes experience in evaluation and patient care, administration, research, teaching, and supervision. It is a participatory experience with limited time spent in observation. The importance of providing positive pediatric clinical education experiences becomes a major issue in increasing the number of pediatric practitioners because many new graduates go to work for facilities at which they previously were affiliated.

Clinical education has been an ongoing topic of focus by the APTA. Numerous workshops and symposia have been sponsored and in the 1992–1994 Comprehensive Plan for Clinical Education the priorities were revisited.[11] The plan was developed by the APTA Task Force on Clinical Education and was based on the following six assumptions;

1. There seems to be no universal truth regarding the best model or method of accomplishing an end product in clinical education.

2. Current and future designs of clinical education should be driven by a structured process that addresses the quality of performance outcomes at each level of clinical experience.

3. In the short term, our current system is not in crisis. There is evidence, however, that it needs attention and additional exploration in specific areas.

4. There is evidence that a model incorporating a longer experience of clinical education that shifts increased responsibility to the clinical setting is evolving and needs further study.

5. Changes in clinical education must be related to: a) greater competence or efficiency of the practitioner (quality), b) increased cost-effectiveness (value), and c) greater availability of services to consumers (access).

6. Optimal outcomes of clinical education must reflect changes not only in the clinical education process but in the prior academic preparation in subsequent employment experiences.

In reviewing the assumptions it becomes clear that the work in delineating the optimal model for clinical education and to answer other related questions is far from complete. Based on the aforementioned assumptions, the priorities of the APTA task force are to increase the number and quality of clinical educators, develop revised standards of clinical education for entry-level programs, develop an accreditation process for clinical education residency programs, and to focus additional resources and research into determining the most effective method of clinical education.[11]

Clinical education for the preparation of students desiring to become pediatric practitioners is the focal point of this section. A brief discussion of clinical education models will be presented, trend changes in clinical education during the past decade discussed and special considerations presented that challenge the entry-level practitioner who chooses pediatric practice.

Models of Clinical Education

In the report of the Task Force to Study Alternative Models for Clinical Education in Physical Therapy, four models of clinical education were identified after a review of eight postbaccalaureate entry-level professions including medicine, dentistry and nursing.[12] The models were classified using the terms integrated, separate, self-contained, and independent.

In the integrated model, clinical affiliations are arranged throughout the curriculum with the degree conferred upon completion of both components. Within the integrated model, there is the possible use of concurrent (part-time) vs nonconcurrent scheduling of clinical experiences. In the concurrent schedule the student is in the clinic for part of the day and in the classroom for the remainder. In the noncurrent schedule, the students are scheduled into full-time clinical experiences varying from 1 day per week up to multiple weeks. The integrated model is widely used in physical therapy education.

The separate model includes affiliations arranged at the end of the didactic curriculum with the degree conferred upon completion of both components. Although there are few programs in physical therapy that utilize this model without any clinical exposure during the didactic component, the percentage of programs that utilize a major final clinical education experience is on the increase.[13]

In the self-contained model, the students complete supervised patient contact experiences with faculty members as advisors along with the didactic coursework. Clinical education experiences outside of the educational setting are not used and the degree is conferred at the end of the program. This model is not utilized in physical therapy education.

And finally in the independent model, the clinical experiences are limited to clinical laboratory activities with the degree conferred upon completion of the program. An independent clinical experience is then required after the didactic program for licensure. Although the independent model is also not utilized in physical therapy education, the concept of completing the didactic component, graduating, and then completing an extended clinical experience or internship is the predominant model in medical education. The model is also being discussed as an option to our current use of the integrated model to allow for a more extensive clinical experience that is not under the supervision of the educational program.[14]

Current Trends in Clinical Education

Pediatric clinical education experiences using either the integrated or separate models vary widely across the country. Factors such as the philosophy of the educational program and availability of clinical sites and personnel often mandate the model of clinical education that is utilized.

The trend in clinical education toward a decrease in concurrent (part-time) clinical education to multiple blocks of 1 to 4 weeks has been reported.[13] The use of multiple blocks provides the student with greater continuity during the clinical experience than the part-time experience. The student is able to participate more consistently in all aspects of the practice's daily schedule. Decreased travel time per day and stress on the student are also significant advantages to a schedule with academic work during part of the day mixed with clinical education.

A slight increase in the percentage of programs that utilize a final full-time block or major portion of full-time clinical education after completion of the didactic coursework has been evidenced.[13] More recent data on the trend since 1985 are not available, however, the trend is gaining wider acceptance in the profession.[15,18]

If the trend toward only a few major clinical blocks at the end of the educational program continues, however, it may not be advantageous to the recruitment of students into pediatrics. The use of a separate model with only a few clinical opportunities at the completion of the didactic curriculum places an educational program in a situation of limited choices for the students. The students may also be less likely to choose a pediatric clinical experience if they view it as too specialized and they are in greater need of a general acute or rehabilitation experience. The use of even short multiple blocks with an integrated model allows more students to participate in all areas of physical therapy practice and therefore receive an exposure to pediatrics.

A more significant change and a positive trend relating to pediatrics, however, is the significant increase in the number and type of facilities offering pediatric experiences to students. Pediatric outpatient facilities, school settings, and pediatric child care facilities have all seen a significant rise in the number of affiliating students over the past 15 years.[11] The increase in the number of pediatric practitioners

and the increasing demand for therapists in pediatrics have assured continued growth in the number of pediatric clinical affiliation sites.

The optimal length of time for clinical education is a topic of ongoing debate that remains unresolved. The trend in clinical education has been to increase the amount of clinical education in curriculums, particularly in the entry-level postbaccalaureate degree programs, and to use multiple full-time blocks. In a survey of academic administrators completed in 1985, the majority of respondents chose 6 to 9 months for the final full-time clinical education experience.[13] Discussion regarding a 1-year final full-time experience has been widely debated in the education community over the past decade. As preliminary research supports the relationship of greater competence, efficiency, and increased cost-effectiveness when clinical education experiences are longer,[19,20] additional study addressing the issue has been identified as an objective in the APTA's plan for development of clinical education.

Perhaps the answer to the question of how long the experience should be is not definable. A competency-based outcome model would allow for varying lengths of clinical education dependent on the student's ability to master the competencies necessary to become an entry-level practitioner.

Use of a competency-based independent model in physical therapy may be a future trend to consider.[14] Using an independent model would require the APTA and educational programs to develop uniform clinical education standards and a mechanism to certify sites. The students could complete their college or university curriculum, receive their degree and then move on to completing clinical education requirements before receiving permanent licensure. The students could then be paid during clinical rotations, as is presently practiced in medicine, and completion of clinical education in a select practice area could coincide with career laddering toward specialization.

Practice Considerations in Pediatrics

Except in the case of practice settings with multiple pediatric therapists, the entry-level practitioner desiring to practice pediatrics may find themselves in an environment where technical assistance or supervision is limited. Physical therapists working in the public schools frequently practice without physician referral, and therefore, are required to practice as a "clinical expert" on the educational team.

The limited educational exposure to pediatrics in many programs has lead to the conclusion by certain clinicians that perhaps pediatrics is not appropriate for the entry-level practitioner, unless the practice situation includes adequate technical assistance and support. Many pediatric competencies have to be obtained through continuing education because of the limited time available in entry-level curricula. The use of standardized tests, specialized evaluation procedures used in pediatrics, familiarization with changing federal and state mandates, development of individualized education plans or individualized family service plans, and inadequate time to develop hands-on treatment skills are but a few of the areas of frequent deficiency in the entry-level practitioner.

Practice in the public schools particularly places unique challenges on the entry-level practitioner and the educational program to develop clinical problem-solving skills. Although the clinical reasoning process used in medicine by physicians has been shown to use the same process used by expert physical therapy clinicians, the experience and support required to develop the skills remains the subject of ongoing research.[21] The development of problem-solving skills will continue to be one of the major challenges for clinical and didactic education for entry-level practitioners.[22,23]

Another area that affords unique challenges to the entry-level pediatric practitioner is their limited understanding of the maturational process and its relationship to normal and abnormal development in children. Children with developmental disabilities rarely outgrow their functional impairments or resulting disabilities. The impairments and disabilities cannot be "treated away" and therefore unique challenges are placed on the clinician to assess treatment need and efficacy in lieu of such factors as maturational changes vs treatment effects, available resources, and use of a team concept to deliver care.

Curricular Considerations for Pediatrics

Introduction of pediatrics early in the didactic or clinical education experience is desired to increase the likelihood of students choosing to practice in pediatrics. Multiple courses that include pediatric content may increase the student's focus toward pediatrics. Pediatric content can be spread across the curriculum in multiple courses such as in the evaluation methods course or clinical medicine in addition to the traditional growth and development and pediatric rehabilitation courses.

The inclusion of a full or part-time faculty with pediatric expertise is desired to increase the focus of pediatrics in the curriculum. In the case of programs without a faculty member with pediatric expertise, utilization of adjunct faculty or local pediatric clinicians in the curriculum may help provide role models for students interested in pediatrics.

If an educational program uses a separate model for clinical education with limited affiliation options, the faculty member responsible for the pediatric curriculum can alternatively use "in class" pediatric demonstrations to increase the exposure of students to pediatric clinical problems in the didactic section of the curriculum. If part-time or multiple block clinical education experiences are utilized in an integrated clinical education model, the availability of pediatrics is essential to promote interest in pediatrics, especially because many curriculums provide limited pediatric information in the didactic coursework.[5]

SUMMARY

Pediatric practice provides unique challenges to the academician and clinician who prepare entry-level practitioners. As most graduates will not choose pediatrics as their full-time practice area, a general goal of providing the student with adequate knowledge to identify common pediatric problems and when to refer to a pediatric clinician is desired.

For the entry-level practitioner who desires to practice in pediatrics, the pediatric background provided in school is only the foundation in developing clinical expertise. Students should not be dissuaded from pediatrics as a first-practice choice, but rather the importance of continuing education and supervision in the practice setting emphasized by academic and clinical faculty. Pediatric practitioners need to take an active role in mentoring entry-level practitioners who desire to become clinical experts in pediatrics because educational programs cannot provide all of the background needed to independently practice in pediatrics.

The health care system is in transition and will continue to demand greater competence and efficiency of the practitioner, increased cost-effectiveness of services, and greater access to services. As is true in so many areas of physical therapy practice, pediatrics is greatly in need of additional practitioners to respond to the changes in the health care system. The faculty and clinical education models reviewed in this article are alternatives that have been developed to meet the unique needs of education programs as they strive to educate practitioners to work in the health care system. The ongoing research, collaboration, cooperation between educational programs, clinical education facilities, and clinicians will assure that the challenges will be met in pediatric practice.

The authors wish to thank Jody Gandy and the Department of Education, APTA for their support in the development of this article.

This work was supported in part by a grant from the Maternal and Child Health Bureau, Health Resources and Services Administration.

REFERENCES

1. American Physical Therapy Association Department of Membership. Alexandria, Va: 1992.
2. Long T. Editorial: academic clinical linkages. *Pediatr Phys Ther.* 1989;1:157.
3. Martin T. Message from the chair: facing the future. Pediatr *Phys Ther.* 1989;1:121–122.
4. Action Plan to Address the Faculty Shortage. Alexandria, Va; APTA; March 1988.
5. Survey on Pediatric Curriculum Structure and Content. Alexandria, Va; APTA; Sections on Pediatrics and Education, 1991.
6. Rothman J, Rinehart ME. A profile of faculty development in physical therapy education programs. *Phys Ther.* 1990;70:310–313.
7. Jensen G. The work of accreditation on-site evaluators: enhancing the development of a profession. *Phys Ther.* 1988;68:1517–1525.
8. Versteeg ML, Strein JW, Fitch DH, Darnell RE. Utilization of rotatory clinical faculty members in physical therapy education. *J Phys Ther Ed.* 1987;1:21–26.
9. Commission on Accreditation in Physical Therapy Education. *Accreditation Handbook.* Alexandria, Va; APTA; August, 1990.
10. Moore ML, Perry JF. Clinical Education in Physical Therapy: Present Status/Future Needs. Final Report of the Project on Clinical Education in Physical Therapy. Section for Education. APTA; 1976;2.
11. Plan for the Development of Clinical Education in Physical Therapy Education. APTA; 1991.
12. Report of Task Force to Study Alternative Models for Clinical Education in Physical Therapy. Section for Education. APTA; 1985.
13. Myers RS. Fact and fantasy from Rose's almanac: or, all that you wanted to know about clinical education and have been asking. In: *Leadership for Change in Physical Therapy Clinical Education,* Department of Education. APTA; 1986;95–107.
14. Gandy JS. Fiscal implications for clinical education. In: *Pivotal Issues in Clinical Education, Present Status/Future Needs,* Section for Education. APTA; 1988;62–72.
15. Barnes M. The optimum design for clinical education: an academic administrator's perspective. In: *Pivotal Issues in Clinical Education, Present Status/Future Needs,* Section for Education. APTA; 1988;130–140.
16. DeMont M. Establishing the optimum design for clinical education: the academic coordinator of clinical education's perspective. In: *Pivotal Issues in Clinical Education, Present Status/Future Needs,* Section for Education. APTA; 1988;141–146.
17. Hislop HJ. Post-graduate education: the internship. *Phys Ther.* 1967;47:271.
18. Jackson D. Establishing the optimum design: the clinical administrator's perspective. In: *Pivotal Issues in Clinical Education, Present Status/Future Needs,* Section for Education. APTA; 1988;120–129.
19. Porter RE, Kincaid CB. Financial aspects of clinical education to facilities. *Phys Ther.* 1977;57:905–909.
20. Lopopolo RB. Financial model to determine the effect of clinical education programs on physical therapy departments. *Phys Ther.* 1984;64:1396–1402.
21. Payton OD. Clinical reasoning process in physical therapy. *Phys Ther.* 1985;65:924–928.
22. Olsen SL. Teaching treatment planning: a problem-solving model. *Phys Ther.* 1983;63:526–529.
23. Slaughter DS, Brown DS, Gardner DL, Perritt LJ. Improving physical therapy student's clinical problem-solving skills: an analytical questioning model. *Phys Ther.* 1989;69:441–447.

The ACADEMIC-CLINICAL
FACULTY EXCHANGE MODEL

By Meredith E. Drench, PhD, PT,
and Jane Toot, PhD, PT

Complex subject matter—coupled with the orchestration of clinical practice and academic theory—results in what often seems to be the Gordian knot of physical therapy education. Untying this knot to produce coherent threads of learning can be a difficult and sometimes frustrating task. Curriculum designers must make certain that the needs of the student are compatible with the practices of both the academic institution and the clinical facility.[1]

The literature is rich with discussions of clinical education in physical therapy, including descriptions of theoretical approaches, models in practice, evaluation techniques for students and faculty, and concerns about the future delivery of clinically based experiences.[2-7] Much thought has been given not only to retaining clinical education in the curriculum but to enhancing the entire process of providing "hands-on" learning opportunities. Current configurations of clinical education, looming financial constrictions, and institutional priorities, however, can make high-quality clinical and academic education seem elusive.[8]

Concerns about clinical education may be said to center around the following three areas.

Tying together practice and theory in clinical education may result in what seems to be a "Gordian knot." This alternative model could help unravel that knot—while helping to contain costs and enhance staff retention.

other's physical or social "turf."[9] Academic and clinical educators may differ, for example, in the amount of value they place on teaching problem solving, clinical competency, and medical ethics. Even though they may develop mutual goals and objectives, they may never feel they *belong* in each other's setting.

Costs Versus Benefits

The issue of the *costs* of clinical education for providers and recipients versus its *benefits* is unresolved. Because the ability of clinical facilities to use funds from Medicare and Medicaid to mitigate the cost of clinical education has been challenged by the US Department of Health and Human Services, many administrators of clinical facilities have had to closely examine the financial implications of clinical education[8] and reassess their roles in this area.[10] Diagnostic-related groups (DRGs), which revolve around patient-care-identified settings, are another factor in the cost-to-benefit ratio.[8] Staffing patterns and duties in hospitals have undergone several changes as a result of DRGs, including changes that have a direct or indirect impact on clinical education: shorter lengths of hospital stay in acute care facilities (resulting in a higher volume of "new" patients), a greater emphasis on cost-effectiveness and volume productivity (reducing the amount of time available for teaching), an expansion in the therapist's role in assessing patient progress and discharge status (which can make teaching more difficult, especially when the student's exposure to the clinic has been limited and when the student has not observed patients throughout the course of treatment), decreased numbers of therapists as hospital employees (which means fewer physical therapy students can be accommodated), and decreased continuing education budgets (which means that clinical educators may not be

The "Guest-In-The-House" Syndrome

Even the most ardent clinical educators (who spend hours planning experiences and creating volumes of procedures) may not be able to dispel the feeling of being a "guest in the house": Despite efforts to engage in dialogue and demonstrate mutual respect, clinical instructors (CIs), academic coordinators of clinical education (ACCEs), and center coordinators of clinical education (CCCEs) alike may feel uneasy on each

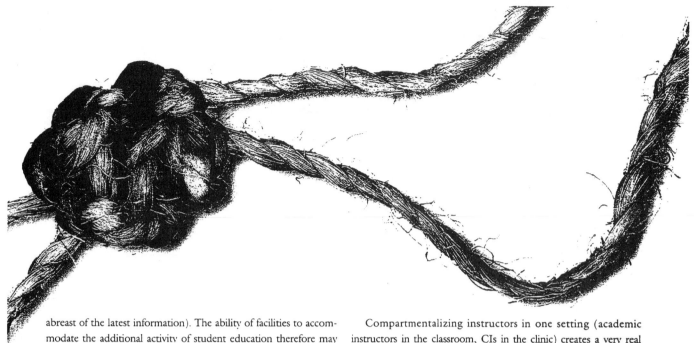

abreast of the latest information). The ability of facilities to accommodate the additional activity of student education therefore may not be realistic.[6,8,11]

The *benefits* of on-site clinical education may include its use as a recruitment tool and as an intrinsic motivator for involved staff members. The challenge of teaching students adds an intriguing dimension to a clinical staff position. Several ancillary benefits, such as vouchers for college courses, access to research facilities and academic faculty, and status as a clinical faculty member of an academic institution, also may accrue for staff.[6]

Administrators for clinical facilities must carefully weigh these and other costs and benefits before determining level of involvement in clinical education. In these difficult economic times, what makes sense in terms of staff development may not make "cents" to the financial officer of a clinical facility. Clinical education also requires the administrator of the academic institution to make financial considerations. For example, the expenses of travel, postage, printing, and telephone can become unwieldy and have a negative impact on: 1) the patterns of supervision provided by the *academic* program, 2) the ability of academic faculty members to work with clinically based faculty, and 3) the student's educational support system.

Academic-Clinical Compatibility

As with the "Telephone Game"—in which messages change by the time they make their way around the circle of players—the effect of a classroom lesson, of an objective written in a clinical education book, or of a technique demonstrated with a classroom "patient" can change when the lesson or technique is applied to actual experiences in the clinic.

The result of alterations to mold classroom theory into clinical practice may be far different from the original intent; however, the need for change may be obviated if the academic instructor accompanies the student into the clinic.[1,9] Similarly, the CI may have a rationale (for selecting a particular treatment approach) that can withstand theoretical analysis during *classroom* discussion.

Compartmentalizing instructors in one setting (academic instructors in the classroom, CIs in the clinic) creates a very real barrier to the fusion of academic and clinical learning. ACCEs and CCCEs may develop formal and informal lines of communication through clinical education manuals, jointly sponsored seminars, conference calls, and collaborative articles; however, the support and knowledge gained through the association between students and instructors may be fragmented or lost across environments because of poor curriculum design or the need to search for available student placements.

One problem inherent in this compartmentalized, or non-concurrent, pattern of clinical education is that students typically do not see the on-site educator in multiple roles. They may erroneously assume that the classroom instructor does not understand the reality of the clinic and that the CI would not be able to meet the theoretical and scholarly demands of the classroom (assumptions that may be made not just by students but by academic and clinical instructors themselves). The result: *The student may perceive the professional role to be a narrow path, not recognizing the broad matrix in which a professional career in physical therapy can develop.*[12]

Physical therapy clinical education models often assign one CI to each student. The CI typically is prepared to engage in clinical education through the use of manuals and on-site training sessions. Communication between the academic institution and the clinical facility frequently begins before the student arrives in the clinic and continues throughout the affiliation, and extensive information detailing the academic curriculum through course descriptions and syllabi is sent to the clinics; however, because the academic and clinical worlds touch but may not interconnect, the integration of both cultures may be difficult to achieve.

Some Proposed Solutions

The concurrent pattern. In an effort to achieve better integration, a clinical education program may adopt a concurrent pattern, interweaving experiential and didactic learning—for example, a student may spend 2 days a week in the clinic and 3 days a week in the

Two Clinical Education Programs in Action

The University of Vermont

The Physical Therapy Department at the University of Vermont (UVM) in Burlington has traditionally reflected the working relationship between clinicians and academicians. University regulations allow academic faculty to practice clinically, much as they do at UVM's medical school. Each faculty member is permitted release time to treat patients at the off-site faculty practice (The Associates), at the Medical Center Hospital of Vermont (MCHV), or at other facilities as well as to teach at UVM. Clinical faculty are given the same latitude.

According to Sam Feitelberg, MA, PT, UVM's Chairperson and Director of Clinical Services, "Each person, depending on his or her role and initial appointment at the University, has the ability to conduct research, teach, or practice. The three organizations—the Department of Physical Therapy, The Associates, and MCHV—are drawn together for mutual benefit. Although they are separate entities, they work together, with decision making at the level of staff and faculty."

With 33 physical therapists based at UVM's hospital and 20 based at The Associates, the key objective is access, says Feitelberg. "In today's clinical delivery system, the classic professional lines of communication are changing. We now are structuring our program so that therapists have a multitude of opportunities to interact and contribute as professionals in a more integrated system."

Feitelberg emphasizes that UVM regulations are structured to grant clinical appointments as high as the level of clinical professor—the equivalent of professor. Explains Feitelberg, "If we as academicians believe that the nature of clinical experience is an academic lesson in itself—the objectives, the outcomes, the measurements—then it's important to appropriately appoint clinicians in the univer-

sity setting. Otherwise we make them second-rate."

In fostering this model, the University carefully looked at what has happened in other models, he adds. "We tried to take the best of the models and apply that to physical therapy," says Feitelberg. "In the medical model, faculty members are important income-generating persons, and that creates a lot of pressure. On the one hand, that model provides a rich mix of access to academia and the clinic, but there are violations as well, for instance, when the university benefits from the productivity of the physician/teacher in a way that drives the financial capability of a department."

The UVM Department of Physical Therapy is now involved in a movement toward an academic medical center, with an emphasis on integrated systems and primary care, goals that Feitelberg predicts will be reached "in the not-too-distant future. We're enjoying, and we will continue to enjoy, our native right as practitioners to have full access to the clinic and classroom and to become more involved with our colleagues at all levels."

Temple University Hospital

Close proximity no doubt had a hand in building the close working relationship that has evolved between Temple University Hospital and Temple University over the last 3 years. "We made a conscious decision to build on their curriculum when we developed our program," says Joyce Adcock, Chief Physical Therapist for Temple University Hospital. "It seemed like the most logical relationship because we work right across the street from one another."

Depending on the curriculum being offered each semester, clinical faculty members are involved in a number of activities to enhance

students' learning experiences: They assist in teaching the basic skills course (a third of which is taught at the hospital); they conduct lab instruction for orthopedics, neurology, and kinesiology courses; and they offer a student "extern" program as part of the hospital's formal clinical education program.

"We feel our ongoing relationship with the PT faculty benefits students in that it exposes them early on to the different approaches of clinicians and academicians, that is, the functional versus theoretical," says Adcock. "We can take what students have learned in the classroom and immediately apply it to a real-life situation."

The University also participates in the hospital's extern program for students at neighboring schools. "The program allows a student to have employment during the school year, and it offers something unique as well," says Adcock. "We involve our externs in more 'nuts and bolts' operational duties, such as inventory, ordering equipment, paperwork for new patients, staff meetings, educational programs, etc. Our aim is to give externs an overall experience working in a PT department, not just have them work with patients. We try to demonstrate the full spectrum of roles a health professional plays in a community environment like a university."

Adcock predicts an increased involvement with Temple's academic faculty in years to come. "Today, we provide the hands-on practical skills, and they provide the didactic skills, which together fulfills our professional obligation to give students a well-balanced education. In the future, we hope to get to the point where the lines of distinction between academicians and clinicians are blurred. That would be the ultimate kind of melding for our profession."

—Beth Monahan

classroom—but difficulties with this model can include scheduling and ensuring continuity of patient care.[13]

The preceptor model. The preceptor approach is not a new idea. Nursing has incorporated the preceptor model of clinical experience into its educational programs: Academic nursing faculty routinely accompany nursing students into the clinical setting as tutors and supervisors.[9] Respiratory therapy also has used this model, with academic faculty members serving as

full-time preceptors and accompanying students into the clinic.[14]

The nursing education literature has long documented this model's advantages (eg, education takes place in clinical sites with actual patients versus in the classroom through exercises; there is onsite involvement with other staff members as well as with the preceptor; it is the preceptor's responsibility, not the staff clinician's responsibility, to discuss patient issues, coordinate learning experiences and evalu-

ate competencies, which promotes better time management and cost-effectiveness) and disadvantages (eg, students continue to be associated with and accountable to a "teacher" rather than to a "colleague," the continuity of patient care cannot always be ensured when the student does not work with the same patients on a consistent basis). In brief, the preceptor model does encourage continuity for both faculty and students—but it demands intensive faculty and institutional commitment.[15]

During the past several years, alternative patterns of supervision that utilize a variety of staffing profiles have been implemented to provide valid clinical experiences for students while also minimizing costs for the providers. In 1986, one such alternative pattern was developed at Northeastern University, Boston, Mass.

The Academic-Clinical Faculty Exchange Model

Placing students in qualified clinical facilities had become increasingly difficult with the growing enrollment of students in Northeastern University's physical therapy program, one of three programs in Boston and one of five in the state. Assignments of 160 to 180 junior and senior students within a 12-month period were complicated by saturated clinical sites, a lack of transportation to and affordable housing in affiliated off-campus sites, and the need for junior students to be located within reasonable traveling distance of the university to accommodate course work on campus. In addition, physical therapy staff shortages created a dearth of available CIs.

The designers of what would be the Academic-Clinical Faculty Exchange Pilot Project reviewed the literature on the effectiveness of current methods of clinical education for nurses, physical therapists, and other health professionals in the effort to create a program that would address the staffing and site shortage while also addressing the three areas of concern detailed above. The designers concluded that the exchange model would emphasize a sense of belonging: Academic team members would have the opportunity to engage in clinical practice; clinical faculty team members would have the opportunity to develop didactic teaching skills in the classroom. The team members would combine theoretical and practical educational components in a professional experience. The goal would be to provide a valid experience for the student while also minimizing costs and meeting institutional and facility parameters of both efficiency and quality.

The pilot project. In February 1985, a proposal for an academic-clinical faculty exchange model was presented to the Chairperson of the Department of Physical Therapy and to the Dean of Boston-Bouvé College of Human Development Professions at Northeastern University. Upon approval, the Department of Physical Therapy's Clinical Education Committee and the CCCEs of four affiliating Boston hospitals began discussing the project. All CCCEs believed that the potential advantages (enhanced staff morale, motivation, and retention) outweighed any potential disadvantages (eg, staffing changes necessitate patient coverage when clinical faculty are teaching at the university, an increase in personnel may result in congestion in the treatment area, concurrent involvement with other academic programs may decrease, more time and energy would be expended by clinicians working in dual roles). All team members believed that the daily presence of the academic instructor in the clinic was imperative.

Tufts-New England Medical Center (NEMC) and Northeastern University mutually agreed on a pilot project to test the model. An Agreement for Faculty Exchange was signed, which described the joint planning and conducting of the program for the purpose of providing physical therapy education; the responsibilities of the university and the affiliating center; and the duration of the project. The academic faculty member, as an employee of the university, received no remuneration from the hospital; the clinical faculty members, as employees of the hospital, received no payment from the university. The university ensured that the academic faculty member was covered by general liability insurance.

In 1986, during the university's winter and spring quarters, a clinical supervisor from the Department of Physical Therapy at Northeastern University worked as a supervisor-preceptor ("super-preceptor"), or CI, with six physical therapy students on clinical affiliation in the physical therapy department at NEMC. The students would work with patients with a wide range of conditions (eg, related to amputation, spinal cord injury, traumatic brain injury, stroke, ventilator dependence).

During the first block of winter affiliations, the super-preceptor was oriented to the facility by the clinic staff and assumed a caseload. When the first student arrived 2 weeks later for block 1, the super-preceptor served not only as the supervisor responsible for the caseload but also as a preceptor and CI. During block 2, the senior student continued in the affiliation (for 6 weeks), joined by one new senior student. In block 1 of the spring affiliations, two junior students would have a 5-week clinical experience; in block 2, two new junior students would have a 5-week clinical experience. The super-preceptor established learning objectives for each student, planned learning experiences based on each student's clinical education needs and level of learning, monitored and assessed the students' clinical work, and evaluated the students' performance outcomes. This concept differed from the traditional model of one CI for each student, which had become a historic luxury rather than a pragmatic solution to current problems.

As part of the department's organizational hierarchy, the super-preceptor was to be responsible both for the students' actions and for the well-being of patients. The CCCE was to be responsible for all clinical education within the department of physical therapy. It was critical that the patients did not serve as "laboratory subjects" for the students. All project members were cognizant of the need to provide high-quality patient care within the time constraints of the facility and the external payment systems.

While the academic faculty member worked in the clinic as a super-preceptor, two clinical faculty members taught the university courses for which the super-preceptor previously had been responsible. The super-preceptor's delineated responsibilities in the hospital included student instruction and supervision, whereas the clinical faculty members were responsible for teaching courses in therapeutic exercise at the university.

How Well Did It Work?

Students evaluated their clinical experiences in this pilot project by completing the Student's Evaluation of a Clinical Experience from *Standards for Clinical Education in Physical Therapy: A Manual for Evaluation and Selection of Clinical Education*
(continued on page 112)

(continued from page 77)

Centers.[16] The Student Evaluation of Clinical Instructor form, an assessment tool designed by the super-preceptor to meet departmental merit review goals and university documentation requirements, also was completed by each student. Because it was the intent of the pilot project to determine whether the model was a viable alternative to clinical education, the Clinical Evaluation form used for all students in the Department of Physical Therapy also was used to evaluate the students in the pilot project. Three questionnaires for the ACCE, CCCE, and student were designed to further evaluate the exchange model. In addition, formal interviews were conducted by the ACCEs with the CCCE and staff of the affiliating center, the super-preceptor, and the students to obtain their perceptions of the benefits and concerns. Some of the evaluation results are contained in detail in the Appendix.

The quality of the clinical experience. Overall, the CCCE and staff of the affiliating center, the super-preceptor, and the students indicated that this model was viable and valuable. The project aided in the regulation and control of the learning experiences; facilitated peer review and discussion, decision making, and problem solving; enhanced the teaching and learning process through specific, planned learning experiences with group and individual work; and provided an opportunity for academic faculty to develop firsthand knowledge of the students' proficiency in the clinical setting. The super-preceptor's current clinical expertise also was enhanced—which could supplement classroom teaching.

The super-preceptor asserted that the exchange model was "at least as effective as our current model [one CI working with one student] in allowing students to work on clinical competencies." All students performed competently (as documented on the Clinical Evaluation form), achieving growth and improvement over the course of the clinical education experience. In the Student's Evaluation of a Clinical Experience, the students consistently indicated they believed that, more than 80% of the time, the super-preceptor: 1) planned,

implemented, and coordinated learning experiences that met their needs in achieving entry-level competencies; 2) demonstrated effective and efficient utilization of time; 3) followed the teaching-learning process in planning and implementing learning experiences; and 4) demonstrated teaching effectiveness during the implementation of learning experiences.

Occupants, not visitors. Because this model was integrated into the hospital department, the super-preceptor and the students developed a sense of belonging in the clinic, which helped reduce the "guest-in-the-house" syndrome. Clinical faculty, however, did not report having the same sense of belonging in the university setting.

Continuity of patient care. Critical to this model was an emphasis on providing high-quality care to patients and on realizing optimal therapeutic goals within a reasonable timeframe. The super-preceptor was responsible for supervising all patient-related activities and for ensuring that patient needs were addressed. The students worked with specific patients on a consistent basis throughout the course of their affiliation, which also helped ensure continuity of care.

Placement and staffing. The exchange project helped facilitate the placement of students in a high-quality facility because it was possible to assign multiple students during consecutive blocks of clinical affiliations (ie, 6 students within 4 blocks). The project also contributed to physical therapy staffing through the super-preceptor's coordination of a caseload. Because the project provided a change of environment and presented stimulating challenges to both academic and clinical faculty, a new mechanism for staff retention was established. In addition, the project helped enhance the educational program at the clinical facility because the project supported the staff, provided a role model for other clinical faculty, and became an educational resource.

The Bottom Line

This project required intensive commitment from both academic and clinical fac-

ulty members and therefore diminished personnel resources in both domains—which could be said to be the academic-clinical faculty exchange model's highest cost. And although academic and clinical faculty members practiced in dual roles, neither completely participated in meeting each other's responsibilities. In addition, students were unable to manage a full caseload of patients, a cost that primarily was offset by the breadth and depth of the patient care they did provide.

Did the benefits of the model outweigh the costs? This project provided the students with an effective learning experience, a continuous interweaving of theory and clinical practice, and an opportunity for team building, individual and group problem solving, and peer review. The relationship between the clinical facility and the university was strengthened. Professional development and intrinsic motivation for academic and clinical faculty were additional by-products of the project. In their dual roles, academic and clinical faculty members were positive role models, showing the breadth of their profession. The ratio of super-preceptor to students in contiguous blocks of affiliation time, the addition of a full-time staff member to the hospital, and the utilization of the clinical faculty members (when they were not teaching at the university) allowed for more effective use of resources. Academic and clinical compatibility was evidenced by the effective blending of components of the curriculum in the clinic and in the classroom. A crossing-over of faculty from one domain to another occurred without compartmentalizing instructors or fragmenting knowledge, and the project facilitated continuity both for faculty members and for students.

Recommendations

Recommendations for future development and application of this alternative model would include conferring clinical faculty appointments on the clinicians who exchange roles with the academic faculty members, providing an uninterrupted work schedule, and eliminating frequent travel between clinic and university. Clinical faculty could serve on committees and assume advisory duties, filling the void left by the

Appendix.
Participant Feedback Regarding the Academic-Clinical Faculty Exchange Model

Perceived Benefits

From the perspective of the CCCE and staff members of the affiliating center:

- Time commitment was reduced. The CCCE needed to be involved in a one-time facility orientation—not in training the CI.
- More patients could be accommodated through the addition of a full-time staff member and through the retention of the clinical faculty members (when they were not teaching at the university).
- Intrinsic motivation was developed through new assignments and responsibilities.
- Professional development was enhanced by the opportunity to teach in an academic setting.
- Students and the super-preceptor were integrated into clinical staff, becoming professional occupants rather than visitors.
- The ratio of one super-preceptor to two students allowed for more efficient clinical education.

From the perspective of the super-preceptor:

- Intrinsic motivation was developed through new assignments and responsibilities.
- Professional development was enhanced by the opportunity to update clinical skills.
- Students and the super-preceptor were integrated into the clinical staff.
- Relationship between the university and the clinical site and staff was strengthened, augmenting possible resources for classroom teaching, patient demonstrations, and videotapes.
- Concurrent involvement of two students allowed efficient use of the super-preceptor's time while providing an appropriate learning experience.
- Continuity between classroom theory and clinical practice was achieved when the same instructor held dual roles.
- The model could be adapted to other types of facilities, particularly those with clinical rotations that group patients with similar needs and problems.
- Working in teams provided the students with peer support and encouraged independence from the super-preceptor.

From the perspective of the students:

- Problem solving and independent work were encouraged.
- Adequate feedback was received.
- Students were able to begin developing the competencies expected of them upon completion of clinical education.
- Individual objectives were included in planned learning experiences.
- Learning experiences were based on students' level of competency.
- Supervision was commensurate to level of competency.
- Students were able to use time more efficiently.
- Academic and clinical components of the curriculum were effectively blended.
- Peer observation was an educational advantage.
- Students felt that they belonged in the clinic as a part of the clinical staff.
- Observation of the academic faculty member effectively interacting with the clinic staff was a positive experience, and the academic faculty member served as a role model.
- Senior students perceived that they received the same degree of attention during this affiliation that they had received during previous affiliations that used the one-CI-to-one-student model.

Suggestions and Concerns

From the perspective of the CCCE and staff members of the affiliating center:

- Grouping university assignments, which would allow clinical faculty members to be on campus for entire workdays, could reduce stress and enhance integration into the university environment; this in turn would allow preparation time for course work and committee and advisory assignments.
- Travel expenses (fares, mileage, parking) were assumed by the clinical and academic faculty; they *should* be assumed by the host facility.
- Using a clinical team to teach a course could lessen the stress of an unfamiliar work situation; such a team should include no more than one *senior* clinical staff member to avoid the depletion of the clinic's manpower resources.
- Academic and clinical faculty, as well as students, need to be flexible, capable, and committed to the model.
- The number of students assigned to the super-preceptor must be carefully considered, based on the type of clinical rotation and the size of available treatment space; two students would be appropriate for the super-preceptor.
- The ratio of two students to one super-preceptor may alter the ability of the clinic to accommodate students from other academic programs.

From the perspective of the super-preceptor:

- The university department "loses" the super-preceptor for other responsibilities (ie, clinic visits, committees, student advising).
- The role of the super-preceptor could become overwhelming unless allowances are made for time constraints, a limited number of students, and individual differences among students.
- This model is most suitable for accelerated learners.

From the perspective of the students:

- A student peer at the same facility might be perceived as competition rather than as support.
- Because it was not possible for each student to carry a full caseload, this model is recommended for use for only one of the student's affiliations.
- This model is more suitable for "average" learners than for slower learners.

academic faculty member and engaging the clinical faculty more fully in the university environment. Academic faculty in the clinic could have similar responsibilities. Staff members who participate in the exchange model could be rotated, providing opportunities for other individuals who could benefit from the experience.

Questions for Clinical Education Research

More research is needed on clinical education generally and on this alternative pattern specifically. Would the familiarity between the students and academic faculty members in the clinical setting increase the efficiency of teaching and learning? Would differences in job satisfaction exist between participants in the one-to-one clinical education model and participants in the super-preceptor model? Project participants believed that this model was not particularly appropriate for slower learners (Appendix). Comparisons among a random sample, a group of learners with like abilities, and a purposeful mix of students might prove to be insightful. Would it be effective to group clinical education students according to ability? *PT*

Meredith E Drench, PhD, PT, is Director, Adaptive Health Associates, Inc, East Greenwich, RI. Jane Toot, PhD, PT, is Chairperson, Department of Physical Therapy, Grand Valley State University, Allendale, Michigan. Drench gave a presentation on the academic-clinical faculty exchange model at APTA's Annual Conference held in Cincinnati, Ohio, June 12-16, 1993.

The authors acknowledge Ruth P Hall, former Associate Professor and ACCE, Department of Physical Therapy, Northeastern University, and Nancy Gilberti, former Clinical Supervisor, CI, and Super-Preceptor at the time this program was conducted.

Although all who participated in the academic-clinical faculty exchange project agreed that it should be further developed, political reorganization at the university prevented the implementation of any new programs. The model is being partially implemented this year at Grand Valley State University, *with academic faculty accompanying students into the clinic. The authors hope that other facilities and universities will consider using this model in its entirety.*

References

1 Balla JI, Gibson M, Biggs JB. Problems with curriculum implementation in in-service clinical education. *Med Educ.* 1989;23:282-289.

2 Gwyer J. Resources for clinical education: current status and future challenges. *Journal of Physical Therapy Education.* 1990;4(2):55-58.

3 Deusinger S. Establishing clinical education programs: a practical guide. *Journal of Physical Therapy Education.* 1990; 4(2):58-61.

4 Foord L, DeMont M. Teaching students in the clinical setting: managing the problem situation. *Journal of Physical Therapy Education.* 1990;4(2):61-66.

5 Deusinger S. Evaluating the effectiveness of clinical education. *Journal of Physical Therapy Education.* 1990;4(2):66-70.

6 Gandy J, Sanders B. Cost and benefits of clinical education. *Journal of Physical Therapy Education.* 1990;4(2):70-75.

7 Deusinger S. Summary and future initiatives. *Journal of Physical Therapy Education.* 1990;4(2):75.

8 Holder L. Paying for clinical education: fact or fiction. *J Allied Health.* 1988;17:221-229.

9 Heyrman KS, Phillips KM, Lessner JR. Collaboration: clinical education and hospital orientation. *Nursing Management.* 1987;18:64,66.

10 *Clinical Education in Physical Therapy: Considerations for Alternative Models.* Alexandria, Va: American Physical Therapy Association; 1985.

11 Graham CL, Catlin PA, Morgan J, et al. Comparison of 1-day-per-week, 1-week, and 5-week clinical education experiences. *Journal of Physical Therapy Education.* 1991;5:18-23.

12 Shepard KF, Jensen GM. Physical therapist curricula for the 1990s: educating the reflective practitioner. *Phys Ther.* 1990;70:566-573.

13 Walish JF, Olson RE, Schuit D. Effects of a concurrent clinical education assignment on student concerns. *Phys Ther.* 1986;66:233-236.

14 Hammersberg SS. A cost/benefit study of clinical education in selected allied health programs. *J Allied Health.* 1982;11:35-41.

15 Carpanito L, Duespohl TA. *A Guide for Effective Clinical Instruction.* Wakefield, Mass: Nursing Resources Concept Development; 1981.

16 Student's Evaluation of a Clinical Experience. In: *Standards for Clinical Education in Physical Therapy: A Manual for Evaluation and Selection of Clinical Education Centers.* Alexandria, Va: American Physical Therapy Association; 1981.

A Model for Faculty Practice Teaching Clinics Developed at the Oregon Health Sciences University

MARK T. O'HOLLAREN, M.D., CAROLE L. ROMM, R.N., M.P.A.,
THOMAS G. COONEY, M.D., EMIL J. BARDANA, M.D., JAMES WALKER, and
CAROLYN MARTIN

Abstract—In 1988 the Oregon Health Sciences University established its first faculty practice teaching clinic wherein physicians in training were incorporated into a faculty private practice clinic; this pilot project proved very successful and has been subsequently adopted as the model for essentially all outpatient clinics (both medical and surgery) in the university system. The model encourages efficiency, overhead control, and appropriate staffing; it also compensates faculty members for their additional time spent teaching. The authors conclude this model may help other academic training centers adapt to the changing demands of medical education. *Acad. Med.* 67(1992):51–53.

Teaching in the outpatient setting began with Hippocrates,[1] according to the hospital record, and dominated medical education until the rise of the teaching hospital at the end of the nineteenth century.[2] Today, economic and technological forces are creating an increasing demand for training in the ambulatory setting. Among these forces are the sharp decrease in the average patient's length of stay in the hospital, the increasing severity and complexity of illnesses in hospitalized patients, and the shift in patient care to the outpatient setting.[1-3]

Inpatient-based residencies often fail to reflect patient care in a typical medical practice.[3,4] For example, Byyny[5] reports that internists spend half of their time with ambulatory patients. Schroeder[2] has noted the reduced opportunities for residents to interact with and observe patients in the inpatient setting as the average inpatient's length of stay decreases,[2] and some authors[1,2] have emphasized the need for residents to learn skills that are now being taught only in the outpatient setting.

Despite the forces propelling the emphasis in medical education toward ambulatory care, strong financial disincentives remain. Most notable, reimbursement from third-party payers is considerably less for outpatient services than for inpatient services.[2,4] As a result, education in outpatient care often remains subsidized by payments for inpatient services.[2,6] In addition, in the increasingly competitive environment of health care, university clinics are at a disadvantage because of their greater percentage of indigent patients and their resultant greater share of uncompensated care.[2,7]

Medical school clinical faculties have always provided direct patient care, but before the advent of Medicare and Medicaid in the 1960s, this care was largely unreimbursed. Faculty practice organizations were developed for billing and accountability purposes, and, most important, so that income derived could be redistributed in proportional amounts to the university, department, and faculty member, according to the plan in effect. MacLeod and Schwarz[8] note the growth of faculty practice plans to supplement medical education funding, and Bentley and colleagues[3] recommend support of resident education by faculty practices.

The Model

In 1988, the Oregon Health Sciences University (OHSU) acted to expand the outpatient-based education of physicians in training while continuing to encourage the operation of successful faculty practice plans. The OHSU implemented a faculty practice teaching clinic as a pilot project for a three-year trial period in a medical subspecialty outpatient clinic; this model proved very successful and has been adopted by nearly all the outpatient clinics (in both medical and surgery subspecialties) at the university. As a model for a teaching clinic in which faculty members integrate four types of physicians in training (medical students, interns, residents, and fellows) into their academic private practice, it endeavors to expand teaching time in the clinics as well as the available base of patients for teaching purposes. Such a plan requires a commitment from the hospital and/or clinic administration to support teaching.

Using this model, one faculty physician is identified as the director of each clinic and is expected to play a leadership role in its efficient operation and supervision. A key feature of this model is that the director (and

Dr. O'Hollaren is director of the allergy and asthma clinic and assistant professor of medicine, Division of Allergy and Clinical Immunology; Ms. Romm is coordinator of ambulatory care quality assurance, University Hospitals and Clinics; Dr. Cooney is internal medicine residency program director and professor of medicine, Department of Medicine; Dr. Bardana is chair, Division of Allergy and Clinical Immunology, and professor and assistant chair, Department of Medicine; Mr. Walker is associate hospital director, University Hospitals and Clinics; and Ms. Martin is clinic administrative director, Medicine Clinics, University Hospitals and Clinics; all are at the Oregon Health Sciences University, Portland.

Correspondence and requests for reprints should be addressed to Dr. O'Hollaren, Division of Allergy and Clinical Immunology, Oregon Health Sciences University, 3181 S.W. Jackson Park Road, L329, Portland, OR 97201.

Reprinted with permission from *Academic Medicine*.
O'Hollaren MT, Romm CL, Cooney TG, Bardana EJ, Walker J, Martin C. 1992;67(1):51–53.

other faculty participants, if any) assumes partial financial responsibility for the operation of the clinic and is reimbursed a portion of the profit generated by that clinic. The share of expenses involved in running the clinic that must be reimbursed to the university is inversely proportional to the amount of teaching that is done in that clinic, as described in the present report.

We have found that in attempting to structure a compensation formula for a faculty practice teaching clinic, several important principles need to be incorporated. First, an optimal system should encourage efficiency and productivity in the operation of the clinic, while encouraging the active involvement of the physicians in training. The financial commitment of the faculty member(s) should promote an interest in the efficient operation of the clinic. The system requires involved faculty participation to ensure continuity of care despite rotating coverage by the physicians in training in the clinic. Close faculty supervision is crucial to the success of such a system.

Second, an optimal system should recognize the diversity of supervision required for medical students, interns, residents, and fellows. Both level of training and prior exposure to the specialty create different needs in learners.

Third, a procedure should be established to provide feedback to the faculty member(s) on the evaluations performed by the residents, interns, and students who have rotated through the clinic. This feedback should provide information to improve the educational experience of the clinic, and encourage a high level of commitment from the physicians in training.

Fourth, the system should recognize the specific teaching load of each faculty member. For example, three faculty members seeing patients in conjunction with one fellow is quantitatively and qualitatively different from one faculty member supervising a fellow, a resident, and two students.

In any institution, systems of this type should undergo continuous evaluation and be modified appropriately. The model must be flexible, and modification is inevitable as it is applied to diverse specialties in a variety of academic settings. As experience is gained, changes should be made to accommodate new knowledge acquired by working with the model.

Certain patients may prefer to see faculty physicians alone, without physicians in training. Thus, this model is not intended to replace all faculty practice plans but to present an option that may be applicable in certain settings.

The advantages of a successful model of this type are many, and are in part reflective of the director's closer supervision of the operation of the clinic. Clinic efficiency and productivity may be improved by the closer scrutiny of appointment scheduling practices and utilization of services and supplies, as well as physician and ancillary staffing.

This system may provide physicians in training with experience concerning the operation of a private office, an area of their education that is seldom adequately addressed in their training. In such a setting, faculty members could continue to meet the dual goals of teaching and generating income for the practice plans upon which both their reimbursements and the university's funds for medical education are often dependent.

Currently, each outpatient teaching clinic at the OHSU generates a gross revenue figure each month, from which direct expenses are subtracted. Direct expenses include the salaries of personnel, the costs of services and supplies, and the rental fees for space.

Gross revenue refers to all charges generated by that clinic, including revenue from visits to a physician, as well as procedures performed in that clinic by or under the supervision of the faculty member(s) in the clinic. These charges do not include charges for lab or X-ray tests, unless the tests are performed in the clinic by the physician(s) or nurses. The physician(s) usually bills for those services.

The model of the faculty practice teaching clinic assigns a "teaching credit" to a given clinic, which is based on the supervisory responsibilities of that clinic's faculty member(s). If the faculty member(s) has a particularly heavy teaching load, then the overhead expenses for that faculty member(s) are appropriately reduced to compensate for the loss in efficiency and productivity. The teaching credit is arrived at by compiling the number of students, interns, residents, and fellows that are regularly present in the clinic. Each of these physicians in training is given a relative teaching-point score.

Those physicians in training who require more supervision are given a greater teaching-point score than those who require less supervision. At the OHSU, medical students are given the highest score (three points) because they require the greatest supervision and take the largest amount of faculty time. Interns generally require less faculty supervisory time than students, and are given a value of two points. Residents require the least faculty time in a teaching clinic setting, and are given a one-point value. Fellows in the same subspecialty as the faculty member(s) are generally thought to help speed the clinic's operation and are not given a teaching-point score.

The scores of the physicians in training are totalled and divided by the number of faculty members who regularly staff the clinic in order to obtain the numerical value of that clinic's teaching credit(s). One credit translates into a reduction of total overhead expenses by 10%, whereas three credits decrease overhead by 30%.

A clinic, of course, may operate with varying numbers of personnel on different days of the week. For example, a clinic that has two half-day sessions a week may be staffed during session one by only one physician and no physicians in training. The clinic would receive no teaching credit for that session. During session two, the same clinic may be staffed by two physicians, one resident (one point), one intern (two points), and one student (three points) for a total of six teaching points. Thus, the clinic would receive three teaching credits for session two (the six teaching points divided by the number of physicians—two—in the clinic that session). The three teaching credits entitle the clinic to a 30% reduction in its overhead expenses for that session. The following example contrasts the monthly financial summaries of the two sessions of the clinic:

	Session One	Session Two
Nurse 1	$284*	$284*
Nurse 2	$342*	$342*
Nurse 3	—	$284*
Receptionist	$155*	$155*
Benefits, vacations, etc.	$328	$447
Services and supplies (flat fee)	$40	$40
Space rental fees (flat fee)	$150	$150
Total direct expenses	$1,299	$1,702
Teaching credits	0	3
Reduction due to teaching credits	0%	30%
Expenses minus reduction	$1,299	$1,191

*0.1 FTE.

Thus, the total direct expenses for both sessions are $1,299 + $1,191 = $2,490. If the gross revenue from charges to patients for both sessions is $4,800, then the total due the faculty members for deposit into their practice plan would be $4,800 − $2,490 = $2,310. (The ancillary service income generated by the private faculty practice is assumed to offset the indirect costs not included in this formula.

This system tends to be equitable and encourages the incorporation of all levels of students and housestaff into the outpatient clinic setting. In order to encourage an efficiently managed clinic, the model does not permit a faculty member to reach a zero-overhead situation. The maximum reduction of overhead expenses possible in our model is 30%. This cap also discourages understaffing in a teaching clinic, and is consistent with maintenance of enough faculty supervision to ensure quality of care. Individual teaching credit scores, as well as the maximum teaching allowance, can be adjusted to meet the needs of an individual clinic or institution.

It is recognized that it may take a variable period of time for each director of a clinic to adapt the teaching clinic to a faculty practice model. This process involves time, and must start with an assessment of the current financial status of the clinic, followed by an analysis of areas that may need to be changed or improved.

It is therefore recommended that there be a gradual phase-in period, during which time the faculty member(s) assumes increasing financial responsibility for overhead expenses involved in the operation of the clinic. For example, in year one, the faculty member(s) assumes only 50% of the actual costs of running the clinic, and in year two, 75%, and all of the appropriate expenses in year three, minus the teaching credit(s). Thus, a faculty member in a clinic using this system, with a 20% teaching credit, would actually be responsible for 80% of the overhead expenses of that clinic. The remainder of the costs involved in running that clinic (20%) would be absorbed by the university hospitals and clinics.

The pilot project for this system was begun as a medical subspecialty clinic with two faculty members, one fellow, one resident, and one student. The faculty members in the pilot project were one 0.5 full-time equivalent (FTE) university faculty member as well as one 0.95 FTE faculty member who helped periodically in the clinic. The physicians in training, with the exception of the fellow, rotated through the clinic on one-month rotations. The fellow stayed throughout the year.

The pilot clinic provided a teaching syllabus containing core reading material, which was forwarded to the physicians in training several weeks before their rotation, with instructions to read several key references prior to beginning the rotation. This process familiarized the student or resident with pertinent clinical material in order to ease his or her transition into the clinic. The syllabus has been very useful in its subsequent applications in other clinics using the system, especially when the clinics have been subspecialty clinics.

Summary

The faculty practice teaching clinic developed at the OHSU is a successfully functioning system that strives to adapt existing resources to the changing demands of medical education. Use of this system encourages efficiency, overhead control, and appropriate staffing. Moreover, it provides a useful and relevant learning experience in the ambulatory care setting for physicians in training. It compensates faculty for the extra time involved in teaching, and it does so in a way that is commensurate with the level of training of the physician in training. The overall goal is to provide an opportunity for faculty physicians who wish to be involved in clinical teaching to do so in more efficient teaching clinics. It is hoped that models such as this will result in continued growth in the outpatient-based teaching of physicians in training while maintaining optimal care for patients.

References

1. Federman, D. Medical Education in Outpatient Settings. *N. Engl. J. Med.* **320** (1989):1556–1557.
2. Schroeder, S. Expanding the Site of Clinical Education: Moving beyond the Hospital Walls. *J. Gen. Intern. Med.* **3**, Supplement (March–April 1988):S5–S14.
3. Bentley, J., Knapp, R., and Petersdorf, R. Education in Ambulatory Care—Financing is One Piece of the Puzzle. *N. Engl. J. Med.* **320**(1989):1531–1534.
4. Eisenberg, J. How Can We Pay for Graduate Medical Education in Ambulatory Care? *N. Engl. J. Med.* **320**(1989):1525–1531.
5. Byyny, R. Challenges in the Education of the General Internist. *Arch. Intern. Med.* **148**(1988):369–372.
6. Delbanco, T., and Calkins, D. The Costs and Financing of Ambulatory Medical Education. *J. Gen. Intern. Med.* **3**, Supplement (March–April 1988):S34–S43.
7. Schwartz, W., Newhouse, J., and Williams, A. Is the Teaching Hospital an Endangered Species? *N. Engl. J. Med.* **313**(1985): 157–162.
8. MacLeod, G., and Schwarz, R. Faculty Practice Plans. *JAMA* **256**(1986):58–62.

Using "Standardized Students" to Teach a Learner-centered Approach to Ambulatory Precepting

Linda G. Lesky, MD, and Luann Wilkerson, EDD

Many medical schools are in the process of developing required clerkships in ambulatory care and are looking to faculty-group practices, managed care settings, and private offices as potential training sites for students.[1] The clinical inexperience of third-year medical students, the one-on-one nature of the precepting process, and a geographically dispersed network of physician preceptors create new challenges for those who are involved in faculty development. In this article, we describe the development of a faculty development program for a required ambulatory care clerkship in which students were assigned to over 20 training sites. We discuss how we worked with students to define the competencies of an ambulatory preceptor, how we designed a workshop to help clinical teachers develop these competencies, and how we implemented the workshop in the community.

Clerkships are often loosely organized events, in which the student's experience is dictated to a large extent by the types of patients he or she encounters. Even when a clerkship planning committee has defined the expected content of students' educational experiences, including the knowledge, skills, and attitudes that they should possess at the conclusion of a clerkship, little of this structure is successfully communicated to the actual clerkship teachers. In addition, few clinical teachers have had assistance in developing the knowledge and skills needed to be an effective teacher. Ambulatory clerkships pose a particular problem given the wide variety of clinical sites and the involvement of diverse community physicians, some of whom have limited experience in teaching medical students.

Our goal in designing this faculty development program was to assist physicians teaching in a new ambulatory clerkship for third-year medical students in adopting a learner-centered precepting process.[2] Although few studies have been conducted of the specific ways in which students and teachers interact in the ambulatory setting, a study of resident and preceptor interactions in a family medicine program had suggested that ambulatory teachers were more likely to engage in patient care rather than teaching activities given the press of time.[3] Our own observations of residents and fourth-year students in the hospital-based clinics suggested that the pace of patient care in the ambulatory setting often encouraged a more teacher-directed style,[4] a view supported by a recent study of family medicine residents.[5] To help clarify what a learner-centered experience might look like in this setting and what teaching skills would help to foster it, we met with a group of second- and third-year medical students who had worked with preceptors in an ambulatory setting in learning clinical skills or during their medicine clerkships. All had experience in the use of student-directed discussion as part of problem-based learning.

This initial meeting with the students yielded three basic principles that guided the development and focus of the faculty development program:

1. Clinical teachers rarely articulate their expectations of students. On inpatient wards, this may be less problematic, since housestaff contribute significantly to student teaching and tradition dictates appropriate student behaviors. But in the ambulatory setting, students usually must rely on the faculty member for instruction and supervision with no residents or tradition to use as guides. Students reported feeling particularly unsure of what was expected of them in the ambulatory setting.

2. Third-year students are a very diverse group with a wide range of prior experiences and personal goals. Teachers in ambulatory settings have little experience in estimating what students at this level already know and what a particular student needs to learn. They understand little about the learning goals for the ambulatory experience and often assume that it is sufficient for the student to shadow them as they see patients. Recognizing a student's level of competence and knowledge is critically important to determining when and how to move beyond simple observation. Aiming too high or too low results in lost teaching opportunities or possible disruption in patient care. The students' most frequent complaint about their previous ambulatory experiences was a lack of meaningful participation in patient care.

3. Third-year medical students want to be educationally challenged. For example, they do not mind presenting cases or being asked questions in a patient's presence (especially if it means that the time saved will be used for other teaching), so long as this is done sensitively. Given their experience in problem-based learning, these students expected patient encounters to raise questions that they could not answer without subsequent reading and research. However, they expected to have the opportunity to discuss their research and to receive feedback on their efforts. They did not necessarily expect didactic teaching in this setting.

These student-derived principles led us to conclude that preceptor training would be needed if the new ambulatory clerkship were to promote a learner-centered approach to education. From the students' comments, we identified three opportunities for teaching in the ambulatory setting that seemed to be frequently missed or misused: the first meeting between the student and the preceptor, where expectations and goals are discussed; supervision and teaching around a specific patient; and brief meetings for purposes of giving formative feedback on a student's strengths and weaknesses.

Learning a new way of teaching, like the adoption of any change, is a complex process that is facilitated if certain conditions are met.[6] First, the change must be perceived as meeting a need and producing a rewarding outcome. Second, the recommendation for change must come from and be supported by a credible source. Third, the change must be compatible with what preceptors believe about teaching and learning as well as with the skills that they possess. Activities designed to teach new ways of precepting would need to connect attitudes and skills, prior experience and future opportunities, theory and practice.[7]

Two conditions created a need to know more about ambulatory teaching among those physicians who volunteered as preceptors. This new required clerkship was unlike anything these physicians had experienced in their own education. There was no tradition to suggest what students should be doing and how preceptors should be teaching. Then there was the concern that having a third-year medical student in one's practice would have a negative impact on productivity. Since many physicians volunteer to teach because they enjoy working with students, we decided to continue the involvement of the medical stu-

Reprinted with permission from *Academic Medicine*. Lesky LG, Wikerson L. 1994;69(12):955-957.

dents as faculty developers with the expectation that their suggestions and feedback on teaching would be particularly credible. Finally, to connect personal beliefs and skills and to create awareness of a need for change, we developed a set of simulated teaching situations in which each preceptor met with a *standardized student* to analyze and respond to the learner's needs. We organized these simulations into a multiple-station exercise that we called an objective structured teaching exercise (OSTE). The OSTE formed the core of a faculty development workshop, which was offered in a conveniently located site in the community for a specific group of preceptors just prior to their having students join their practices. The session began with a review of the objectives and required activities of the new clerkship. The participants were then introduced to the format of the OSTE and proceeded through the stations as individuals before reconvening to discuss strategies for teaching in each of the proposed situations.

The OSTE simulations were designed to provide models for precepting by underlining the importance of the three teaching opportunities mentioned earlier: the first meeting, a case presentation, and a feedback discussion. For example, a preceptor was given the following introduction to the case presentation station:

Objective: To provide teaching and supervision to a third-year medical student in the outpatient setting.

Task: This is the second week of an ambulatory medicine clerkship for a third-year student. She has recently completed a two-month core clerkship in internal medicine. Among the patients that she is seeing today is Ms. Janet Jones, a patient of yours for several years. You have not seen her for some time and she presents today with an acute problem.

You speak with Ms. Jones very briefly to determine the nature of her problem (pain on urination) and to ask her whether the student who is working with you might conduct the initial history. She readily agrees. You suggest to the student that she take the history and then come to find you before proceeding further.

The role play begins after the student has completed the history. You have only ten minutes to discuss the case since other patients are waiting to see you. There is a patient available should you wish to conduct any portion of the teaching exercise with the patient.

The student was trained to provide a somewhat incomplete case presentation and to ask questions or offer opinions on the case only if invited to do so. Whatever knowledge that the student actually possessed relevant to the patient's problems was to be used to ask or answer any questions. In addition, the student was trained to recognize whether the preceptor used any of a specific set of teaching behaviors during the encounter (e.g., asked one or more questions to establish the student's assessment of the patient's problem) and to respond in ways that rewarded these teaching behaviors.

Each station was limited to ten minutes to match the fast pace of the ambulatory setting. Since the simulations came prior to any direct instruction on learner-centered precepting, we expected the preceptors to rely on their previous experiences as attending physicians in inpatient wards and their unexamined belief that teaching is telling in deciding how to address the opportunity or dilemma presented by the student. In addition, we expected the ten-minute time limit to encourage the use of brief lectures and questions directly related to accomplishing patient care. During the post-OSTE discussion, individuals were encouraged to examine their teaching beliefs and skills in light of the comments of other preceptors, the educator (LW), the faculty member experienced in ambulatory teaching (LGL), and the standardized students. The focus of the discussion was on moving from a teacher-directed to a learner-centered approach as a strategy for optimizing time and learning. Preceptors were given a brief handout at the end of the session, with concise suggestions for learner-centered responses in each of the three situations.

Informal feedback from the preceptors indicated that the experience encouraged them to examine their teaching beliefs and skills and to recognize the need for new strategies for ambulatory teaching. They learned that they could not conduct lengthy discussions of each case, as they might when teaching in an inpatient ward. Lacking a workable, alternative teaching approach and faced with limited time, they simply told students what to do to care for the patient, asked questions related to data collection, or delivered brief lectures. Most preceptors indicated that the workshop experience had made them more aware of their teaching behaviors and that they would be inclined to try the suggestions offered by the students and the handout. The standardized students were particularly pleased that they could contribute to a faculty development effort that would improve their own learning experiences in the ambulatory setting and were gratified during the workshops to see many of the preceptors arrive at new insights and understandings about teaching. A more formal study of the effect of participating in the OSTE is under way.

The ambulatory clerkship was introduced at approximately 20 sites over a two-year period. During that time we and our students visited each community at least once to provide an opportunity for preceptors from the neighborhood to experience and discuss the OSTE. The workshops occurred either during a regularly scheduled meeting time for the staff or in the evening and lasted approximately two hours. Four to eight preceptors participated in each session.

In subsequent workshops, we have used the standardized students or standardized residents and ambulatory simulations in a small-group setting in a manner similar to that described by Simpson, Lawrence, and Krogull.[8] Although still a useful tool for stimulating discussion of teaching beliefs and practices, this approach provides fewer participants with the opportunity to make individual teaching decisions and to practice essential skills. What one says or intends to do may not be the same as what one actually does when faced with a student waiting to be taught.

Academic institutions need ambulatory training sites in the community. In order to avoid a return to an apprenticeship model of training, the ties between the ambulatory sites and the parent academic institution need to be apparent to students and preceptors alike. These links are critical to ensure appropriate curricular exposure and high-quality teaching. Faculty development is an important link, tying the community preceptors to the faculty and students of the medical school and supporting their efforts to be the best teachers possible.

Dr. Lesky is director of Faculty Development for the Ambulatory Care Clerkship in the Office of Educational Development and assistant professor of medicine, Harvard Medical School. Dr. Wilkerson is director of the Center for Educational Development and Research and associate professor of medicine, University of California, Los Angeles, School of Medicine.

References

1. Feltovich, J., Mast, T. A., and Soler, N. G. Teaching Medical Students in Ambulatory

Settings in Departments of Internal Medicine. *Acad. Med.* **64**(1989):36–41.

2. Harden, R. M., Sowden, S., and Dunn, W. R. Educational Strategies in Curriculum Development: The SPICES Model. *Med. Educ.* **18**(1984):284–297.

3. Glenn, J. K., Reid, J. C., Mahaffy, J., and Schurtleff, H. Teaching Behaviors in the Attending–Resident Interaction. *J. Fam. Pract.* **18**(1984):297–304.

4. Lesky, L. G., and Borkan, S. C. Strategies to Improve Teaching in the Ambulatory Medicine Setting. *Arch. Intern. Med.* **150**(1990): 2133–2137.

5. Taylor, C. A., Dunn, T. G., and Lipsky, M. S. Extent to Which Guided-discovery Teaching Strategies Were Used by 20 Preceptors in Family Medicine. *Acad. Med.* **68**(1993): 385–387.

6. Rogers, E. M. *Diffusion of Innovations.* 3rd Edition. New York: Free Press, 1983.

7. Wilkerson, L., Armstrong, E., and Lesky, L. Faculty Development for Ambulatory Teaching. *J. Gen. Intern. Med.* **5**(January/February Supplement 1990):S44–S53.

8. Simpson, D. E., Lawrence, S. L., and Krogull, S. R. Using Standardized Ambulatory Teaching Situations for Faculty Development. *Teach. Learn. Med.* **4**(1992):58–61.

EVALUATION
AND
RESEARCH

Methods of Evaluation and Assessment of Student Competence

Model for Ability-Based Assessment in Physical Therapy Education

Warren W May, PT, MPH
Barbara J Morgan, PhD, PT
Janet C Lemke, MA, PT

Gregory M Karst, PhD, PT
Howard L Stone, PhD

ABSTRACT: An ability-based assessment program was developed to facilitate the transition of physical therapy students from classroom to clinic. Generic abilities critically important to physical therapy practice were identified by surveying selected clinical educators using the delphi technique. Evaluation criteria then were developed to define behaviors representing competence in each generic ability. Formal introduction of the program into the curriculum occurred in the fall of 1993. Exercises were developed to assess progress and to provide immediate feedback to students throughout the professional curriculum. Based on feedback from students and clinicians, we believe that we have developed an assessment program critically important to physical therapy practice. Ability-based assessment does not replace knowledge and skill-acquisition assessment. It complements these more traditional assessment forms in helping students develop the repertoire of behaviors essential for clinical success.

INTRODUCTION

Transition from the classroom to the clinic is one of the most challenging experiences faced by physical therapy students. When the University of Wisconsin-Madison physical therapy faculty questioned clinical instructors about why some students fail to make this transition smoothly, lack of knowledge or inadequate psychomotor skills were rarely implicated. Instead, difficulty often arose from underdevelopment of certain professional behaviors that facilitate the use of knowledge and psychomotor skills in the clinical set-

Mr May is Academic Coordinator of Clinical Education, Physical Therapy Program, Department of Kinesiology, University of Wisconsin-Madison, 1300 University Ave, Madison, WI 53706-1532. Dr Morgan and Ms Lemke are Assistant Professors, Physical Therapy Program, University of Wisconsin-Madison. Dr Karst is Assistant Professor, Division of Physical Therapy Education and Department of Physiology and Biophysics, University of Nebraska Medical Center, Omaha, NE. Dr Stone is Professor Emeritus and Director, Office of Educational Research and Development, University of Wisconsin Medical School.

ting.[1] These behaviors reflect abilities that often are modeled by faculty rather than taught explicitly in the curriculum.[2]

Many clinical instructors associated with our program have alluded to these professional behaviors, such as effective communication, time management, and responsibility, when they provided narrative evaluations of students. They have expressed frustration that the existing evaluation tool does not provide the structure to assess these more universal or "generic" abilities as well as it does professional knowledge and technical skills. They also have reported difficulty in assessing these behaviors in their narrative evaluations.

To bridge this gap, the physical therapy faculty at the University of Wisconsin-Madison embarked on a program to identify important generic abilities for physical therapy graduates and to establish behavioral criteria by which to measure them. The approach we chose was ability-based assessment, a program developed at Alverno College in Milwaukee, Wis, during the 1970s.[1]

We first became aware of ability-based assessment through interaction with members of the University of Wisconsin Medical School faculty who have been involved in an ability-based assessment program since 1988.[3,4] Using the medical school experience as a template, we adopted an approach that would identify and assess professional behaviors essential to developing competency as a physical therapist. The ultimate goal of this project is to incorporate into the didactic curriculum many opportunities for students to practice and perfect these abilities, thereby facilitating their transition to the clinical setting.

Ability-Based Assessment

Ability-based assessment involves multidimensional observation and appraisal, based on explicit behavioral criteria, of the individual learner in action. This concept evolved from the recognition by educators in medicine, law, pharmacy, veterinary medicine, optometry, and the liberal arts that, in addition

to a core of knowledge and skills, a repertoire of behaviors is required for success in any given profession. Mastery of this repertoire of behaviors facilitates the ability to (1) generalize from one context to another; (2) integrate information from different sources; (3) apply knowledge and skills in the practice setting; (4) synthesize cognitive, affective, and psychomotor behaviors; and (5) interact effectively with clients, families, the community, and other professionals.[1]

Ability-based assessment has as its foundation the identification of generic abilities expected of entry-level practitioners. Generic abilities are attributes, characteristics, or behaviors that are not explicitly part of a profession's core of knowledge and technical skills but nevertheless are required for success in that profession. These abilities must be systematically developed, have explicit behavioral criteria, be reinforced, and be practiced and assessed at varying levels of complexity.[3]

Ability-based assessment provides information about the student's ability to analyze and apply information, whereas more traditional formats (eg, multiple choice, fill in the blank, true-false) assess only recall or recognition of information.[5] Ability-based assessment provides the student with clear guidelines about instructor expectations[6] and reflects real-life situations.[7] Assessment is considered an integral part of the learning experience. Explicit criteria and timely feedback help students develop the ability to self-assess, self-correct, and self-direct their own development.

Reliability and Validity

The reliability and validity of ability-based assessment has been studied by several researchers. Studies have demonstrated interrater reliability of content-specific assessments.[5,8] In addition, several studies have found the interrater reliability of ability-based assessments to be high.[5] Establishing the validity of ability-based assessment is more difficult. Although performance assessments are considered to have strong face

Reprinted with permission from the *Journal of Physical Therapy Education*, Vol 9, No 1, pp 3-6, 1995.

Figure 1.

Generic abilities important to physical therapy listed in rank order.

Generic Ability	Definition
1. Commitment to learning	The ability to self-assess, self-correct, and self-direct; to identify needs and sources of learning; and to continually seek new knowledge and understanding.
2. Interpersonal skills	The ability to interact effectively with patients, families, colleagues, other health care professionals, and the community and to deal effectively with cultural and ethnic diversity issues.
3. Communication skills	The ability to communicate effectively (ie, speaking, body language, reading, writing, listening) for varied audiences and purposes.
4. Effective use of time and resources	The ability to obtain the maximum benefit from a minimum investment of time and resources.
5. Use of constructive feedback	The ability to identify sources of and seek out feedback and to effectively use and provide feedback for improving personal interaction.
6. Problem solving	The ability to recognize and define problems, analyze data, develop and implement solutions, and evaluate outcomes.
7. Professionalism	The ability to exhibit appropriate professional conduct and to represent the profession effectively.
8. Responsibility	The ability to fulfill commitments and to be accountable for actions and outcomes.
9. Critical thinking	The ability to question logically; to identify, generate, and evaluate elements of logical argument; to recognize and differentiate facts, illusions, assumptions, and hidden assumptions; and to distinguish the relevant from the irrelevant.
10. Stress management	The ability to identify sources of stress and to develop effective coping behaviors.

Figure 2.

Behavioral criteria for generic ability 1: Commitment to learning.

Beginning Level
Identifies problems
Formulates appropriate questions
Identifies own needs based on life experiences
Identifies and locates appropriate resources
Demonstrates positive attitude (motivation) toward learning
Sets personal and professional goals
Offers own thoughts and ideas
Identifies need for further information

Developing Level
Prioritizes information needs
Takes collaborative approach
Analyzes and subdivides large questions into components
Monitors own progress
Initiates own learning projects
Accepts learning as a lifelong process
Accepts that there may be more than one answer to a problem
Recognizes the need to and can verify solutions to problems
Meets all beginning-level criteria

Advanced Level
Questions conventional wisdom
Responds appropriately to unexpected or entirely new experiences
Reconciles conflicting information
Seeks additional learning opportunities
Applies new information and reevaluates performance
Formulates and reevaluates position based on available evidence
Plans and presents in-service program during clinical internship
Meets all beginning- and developing-level criteria

validity, which means that the assessment appears to measure what it is supposed to, some researchers warn that face validity is not sufficient.[9] Gathering evidence to confirm that ability-based assessments do in fact measure performance is quite difficult.[5] Therefore, more research is needed to determine the validity of ability-based assessment.

METHOD

Identifying Generic Abilities

A rank-ordered list of generic abilities deemed important for physical therapy graduates was generated based on input from a subset of clinical instructors associated with our program. The delphi technique[10] of soliciting and collapsing responses until consensus is achieved was used to develop the list of abilities. Selection criteria for sampling of clinical sites were (1) the clinical site had been affiliated with our program for at least the past 3 years and (2) the clinical site offered both short- and long-term clinical experiences. In addition, a few clinical sites were chosen because clinicians who had supervised our students for many years had recently relocated to that facility. Both small and large clinical sites across the country were represented. Eighty of the program's 200 clinical sites met the criteria and were surveyed in April 1991. Clinical educators from 76 clinical sites responded and identified the abilities they expected of physical therapy graduates. The responses were collapsed, and the refined list was returned to the clinical sites for comments, additions, and ranking. Consensus was achieved after four mailings. Ten generic abilities emerged from the survey of clinical sites as the most important abilities for graduates to possess (Fig. 1).

Developing Evaluative Behavioral Criteria

We then developed behavioral criteria to provide specific standards by which each generic ability could be assessed. The purpose of the criteria was to define behaviors representative of a given level of competence. Three progressively sequenced levels of complexity for each ability were chosen because attainment of competence in generic abilities is developmental: each level includes criteria from the previous level(s) *in toto* or in summary.[11]

Using the nominal group process[10] to brainstorm ideas, Madison-area clinicians and University of Wisconsin-Madison physical therapy faculty and students began to develop evaluative behavioral criteria in April 1992. A few months later, clinicians at the 76 participating clinical education sites were contacted again and were asked to respond to the criteria that had been developed. They also were asked to categorize each criterion into one of three levels based on complexity:

1. Beginning—behaviors students should demonstrate by the end of the first year of their professional education.

2. Developing—behaviors students should demonstrate by the end of the second year of their professional education.

3. Advanced—behaviors students should demonstrate by the end of their clinical internships.

The delphi technique was used again, and two mailings were required to reach consensus. Although it is not our intention to have a set number of criteria for each level, we expect that as they are refined, four to six representative criteria will emerge as sufficient to determine competency. Figure 2 lists the behavioral criteria for one generic ability, commitment to learning.

The relationship of the three levels to the divisions of the professional program provides the opportunity to assess overall progress towards entry-level competence at key points in the curriculum. In addition to providing standards to assess the level of competency in each generic ability, the criteria can be used by students to direct their efforts to improve. As the program of ability-based assessment develops, we will determine whether students will be required to exhibit competence at the developing level in each generic ability in addition to completing all didactic courses before starting the 18-week clinical internship.

IMPLEMENTATION AND EVALUATION

Ability-based assessment was formally introduced into the University of Wisconsin-Madison physical therapy curriculum in the fall of 1993. During the orientation session for the incoming class in August 1993, the concept of ability-based assessment was explained, and a description was provided in the student handbook. It was stressed that the 10 generic abilities were developed and are valued by clinicians with whom students will be working and that they represent the values and expectations of both clinical and academic faculty. Students in the second year of the professional program were oriented to ability-based assessment and to how it would affect them during their final two semesters and their clinical internships.

Each academic faculty member is responsible for developing assessment exercises for abilities that are appropriate for his or her

Figure 3.
Checklist for rating three generic abilities.

Generic Ability	Behavioral Criteria	Rating Yes/No	Comments
Use of constructive feedback	1. Presenter is receptive and nondefensive to constructive remarks 2. Presenter actively seeks feedback and help 3. Presenter critiques his or her own performance		
Communication skills (speaking)	1. Appropriate English 2. Appropriate body language, poised, good posture 3. Appropriate eye contact		
Problem solving	1. Correct treatment rationale 2. Treatment based on data and goals 3. Treatment rationale well explained 4. Treatment logically sequenced		

courses. The goal is to provide multiple assessment settings for each ability. The following example illustrates how one faculty member incorporated an assessment exercise into her therapeutic exercise course. Students, working in pairs, designed a treatment program for a hypothetical patient, presented the program to classmates and instructors, demonstrated treatment techniques, and responded to questions and comments from the audience. Two instructors and five randomly selected students assessed the generic abilities of communication skills, problem solving, and use of constructive feedback based on behavioral criteria that had been established for each generic ability. Figure 3 lists the criteria for assessing these three generic abilities. To provide assessment in a different context, another faculty member assessed these same abilities during a practical examination.

Evaluating Effectiveness

Introducing ability-based assessment at the beginning of the professional program provides early identification of behaviors requiring development. Students then have ample time in a supportive environment to develop the behaviors required for demonstrating competence in a given ability. Allowing time to practice and receive feedback from faculty and other students is the key to developing competency in the 10 generic abilities. The expected outcome is that students will use their clinical internship experiences to refine abilities that are fairly well developed.

To evaluate the effectiveness of this program, students in the class of 1993 (who had not participated in ability-based assessment) rated their own levels of competency

in each generic ability before and after their 18-week clinical internship. Their clinical instructors in their final clinical rotation also rated them. The following scale was used for ratings by students and clinical instructors: 1=rarely, if ever, demonstrates ability; 2=demonstrates occasionally, needs substantial improvement; 3=not entry-level but making steady progress; 4=entry-level, demonstrates consistently; and 5=exceeds entry-level competency. These ratings will be used as a baseline for assessing the competency outcomes of future students.

Students in the class of 1994 were the first group required to demonstrate advanced-level competency in each generic ability to receive credit for their clinical internships. Clinical instructors were asked to use the generic ability as a basis for their narrative evaluations at midterm and at the end of each 6- or 9-week rotation and to complete a rating form (Fig. 4.). This process will be evaluated and refined, and its reliability and validity will be studied.

DISCUSSION

Ability-based assessment differs from knowledge-acquisition assessment in at least two ways: the timeliness of feedback and the context in which feedback is provided. Feedback with knowledge-acquisition assessment is delayed because of the time interval required for scoring the examination, and assessment can occur only in the context of classroom or laboratory examinations. Feedback in ability-based assessment is provided immediately after the assessment, is structured, and may occur in a variety of classroom, laboratory, or clinical settings.

Because of its focus on behavior, ability-based assessment does not replace, but rather complements, traditional knowledge-acquisition assessment. This focus provides more diversity in assessing learning fully and fairly and makes assessment an integral part of the instructional process.[12] Whereas knowledge-acquisition–based systems of teaching assessment cultivate the student's ability to recall detailed information, ability-based systems develop the processes of seeking, integrating, and applying knowledge—all of which are essential to function optimally in the health care system.[13] In addition, ability-based assessment provides both formative and summative assessment, informing students of their performance relative to expected standards and directing their efforts to improve that performance.

A potential disadvantage of ability-based assessment is that it requires significant changes in instructional practices. For example, instructors must focus their instruction on outcome performance rather than on the content of standard achievement tests. There is evidence that implementation of ability-based assessment requires such changes[14] and that without adequate changes in instructional practice, improvement in student learning cannot be expected. Thus significant improvements in educational outcomes may hinge not only on embracing the concept of ability-based assessment but also on providing faculty with appropriate professional development opportunities to facilitate successful implementation of this concept.[15]

The generic abilities and associated behavioral criteria presented here are, to our knowledge, the first of their kind derived specifically for the physical therapy profession. Based on feedback from students and clinicians, we believe that we have developed an assessment program critically important to the practice of physical therapy. We are confident that our graduates will be better prepared as a result of their participation in this program.

CONCLUSION

Transition from the classroom to the clinic often is hindered by underdevelopment of generic abilities that facilitate the use of knowledge and psychomotor skills in the clinical setting. The clinical and academic faculty of the University of Wisconsin-Madison Physical Therapy Program identified abilities critically important to the practice of physical therapy and implemented a program to assess those abilities through assessment of specific behavioral criteria. These generic abilities and their behavioral criteria reflect our values and expectations.

Other physical therapy programs have expressed an interest in ability-based assessment and have used our list of abilities and criteria, modified our list to suit their needs, or are developing their own abilities and criteria reflecting their values and expectations. Several clinical facilities also are using generic abilities as a basis for staff-performance appraisal. As we continue to develop and expand our program of ability-based assessment of generic abilities, we are encouraged by the support and affirmation of our academic and clinical colleagues. Ability-based assessment will not replace standard written and practical examinations, but it can be used in conjunction with them to help students develop the repertoire of behaviors essential for success as a physical therapist.

ACKNOWLEDGMENTS

We thank all of the clinicians from the clinical education sites who gave of their time and expertise to develop the generic abilities and evaluative criteria. Without them, this project would have been impossible. We also thank Dr Nancy Patton for reviewing the manuscript and Sharon Ruch, Pat Mecum, and Dorothy Schmidt, who provided valuable secretarial support.

REFERENCES

1. Alverno College Faculty. *Assessment at Alverno College.* Milwaukee, Wis: Alverno College; 1979.

2. Shepard K, Jensen G. Physical therapist curricula for the 1990s: educating the reflective practitioner. *Phys Ther.* 1990; 70:566–577.

3. Stone HL, Meyer TC. *Developing an Ability-Based Assessment Program.* Madison, Wis: University of Wisconsin Medical School; 1989.

4. Friedman M, Mennin S. Rethinking critical issues in performance assessment. *Academic.* 66:390–395; 1991.

5. Marzano RJ. Lessons from the field about outcome-based performance assessments. *Educational Leadership.* 1994; 51:44–50.

6. Berk RA, ed. *Performance Assessment: Methods and Applications.* Baltimore, Md: The Johns Hopkins University Press; 1986.

7. Hart D. *Authentic Assessment: A Handbook for Educators.* Menlo Park, Calif: Addison Wesley; 1994.

8. Shavelson RJ, Gao X, Baxter GR. *Sampling Variability of Performance Assessments.* Santa Barbara, Calif: National Center for Research in Evaluation, Standards and Student Testing, UCLA; 1993. CSE Technical Report 361.

9. Linn R, Baker EL. *Complex, Performance-Based Assessment: Expectations and Validation Criteria.* Los Angeles, Calif: National Center for Research in Evaluation, Standards and Student Testing, UCLA; 1991.

10. Delbecq AL, Van de Ven A, Gustafson DH. *Group Techniques in Program Planning: A Guide to Nominal Group and Delphi Processes.* Dallas, Tex: Scott, Foresman and Co; 1975.

11. Stone HL. A review of the ability-based assessment program in medical education at the University of Wisconsin Medical School. *Assessment Update.* Spring 1991; 13:1–4.

12. Wiggins G. Teaching to the (authentic) test. *Educational Leadership.* 1989; 46:41–47.

13. Stone HL. Developing and implementing an ability-based assessment program at the University of Wisconsin Medical School. *Outcomes.* 1991;10(1):17–30.

14. Vitali G. *Factors Influencing Teachers' Assessment and Instructional Practices in an Assessment-Driven Educational Reform.* Lexington, Ky: University of Kentucky; 1989. Dissertation.

15. Guskey TR. What you assess may not be what you get. *Educational Leadership.* 1994;51:51–54.

Figure 4.
Generic abilities assessment rating form.

SHORT PAPERS

Use of a Group Objective Structured Clinical Examination with First-year Medical Students

DIANE L. ELLIOT, MD, SCOTT A. FIELDS, MD, TIMOTHY L. KEENEN, MD, ARTHUR C. JAFFE, MD, and WILLIAM L. TOFFLER, MD

Purpose. To evaluate the implementation of a quarterly group objective structured clinical examination (GOSCE) to assess the patient-evaluation abilities of a medical school class. **Method.** The study subjects were 94 first-year students participating in the Principles of Clinical Medicine course at the Oregon Health Sciences University School of Medicine in 1992–93. To create the GOSCE, the authors modified the format of the quarterly objective structured clinical examination by making each standardized-patient station the site of an interaction between a standardized patient and a group of four or five students. The GOSCE's reliability, content and face validity, and expense were evaluated. Student feedback was obtained using a structured questionnaire. **Results** Performances varied both among the five stations of the GOSCE and among the 23 student groups: the mean percentage of items performed correctly per station was 83%, with a range of 73–97%. The reliability of the GOSCE's stations was low, with intraclass correlations during the three consecutive quarters of .29, −.05, and .12. Despite no prior experience with this type of testing, the students' mean rating of the GOSCE's appropriateness was 3.8 (on a Likert scale of 1, poor, to 5, excellent), compared with 2.5 for the appropriateness of the written examination also used for quarterly assessment. The expense of the GOSCE was much less than the costs reported for the OSCE format. **Conclusion.** The use of the quarterly GOSCE favorably influenced the students, faculty, and curriculum. The GOSCE format made possible the assessment of a large number of students abilities, without the time and expense needed to evaluate students individually. *Acad. Med.* 69(1994):990–992.

The objective structured clinical examination (OSCE) is a form of assessment during which an individual interacts with a series of standardized patients. The method has been employed to evaluate clinical skills of medical students, house officers, and physicians seeking licensure.[1] Despite an OSCE's many advantages, the time, expense, and number of stations required to reliably assess an entire medical school class limit its feasibility. The group objective structured clinical examination (GOSCE) is a modification of the format, in which a group of trainees is involved at each station.[2] We describe use of a quarterly GOSCE to evaluate first-year medical students.

METHOD

At the Oregon Health Sciences University School of Medicine first-year students are introduced to interviewing, physical examination, and behavioral science issues during weekly two-hour sessions with a faculty member and four or five students. Students are reassigned to a new learning group each quarter. These sessions are one component of the Principles of Clinical Medicine (PCM) course. At each quarter's conclusion, students' learning is assessed by both a written examination and a clinical skills examination. In 1992–93 the GOSCE was introduced as the clinical skills examination. It constituted 25% of the total grade. The written examination (12.5% of the total) and other assessment components (an essay, preceptor's evaluation, and small-group leaders' evaluation) comprised the other portions of the final grade.

The GOSCE was structured as two parallel tracks, each consisting of six assessment stations. For two hours, working in their four- or five-student groups, one-fourth of the class rotated through one track, while another fourth rotated through the other track. During the same interval, the other half of the class completed the written examination. Following this session, the students traded places and completed the alternative forms of testing. The entering class of 1992 consisted of 94 students, who participated in 23 four- or five-student groups.

The stations assessed circumscribed interpersonal and physical examination abilities, and unique scenarios were used each quarter. At each station, a different group member was assigned to act as the *student–doctor*. A faculty observer was present and completed a performance checklist during the interaction. The score sheet contained items referable to interpersonal abilities, appropriate data gathering, and explicit physical examination skills. For example, one station was a focused interaction involving a patient whose antihypertensive medications had been changed the previous week. The students were evaluated on abilities to open the encounter, obtain relevant historical data, and determine vital signs. Prior to testing, the two faculty observing the same station on

Dr. Elliot is professor, Department of Medicine; Dr. Fields is assistant professor, Department of Family Medicine; Dr. Keenen is assistant professor, Division of Orthopedic Surgery; Dr. Jaffe is associate professor, Department of Pediatrics; and Dr. Toffler is associate professor, Department of Family Medicine; all with the Oregon Health Sciences University School of Medicine, Portland

Correspondence should be addressed to Dr. Elliot, Oregon Health Sciences University, 3181 S. W. Sam Jackson Park Road, L475, Portland, OR 97201-3098. Reprints are not available.

Reprinted with permission from *Academic Medicine*.
Elliot DL, Fields SA, Keenen TL, Jaffe AC, Toffler WL. 1994;69(12):990-992.

the two tracks conferred to clarify their interpretations. Because faculty observers were present, the standardized patients required training only about their scenarios, which necessitated less than one hour.

Each station was allocated 18 minutes. During the initial three minutes, a group reviewed the station's scenario, discussed which history and physical examination components to emphasize, and developed a plan for the interaction. Next, the designated student–doctor for that station had seven minutes for her or his interaction, after which the other students had three minutes to correct or add components. During the final five minutes, the faculty observer and standardized patient provided immediate feedback on the group's performance.

We calculated the percentage of items completed correctly for each interaction, including observations from the student–doctor encounter and additions by others in the group. Prior to assigning scores, the overall results of the two parallel stations and of the early and later afternoon sessions were compared to ensure comparable scoring. Each quarter, one of the six stations had significantly different mean scores when the two tracks were compared. This suggested that observers' assessment criteria differed. These stations were not included in scoring, resulting in five stations comprising each GOSCE.

The stations were written by faculty involved in preparing the course curriculum. Items selected for the checklists were skills that faculty felt students should be able to perform. To arrive at a station's grade, the distribution of scores for the 23 groups was determined. Based on the groups' performances, either domain-assigned or norm-referenced scoring was used to define grades. We used preset criteria for the domain-assigned grades (more than 90% of items performed correctly was honors, 80% to 89% was near honors, 66% to 79% was satisfactory, 51% to 65% was marginal, and less than or equal to 50% was failure). For stations where performance was less than expected, scoring was norm-referenced. For these stations, the mean plus or minus one standard deviation was used to determine grades. All students in a group received the same score for a station. A student's composite GOSCE grade was the average for the five stations.

Overall test generalizability was assessed by calculating the intraclass correlation coefficient for each GOSCE.[3] The students' perceptions about the GOSCE were determined with a survey administered at the year's conclusion. The instrument contained items that asked for agreement with explicit statements using a five-point Likert scale and open-ended questions to solicit opinions concerning the PCM course.

RESULTS

Twenty-three student groups completed each quarter's GOSCE. The performances varied both among student groups and across stations. The mean percentage of items performed correctly per station was 83%, with a range of 73% to 97%. Most interactions resulted in normal distributions of group performances, and the distribution of the groups' overall GOSCE grades (the averages of the five individual stations) followed a similar pattern.

We were able to implement the testing with only limited expense. The cost for each GOSCE was approximately $1,100, excluding faculty and support staff time. This amount included $130 for supplies, with the remainder for standardized patients' stipends. The reliability of the quarterly GOSCE's stations was low. The intraclass correlations during the three consecutive quarters were .29, −.05, and .12.

The students were asked whether they felt that different components of their assessment had been "appropriate." Despite no prior experience with this type of testing, the students rated the GOSCE's appropriateness as 3.8, SD, 1.1, using a scale of 1, poor, to 5, excellent. This was significantly higher ($p < .0001$) than the 2.5, SD, 1.2, rating of perceived appropriateness for the short-answer written examination.

DISCUSSION

We successfully implemented an efficient and economical quarterly performance-based assessment for first-year medical students. Evaluating abilities using a multistation examination has several benefits. Van der Vleuten and Swanson[4] reviewed performance-based multistation testing and identified three specific dimensions: reliability, validity, and influence on the students, faculty, and curriculum. We assessed the GOSCE for each of these aspects.

Performance-based testing has been shown to influence students' study behavior,[5] and others have noted an OSCE's educational value.[6] Although it is difficult to attribute students' behavior to any single factor, we believe that several aspects of the GOSCE influenced students. First, the need to support the group's overall performance and ensure good individual grades enhanced students' motivation and learning. In addition, the faculty's commitment to the GOSCE reinforced the importance of patient-evaluation abilities. Finally, clinical care often requires working as a team. The GOSCE emphasized the necessity of an effective group, as students had to respond to time constraints and prioritize procedures. The students also reported that learning occurred during the GOSCE. They obtained and bolstered skills as they collaborated on stations, gave and received peer feedback, and heard observations of faculty and standardized patients.

Our faculty benefited from writing and administering the GOSCE. The stations were developed by individuals responsible for different aspects of the course. The writing of case scenarios and performance checklists necessitated that faculty from several departments collaborate to review the curriculum, define explicit performance standards, and clarify course objectives. Consequently, the GOSCE was congruent with course objectives and had content validity (comprehensive coverage) and face validity (measured important features). By observing stations, faculty strengthened their belief in the value of watching performance and providing immediate feedback. The GOSCE outcomes also influenced course content. When students repeatedly made certain errors, faculty identified skills to be reemphasized in the curriculum.

We calculated reliability to measure the expected correlation between the GOSCE scores and those from a similar examination that uses different stations drawn from the same larger set. The minimally acceptable reliability level is .8. Although the GOSCE had several favorable outcomes, the five stations did not reliably assess a group's performance. This finding was not unexpected. In other settings, three to four hours was needed for acceptable reliability from multistation examinations.[6,7] Each station seems to assess unique abilities, and individuals demonstrate little consistency across skills.[8,9] The GOSCE's one hour of direct patient interaction produced a reliability comparable to the .19 to .59 levels reported for examinations of this length.[4] Reliability may be enhanced by breaking down a station into subscales, e.g., questioning skills or cardiac auscultation. In subsequent GOSCEs, refining scenarios and checklists may allow better representation of underlying ability constructs, and analysis using these subscales may increase reliability without lengthening the examination. When assessed, the number of OSCE stations to achieve reliability for pass–fail or mastery was less than half that needed to stratify perfor-

mance.[8,9] The GOSCE was able to identify student groups needing additional work to achieve a minimum skill level.

Expense is a major limitation of performance-based assessments. In 1993, Reznick et al. reported the estimated costs for different OSCE examinations.[10] The costs of a four-hour examination for 120 students ranged from $60,000 to $100,000. While the GOSCE was an inexpensive means to assess students' abilities (approximately $1,100 per quarter), our calculated expense underestimated the true cost. Test production and administration and data-analysis reporting account for 35% to 60% of an examination's total expense,[10] and we did not include these in our estimates. Although our total did not include these expenses, even doubling the GOSCE's price would have resulted in true expenditures considerably less than $10,000 per year.

We found that a GOSCE format made a quarterly multistation skill examination feasible for a class of medical students. The GOSCE was accomplished without the time and resources required to separately evaluate each individual. Although unreliable for stratifying performance, the examination identified students who had not achieved mastery of basic abilities. The GOSCE's content and face validity were high, and its use favorably influenced the curriculum, students' learning, and the faculty involved in teaching clinical skills.

This study was supported in part by grants from the Josiah H. Macy, Jr. Foundation and the Robert Wood Johnson Foundation.

References

1. Barrows, H. S. An Overview of the Uses of Standardized Patients for Teaching and Evaluating Clinical Skills. *Acad. Med.* **68**(1993):443–451.
2. Biran, L. A. Self-assessment and Learning through GOSCE (Group Objective Structured Clinical Examinations). *Med. Educ.* **25**(1991):475–479.
3. Shrout, P. E., and Fleiss, J. Intraclass Correlations: Uses in Assessing Rater Reliability. *Psychol. Bull.* **86**(1979):420–428.
4. van der Vleuten, C. P. M., and Swanson, D. B. Assessment of Clinical Skills with Standardized Patients: State of the Art. *Teach. Learn. Med.* **2**(1990):58–76.
5. Newble, D. I., and Jaeger, K. The Effects of Assessments and Examinations on the Learning of Medical Students. *Med. Educ.* **17**(1983):165–171.
6. Hodder, R. V., Rivington, R. N., Calcutt, L. E., and Hart, I. R. The Effectiveness of Immediate Feedback during the Objective Structured Clinical Examination. *Med. Educ.* **23**(1989):184–188.
7. Barrows, H. S., et al. *The Clinical Practice Examination: Six Years Experience.* Springfield, Illinois: Illinois University School of Medicine, 1991.
8. Roberts, J., and Norman, G. Reliability and Learning from the Objective Structured Clinical Examination. *Med. Educ.* **24**(1990):219–223.
9. Colliver, J. A., Vu, N. V., Markwell, S. J., and Verhulst, S. J. Reliability and Efficiency of Components of Clinical Compliance Assessed with Five Performance-based Examinations Using Standardized Patients. *Med. Educ.* **25**(1991):303–310.
10. Reznick, R. K., et al. Guidelines for Estimating the Real Cost of an Objective Structured Clinical Examination. *Acad. Med.* **68**(1993):513–517.

Evaluation of Clinical Sites and Clinical Faculty

Implementation and Evaluation of a New Approach to Clinical Instruction

Susan J. Beck
Patricia Youngblood
Frank T. Stritter

ABSTRACT: An approach to clinical instruction based on the Learning Vector model was introduced in a hospital laboratory during the 1985-86 academic year. Fifteen clinical instructors and nine medical technology students participated in the study. Clinical instructors attended an initial workshop on the model and met monthly during the academic year with the project directors to discuss their progress. The implementation of the model and the reactions of students and instructors to the model were evaluated using attitudinal questionnaires, interviews, and observations. Instructors were most successful using the model during the learning activities component of clinical instruction and were less consistent in implementing the model in the expectation-setting and evaluation components of instruction. According to instructors and students, advantages of this approach included improved communication, guidance and organization of instruction, and an increased emphasis on feedback and evaluation. The major constraint to implementation was a limited amount of time spent with students, due to scheduling or workload.

Research on clinical instruction in the health professions has focused on identifying the characteristics of effective instructors and on assessing the effectiveness of specific teaching strategies.[1,2,3] Some authors have also described common problems and the approach to their resolution.[4,5] Although these studies provide suggestions for improving specific teaching strategies, additional guidance is needed for the overall organization of clinical instruction. Such guidance is needed because most clinical instructors have received the majority of their formal education in the theoretical and technical aspects of their profession and little training in education. This study was undertaken to implement and evaluate a new approach to organizing clinical instruction. The approach is based on the Learning Vector model[6] which provides guidance for each of the major components of clinical instruction: expectation-setting (objectives), designing learning activities, providing feedback, and evaluating performance. This approach to instruction is applicable to any educational program preparing students for a career in the health professions with a significant clinical component.

This study addressed the following questions regarding the implementation of the Learning Vector model in a clinical setting:

1) Would clinical instructors be receptive to the model?
2) Would clinical instructors be able to implement the model in their clinical teaching situations?
3) How would students and instructors react to the use of the Learning Vector model?

THE LEARNING VECTOR MODEL

The Learning Vector model (Figure 1) is based on developmental psychology and describes the passage of students through three successive stages of professional development: exposure, acquisition, and integration.[7,8] The clinical

FIGURE 1

The Learning Vector

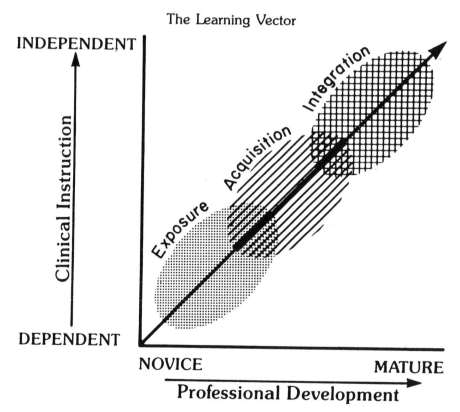

From: Beck SJ, Stritter FT: Applying developmental instruction in the clinical laboratory, in Beck SJ and LeGrys VA (eds): *Clinical Laboratory Education*. Norwalk, Connecticut, Appleton-Lange, 1988. Used with permission.

instructor modifies the way expectations are set and how learning activities are conducted. Evaluation is provided as students pass through each developmental stage. The instructor gradually and systematically gives each student more responsibility for his/her learning so that the student will develop self-directed learning skills.

In the exposure phase, the student is a novice in the clinical setting and is dependent on the instructor for all aspects of instruction. The instructor sets expectations and plans the learning activity, usually a demonstration of a procedure, and then involves the student by asking questions. The student then receives feedback from the instructor on how well he/she has answered the questions.

By the acquisition stage, the student is more experienced in the clinical setting, and the instructor begins to give the student more responsibility for learning by asking the student to participate in planning and evaluating the learning experience. The student is given options in selecting at least a portion of the learning activities. For example, a student learning about the quality control and maintenance of laboratory instruments might be asked to choose the particular instrument for the learning activity. After completing the learning activity, during which the instructor provides guidance and supervision, the student is asked to evaluate the work that was performed. The instructor then provides feedback on the student's work and on the student's ability to evaluate that work.

By the integration stage, the student has matured in a particular clinical learning experience and is given even greater responsibility for the planning, implementation, and evaluation of the learning. The student is asked to participate in the design of the learning activity and the criteria for evaluating the work. The instructor responds to the student's suggestions and modifies them when necessary. The student then performs tasks independently while the instructor serves as a consultant to the student. In the evaluation component of clinical instruction, the student is again asked to evaluate his/her own work and, additionally, asked to seek evaluation from fellow students, practitioners, or supervisors. The instructor then provides feedback on the student's work, the student's self-evaluation, and on the student's ability to integrate evaluative data from other sources.

METHODS

Subjects

This study included the senior class of nine students in the baccalaureate medical technology (clinical laboratory science) program at the University of North Carolina at Chapel Hill, and 15 clinical instructors scheduled to teach the students during the 1985-86 academic year. The class size was similar to the national mean of 8.7 students for medical technology classes.[9] Each clinical instructor was a certified medical technologist (ASCP) or clinical laboratory scientist (NCA).

Implementation

Prior to the start of the academic year, the clinical instructors attended a one-day workshop on the use of the Learning Vector model in clinical teaching. The instructors watched a videotape that illustrated the application of the model in each developmental stage,[10] and role-playing situations were used to practice new instructional techniques. Instructors made specific plans to implement the Learning Vector model in their clinical teaching situations, while the students were informed of the study and attended a presentation on the Learning Vector model at the beginning of the academic year. As instructors worked with students in clinical rotations, they attempted to assess each student's developmental stage and to organize the instruction to match the student's stage of development. The assessment of a student's stage was based on the mastery of the cognitive, psychomotor, and affective objectives for that clinical rotation. During the academic year, the instructors met monthly with the project directors to discuss their progress.

Data Collection

The success of the implementation of the Learning Vector model was based on the answers to the following questions:

1) Would clinical instructors be receptive to the model?
2) Would clinical instructors be able to implement the model in their clinical teaching situations?
3) How would students and instructors react to the use of the Learning Vector model?

Three methods of gathering data were used: attitudinal questionnaires, interviews, and observations. The first method entailed clinical instructors being given the Attitude Toward Increasing Responsibility for Learning (ATIRL) questionnaire[11] both at the beginning of the academic year and at the conclusion of the study. The questionnaire assessed an instructor's receptivity to giving students more responsibility for their learning: this is the underlying premise of the Learning Vector model. The second method involved standardized open-ended interviews[12] with students and instructors at the end of the clinical instruction. Interview questions were designed to assess the implementation of the model and to gather the students' and instructors' reactions to the use of the model in clinical instruction. Observations of the interactions between instructors and students provided the third method of gathering data on the context of the learning environment, and served to validate the responses made by students and instructors in interviews. Interviews and observations were conducted by an educational researcher who was neither associated with the medical technology program nor the implementation of the model.

Two approaches were used to validate the results of the study: 1) comparing the findings obtained from the three different data collection methods and 2) comparing the perspectives of students with those of instructors on the same questions.

RESULTS

The first question regarding the instructors' receptivity to the model was addressed by comparing the instructors' responses on the ATIRL questionnaire at the beginning and conclusion of the study. A score of 60 or greater on the ATIRL was chosen by the investigators to indicate instructor receptivity to increasing student responsibility for learning. The mean score of the 15 instructors was 67.8 at the beginning of the study and 70.5 at its conclusion. This was not a statistically significant change in mean scores.

The second question concerning the ability of the instructors to implement the Learning Vector model in their clinical settings was addressed by reviewing data collected from interviews and observations of clinical teaching interactions. Observed and reported instructor behaviors were compared to the behaviors suggested by the model. The components of clinical instruction that were implemented according to the Learning Vector model are identified in Table 1.

The third question concerning the instructors' and students' reactions to the Learning Vector model was addressed by reviewing their responses to interview questions. Their comments are ranked based on frequency of response in Tables 2 and 3.

DISCUSSION

The central focus of this study was to determine whether the Learning Vector model could be applied in a clinical setting. The first step in implementing any new clinical approach is to obtain the interest and support of the clinical instructors. The instructors' responses to the ATIRL questionnaire indicated that they were receptive to the major premise of the Learning Vector model both at the beginning and at the end of the study. The instructors' experiences using this approach did not alter their initial receptivity to the model.

The analysis of the data pertaining to implementation of the model indicates that the instructors were able to implement the Learning Vector in most situations; however, all of the components of clinical instruction were not implemented consistently according to the model. The data in Table 1 indicate that the instructors were most successful in using the model during the learning activities component of clinical instruction. In many cases, the instructional techniques needed for learning activities according to the model were similar to techniques that the clinical instructors had already been using. Therefore, most instructors only had to alter their teaching behaviors slightly to implement learning activities according to the model.

Applying the Learning Vector model to the expectation-setting component of clinical instruction called for a greater change in the instructors' behaviors and, in some instances, the instructors appeared to have difficulty. In the acquisition and integration stages, the instructor was asked to give the student more responsibility for deciding what would be learned and how the learning would be evaluated. This interaction between the instructor and the student was not generally observed or reported in the integration stage. Instructors were apparently

TABLE 1

Clinical Instructor Behaviors Consistent with the Learning Vector Model

Developmental Stage	Component of Clinical Instruction	Instructor Behavior	Verified by		
			Observation	Instructor	Student
EXPOSURE	Expectation Setting	Asked questions to assess student's background, listed objectives	+	+ +	+
	Learning Activities	Demonstrated procedure, asked questions of student	+ +	+ +	+ +
	Evaluation	Gave feedback on how well questions were answered	N	N	N
ACQUISITION	Expectation Setting	Listed required objectives	+	N	+ +
		Gave student choices in learning activities	+	N	+ +
	Learning Activities	Supervised and guided student performance	+ +	+ +	+ +
	Evaluation	Gave student feedback on performance	+	+ +	+ +
		Asked student for self evaluation	+	+	+ +
INTEGRATION	Expectation Setting	Asked student to set expectations, plan learning activities and plan evaluation	N	N	N
	Learning Activities	Allowed student to perform independently, served as consultant	+ +	+ +	+ +
	Evaluation	Gave student feedback on performance	+	+ +	+ +
		Asked student for self evaluation	+	+	+ +
		Asked student to gather evaluative information from other sources	N	N	N

+ = behavior occurred occasionally   N= behavior not observed or reported
+ + = behavior occurred consistently

TABLE 2

Instructors' Reactions to the Learning Vector Model*

Advantages of using a model:

---

1. Students progressed to a more independent level of performance
2. Students received daily feedback
3. Communications between instructors and students improved
4. Objectives were clarified on a daily basis
5. The model helped instructors improve their teaching
6. Communications between clinical instructors improved

Problems encountered with the model:

---

1. Insufficient time to work with students when the workload was heavy
2. Difficult to identify a student's developmental stage
3. Some technologists do not like to teach
4. Lack of time with students due to frequent changes in work schedules
5. Amount of material that must by covered in a short period of time
6. A particular student's enthusiasm for learning influenced the effectiveness of the model

---

*Instructors' comments are ranked according to frequency of response

willing to give the student responsibility during learning activities but were not seeking the student's input in planning those activities.

The instructors generally agreed that implementing the Learning Vector model was the most difficult for the evaluation component of clinical instruction. In the exposure phase, there was little evidence that the instructors gave the students feedback. Although they demonstrated procedures and asked questions, they did not consistently give students feedback on how well they had answered questions. The instructors seemed to assume that the student was aware of how well he/she was doing at that point and generally continued on to the next learning activity. In the acquisition and integration stages, the instructors gave the students specific feedback on their performance but were not consistent in asking the students to evaluate their own work. Students reported that they were asked to evaluate their own work, but observations and instructor interviews indicated that this behavior occurred only occasionally (Table 1). Because self-evaluation was difficult for the students (Table 3), it may have seemed to the students that it occurred frequently. In the integration stage, the instructors were not able to help the students seek evaluative information from other

TABLE 3

Students' Reactions to the Learning Vector Model[*]

Advantages of the model:

1. Daily feedback and evaluation on progress
2. Opportunity to choose learning activities or sequence of activities
3. Increased opportunity for independent work
4. Opportunity to attempt self-evaluation
5. Improved communication between students and instructors
6. Instruction was more organized and structured

Problems encountered with the model:

1. Lack of time for feedback on student performance due to workload
2. It was difficult to make choices concerning learning activities
3. Self evaluation was difficult
4. Too much responsibility was occasionally given to students
5. Difficult to apply the model in short rotations
6. Amount of material to cover with insufficient time for practice

[*]Students responses are ranked according to frequency of response

sources. This step seemed difficult for both the instructors and the students, as it was so different from evaluative techniques used previously.

The instructors stated several advantages to using the Learning Vector model in their clinical settings (Table 2). They felt that using the model had improved their communication with the students and with other clinical instructors. New instructors liked the guidance that the model provided and the more experienced teachers welcomed the opportunity to improve. Although the model was not fully implemented in the evaluation component, the instructors felt that the emphasis on evaluation was important and that their ability to evaluate students had improved. They also felt that the students developed greater independence using the model.

Instructors encountered several problems in implementing the model. Some of these problems, such as lack of time for teaching due to heavy workload, are applicable to clinical teaching in general. Other problems were more specific to the Learning Vector model. For example, limited time with a particular student made it difficult for an instructor to assess the developmental stage of the student and facilitate the student's progression to the next stage.

The students' reactions to the Learning Vector model are listed in Table 3. Students liked the emphasis on daily feedback and the organization that the model provided for their clinical experiences. They commented that the opportunities to work independently, choose learning activities, and practice self-evaluation were advantages of this approach. The students agreed with the instructors that time limitations and the amount of material to be covered in a clinical rotation were concerns.

A major concern of the students involved the choices they were asked to make. Although many students liked the responsibility involved with making choices, others preferred to have the instructor direct their activities. These students were concerned that they would miss an important part of their clinical coursework by making a wrong choice. Instructors should, therefore, plan the student's options so that they clearly allow the student to meet the expectations for a clinical experience. Because the student's comfort with making choices seemed to be related to their developmental stage, the instructor should first assess the student's progress and then plan the options for the student based on his/her stage of development.

In conclusion, the Learning Vector model was well-received by the clinical instructors and was implemented to some extent in the clinical laboratory. The expectation-setting and evaluation components of clinical instruction were the most difficult for the instructors to implement according to the Learning Vector model. Immediate benefits for the instructors included guidance for all aspects of clinical instruction and increased confidence in their clinical teaching skills. Although the investigators believe that the model is applicable to any educational program in the health professions with a clinical component, additional studies are needed to assess the effectiveness of the model in other settings. Further study is also needed to assess the contribution of each component of clinical instruction to a student's professional development, and to determine the long-term significance of the model in facilitating the development of self-directed learning skills.

REFERENCES

1. Daggett CJ, Cassie JM, Collins GF: Research on clinical teaching. *Rev Educ Res* 1979;49(1):151-169.
2. Dinham SM, Stritter FT: Professional education, in Wittrock MC (ed): *Third Handbook of Research on Teaching.* New York, MacMillan Publishing Co, 1986, pp 952-970.
3. Irby D, Rakestraw P: Evaluating clinical teaching in medicine. *J Med Educ* 1981;56:181-186.
4. Crocker LM, Muthard JE, Slaymaker JE, et al: A performance rating scale for evaluating clinical competence of occupational therapy students. *Am J Occup Ther* 1975;29:81-86.
5. Snyder JR, Cooper JT, Wilson PC: Satisfactory/unsatisfactory versus traditional letter graders for reporting student achievement. *J Med Tech* 1985;2(10):659-662.

6. Stritter FT: Clinical instruction for students in the laboratory. *Lab Med* 1983; 14:795-798.

7. Stritter FT, Beker R, Shahady E: Clinical instruction, in McGaghie WC, Frey JJ (eds): *Handbook for the Academic Physician.* New York, Springer-Verlag, 1986, pp 98-124.

8. Beck SJ, Stritter FT: Applying developmental instruction in the clinical laboratory, in Beck SJ, LeGrys VA (eds): *Clinical Laboratory Education.* Norwalk, Connecticut, Appleton-Lange, 1988.

9. Rolen-Mark HB, Castleberry BM: Survey of educational programs. *Lab Med* 1986; 17(7):415-418.

10. Beck SJ, Cowan D, Stevens RC, et al: *Applying Developmental Instruction in the Clinical Laboratory,* videotape. Chapel Hill, North Carolina, Health Science Consortium, 1987.

11. Beck SJ, Stritter FT: Clinical instructors' attitudes toward increasing learning responsibility, abstracted. *J Med Tech* 1986;3(4):249.

12. Patton MQ: *Qualitative Evaluation Methods.* London, Sage Publications Inc, 1980, p 203.

Susan J. Beck, MS, CLS (NCA), is assistant professor, Division of Medical Technology, Department of Medical Allied Health Professions; Patricia Youngblood, MEd, is instructional development consultant, Office of Research Development for Education in the Health Professions; and Frank T. Stritter, PhD, is professor, all in the School of Medicine, The University of North Carolina at Chapel Hill, Chapel Hill, North Carolina 27599.

Manuscript received October 30, 1987; accepted April 25, 1988.

Research Report

Clinicians' Perceptions of Self-assessment in Clinical Practice

Background and Purpose. *Self-assessment may be a way for clinicians to focus on continued clinical competence. Self-assessment is the clinicians' ability to assess their skills, identify their educational needs, evaluate their progress, and determine the strengths and weaknesses of their performance. The purpose of this study was to describe selected physical therapists' perceptions of self-assessment in their clinical practice.* ***Subjects.*** *The subjects were four practicing physical therapists who were willing to discuss the topic of self-assessment.* ***Methods.*** *A qualitative methodology using in-depth interviews generated the data for analysis.* ***Results.*** *The themes related to self-assessment of competence, patient outcome, and professional development were identified as a result of this study.* ***Conclusion and Discussion.*** *Within these three themes of self-assessment, the subjects wanted to improve themselves as clinicians to be better able to serve their patients.* [*Orest MR. Clinicians' perceptions of self-assessment in clinical practice. Phys Ther. 1995;75:824–829.*]

Key Words: *Competence, Patient outcome, Professional development, Self-assessment.*

Marianne R Orest

Self-assessment is the clinicians' ability to assess their own skills, to identify their own educational needs, to evaluate their progress, and to determine the strengths and weaknesses of their performance.[1] Clinicians who self-assess are said to be more likely to become "more questioning, more analytical, more self-challenging, more self-motivated, and more curious."[2(p140)] Clinicians who do not self-assess may be sliding toward incompetent practice and may easily become "careless or out of date without realizing it, and may waste valuable energy in efforts to learn."[1(p214)]

Self-assessment may have a number of clinical applications. A competent professional has the ability to exhibit knowledge and demonstrate behaviors that meet the accepted standards of the profession,[3] yet is in the opinion of one author "not merely one who minimally qualifies, but one who seeks an ever more perfect understanding and performance of his or her work."[4(p24)] The clinicians' self-assessment may assist in developing and maintaining competence.[5]

If self-assessment is a method of seeking clinical excellence, patient outcome may be a stimulus for continual self-assessment. Self-assessment is a method professionals have to help ensure quality care.[6] Clinicians make many judgments while providing care to their patients, and the ability to self-assess may result in "superior work and better critical judgment."[2(p140)]

This process of obtaining feedback on knowledge base and performance may contribute to professional development.[7] The four prerequisite characteristics of self-assessment of "self-starting, self-directed, self-paced, and self-steering"[1(p214)] may be helpful for independent learning. Self-assessment is integral to determine the direction

MR Orest, PT, is Advanced Clinician, Department of Physical Therapy, Fletcher Allen Health Care/ Medical Center Hospital of Vermont Campus, Burlington, VT 05401 (USA).

This study was completed in partial fulfillment of the requirements for Ms Orest's Master of Education degree in the Interdisciplinary Program at the University of Vermont, Burlington, VT.

This study was approved by the Committee on Human Research at the University of Vermont.

This article was submitted May 19, 1994, and was accepted April 26, 1995.

of the lifelong learning process.[8] Self-assessment may assist clinicians in remaining current with the changes in practice.[9]

The purpose of my study was to describe selected physical therapists' perceptions of self-assessment in their clinical practice.

Method

Subject Selection

The subjects were licensed physical therapists in the state of Vermont who spent most of their workday treating patients and were willing to discuss the topic of self-assessment.[10] The selection criteria also required that the sample include at least one subject who was female, male, had less than 2 years of experience, and had greater than 7 years of experience. This purposive sample was obtained in an attempt to ensure some diversity on the dimensions of gender, age, and experience.[11]

Three subjects were female, and one was male. The age range was 24 to 42 years, with a mean age of 30.7 years. Three subjects had bachelor degrees, and one subject had an entry-level master's degree. The practice experience range was 0.75 to 12 years, with a mean of 7.31 years. Current practice settings included private practice, outpatients, inpatient rehabilitation, and nursing home, and past practice settings included long-term rehabilitation and acute care inpatients.

Through her experience as a physical therapist, the investigator knew the subjects by various interactions with them in the community. None of the subjects felt that his or her specific relationship with the investigator interfered with or changed the answers to the questions during the interview, and the investigator agreed with this. The subjects read a summary of the research study and signed a statement of consent before their participation in the study.

Data Collection and Analysis

A qualitative methodology utilizing in-depth interviews was chosen to ask exploratory questions to discuss perceptions about self-assessment.[12] An interview guide (Appendix 1), which was developed during the literature review, was used to facilitate discussion with the subjects. Self-assessment was defined, and a framework for the responses was provided. The interview guide was not tested prior to using it with the subjects.

The interviews were tape-recorded, and the tapes were then transcribed. The transcribed interviews were sent to each subject, and the subject was requested to add any ideas, check the accuracy of the transcription, and clarify stated thoughts. None of the subjects returned any comments.

The raw data in the transcripts were coded into categories generated by the information provided by the subjects and the literature review. These initial coding categories were grouped by processes and outcomes of self-assessment (Appendix 2). The Ethnograph™ computer program* was used to sort the coded data, and the coding categories that contained the most content across subjects were selected. The coded data were then analyzed, and the three themes of competence, patient outcome, and professional development evolved. These three themes of self-assessment will each be discussed in the "Results and Discussion" section.

Results and Discussion

Competence

The subjects each discussed the need to remain competent as physical therapists. Subject 1 discussed the relationship between self-assessment and remaining competent. He said that he believed all physical therapists need to self-assess. The subjects said that even if physical therapists are only beginning to learn how to self-assess and are working toward improving in this area, they are in a much better position than a physical therapist who does not self-assess.

> I think anybody that doesn't do some sort of self-assessment is going to be stagnant unless of course they're in a position where they have somebody looking over their shoulder all the time, which doesn't occur in our profession. (Subject 1, Line 96)

> I think there is the potential for a person to stagnate. I can see individuals within the profession who, for whatever reason, have not progressed their skills as well as they should have. (Subject 1, Line 234)

> There is always something new to learn about something, and to get feedback from a peer, you may learn, "Gee, I guess there was something else I could have done or can add." (Subject 3, Line 311)

> I think if I didn't look back at what I was doing, I would just keep doing the same things all the time. (Subject 2, Line 112)

Even though the subjects discussed the need to remain competent as physical therapists, they were not sure how they would know whether they remained competent.

> I think if your peers are telling you that you are doing a good job, then your self-assessment must be competent. I mean, I think that is one portion of it and, as I said, patient outcome...if the third-party payers are telling you that you are doing a good job; you're going to be getting feedback from outside as well as feedback from inside, and I think it all goes together. (Subject 4, Line 132)

External feedback comes from peers, patient outcome, and third-party payers, whereas the internal feedback comes from the physical therapist who is providing the treatment. Subject 4 said that comparing the external feedback with the internal feedback assured her that she remained competent.

---

*Qualis Research Associates, PO Box 3129, Littleton, CO 80161.

Subject 4 said that the level of importance of self-assessment was different depending on whether a physical therapist worked alone or with other physical therapists. Working alone was when there was only one physical therapist working in the clinic, according to subject 4. When a physical therapist was working alone in a setting, other physical therapists were not available to provide feedback that can be helpful in remaining competent.

> I think it makes a difference whether you are working alone or you're working with others. If you're working alone, I think it's [self-assessment] more important. If you are working with others so that you can get feedback from somebody else as well, either your peers or a supervisor, it may not be as important...I think it's critical when you are working alone that you be able to self-assess. (Subject 4, Line 97)

Patients and other professionals can provide feedback, but subject 4 said that this feedback may be different from the feedback received from another physical therapist. Some feedback from other physical therapists may be necessary to ensure the accuracy of self-assessment, but other physical therapists are not available for constant feedback in the field of physical therapy.

Subject 3 said that trusting the literature was also an important aspect of remaining competent. She realized the importance of questioning what she read instead of just believing everything she read.

> Granted, you don't have to trust everything you read, but at least you know there is background on it...if you can feel comfortable because of the input you've gotten from your peers and from the readings, I guess you can feel like you're staying on top of your ability to self-assess and that competency will continue. (Subject 3, Line 294)

The subjects also commented on the patients' perception of clinical competence. Subject 3 said that she thinks patients can tell when a physical therapist who is working with them is not competent.

> We [physical therapists] don't want a therapist working with someone [a patient] if they don't feel competent, because it definitely shows. (Subject 3, Line 1172)

In these cases, the patients may not be receiving quality care.

Patient Outcome

During the interviews, patient outcome was discussed as a stimulus for self-assessment. Subject 4 said that the field of physical therapy has changed in the area of assessing patient outcome due to the need to justify intervention.

> Learning to assess a patient gives you a leg up on being able to assess yourself and understanding the whole concept of assessment and goal setting. (Subject 4, Line 418)

> I think to strive to get the best outcome, one needs to self-assess, and I think therapists strive to do that and we are very goal oriented. (Subject 3, Line 205)

The subjects looked at how patients improved and decided whether progress was being made. If the patient's progress was not leading toward the intended outcome, the subjects realized that the treatment needed to be modified.

> I think a lot of times I kind of assess my abilities by looking at how well or not well my patients are doing, and that is a way which I get feedback. (Subject 1, Line 57)

> If what I do gets the results that I am looking for, then I must be doing it right. (Subject 4, Line 116)

> If the outcomes are slow, I might question my abilities. (Subject 3, Line 448)

> If mobilization or traction isn't working for this individual, and I change to a different style of treatment or a different modality of treatment and they start to get better, I know that that change was warranted or correct. (Subject 1, Line 292)

The goal was to help patients in achieving their outcomes. These physical therapists said they needed to do the best they can for the patient.

That's really the bottom line or even more importantly when I had to stand there and talk to so-and-so and say I have done everything within my abilities and you still hurt. I think that is really the bottom line. (Subject 1, Line 417)

> I think, for therapists in general, we want the best outcome for our patients.... I think it is because we have a genuine concern for our patients. The caring goes along with it. (Subject 3, Line 224)

Patient outcome can be a stimulus for engaging in the process of self-assessment.

Professional Development

The subjects said they wanted to develop as professionals. They used self-assessment to decide the goals to set and to figure out the steps to take to achieve the goals. Goals helped them decide the direction they wanted to take in their careers.

> In terms of professional goals, [I want] to be the best therapist I can be. (Subject 4, Line 362)

> I think if you set goals for yourself, then you need to be able to look at that and figure out where you are going with it. (Subject 4, Line 422)

> I use self-assessment to realize if I am getting closer to achieving that goal.... I think that when I achieve one goal, I'm probably going to want to achieve another goal. (Subject 3, Line 844)

Subject 1 also used self-assessment to help with his development. He self-assessed to determine the questions he had regarding patient care and was constantly determining these questions and looking for ways to broaden his clinical skills.

> You need the question before you can seek the answers.... I think it's really made rather easy in our profession. We are bombarded with stuff. Always getting pamphlets in the mail with come to my course and learn how to do this. The APTA [American Physical Therapy Association] sponsoring this...we are really encouraged to interact with one another. (Subject 1, Line 597)

Appendix 1. Interview Guide

Self-assessment is defined as the clinicians' ability:

A. to assess their own skills;

B. to identify their own educational needs;

C. to evaluate their progress; and

D. to determine the strengths and weaknesses of their performance.[1]

1. In your practice, do you recognize anything like this?

2. Do you think self-assessment is important for you to be a competent professional? If yes, why? If no, why not?

3. Are there any barriers in your work to doing self-assessment? Are you encouraged openly to self-assess by peers, by superiors? If yes, how? Are you discouraged either explicitly or implicitly to self-assess?

4. Assuming that you agree that self-assessment is important, do you think formal training would help you to be a better self-assessor? If yes, what kind of training would be helpful?

Subject 3 said she thinks there is more awareness of the concept of self-assessment in the profession now than there was 5 years ago. She stated that her peers now encourage more self-assessment by not providing her with direct answers to her questions. They ask her questions so that she would figure out the answer herself. She said she does not remember discussing the concept of self-assessment 5 years ago.

> But I can't think of a time...that as a student or as a graduate, a clinician, one day that I haven't self-assessed in one way, but I didn't know I was self-assessing, and now I do because now I know what it is all about. (Subject 3, Line 251)

She said she became aware of this by just more discussion of self-assessment in the clinic. Subject 2 said that she used self-assessment to develop in professional relationships as well as patient care.

> It's not just patient care. Your relationship with other therapists and doctors and all that. I think you have to assess, and I think it will help. (Subject 2, Line 380)

The more physical therapists self-assess, they may find that there may be many more areas to develop in the profession. In order to keep improving, subject 3 constantly self-assessed to determine another goal to work toward achieving. Subject 2 explained that one of her goals was to constantly

self-assess. She said that she thinks the only way to become better at self-assessment is to self-assess as much as possible through practice.

> How else could you do it besides assessing how you are now and trying to change? (Subject 2, Line 399)

> Maybe pay more attention to it. I think that personally I tend to get more thinking about self-assessment when things aren't going well. If I am having a problem with something, then the first question I ask myself is, "Okay, what am I doing wrong?"... If things are going along fairly smoothly, then I don't tend to think about it so much. (Subject 4, Line 149)

A negative outcome may be a powerful stimulus for self-assessment. Subject 4 also said that the other physical therapists could pay more attention to self-assessment and encourage each other to look at what they were doing to ensure that they are all delivering quality care.

According to the subjects, self-assessment is not always an easy process. Physical therapists who self-assess may choose to deal with situations that are difficult or uncomfortable. The ability to deal with these situations may be different for master clinicians and novices. Though it is not easy, self-assessment is necessary for professional development.

> I think a big part of it comes with maturity and being comfortable with yourself. (Subject 4, Line 400)

> To be a good physical therapist, in my opinion, you can't operate in a vacuum. (Subject 1, Line 611)

If a patient had a diagnosis that the physical therapist was unfamiliar with, it created an ideal time for professional development. The physical therapist could look in the literature or talk with another physical therapist to gain more information to work with that patient.

To develop professionally, resources are available for the physical therapist to use. Subject 1 knew what and who his resources were.

> By reading, by speaking to other physical therapists, by speaking to other health care professionals, by practicing. (Subject 1, Line 591)

Peers are a valuable and readily available resource. If she were in a situation in which she was unsure, subject 3 said she was comfortable discussing the situation with another physical therapist or having that person watch what she was doing. She knew who to go to for different situations.

> Working here you kind of have an idea of what people like to do and where their interests are, given their caseloads and their background. (Subject 3, Line 1103).

If the person she sought out was not the appropriate person for the information she needed, subject 3 found that that person was willing to say so and point her in the right direction to the appropriate resource.

In her department, subject 2 was not as comfortable in seeking out peers as a resource due to the competitive feeling she perceived among the physical therapists. She was not as comfortable asking some physical therapists for help because they did not seem to want to help her or she did not obtain good information from them. Subject 2 chose not to use these physical therapists for assistance.

Limitations

The number of subjects may be problematic given the sample size of four.

Appendix 2. Initial Coding Categories

Components of Self-assessment

Self-evaluation
Self-awareness
Reflection
Reflection-in-action
Self-directed learning

Internal Processes of Self-assessment

Motivators	Barriers	Accuracy
Patients	Time	Objectivity
Insecurity/less confidence	Ability/lack of knowledge	Confirmation/feedback from peers
Regulations	Work load	Patient progress
Self-esteem	Competition	Experience
	Risk/comfort	
	Communication	
	Fatigue/burnout	
	Finances for further education	

Educational Outcomes and Processes of Self-assessment

Competence	Professional Development	
Peers/working alone	Resources	Formal training
Reading	Continuing education	Curriculum
Stagnant/rut	Peers	Clinical education
	Books/articles	Structured sessions at work
		Self-assessment workshops

Service Outcome of Self-assessment

Patient outcome

Each subject did not comment on all the coding categories, so the generalizability of the information is limited. Conclusions related to gender, age, and experience also cannot be drawn due to the sample size. Even though the sample size was small, I believe these four physical therapists had valuable information to contribute to the profession. In future studies to extend this topic, more subjects should be interviewed.

Implications

Competence is "the goal of medical education and the expectation of the public."[4(p27)] An essential part of professional competence is self-assessment.[13] Clinicians need to remain competent to provide quality care. Evaluation of competence should be ongoing to ensure safe and effective practice to society.[14]

Clinicians owe it to their patients to provide quality care that will help patients achieve better outcomes. Clinicians who self-assess demonstrate an increased initiative in taking responsibility to develop professionally and seek excellence as a practice goal. From a societal point of view, self-assessment is essential for enhanced professional growth and better utilization of resources to provide efficient and effective patient care.

Self-assessment has implications for professional education in physical therapy. For professional development, the subjects suggested that formal training in the concept of self-assessment is necessary for physical therapists and students in physical therapy programs. Formal training consists of structured instruction in the specific area of self-assessment.

The subjects said that they each had little, if any, formal training in the concept of self-assessment in their schooling or since they have been practicing. They believed formal training should be provided and self-assessment could be learned through the curriculum, through clinical education, by structured sessions at work, or at self-assessment workshops. Each physical therapy program and each clinic would need to decide how formal training of self-assessment can be incorporated into its setting.

Conclusion

This study described selected physical therapists' perceptions of self-assessment in clinical practice. The subjects were constantly trying to improve as clinicians and believed that self-assessment is a continuous process. In talking about self-assessment, the subjects consistently related comments to the patients they treat. Self-assessment benefits the patients as well as the clinicians themselves. The subjects wanted to improve themselves as clinicians to be better able to serve their patients.

Many questions still remain because this study was only the beginning to a better understanding of the topic of self-assessment. Is self-assessment within a person at all times and just needs to be challenged? Is self-assessment teachable, or is it a natural skill that cannot be taught but only nurtured? How can self-assessment be measured? Should the ability to self-assess be a criterion for admission into a physical therapy program? These remaining questions encourage further research in the area of self-assessment.

Acknowledgments

I am grateful to the physical therapists who were willing to take the time to discuss the topic of self-assessment with me. I also thank Dr Ernest Nalette and Vincent Orest for their advice, support, and encouragement during this research study.

References

1 Watts N. *Handbook of Clinical Teaching.* New York, NY: Churchill Livingstone Inc; 1990.

2 Fuhrmann B, Weissburg M. Self-assessment. In: Morgan M, Irby D, eds. *Evaluating Clinical Competence in the Health Professions.* St Louis, Mo: CV Mosby Co; 1978:139–150.

3 Deusinger S, Sindelar B, Stritter F. Assessment center: a model for professional development and evaluation. *Phys Ther.* 1986;66:1119–1123.

4 Jonsen A. *The New Medicine and the Old Ethics.* Cambridge, Mass: Harvard University Press; 1990.

5 Mast T, Bethart H. Evaluation of clinical dental procedures by senior dental students. *J Dent Educ.* 1978;42:196–197.

6 Cochran S, Spears M. Student self-assessment and instructors' ratings: a comparison. *J Am Diet Assoc.* 1980;76:253–257.

7 Henbest R, Fehrsen S. Preliminary study at the Medical University of Southern Africa on student self-assessment as a means of evaluation. *J Med Educ.* 1985;60:66–68.

8 Woolliscroft J, Palchik N, Dielman T, Stross J. Self-evaluation by house officers in a primary care training program. *J Med Educ.* 1985;60:840–846.

9 Windom P. Developing a clinical education program from the clinician's perspective. *Phys Ther.* 1982;62:1604–1609.

10 Raz P, Jensen G, Walter J, Drake L. Perspectives on gender and professional issues among female physical therapists. *Phys Ther.* 1991;71:530–540.

11 Jensen G, Shepard K, Hack L. The novice versus the experienced clinician: insights into the work of the physical therapist. *Phys Ther.* 1990;70:314–323.

12 Shepard K, Jensen G, Schmoll B, et al. Alternative approaches to research in physical therapy: positivism and phenomenology. *Phys Ther.* 1993;73:88–101.

13 Elman S, Lynton E. *Assessment in Professional Education.* ERIC Document Production Service No. ED 260 680. Columbia, SC: American Association for Higher Education; 1985.

14 McGaphie W. Professional competence evaluation. *Educational Research.* 1991;20:3–9.

MIRIAM FRIEDMAN, Ph.D., and STEWART P. MENNIN, Ph.D.

Rethinking Critical Issues in Performance Assessment

Abstract—The recent interest of medical schools and licensure organizations in establishing performance assessment methods in medical education presents new challenges to medical educators. The problems encountered in establishing the reliability and validity properties of performance assessment necessitate rethinking the accepted definitions of reliability and validity. The authors examine the relationship between Classical Test Theory and job performance. They discuss several critical issues: the meanings of reliability and validity in performance assessment and the balance between them (including simple versus complex behaviors), stability of performance, specific versus generic abilities, and the role of experts in clinical performance assessment. The authors call for a critical appraisal of applying Classical Test Theory to the assessment of job-related behaviors. *Acad. Med.* 66(1991):390–395.

Experts in testing methods for assessing clinical performance are grappling with issues of validating patient, computer, and written simulations and establishing reliability estimates that will enable examiners to generalize to the larger universe of the clinical behavior assessed.[1] The problems encountered in this process have drawn medical educators' attention to the measurement aspects of clinical performance, while factors such as content, abilities measured, and the creation of new methods have been somewhat neglected.

Clinical faculty members who teach students and residents in medical schools usually do not have a working knowledge of reliability and validity as they apply to trainee assessment. Consequently, they often design assessment tools that meet their own needs but do not consider reliability and validity issues.

The need to close the gap between the experts in testing methodology and the medical experts in the field has stimulated us to clarify key measurement concepts. Such clarification can enhance clinical faculty members' understanding and working knowledge of reliability and validity

Dr. Friedman is a director of The Learning Center and assistant professor of family, community and emergency medicine, and Dr. Mennin is director of the Primary Care Curriculum and of the Longitudinal Evaluation Project, and associate professor of anatomy, both at the University of New Mexico School of Medicine, Albuquerque, New Mexico.

Correspondence and requests for reprints should be addressed to Dr. Friedman, University of New Mexico, School of Medicine, PCC Curriculum, Albuquerque, NM 87131.

as applied to clinical performance assessment. The authors hope to stimulate medical faculty members to examine their assessment practices. The problems encountered in current performance assessment methods have brought us to challenge some of the accepted definitions of reliability and validity.

Reliability and Validity

Reliability and validity are dealt with mostly in the context of paper-and-pencil tests. We use the analogy of the driver's road test to compare and rethink the meanings of reliability and validity in clinical performance assessment. The driver's test, considered in this context a performance assessment, provides a familiar model to help us rethink which principles from Classical Test Theory (measurement concepts applied to paper-and-pencil tests) are transferable to the assessment of abilities and behaviors in the context of professional performance.

The following critical issues are examined: The meanings of reliability and validity in performance assessment and the balance between them (including simple versus complex behaviors), stability of performance, specific versus generic abilities, and the role of experts in clinical performance assessment.

Underlying Assumptions of the Driver Examiner

An applicant for a driver's license is required to take a driving test; it is not a simulated test, but rather an actual test in the real driving environment. Why? The examiner assumes that in order to become a competent driver one must while driving pay attention and react simultaneously to numerous things—road signs, other drivers, road regulations—while demonstrating coordination and orientation skills, acting under pressure, making quick decisions, and so forth. Ideally, performance assessment should include as many important factors that interplay in real-life performance as possible. In measurement terms, important abilities for job-related behaviors are represented in a job-sample test.[2]

The driving test given to prospective drivers is used here to examine systematically the intuitive assumptions of reliability and validity that underlie the test examiner's behavior. Reliability and validity are often confused with each other. In reliability, we search for the consistency or stability of the measure over time and over situations. In establishing validity, we try to design an appropriate and accurate test of a target behavior that needs to be measured.

In the driving test, the expert examiner is concerned only with the validity of the driving performance, that is, the extent to which the test measures driving behavior in a real situation. The driving test is one tool that assesses many behaviors. It can be viewed as "scaled testing," in which the examiners may assess different skill levels to ensure that those skills meet basic standards. Because this is a single encounter, it implies that the examiner assumes the test is reliable. The examiner believes that the examinee would perform similarly on parallel forms of the driving test concurrent or over time, and that the examinee's performance may be generalized to other driving situations. The expert examiner also assumes that his or her judgment agrees with that of other examiners. A written test of factual knowledge is given as a prerequisite to the driving test; the license is granted only when these two tests are passed.

Is the driving examiner making the right assumptions? Is a valid performance test reliable? In general, yes. A valid performance test is one that has demonstrated its power to detect some real ability and/or behavior assumed to be stable. However, the reverse is not true. To demonstrate that several measures of the same test are consistent is not conclusive evidence that a test is valid.[3] Furthermore, if a test is not reliable, can we conclude that it is not valid too? Indeed, it is possible to have a valid test situation such as the driving test but still find that either the tools we use to measure the performance or the examinees' unstable behaviors produce inconsistent measurements.

Why then is the driving examiner confident that the test is reliable? Probably because the examiner assumes that in real life demonstrating integrated complex driving behaviors indicates stable performance, or that to integrate many behaviors one has to acquire some automatic skills that can be almost unconsciously reproduced. This may not be true, however, for simple behaviors. If the examiner assesses a simple driving behavior, for example, an examinee's getting the car from one point to another in a parking lot without the complexity of the road situation, the examiner may not be able to assume that the driver will adequately perform in other road conditions. Does the complexity of behaviors measured, then, assure generalized ability to other equally or less complex behaviors? It has been suggested that two other mechanisms may enhance transfer and generalizability: (1) automatic skills, which depend on the extensive and varied practice of skills, and (2) the abstraction of principles from the performed behavior and comprehension of the logic behind these principles.[4]

In the case of a driving test, the examiner assumes that the driver's performance can be generalized to the larger universe of actual driving situations by employing validity techniques rather than reliability techniques. For example, the examiner may estimate the extent to which the driving performance meets an external standard; this may be the examiner's expert judgment, a given paradigm, or criterion standards (in a checklist, for example).

One may further assume that if the examinee takes the test many times, that person's performance will still be compared each time with the same criterion standards rather than with his or her previous performances. For the examiner, many similar performances by the same examinee may imply "bad news," since the examinee should perform better each time. The examiner's own frame of reference has been established through extensive experience with many examinees, since the examiner has sampled many behaviors over time. The examiner's norm-referenced or criterion-referenced set is defined by generalizability and validity concepts. Messick defined validity as:

> . . . an integrated evaluation judgment of the degree to which empirical evidence and theoretical rationale support the adequacy and appropriateness of inferences and actions based on test scores or other modes of assessment . . . What is to be validated is not tests but the inference and the implications for action.[5]

The "implication for action" is the provision of a driver's license, based upon the examinee's driving ability. What are the implications for actions in the assessment of clinical performance?

The Underlying Assumptions in Clinical Performance

Medical educators and licensed medical organizations are concerned with both the validity and the reliability of performance measures in order to define the extent of their confidence in decisions to pass students into residency programs and grant licensure and certification to physicians. A real-life performance examination in the medical profession is difficult because real patients must be used. Lack of standardization and sampling limitations are the major problems.[6] The best that medical educators can do is to create simulations that closely approximate real clinical settings.

Simulated patients[7,8] and objective structured clinical examinations (OSCEs)[9] are two current methods for assessing clinical performance that use simulated patients. Whether these simulations are equivalent to the actual clinical encounter remains to be proven. Studies have indicated that examinees cannot tell the difference between simulated and real patients,[10] but the degree to which the simulated encounter represents the real practice setting has yet to be demonstrated. Using the driving test analogy, if we created a simulated road with road signs and other traffic conditions, would that approximate the real road situation? Indeed, differences have been documented between office-based performance with simulated patients and testing-based performance with the same patients by the same physicians.[11]

Because of the difficulty in establishing the validity of clinical performance measures, medical educators have concentrated mainly on reliability issues, emphasizing that the reliability properties of a test are not going to produce a more valid test. However, as much as assessing validity appears to be difficult, establishing reliability seems to be as troublesome.

In reliability, two types of errors are recognized. (1) Systematic error, which stems from predictable variation in performance, may consistently bias the test results in one direction or another, either overestimating or underestimating the test scores. This is usually attributed to examiner or examinee characteristics such as test anxiety, race or gender biases, or other factors. (In the driving test, the examinee may drive a car unfamiliar in either size or gearshift, which may systematically affect driving behavior.) (2) Random error, which accounts for unpredictable variation in the test results, may arise from a number of sources such as subtle variations in the mental and physical efficiencies of the test taker and the examiners or uncontrollable fluctuation in external conditions[12] (in the driving test, occasional road conditions, or behaviors of drivers of other cars, for example).

Both types of errors, systematic and random, affect the test's accuracy and consistency, and both are taken into account in reliability calculations. If behavior is sampled appropriately, one can control for random error. Systematic error, when identified, can be factored out; the main problem exists when sources of systematic error cannot be identified.

Other sources of systematic error are present in the clinical test situation. For example, a measure of diagnostic ability may also measure interviewing ability; thus a systematic error in the measurement of interviewing ability affects the measurement of diagnostic ability. Or, patient examiners' ratings may be affected by "knowledgeable" examinees who correctly diagnose the case. Behaviors that were not intended to be measured may introduce systematic error, thus affecting the reliability as well as the validity of the test. As much as reliability is inversely related to the amount of random error, validity depends on the extent of the systematic error presented[13]; thus, studies that result in inconsistent behaviors across situations or across time may reflect problems of reliability as well as validity.

To increase reliability, most current performance assessment methods attempt to break the complexity of clinical performance into manageable units of clinical skills by using checklists.[14] Norman indicates that checklists are not necessarily more reliable than global ratings.[15] Checklists, which describe the micro-units of an ability, are instrumental in attaining standardized observations of

performance; however, the possible increase in reliability does not establish higher validity, and may even decrease it. For example, fragments or micro-units of clinical performance may be analogous to the assessment of a driver's skill in turning the wheel or parking. If we design a series of tasks for the driver where the car is in a parking lot, and we check separately for parking skills, use of brakes, use of mirror, and use of stick shift, how confident can we be then in licensing the individual? We can, however, obtain consistency of performance per skill unit. Based on multiple micro-units or fragments of skills, will the expert examiner be able to decide that the examinee knows how to drive? Without access to the whole performance picture, examiners may lose some of their expert insight and ability to validate the driving performance and thus to grant the examinee a license.

> When multiple dimensions or components of criterion performance have been identified through job or task analysis or through domain theory, it may be necessary to artificially construct tailored criterion measures to represent the separate dimensions. Such narrowly defined criterion measures are likely to be more interpretable and probably more predictable than global or composite criteria, but they are also only *partial criteria*. Hence, they need to be considered in the context of a comprehensive, representative or critical set of partial criteria or else buttressed by more global measures of remaining criterion aspects.[16]

In establishing the reliability of a clinical test, one opts for a consistency of examinees' performances across units of the test to obtain generalizability to the larger universe of related clinical abilities. However, medical educators have difficulty establishing consistency of performances across cases for problem-solving ability or even for history taking and physical examinations.[17] Are clinical "cases" (which form a "test") equivalent to written multiple-choice items? Can we assume homogeneity of the case domain? Can we assume equivalency in case difficulty? How is

case difficulty defined: by a proportion of examinees passing? by multiplicity of symptoms? by common or uncommon problems? or by the number of variables introduced in the case? (Classical Test Theory defines item difficulty by the proportion of examinees answering an item correctly.) Will variation in case difficulty affect reliability?

One of the reasons for inconsistent performance is probably the complexity of the behavior observed; no matter how much the performance is reduced to small units of behavior, it remains complex. For the sake of reliability, medical educators may be measuring complex behaviors using simple tools. As Messick states:

> Generalizability of the construct measure of test scores across various contexts can not be taken for granted, because numerous factors contribute to interactions and systematic variability in behavior and performance. Generalizability of performance does not require that all of the statistical relationships that a score displays with other variables in one group or context need be duplicated in other groups or contexts. Indeed, scores may interact with different variables in different contexts or with same variables in different ways.[5]

Stability of Performance: The Steady-state Assumption

Classical Test Theory and Generalizability Theory assume that behavior remains constant over time or during the brief time of an examination —the "steady-state assumption."[18] However, if within a short period (one week, for example) examinee behavior still varies across cases, one may seriously question the "steady-state assumption."

Unstable performance may be a function of content-specific behaviors and the rater's performance. Many more factors may be involved, according to Norman:

> Content specificity is addressed primarily by the exploration of the number of encounters necessary for reliable measurement with little evidence of the sources of error variance.[19]

For example, if one perceives that clinical abilities develop from experience, taking the first unit of a test may produce a practice effect, influencing "steady-state" performance. Due to individual differences, some examinees may improve with practice and some may not, thus introducing a source of error that may affect the assumption of stability. Clinical skills are considered to be case-specific.[1] The standardized patient may present individual salient factors that differ from other similar cases and are not part of the presenting problem. Thus, cases with similar problems may appear differently to the examinee because different patients are used. While it may be possible to standardize presenting problems, it is difficult to standardize people's unique behaviors. Since physicians rely on visual perceptions in gathering patient information,[19] these salient behaviors are also considered by the examinee. These nonverbal "errors" may not even have been identified by previous studies of patient accuracy.[20] All of these considerations constitute a dilemma regarding consistency of performance. Furthermore, the natures of clinical abilities are not fully understood.

Medical education researchers are exploring the underlying cognitive processes of diagnostic ability, history taking, patient management, and information-seeking behaviors. Some research studies indicate that diagnostic ability may rely heavily on experience.[19] The differences between novices' and experts' performances of this ability may involve different cognitive processes. Diagnostic ability, for some students, will involve pattern recognition; for others, it may be more related to problem-solving mechanisms, since they may have had little exposure to the given case. The same performance construct (in this case, diagnostic ability) may incorporate different underlying processes. If we use a variety of cases, we introduce more variation, since performance may be a function of familiarity with the case. Thus, many cases may be needed to construct a reliable test.

Consistency of performance across similar or different cases is a serious consideration. Are inconsistent behaviors caused by case-specific criteria? Is it possible that if abilities are defined in general terms, those general terms will transfer to other cases and demonstrate performance consistency?

Specific and Generic Abilities

Research on the transfer of knowledge or skills from one context to another suggests that cognitive skills are used in contextualized ways. Effective critical thinking depends on those skills learned in a specific context and in relation to specific units of knowledge, which may have little application to other domains.[4]

Metacognitive approaches to learning, in which students monitor their progress by analyzing their thinking processes in general terms, may bring about transfer to other contexts.[4] Unfortunately, in medical education, we neither use a metacognitive approach to teaching nor measure performance by using general or generic abilities.[21]

Generic criteria are independent of case or situation and may provide the theoretical basis for consistency of performances across cases. Examples of generic abilities are communication skills such as listening, writing, and speaking.[22] It may be hypothesized that generic abilities can be defined for many professional tasks, but it is questionable whether the whole domain of clinical performance can be assessed with *only* generic abilities. Recently, it was indicated that communication skills appear to be more consistent across cases,[23] implying that those skills may be more generic. This approach may guide researchers who attempt to establish consistency of performance to define abilities in generic terms that could be applied to any content domain. However, in many instances medical educators may be interested in measuring specific behaviors that are relevant to a specific case.

Sampling many specific behaviors over time and in various situations may provide an approximation of the true performance picture. In situations where performance assessments can not be accumulated over time, consistency or generalizability of specific behaviors can be *redefined* by employing the following maneuvers:

1. repeatedly matching of specific behaviors to external standards rather than to previous performances.

2. assessing unidirectional manifestations of specific behaviors within groups such as novices vs. experts, different levels of experience, and different educational programs.

3. establishing consistency among generic behaviors.

To establish reliability in specific behaviors, we use criterion validity (no. 1 above) and construct validity (no. 2 above); consistency across cases refers only to generic behaviors (no. 3 above). The limitations of current methods in establishing reliability and validity focused our attention on the expert's role in judging behaviors and how the judgment is related to measurement principles.

The Expert's Role

Experts may share similar standards of examinee performance. They can agree on checklists as well as on more comprehensive criteria so long as expert training is effective and so long as the experts share similar paradigms of the behaviors being measured. When experts agree, not only do we get interrater reliability, but we also get some form of validity, since the experts judge performances in relation to their understanding of real-life performance as well as the specific criteria generated for the test. Variability among clinical experts is well documented[24]; however, with extensive training and the study of common generic constructs, physicians may interpret clinical performance similarly and generally agree. Reliability estimates can be calculated for few experts observing the same examinee.

Experts can assist us in identifying systematic error and separating it from true ability. Cronbach gives the example of an engineer who had to describe an automobile's performance, which was functionally related to the fuel octane rating. In this example, octane rating was actually related to the engine's design, its cleanness, and driving speed.

> The variation in those parameters (engine design, cleanness and driving speed) does not per se call the validity of octane measurement into question. If the engineer understands the interaction of all those variables he can approach an understanding of the validity of just the octane measure.[25]

This example may imply that expertise enables experts to differentiate the effects of systematic error from those of random error and their influence on the performance outcome. It may demonstrate the experts' ability to make decisions consistent with a standard external criterion. The examiner has to observe the examinee's adjustment to both the random error and the systematic error. Well-trained experts know what they are measuring and understand the interplay of generic and context-specific abilities. The expert evaluates the quality of the behavior and its appropriateness in the given context and does not rely only on identifying whether or not the behavior occurs.

Sampling subjective judgments over time and over raters may provide statistical confidence that the evaluation of clinical abilities is not a matter of an expert's personal judgment but rather reflects the examinee's consistent behavior. In this approach we are not looking for consistent behavior across cases but rather for direction of performances that could be either weighted or averaged to produce a score. Mentkowsky's longitudinal study of liberal arts students at Alverno College found that certain abilities showed curvilinear patterns such that when students face certain learning tasks, they may even regress temporarily.[26] It is reasonable to assume that accumulation of many *subjective* expert judgments, if sampled appropriately over time, may produce an overall *objective* judgment that will

also incorporate the temporary regressions.[27]

Using the criteria for adequate driving performance, the driving examiner takes full responsibility to license the examinee and put that person on the road. This is an important judgment that may have life-or-death consequences; the responsibility for making that judgment is given to an expert who was trained to do so. Incorporating expert judgment into clinical assessment requires the development of a specific or overall criterion-referenced test by which examinees' performances are judged. Such a test must consider as legitimate issues the uncertainty of medicine, in which perfect agreement does not exist for the solution of many problems[28]; case specificity; and the importance of expert judgment.

This approach may allow us to overlook, in some cases, the micro-units of assessment. It may also permit us to look at overall behaviors that stimulate real-life performance and assess simultaneously clinical, ethical, stress management, and other important behavioral components. Let the expert judge this overall performance. Micro-units can be measured to highlight very specific important skills. For some specific skills, one may incorporate lay-person raters. If experts are trained to understand the constructs they use in evaluation and the relationships of these constructs to real practice, we not only may get insight into their thinking (the reflective practitioner) but also may arrive at higher levels of agreement.

Conclusion

The authors suggest that in addition to seeking consistency of performance among cases, medical educators and researchers should address issues of validity and expert judgment. Validation studies are needed to reconfirm what constitutes a minimally competent performance for different test users. For example, how does one set standards using expert judgment in performance assessment? (Use of checklist data, review of performance,

or both?) How does one achieve agreement among judges? How does one control for subjective judgment? Confidence about the validity and the judgment used to assess each case permits us to focus on other important issues, such as content, competence, sampling, and appropriate representation of the job-related behaviors, that are generalizable to real practice. Let the content guide decisions about measurement, rather than letting measurement and reliability guide content. The expert may assist us not only to define the essential behaviors but also to define to what extent they are appropriate for a given context. In performance assessment, the demonstration of behavior should be expressed with the occurrence of behavior and with the appropriateness of the behavior in a given task; the appropriateness of the behavior is a highly expert judgment.

The recent interest of medical schools and licensure organizations in establishing performance assessment methods in medical education is highly desirable. Learning from other fields and thinking more broadly about some of the research issues can bring about important developments in clinical performance assessment. The tendency of medical educators to disregard the constant need to rethink and re-examine reliability and validity principles in clinical performance assessment may suggest a driver who constantly keeps his eyes on the rear-view mirror.

This research was supported in part by a grant from the W. K. Kellogg Foundation (UHZM02R).
The authors acknowledge Howard Barrows and Geoffrey Norman for their helpful and constructive critiques of the manuscript and Sally Margolin for editorial assistance.

References

1. Swanson, D. B., and Norcini, J. J. Factors Influencing Reproducibility of Tests Using Standardized Patients. *Teach. Learn. Med.* 4(1989):158–166.
2. Dunnette, M. D., ed. Basic Attitudes of Individuals in Relation to Behavior in Organizations. In *Handbook of Industrial and*

Organizational Psychology, M. D. Dunnette, ed., pp. 469-520. Chicago, Illinois: Rand McNally, 1976.

3. Morris, L. L., Fitz-Gibbon, C. T., and Lindheim, E. *How to Measure Performance and Use Tests*. Newberry Park, California: Sage Publications, 1987.

4. Perkins, D. N., and Solomon, G. Are Cognitive Skills Context Bound? *Educ. Res.* **18** no. 1 (Jan.-Feb. 1989):16-25.

5. Messick, S. Validity. In *Educational Measurement*, 3rd ed. R. L. Lin, ed., pp. 13-105. New York: American Council on Education, Macmillan Publishing Company, 1989.

6. Miller, G. E. The Assessment of Clinical Skills Competence Performance. *In* Research in Medical Education: Proceedings of the Twenty-Ninth Annual Conference. *Acad. Med.* **65**, Part 2 (September 1990):S63-S67.

7. Stillman, P., et al. Assessing Clinical Skills of Residents with Standardized Patients. *Ann. Intern. Med.* **105**(1986):762-771.

8. Barrows, H. S. *Simulated Patients*, 2nd ed. Springfield, Illinois: Charles C Thomas, 1976.

9. Harden, R. M., and Gleeson, R. G. Assessment of Clinical Competence Using an Objective, Structured Clinical Examination (OSCE). *Med. Educ.* **13**(1980):41-54.

10. Norman, G. R., Tugwell, P., and Feighther, J. W. The Validity of Simulated Patients. In *Research in Medical Education: 1981. Proceedings of the Twentieth Annual Conference*, K. G. Fritz, compiler, pp. 215-220. Washington, D.C.: Association of American Medical Colleges, 1981.

11. Rethan, J. J., Sturmans, F., Drop, R., and Van der Vleuten, G. Performance and Competence of General Practitioners: A Direct Comparison. Paper presented at The Fourth Ottawa Conference on Assessing Clinical Competence, Canadian Association for Medical Education, Ottawa, Canada, 1990.

12. Feldt, L. S., and Brehnan, R. L. Reliability. In *Educational Measurement*, R. L. Linn, ed., pp. 105-147. New York: American Council on Education, Macmillan Publishing Company, 1989.

13. Carmines, E. G., and Zeller, R. A. *Reliability and Validity Assessment*. Series: Quantitative Applications in the Social Sciences, J. L. Sullivan, ed. pp. 13-14. Beverly Hills, California: Sage Publications, 1979.

14. Stillman, P. L., and Mina, A. G. Clinical Performance Evaluation in Medicine and Law. In *Performance Assessment*, R. A. Berk, ed., pp. 393-440. Baltimore, Maryland: The Johns Hopkins University Press, 1986.

15. Van der Vleuten, C. P. M., Norman, G. R., and De Graaf, E. Pitfalls in the Pursuit of Objectivity. Personal communication, 1990.

16. Cronbach, L. J. Test Validation. In *Educational Measurement*, 2nd Ed., R. L. Thorndike, ed., pp. 443-507. Washington, D.C.: American Council on Education, 1971.

17. Swanson, D. B., Norcini, J. J., and Grosso, L. J. Assessment of Clinical Competence: Written and Computer-Based Simulation. *Assess. Eval. Higher Educ.* **13**, no. 3 (1987):220-246.

18. Shavelson, R. J., Webb, N. M., and Rowley, G. L. Generalizability Theory. *Am. Psychol.* **44**(1989):922-932.

19. Norman, G. R. Reliability and Construct Validity of Some Cognitive Measures of Clinical Teaching. *Teach. Learn. Med.* **1**(1989):194-199.

20. Tamblyn, R., Schnalb, G., Klass, D., Kopelow, M., and Marcy, M. How Standardized are Standardized Patients? University of Manitoba, Undergraduate Office, 750 Bannatyne, Winnipeg, Manitoba, Canada R3EOW3. Unpublished (1989).

21. Segall, A. Generic and Specific Competence. Proceedings of the 1979 Association of Medical Education in Europe Conference. *Med. Educ.* **14**, Supplement (1980):19-22.

22. Alverno College Faculty. *Assessment at Alverno College*, Revised ed. Milwaukee, Wisconsin: Alverno Production, 1985.

23. Stillman, P. L., et al. An Assessment of the Clinical Skills of Fourth Year Students at Four New England Medical Schools. *Acad. Med.* **65**(1990):320-326.

24. Friedman, M., Prywes, M., and Benhassat, J. Variability in Doctors' Problem Solving as Measured by Open-Ended Written Patient Simulations. *Med. Educ.* **23** (1989):270-275.

25. Cronbach, L. J. Test Validation. In *Educational Measurement*, 2nd Ed., R. L. Thorndike, ed., pp. 443-507. Washington, D.C.: American Council on Education, 1979.

26. Mentkowsky, M., and Rogers, G. *Establishing the Validity of Measures of College Student Outcomes*. Milwaukee, Wisconsin: Alverno Production, 1988.

27. Eisner, G. W. *The Educational Imagination*. New York: Macmillan Publishing Co., 1979.

28. Katz, J. Why Doctors Don't Disclose Uncertainty. *Hastings Center Rep.* **14** (1984):35-44.

Preparing Optometry Students for Clinical Competency
An Overview

Morris S. Berman, O.D., M.S.

Introduction

Optometry colleges can strive for excellence by continuously evaluating and improving their educational programs. These improvements in teaching and advances in research will accelerate the rate of change for the profession. There are some basic issues in this educational process that merit special attention. The preparation of students for clinical competency is one issue. This complex matter involves decision making prior to the acceptance of students into a professional program and restructuring aspects of clinical teaching programs to evaluate performance, provide feedback to clinicians and assure that patients receive quality care. These challenges are shared by other health professions. Methods to enhance the selection and training of clinicians must be adapted by optometric colleges to meet their individual needs.

Admissions

The process by which applicants are admitted to programs preparing students for different health professions is being viewed with an increased sensitivity to its legal and social implications. Admissions committees are rethinking their task in order to justify the criteria used for standards and processes of admission into colleges. This is particularly important in health professions where admissions committees are asked to select students who will be equipped to handle the academic rigors of a profes-

Morris S. Berman, O.D., M.S. is associate professor and dean of academic affairs at the Southern California College of Optometry

sional program, as well as be suited for clinical practice.

The admission process for applicants to optometry programs generally includes an evaluation of undergraduate transcripts, Optometry College Admission Test (OCAT) scores, reference letters and personal interviews. The pre-optometry grades and the OCAT scores measure general academic ability and scientific knowledge. The extent to which the test results are used in deciding whether or not an applicant will be admitted to a college of optometry varies little from one school to another.

Widespread admission trends and practices in the health professions in the United States have been summarized as follows[1]: a) The selection in all health professions continues to depend on prior academic achievement and test scores measuring academic aptitudes or achievement. This practice is of long standing in dentistry, medicine, pharmacy and optometry. It appears that the best single predictor of first year academic scores, in all professional programs, continues to be the entry grade point average based on pre-professional grades. b) The wisdom of relying exclusively on pre-professional grades to validate selection continues to be questioned. Studies in the health sciences including optometry have indicated that pre-clinical grades are unrelated to clinical grades or to professional performance.[1,2] If clinical competence is defined as the application of knowledge and interpersonal effectiveness with patients, then personality and attitude measures of applicants may be a useful technique for predicting clinical performance.[1]

One of the most important tasks for future researchers will be to develop multiple criterion measures, ranging from clinical application of knowledge to specific clinical skills. Measures of interpersonal skills should be developed within the framework of student interviews in health care fields. Without the development of sound clinical criterion measures, selection of students for clinical roles will remain largely speculative. If optometric institutions are to develop criterion measures to be used as predictors of clinical performance, it will be necessary to define desired student outcomes. The curriculum must then be examined to determine whether the qualities sought in the student clinician are being encouraged and reinforced in the teaching program.

Clinical Preparation

Certain factors should be considered by institutions seeking to better prepare students for their clinical participation:

• When gaining skills relevant to the practice of optometry, students should be allowed sufficient time for learning, practice and feedback from instructors.

• The optometric relevance of techniques must be explained and students should understand the processes of scientific inquiry including observation and measurement, interpretation of data, identification of problems and the ability to solve problems. Scientific knowledge must be applied to methods of optometric practice. In the laboratory, the work must be related to body and health functions. Students must also be provided with case studies for practical application of knowledge of didactic information and laboratory techniques.

• The faculty should serve as role models and mentors for students. Teaching techniques necessary in a clinical setting include the use of a standard format for data collection including history taking and the examination records, e.g. problem-oriented records, and the use of a problem-solving approach for patient management.

• In optometry, as with medicine, passive education (rote memorization and fact recall) should be superseded by independent learning and critical thinking. Students must learn to become problem-solvers and should be prepared for a lifetime of learning experiences.[3]

There are many newer techniques available to better prepare students for clinical responsibilities. The use of audio-visual aids, video recordings, computer assisted learning and clinical simulations have expanded the techniques used by instructors to teach in the laboratory, clinic, library and workstation.[4]

Another recent teaching innovation is a paper and pencil task referred to as a patient management problem (PMP).[5] PMP's are designed to measure problem solving skills based on a standard patient data base. This technique can measure clinical performance while serving as an additional learning opportunity for students.[6] PMP's tend to have low correlations with multiple choice tests which may indicate that they measure a different type of cognitive or learning skill than multiple choice techniques.

Recently schools in several professions including optometry have developed courses to improve communication and interpersonal skills of students.[7] The purpose of these courses is to develop the clinician's self awareness when interacting with patients who present different problems.[8] A course of this nature should include appropriate interviewing techniques, and communication with different types of patients in a variety of situations.

Good interviewing skills can make a significant difference in the ability of the practitioner to obtain useful information on the nature of the patient's complaint.[9] Szasz and Hollander have described three models of the doctor/patient relationship.[10] The first model, termed "active/passive," originated in medical emergency centers. In this model, control and responsibility are maintained by the health care professional. The second model is "guidance/cooperation," which is typical of a relationship where the circumstances are less acute than in an emergency center. This model typically occurs in an optometric practice along with the third model of "mutual participation." In the third model, management of chronic illness occurs with the patient carrying out a treatment regimen without frequent consultation with the health care provider. In this case, responsibility shifts away from the health care provider towards the patient. It is important for optometry students to have an understanding of these different modes of interaction, so that they are better able to relate to and communicate with patients.

The attitude of the health care professional is important to each patient. Many urban patients are critical of their health care practitioner's behavior, particularly the lack of human warmth and failure to demonstrate real concern.[11] The relationship between the doctor and patient plays an important part in the delivery of health care. Patients who participate in a mature and understanding relationship with their practitioner are generally more cooperative and take greater responsibility for their own care. Patients will tend to gravitate toward practitioners who not only have the clinical skills, but more importantly, show care and concern for their patients.

Most patients accept the role of student doctors and understand that the training in health care fields is performed under the supervision of licensed, experienced health care professionals. Youth and inexperience are not as much a barrier in establishing relationships as many students think. Older patients may respond favorably to a young doctor and may take pleasure in the clinician's performance as they may see the student being similar to their own child. In another situation, an adolescent patient may communicate better with a young clinician than with an older doctor.

Clinical Performance

The evaluation of student clinical performance is one of the more complex areas of the educational process in the health professions. The clinical instructor must consider the purpose of the evaluation, the goals and objectives of the program and the instructional sequence. In using these guidelines, an instructor can design an effective and efficient evaluation which will provide data for decision making. The utilization of an evaluation program will be based on the quality of the instruments used to collect the data and the ability of faculty to use this information to enhance the performance of students.

One method of evaluating clinical competence is the "Critical Incident Technique" used to determine essential competencies.[12] Many health care professions have adopted this technique which relies on the profession providing specific examples of behaviors that are particularly effective or ineffective in a given situation. This technique does not necessarily assure, however, that an adequate or representative sample of incidents is included.

A second model of evaluating clinical competence is the professional performance situation model (PPSM) which is based on the premise that appropriate behavior varies for each situation.[13] To determine a full range of competencies, it is necessary to develop a full range of professional situations. This approach is similar to that described earlier by Gross[5] and has been used to define entry level competencies for several allied health professions.

A recent trend in clinical evaluation is the use of behavioral objectives. This methodology seems to work best when students are involved in developing the objectives. Current literature also indicates that clinical instructors need greater expertise and training in observation skills to improve the reliability of their evaluations.[14] Clearer criteria and training of the faculty observers/evaluators need to be undertaken in order to increase reliability.

Students can be evaluated in a number of ways including direct observation video recording and discussion of records. The problem oriented record (POR) provides an objective method for verifying the student's ability to identify and solve the patient's problems. This system was devised by Weed and is accomplished by defining the data base, completing a problem list, numbering the type of treatment plans and numbering the progress.[15]

The validity and reliability of these criterion measures continue to be questioned by researchers, faculty and students. The difficulty of evaluating clinical competence was addressed by Woolliscroft.[16] The report showed that it required considerable faculty time and training to develop inter-rater reliability while raising questions as to the validity of clinical evaluation exercises.

A clinical model of effective assessment should:
- state objectives
- screen problems
- clarify problems
- assess specific behaviors
- provide assistance and support
- determine seriousness of problem
- inspect performance
- describe administrative actions

Once the stating of effective objectives has been completed, and the screening for potential behavior problems is in operation, nothing more needs to be done until a behavior or performance problem arises. Providing feedback to students is most useful at the earliest opportunity after a given performance. The feedback should be descriptive rather than judgemental. Guba and Lincoln[17] have stated that multiple data sources are a key to judging a student's performance. Because of differences that are inherent among faculty members, evaluations from a single faculty member should not be relied upon.

Clinical Teaching

A vital component in the process of preparing clinicians is the instructor. Yet clinical teaching is one of the most neglected of all areas of teaching. Clinical faculty are key persons because they are directly responsible for many aspects of the health education process.[18] Attributes of effective teaching include enthusiasm, dynamism and energy. Negative characteristics include arrogance, dislike of teaching, lack of self confidence, dogmatism and disorganization. Meleca[19] reported that skills needed for clinical teaching can be improved when it is recognized that these skills may differ from those needed in the classroom or laboratory and may have to vary considerably from one clinical teaching environment to another.

For effective teaching and learning to occur, the cooperation and endorsement of both the students and the clinical faculty is necessary. In order to maintain and improve the skills of all clinical teachers, it has become imperative in health education teaching environments for the faculty to participate in educational development programs. These programs should allow the faculty to meet the needs of students, their own personal needs and those of the clinical environment in which they

work. Effective development programs, whether seminars, educational workshops or self instructional materials, should include competency evaluations.[8]

Successful clinical teachers should be able to teach applied problem solving, integrate clinical results with basic sciences, closely supervise students during the patient interview and examination, present effective feedback on performance and be role models particularly in the area of interpersonal relationships.[18] Certain characteristics of a clinical instructor's style enhance teaching interaction and will have a positive influence on what and how the student learns. Therefore, the instructor should be sensitive to the relationship with the student in a clinical teaching environment. The instructor must observe the student frequently and should not have

---

"Attributes of effective teaching include enthusiasm, dynamism and energy."

---

to rely heavily on patient records to evaluate the student's performance.

Summary

As the scope of optometry continues to expand, educational institutions must continue to strive for excellence in their programs. The clinical preparation of students must be strengthened so that graduates will have the training to practice full-scope optometry.

The admissions process needs to be reviewed as the standard academic indicators used to select students do not successfully predict clinical performance. The health education literature suggests that personality and attitude measures show the most promise for this purpose.

Clinical training of students must be expanded to include meaningful presentation of coursework in interpersonal and patient communication skills. The educational process should emphasize

the development of problem solving abilities and critical thinking in addition to the recall of factual knowledge. Faculty members should be role models for clinicians and therefore must be effective teachers.

The training of clinicians must include evaluation tools to stimulate learning as well as to assure quality of care rendered to patients. Various newer techniques should be considered for incorporation in a clinical training program to determine whether or not students meet essential competencies. □

References

1. McGuire C, Foley R, Gorr A, Richards R: *Handbook of Health Professions Education.* Jossey-Bass, 1983, pp 202-233.
2. Flom P: The forecast of clinical performance in optometry school. Am J Optom 51(2): 103-115, Feb 1974.
3. Medical schools urged to stress critical thought. Chronicle of Higher Education XXIX (5): Sept 26, 1984.
4. Cox KR, Ewan EF: *The Medical Teacher.* Churchill-Livingston, 1982, pp. 160-192.
5. Gross L: The standardized two-dimensional PMP. J. Optom Ed. 9(1):8-10, Summer 1983.
6. Page G, Fielding D: Performance on PMP's and performance in practice: Are they related? J Med Ed 55(6):529-537, June 1980.
7. Bennett ES: A mini-course on patient communication for optometry students. J Optom Ed 8(2): 10-18, Fall 1982.
8. Morgan MK, Irby DM: *Evaluating Clinical Competence in the Health Professions.* CV Mosby, 1978, pp. 69-88.
9. Bernstein L, Bernstein R, Dana R: *Interviewing: A Guide for Health Professionals.* Appleton-Century-Crofts, N.Y., 1974, pp. 28-45.
10. Szasz TS, Hollander MH: A contribution to the philosophy of medicine: The basic models of the doctor/patient relationship. Arch Int Med 97:585-592, 1956.
11. Koos EL: What city people think of their medical services. Am J Pub Health 45: 1551-1557, 1955.
12. Flanegan JC: The critical incident technique. Physiol Bulletin 51:327-358, 1954.
13. LaDuca A, Engel JD, Risley ME: Progress toward development of a general model for competent definition in health professions. Allied Health 7:149-156, 1978.
14. Holt T: Case presentation in: some objective approaches to evaluation of case presentations, league exchange #98, National League for Nursing, N.Y., 1972.
15. Weed L: Medical Records, *Medical Education and Patient Care.* Year Book Medical Publishers, Chicago, 1969, pp. 3-14.
16. Woolliscroft J, Stross J, Silva J: Clinical competence certification: A clinical appraisal. J Med Ed 59(10):799-805, Oct 1984.
17. Guba E, Lincoln Y: *Effective Evaluation.* Jossey-Bass, San Francisco, 1981.
18. Werner L: Teaching clinical teachers. J Optom Ed 9(4):8-12, Spring 1984.
19. Meleca C: Clinical instruction in medicine: a national survey. J Med Ed (58):395, 1983.

ACADEMIC
RESOURCES

Predictors of Student Clinical Performance

Predictors of Student Success in an Entry-level Master in Physical Therapy Program

Grace L Kirchner, PhD
Margo B Holm, PhD, OTR/L
Ann M Ekes, MEd, PT
Roger W Williams, MPH, PT

ABSTRACT: *The independent and incremental validity of predictors commonly used to screen applicants for entrance into physical therapy programs were examined. Three dependent variables were used to gauge student success: (1) professional grade-point average (GPA), (2) scores on a comprehensive written examination, and (3) patient attendance at an on-site teaching clinic. Support was found for use of two of the five independent variables— undergraduate GPA and scores on the Graduate Record Examination—to predict professional GPA and scores on the written examination. Findings were mixed concerning the effectiveness of the other three independent variables (essays, letters of reference, and on-site writing samples). The third dependent variable, patient attendance, proved generally difficult to predict.*

INTRODUCTION

Several authors have commented on the desirability of predicting the success of physical therapists on the basis of screening criteria for entry-level education programs. This prediction is especially important because the number of applicants is high relative to the number of available positions, a condition that provides opportunity to be selective and mandates careful thinking about the basis on which admission decisions are made.[1-5]

Two steps must be taken initially when investigating this issue. One is to identify the criteria by which both long-term and short-term success in physical therapy can be defined and measured. Another is to identify the variables that might serve as predictors of success.

Dr Kirchner is Professor, School of Education, University of Puget Sound, Tacoma, WA 98416. Dr Holm is Professor, School of Occupational Therapy and Physical Therapy, University of Puget Sound. Ms Ekes is Clinical Assistant Professor, School of Occupational Therapy and Physical Therapy, University of Puget Sound. Mr Williams is Director of Clinical Education, School of Occupational Therapy and Physical Therapy, University of Puget Sound.

A trade-off often exists between the accessibility of a criterion used to gauge success and its meaningfulness. Criteria of undisputed significance, such as ability to treat patients in an actual clinical setting, usually are difficult to define operationally. The time lapse between collection of data on the predictors and assessment of postgraduate performance in the clinic also creates practical problems.

The most accessible criteria by which success can be defined and measured are based on data gathered during and at the time of graduation from training programs. Examples include grades in professional courses, performance in field experiences, and scores on professional licensing examinations.

Identification of relevant predictors is more straightforward than identification of criteria that connote success. Predictors that can be collected before admission to training programs have practical utility. Very few new predictors, however, have been identified and added to those already in use in screening candidates. Predictors in common use include preprofessional grade-point average (GPA), interviews, letters of recommendation, essays, and scores on various standardized tests.

The most consistent finding to date is that preadmission grades and, to a lesser extent, standardized-test scores predict professional grades quite well, particularly when both are considered in the aggregate.[3,6-12] A second tier of predictors, including such variables as essays, interviews, letters of recommendation, and personality tests, has been investigated less frequently and with less consistent results: correlations between these variables and professional grades usually are low or nonexistent.[3,6,10]

Performance in clinical settings as measured by grades, supervisor ratings, or examinations apparently is more difficult to forecast. Positive correlations between performance in clinics and grades in academic courses have been found by some investigators[1,11,13] but not by others.[3,12] The evidence supporting the usefulness of the second tier of predictors that includes essays, interviews, recommendations, and personality tests is inconsistent.[1,3,10]

Although receipt of a passing score is required for entry into the profession, very few investigators have used scores on the physical therapy licensure examination as a criterion. Gross and Roehrig found that preprofessional grades and scores on standardized tests were positively correlated with scores on the licensure examination.[3,14] Roehrig also found that interview ratings but not recommendation ratings could be used to predict scores.

One objective of this study was to examine a novel measure of student physical therapists' performance, the percentage of times that students' patients appeared for scheduled appointments at an on-site teaching clinic. This measure was suggested in the literature on predicting success as a counselor. White and Pollard found that psychotherapist competence as measured by peer and supervisor ratings was correlated positively with client attendance.[15] Tryon and Tryon found that the *engagement quotient,* a measure based on whether clients returned after the first session, correlated positively with several predictors, including student counselors' scores on the verbal section of the Graduate Record Examination (GRE).[16] Many factors influence patient attendance, but we reasoned that the student physical therapist's ability to engage his or her patient might be one of them. Certainly patient attendance is a prerequisite for successful treatment.

A second objective was to extend this area of research to entry-level Master in Physical Therapy programs. All of the research done to date, with the notable exception of a study by Day,[7] focused on undergraduate programs. Some predictors relevant in that context, such as Scholastic Aptitude Test scores, are not pertinent to postbaccalaureate programs.

A third objective was to examine systematically the incremental validity of various predictors so that their cost-effectiveness could be evaluated. Most regression analyses in which incremental validity has been examined have been stepwise, a procedure in which the predictors are entered successively and automatically into the regression on the basis of the strength of their overall contribution to the prediction. This approach overlooks the fact that some predictors are more easily acquired than others. Grade-point average, for example, requires a minimal amount of time and expense to acquire, whereas an in-house writing sample requires considerable staff time to acquire and evaluate. Because it is not uncommon for many predictors to be highly correlated with each other, the decision to enter one rather than another may be based on rather small actual differences in effectiveness. The three subtests of the GRE often are entered separately into the regression equation, although, from a practical standpoint, this approach makes little sense. Not only are the subtests highly correlated with each other, but they always are administered as a package; it is not possible to take one without taking the other two. In a hierarchical regression analysis, the method of analysis chosen for this study, predictors or sets of predictors are entered into the equation in a predetermined sequence.[17]

METHOD

This research study and method of data collection met the criteria for expedited review established by the Institutional Review Board of the University of Puget Sound in Tacoma, Wash.

Subjects

Data were collected from a sample of convenience consisting of 46 students who had graduated during a 2-year period from the Master in Physical Therapy Program at the University of Puget Sound, a small, primarily undergraduate, liberal arts college. The sample consisted of 17 men and 29 women, 89% of whom were white. Students ranged in age from 21 to 42 years, with a mean age of 26. Students had been previously selected from a larger applicant pool.

Data Collection

Predictor variables included in the analysis were undergraduate GPA (U-GPA); scores on the verbal, quantitative, and analytical sections of the GRE (GRE-V, GRE-Q, GRE-A); scores on letters of reference (reference);

Table 1
Descriptive Statistics

Variable	Mean	SD	Range
Examination	97.761	10.539	77–121
PT-GPA[a]	3.552	.225	3.09–3.96
Patient attendance	.974	.055	.67–1.0
Undergraduate GPA	3.401	.394	2.30–3.98
GRE-V[b]	508.913	90.805	350–800
GRE-Q[c]	558.913	93.458	400–780
GRE-A[d]	583.696	94.148	380–800
Reference	.937	.066	.74–1.0
Essay	14.717	4.408	9.00–20.00
Write	13.652	4.408	6.00–19.5

[a]Graduate (professional) grade-point average.
[b]Score on verbal Graduate Record Examination.
[c]Score on quantitative Graduate Record Examination.
[d]Score on analytical Graduate Record Examination.

Table 2
Correlation Matrix

Variable	U-GPA[a]	GRE-V[b]	GRE-Q[c]	GRE-A[d]	Reference	Essay	Write	PT-GPA[e]	Patient
Exam	.50[f]	.43[f]	.44[f]	.32[g]	−.16	.41[f]	.38[f]	.61[f]	.12
U-GPA		.36[f]	.41[f]	.40[f]	.01	−.20	.07	.69[f]	.21
GRE-V			.29[g]	.48[f]	.06	.18	.30[g]	.27[g]	.20
GRE-Q				.66[f]	−.23	.05	.12	.27[g]	.15
GRE-A					.03	.08	.31[g]	.36[f]	
Reference						−.04	.08	.10	.04
Essay							−.16	−.08	−.22
Write							.91[f]	−.09	−.28[g]
PT-GPA									.23

[a]Undergraduate grade-point average.
[b]Score on verbal Graduate Record Examination.
[c]Score on quantitative Graduate Record Examination.
[d]Score on analytical Graduate Record Examination.
[e]Graduate (professional) grade-point average.
[f]$P<.01$.
[g]$P<.05$.

and two measures of writing ability, one submitted with the application (essay) and one collected under controlled conditions (write) in which applicants had 30 minutes to address a topic not known to them in advance. There were three dependent variables: (1) a comprehensive, multiple-choice examination created by the physical therapy faculty (exam), (2) graduate (professional) GPA (PT-GPA), and (3) patient attendance at the on-site teaching clinic (patient). None of the dependent variables had any direct bearing on any of the others.

All data, with the exception of patient attendance, were collected directly by retrospective examination of written records. The letters of reference, essays, and writing samples had been rated previously by members of the physical therapy faculty.

For the essays and writing samples, faculty used a 10-point ordinal scale, with 10 being the highest rating and 1 the lowest. A single

faculty member assigned each student two scores for each piece of writing, one for writing ability based on grammar, style, and syntax and another for writing content based on reasoning ability and ability to develop an argument. (Interrater reliabilities had been checked on two different occasions. Correlations of .91 and .89 were found for both sets of scores.) The four scores available for each student were combined to yield two mean scores, one for the essay and one for the writing sample.

The three reference forms that had been submitted for each student were scored by one faculty member. For some of the sample, a 6-point ordinal scale (6 was the highest and 1 was the lowest) was employed, and for others, a 4-point ordinal scale was used (4 was high and 1 was low). These three scores then were averaged to produce a single score for each student. Each score was converted to a proportion (with 1 being a perfect score) to accommodate the different scales. (No interrater reliabilities were calculated.)

During the last term of their education program, all students participated in an on-site physical therapy teaching clinic attended by patients from the community. Most students saw a total of three or four patients. A student research assistant examined clinic files to obtain patient-attendance information from the beginning to the end of treatment. Data were combined so that each student received a single score, a proportion representing the total number of times that all of his or her patients kept scheduled appointments.

Data Analysis

Data for the three dependent variables, PT-GPA, patient attendance, and exam, were analyzed using separate hierarchical multiple regression analyses. Each independent variable or set of variables was forced into the equation in the same preestablished sequence: U-GPA, GRE, reference, essay, and write.[17] Because gender has not been found to be a statistically significant predictor of professional grades, it was not considered.[7,11] The first variable entered was U-GPA, because it is obtained automatically when we verify that the applicant has completed an undergraduate degree and certain prerequisite courses. The GRE, however, requires additional expense and student time, so it was entered second. The three scores for the verbal, analytical, and quantitative sections of the GRE were entered as a set because they must be taken together and because they tend to be highly correlated. References, essays, and writing samples require not only student time but considerable staff time to read and score. The writing sample also involves staff time to administer and was considered the most costly. Reference was entered third, essay fourth, and write fifth. The decision to enter the reference before the essay was arbitrary.

RESULTS

Descriptive statistics are shown in Table 1, and the intercorrelations among all variables are presented in Table 2. Most variables were positively correlated with each other. Two dependent variables, PT-GPA and examination, were positively correlated with U-GPA and scores on all three sections of the GRE at a statistically significant level ($P<.05$). Essay and write also were positively correlated with examination scores ($P<.01$) but were negatively correlated with PT-GPA and patient attendance. The correlations with PT-GPA were trivial, but the negative corre-

lation between patient attendance and write was statistically significant ($P<.05$). The correlations between patient attendance and all of the other variables, although positive, were modest, and only the correlation with

the analytical section of the GRE was statistically significant ($P<.01$).

Results for the three multiple regression analyses are shown in Tables 3, 4, and 5. All of the overall f statistics were significant at $P<.05$.

Table 3

Regression Analysis for Graduate Grade-Point Average (PT-GPA)[a]

Effect	Total R^2	Increase in R^2	f for Increase in R^2	P	ß
U-GPA[b]	.4596	.4596	37.418	.000	+.6779
GRE[c]	.4639	.0043	.110	.954	
GRE-V[d]					+.0318
GRE-Q[e]					−.0154
GRE-A[f]					+.0832
Reference	.4710	.0071	.538	.467	+.0899
Essay	.4710	.0000	.000	.987	+.0021
Write	.5869	.1159	10.666	.002	−.9230

[a]Overall f=7.714; P=.000.
[b]Undergraduate grade-point average.
[c]Graduate Record Examination score.
[d]Score on verbal Graduate Record Examination.
[e]Score on quantitative Graduate Record Examination.
[f]Score on analytical Graduate Record Examination.

Table 4

Regression Analysis for Examination[a]

Effect	Total R^2	Increase in R^2	f for Increase in R^2	P	ß
U-GPA[b]	.2485	.2485	14.548	.000	+.4985
GRE[c]	.3778	.1295	2.839	.050	
GRE-V[d]					+.2872
GRE-Q[e]					+.2351
GRE-A[f]					−.1660
Reference	.3885	.0107	.703	.407	−.1105
Essay	.5239	.1354	11.095	.002	+.3910
Write	.5744	.0505	4.508	.040	−.6091

[a]Overall f=7.327; P=.000.
[b]Undergraduate grade-point average.
[c]Graduate Record Examination score.
[d]Score on verbal Graduate Record Examination.
[e]Score on quantitative Graduate Record Examination.
[f]Score on analytical Graduate Record Examination.

Table 5

Regression Analysis for Patient Attendance[a]

Effect	Total R^2	Increase in R^2	f for Increase in R^2	P	ß
U-GPA[b]	.0445	.0445	2.049	.159	+.2109
GRE[c]	.1529	.1084	1.750	.172	
GRE-V[d]					+.1439
GRE-Q[e]					+.0527
GRE-A[f]					+.4348
Reference	.1533	.0004	.019	.891	−.0214
Essay	.1930	.0397	1.919	.174	−.2117
Write	.3214	.1283	7.185	.011	−.9710

[a]Overall f=2.571; P=.029.
[b]Undergraduate grade-point average.
[c]Graduate Record Examination score.
[d]Score on verbal Graduate Record Examination.
[e]Score on quantitative Graduate Record Examination.
[f]Score on analytical Graduate Record Examination.

Findings regarding the incremental contributions of the independent variables were mixed. Only the write variable contributed at a statistically significant level to all three prediction models ($P<.05$). This result is particularly surprising given that write was entered last in every case. Less surprisingly, undergraduate GPA, which was entered first, contributed significantly to the prediction of both examination scores and PT-GPA ($P<.001$) but not to patient attendance. Both GRE, which was entered second, and essay, which was entered fourth, contributed incrementally to the prediction of examination scores ($P<.05$) but not to the predictions of PT-GPA or patient attendance. The letters of reference did not contribute significantly to any prediction.

DISCUSSION

These results were consistent with those of other studies. Preprofessional grades were a powerful predictor of professional GPA and scores on a comprehensive examination. Both the GRE and essay were useful in predicting examination scores, even when the variance attributable to undergraduate GPA was accounted for. Thus there is evidence for relating all three traditional screening devices for admission into physical therapy programs.

The status of other predictors is less clear. No evidence supported the continued use of letters of reference, at least as evaluated for use with this sample. This finding was not surprising, given the limited variability of the ratings associated with that measure. That situation might be improved if a more sensitive and demonstrably reliable scale were developed to rate reference letters, or it may be a reflection of their inherently limited discriminatory power.

After all other predictors had been entered into the regressions, the writing sample made a significant contribution to the prediction of all three dependent variables, but it was weighted in the negative direction in each equation. This outcome may be of interest from a technical standpoint but is unlikely to be of much practical utility. Even if this result were replicated with sufficient consistency to instill confidence in its validity, we would question whether assigning a negative weight to the writing sample could be justified. It would be difficult to explain to various constituencies, including program applicants and admissions personnel, why students who do well on a writing sample should be "penalized." We also must consider the possibility that the writing-sample variable may be positively correlated with other desirable characteristics or outcomes, such as the ability to write clear charts and case notes.

Perhaps the most disappointing finding was that the model used to predict patient attendance, although statistically significant, was relatively weak. As was true for the letters of reference, very little variability existed in patient attendance, which may have accounted for these results. Another possibility is that patient attendance is not an appropriate measure of therapist effectiveness, and powerful prediction models are not to be expected. These results, although inconclusive, merit further study.

REFERENCES

1. Balogun JA. Predictors of academic and clinical performance in a baccalaureate physical therapy program. *Phys Ther.* 1988;68:238–242.
2. Guthrie MR. Physical therapy student selection: analysis of the variables. *Journal of Physical Therapy Education.* Spring 1990:31–36.
3. Gross MT. Relative value of multiple physical therapy admissions criteria on predicting didactic, clinical, and licensure performance. *Journal of Physical Therapy Education.* 1989;3:7–14.
4. McGinnis ME. Admission predictors for pre-physical therapy majors. *Phys Ther.* 1984;64:55–58.
5. Olney SJ. Prediction of clinical competence of students of physical therapy. *Physiotherapy Canada.* 1977;29:254–258.
6. Balogun JA, Karacoloff LA, Farina NT. Predictors of academic achievement in physical therapy. *Phys Ther.* 1986;66:976–980.
7. Day JA. Graduate record examination analytical scores as predictors of academic success in four entry-level master's degree physical therapy programs. *Phys Ther.* 1986;66:1555–1562.
8. Cocanour B, Peatman N. Predictors of success in a baccalaureate physical therapy program. *Journal of Physical Therapy Education.* 1988;2(1):27–29.
9. Schimfhauer FT, Broski DC. Predicting academic success in allied health curricula. *J Allied Health.* 1976;5:34–36.
10. Levine SB, Knecht HG, Eisen RG. Students, interviews and academic predictors. *J Allied Health.* 1986;15:143–151.
11. Peat M, Woodbury MG, Donner A. Admission average as a predictor of undergraduate academic and clinical performance. *Physiotherapy Canada.* 1982;34:211–214.
12. Rheault W, Shafernich-Coulson E. Relationship between academic achievement and clinical performance in a physical therapy education program. *Phys Ther.* 1988;68:378–380.
13. Tidd GS, Conine TA. Do better student perform better in the clinic? Relationship of academic grades to clinical ratings. *Phys Ther.* 1974;54:500–505.
14. Roehrig SM. Prediction of licensing examination scores in physical therapy graduates. *Phys Ther.* 1988;68:694–698.
15. White GD, Pollard J. Assessing therapeutic competence from therapy session attendance. *Professional Psychology.* 1982;13:628–633.
16. Tryon GS, Tryon WW. Factors associated with clinical practicum trainees' engagements of clients in counseling. *Professional Psychology: Research and Practice.* 1988;17:596–589.
17. Cohen J, Cohen P. *Applied Multiple Regression/Correlation Analysis for the Behavioral Sciences.* 2nd ed. Hillsdale, NJ: Erlbaum; 1983.

Assessing Learning-Style Inventories and How Well They Predict Academic Performance

LISA I. LEIDEN, Ph.D., ROSS D. CROSBY, Ph.D., and HUGH FOLLMER, M.D.

Abstract—In the fall of 1988, 79 students at the University of Nevada School of Medicine were administered two learning-style inventories: the Lancaster Approaches to Studying Inventory (LASI) and the Inventory of Learning Processes (ILP). Students' scores on these scales were examined in terms of the theoretical distinction between deep and surface approaches to learning. The data provided strong support for this distinction, with the scores on learning-style measures correlating as expected. The relationships between the students' inventory scores and their scores on two measures of academic performance were also examined. Correlations between measures of learning style and academic performance yielded low, nonsignificant positive correlations and were found to be inadequate predictors of academic performance. Implications and possible explanations for these findings are discussed. *Acad. Med.* 65(1990):395–401.

Helping medical students improve their learning and thus facilitate the acquisition of information is of interest to every medical school. Whether it is the case of an above average student striving to be above average or a student in difficulty struggling just to pass, educators have applied the findings of learning-style research in an

Dr. Leiden is director, office of evaluation and curriculum services, and interim assistant dean for curricular affairs, and Dr. Follmer is clinical assistant professor, Department of Surgery; both at the University of Nevada School of Medicine, Las Vegas. Dr. Crosby is research coordinator, Department of Psychiatry, University of Minnesota Medical School—Minneapolis.

Correspondence and requests for reprints should be addressed to Dr. Leiden, University of Nevada School of Medicine, Office of Evaluation and Curriculum Services, Manville Medical Sciences Building, Reno, NV 89557-0046.

effort to identify patterns of learning that might help students increase both their understanding of information and their performance levels.

Perhaps the most obvious advance in knowledge that learning-style research has provided is the appreciation of individual differences in how people learn. What also appears to be true is that the style a student adopts affects how well he or she learns and understands the material.

Educators interested in applying the findings of learning-style research must select from a variety of scales.[1-8] The instruments vary not only in their reliabilities,[3] but also with regard to the purported theoretical orientations.[1] An interesting and useful theoretical framework from which to describe (and hence select) learning-style inventories was proposed by Curry.[1] Within this model, learning-style instruments are differentiated

by the extents to which they reflect personality characteristics, information-processing characteristics, or preferences for different types of instruction. The Myers-Briggs Type Indicator[8] represents an example of a cognitive-personality learning-style instrument; the Inventory of Learning Processes[3] is an example of an information-processing instrument; and the Learning Preference Inventory[5] represents an instructional-preference instrument.

Two learning-style inventories were selected for examination within this study: the Inventory of Learning Processes (ILP), first developed by Schmeck and colleagues[3] and later revised and reported on by Vu and Galotre,[9] and the Lancaster Approaches to Studying Inventory (LASI).[6,7]

The ILP is divided into four major learning processes. (See the boxed text titled ILP for a detailed descrip-

---

LASI (Lancaster Approaches to Studying Inventory)*

Scale	Description
Meaning	Focuses on the intent to understand what is being studied
Deep approach	Looking for meaning in what is being studied
Relating ideas	Actively relating new information to previous knowledge
Use of evidence	Critically relating evidence to conclusions
Intrinsic motivation	Interest in learning for learning's sake
Reproducing	Focuses on the intent to reproduce what is being studied
Surface approach	Reliance on rote learning
Syllabus boundness	Restriction of learning to defined tasks
Fear of failure	Pessimism and anxiety about assessment requirements
Improvidence	Over-reliance on details
Strategic	Focuses on the intent to achieve high grades fueled by a sense of competition
Strategic approach	Actively seeking information about assessment requirements
Achievement motivation	Competitive drive for success
Extrinsic motivation	Interest in courses for the qualifications they offer
Non-Academic	Lack of concern for academic performance
Disorganized study	Lack of organization and planning
Negative attitudes	Disenchantment with education
Globetrotting	Tendency to jump to conclusions without evidence
Comprehension Learning	Building a general picture of what is being learned
Operation Learning	Concentration on details and logical analysis

*Ramsden, P. *The Lancaster Approaches to Studying and Course Perceptions Questionnaire.* Oxford, England: Educational Methods Unit, 1983.

ILP (Inventory of Learning Processes)*

Scale	Description
Synthesis Analysis	The ability to synthesize and reorganize study material
Study Methods	The extent to which one adheres to traditional study techniques and behaviors
Fact Retention	The ability to retain detailed factual information
Elaborative Processing	The ability to relate new and old information using a variety of techniques

*Schmeck, R. R., Ribich, F., and Ramaniah, N. Individual Learning Style: The Development of a Reliable Instrument. *Res. Med. Educ.* (1984):97–102.

---

tion.) *Synthesis Analysis* assesses "deep" (that is, semantic) information-processing habits and organizational processes; *Study Methods* assesses adherence to traditional study techniques; *Fact Retention* involves the ability to retain detailed, factual information; and *Elaborative Processing* involves reorganizing and relating information to one's own experience.

The LASI is based upon learning-style research conducted in Europe and Australia. The LASI characterizes students' preferences for how new information is learned, and, using Curry's[1] model, may reflect environmental influences rather than internal, cognitive-personality characteristics. The LASI contains four major factors and 16 underlying subscales. (See the boxed text titled "LASI" for a detailed description.) The first factor, *Meaning Orientation* (also known as the "deep approach"), made up of four subscales, focuses on the intent to understand what is being studied. The *Reproducing Orientation* (also known as the "surface approach"), made up of four subscales, involves the intent to reproduce what is being studied. The *Strategic Orientation*, made up of three subscales, involves the intent to achieve high grades, an intent said to be fueled by a sense of competition. The final factor, the *Non-Academic Orientation*, made up of three factors, involves a lack of concern for academic performance. The LASI also has two additional subscales not included in these four major factors: *Comprehension Learning*, which involves the use of illustrations, analogies, and intuition to build a general picture of what is being learned, and *Operation Learning*, which involves the use of details and logical analysis.

These two instruments were selected in order to explore the relationships of the LASI's deep and surface learning factors to the four factors of the ILP. The authors were interested in investigating these relationships first by reviewing the underlying scaling of the measures and second by comparing the performances of medical students on the two inventories. In addition, they wished to ascertain the relationships that the students' learning styles disclosed by these two inventories have to their academic performances in medical school—in this case measured by the grade-point average (GPA) and the total National Board of Medical Examiners (NBME) Part I score—in an effort to determine the extent to which these two scales would be useful in identifying students' academic problems. A third purpose was to describe how the medical students at the University of Nevada learn as measured by these two scales.

Several relationships between scales of the two learning-style inventories were predicted. First, it was predicted that the Meaning Orientation scale on the LASI, characterized as the "deep approach" to learning, would be positively related to all four scales on the ILP. Both the Elaborative Processing and the Synthesis-Analysis scales on the ILP have been characterized as involving deep processing strategies.[10] It was also felt that the Meaning Orientation scale, involving the intent to understand the material, would be related to an adherence to traditional study methods (Study Methods on the ILP) and the ability to retain factual information (Fact Retention on the ILP). Conversely, it was predicted that the Reproducing Orientation on the LASI, involving a "surface approach" to learning, would be negatively related to the two ILP scales involving deep processing strategies (Elaborative Processing and Synthesis-Analysis), but positively related to the Fact Retention scale on the ILP. Presumably, the intent to reproduce what is being studied (the Reproducing Orientation on the LASI) should be related to the ability to retain detailed factual information (Fact Retention on the ILP). It was also predicted that the Strategic Orientation on the LASI, based on a sense of competition and accomplishment, would be positively related to the Fact Retention and Study Methods scales on the ILP, but unrelated to those ILP scales involving deep processing strategies. Finally, it was predicted that the Non-Academic Orientation scale on the LASI would be negatively related to all four scales on the ILP.

In considering predictions regarding the relationships between learning-style measures and academic performance, the nature of the academic performance measures must be considered. Objective examinations in the first two years of medical school (upon which grade-point averages are largely based) are such that, given the frequency of testing, a student might succeed on the basis of short-term memory and external motivation to achieve. The NBME Part I exam, while also an objective, paper-and-pencil exam, is of sufficient breadth that students cannot use last-minute surface approaches to pass. They must enter the test with in-depth, comprehensive knowledge, which, if nothing else, allows them to make reasonable guesses on many of the items for which they do not know the answers. Based on this reasoning and LASI data reported for British students,[6] it was predicted that the Meaning Orientation and Strategic Orientation scales of the LASI would be positively related to grade-point averages (GPAs), but only the former would be positively related to NBME scores. Further, it was expected that Reproducing Orientation and Non-Academic Orientation scores would be negatively related to both measures of academic performance, but more strongly (negatively) related to NBME scores.

Predictions were also made regarding the relationship between scales of the ILP and measures of academic performance. It was predicted that three of the ILP scales—Synthesis-Analysis, Elaborative Processing, and Study Methods—would be related to both measures of academic performance. Schmeck and colleagues[3] report positive correlations between these scales and knowledge and comprehension scores on an objective examination. Finally, a positive relationship between Fact Retention scores and GPA scores was predicted. It was felt, however, given the breadth of the NBME examinations, that Fact Retention would not be strongly related to this measure of academic performance.

Method

The study subjects were 79 medical students at the University of Nevada

School of Medicine (UNSOM). The sample consisted of 32 first-year students, 32 second-year students, and 15 third-year students.

The two measures of learning style just described were used:

1. A version of the Inventory of Learning Processes (ILP) specifically modified for use with medical students.[9] This questionnaire is a 53-item true-false scale divided into four major learning processes. (See the boxed text titled "ILP" for details.)

2. The Lancaster Approaches to Studying Inventory (LASI.)[6-7] This is a 63-item self-report questionnaire. Subjects respond to each question on a five-point scale ranging from "definitely agree" (5) to "definitely disagree" (0). Items are grouped into 16 subscales. Fourteen of these subscales combine to form four major orientations. (See the boxed text titled "LASI" for details.)

Two indicators of academic performance were used:

1. The medical school GPA on a four-point system. GPAs were based on one semester of academic performance for first-year students, three semesters for second-year students, and five semesters for third-year students.

2. The National Board of Medical Examiners (NBME) Part I Total Score. Scores were available for second- and third-year students only.

The inventories were administered to groups of first-, second-, and third-year students in the fall of 1988, a total of 105 students. For the first- and second-year students, inventories were distributed at the end of a lecture and an appeal was made to students to complete and return them on a voluntary basis. For the third-year students, inventories were distributed to students involved in a surgery clerkship.

Results

Response rates were 72.7% (32 of 44) for the first-year students and 71.1% (32 of 45) for the second-year students. The response rate for the third-year students was 93.8% (15 of

Table 1

Students' Mean Scores on the Lancaster Approaches to Studying Inventory, from Both the Present Study (1988) and an Earlier Study (1983)*

Component of Inventory	Present Study (n = 79)		Ramsden Study (n = 2,208)	
	Mean	SD	Mean	SD
Meaning	44.8	7.61	38.5	9.79
Deep approach	11.2	2.54	10.6	3.10
Relating ideas	12.0	2.50	10.1	3.10
Use of evidence	11.1	2.47	9.6	2.89
Intrinsic motivation	10.5	3.14	8.2	3.85
Reproducing	31.7	9.66	34.9	9.59
Surface Approach	12.7	4.43	13.1	4.33
Syllabus-Bound	7.5	2.64	8.3	2.67
Fear of Failure	4.9	2.67	5.9	3.06
Improvidence	6.7	3.24	7.6	3.25
Non-Academic	18.1	7.69	22.7	8.03
Disorganized Approach	8.3	4.14	9.5	4.18
Negative Attitudes	3.4	2.76	5.4	3.94
Globetrotting	6.5	3.14	7.7	3.07
Strategic	23.0	4.73	25.6	7.47
Achievement motivation	5.8	3.07	9.7	3.59
Extrinsic motivation	5.4	2.87	5.9	4.36
Strategic approach	11.9	2.39	10.3	2.95
Comprehension Learning	8.2	3.15	8.6	3.87
Operation Learning	9.3	2.75	10.1	3.16

*In 1988, 79 students at the University of Nevada School of Medicine were administered two learning-style inventories. The table shows their mean scores and the corresponding scores achieved by students in an earlier study. (See the text and reference 6 for details of those studies; see the Results section for an analysis of the comparisons presented in the table.)

Table 2

Students' Mean Scores on the Inventory of Learning Processes, from Both the Present Study (1988) and an Earlier Study (1983)*

	Present Study (n = 79)		Vu and Galofre Study (n = 254)†	
	Mean	SD	Mean, Students Using OBM Curriculum‡	Mean, Students Using Traditional Curriculum
Synthesis-Analysis	12.68	2.48	13.25	11.55
Study Methods	10.46	4.05	11.09	10.18
Fact Retention	4.59	1.27	4.34	4.46
Elaborative Processing	7.20	1.74	7.23	6.37

*In 1988, 79 students at the University of Nevada School of Medicine were administered two learning-style inventories. The table shows their mean scores and corresponding scores achieved by students in an earlier study. (See the text and reference 9 for details of those studies; see the Results section for an analysis of the comparisons presented in the table.)
†Standard deviations were not calculated for these mean scores.
‡Objectives-Based Mastery Curriculum.

16); overall, the response rate was 75.2% (79 of 105).

Learning Styles

Separate multivariate analyses of variance were used to compare class differences on the LASI and ILP. No significant difference was found on the multivariate test of the 16 subscales of the LASI. Univariate tests revealed only one significant difference. Classes were found to differ on the Strategic Approach subscale ($F = 3.57$; df = 2,76; $p = .033$), with the third-year students scoring higher (mean score = 12.67) than the first- or second-year students (mean scores of 12.37 and 11.06, respectively). A multivariate analysis of variance failed to reveal significant class differences in performances on the four scales of the ILP. Results of univariate tests of individual scales also were not significant. Given the lack of evidence for class differences on learning-style measures, the data were combined across classes for subsequent analyses.

The score means and standard deviations were computed for the 16 subscales and four major factors of the LASI. These data are presented in Table 1 along with those from Ramsden[6] based on the scores of students at two universities in Lancaster, England, where much of the original work on the LASI was done. As can be seen, the medical students in the Nevada sample had much more academically oriented learning styles than did those students in Ramsden's original sample, scoring significantly higher on the Meaning Orientation ($t = 5.66$; $p < .001$), and significantly lower on the Reproducing Orientation ($t = 2.91$; $p < .01$), the Non-Academic Orientation ($t = 5.01$; $p < .001$), and the Strategic Orientation ($t = 3.07$; $p < .01$).

For comparison, Table 2 presents means and standard deviations for the scores on the four scales of the ILP. Also presented are data from Vu and Galofre[9] showing the means (no standard deviations are reported in the Vu and Galofre paper) for scores of medical students who used an Objectives-Based Mastery (OBM) curriculum at Southern Illinois University School of Medicine and those who used a traditional curriculum at St. Louis University School of Medicine. Although statistical comparisons are not possible, data from the current sample (a traditional curriculum) appear comparable to those from the original sample, with means falling between the original groups on the Synthesis-Analysis and Study Methods scales. Scores on Fact Retention were slightly higher for the current sample, and Elaborative Processing scores were virtually identical to those of the OBM group in the original sample.

In order to examine the reliability of the learning-style measures on the current sample, alpha coefficients, a measure of internal consistency, were computed for all scales and subscales. Coefficients for the 16 LASI subscales ranged from low (Fear of Failure = .26) to adequate (Disorganized Approach = .76) and were generally consistent with those reported by Ramsden.[6] Coefficients for three of the major factors were adequate, ranging from .74 (Non-Academic Orientation) to .76 (Reproducing Orientation). However, the coefficient for the Strategic Orientation (.37) was extremely low, casting some doubt on the reliability and validity of this factor. Internal consistencies for the ILP ranged from a questionable .41 (Fact Retention) to an adequate .75 (Study Methods). Although the low coefficient for Fact Retention raises some question as to the reliability of this scale, those reported by Vu and Galofre[9] were much higher, ranging from .53 to .65.

In order to examine similarities between learning-style measures, correlations were computed between scores on the LASI and the ILP. The observed pattern of correlations was generally as predicted. The Meaning Orientation on the LASI showed a significant positive correlation ($p <$ .05) with three of the four ILP scales, correlating most highly with Study Methods ($r = .55$; $p < .01$). The Reproducing Orientation revealed significant negative correlations with

both Synthesis Analysis ($r = -.63$; $p < .01$) and Elaborative Processing ($r = -.44$; $p < .01$). Similarly, the Non-Academic Orientation had significant negative correlations with both Synthesis Analysis ($r = -.45$; $p < .01$) and Study Methods ($r = -.57$; $p < .01$). Interestingly, the scales on the learning style measures with the lowest coefficients of internal consistency, the Strategic Orientation on the LASI and the Fact Retention scale on the ILP, failed to correlate significantly with any other measures.

Academic Performance

The classes did not differ significantly in terms of GPA. The mean GPA for the sample was 3.17 (SD = .42). GPAs ranged from 2.13 to 4.00. The NBME total scores were available for the second- and third-year students only ($n = 47$). The classes did not differ significantly in terms of their NBME scores. The mean NBME score for the sample was 479.79 (SD = 84.35). Scores ranged from 315 to 630.

Learning Styles and Academic Performance

Correlations were computed between learning-style scores and measures of academic performance. While the pattern of results was generally as predicted, quite surprisingly, none of the correlations reached statistical significance. In terms of the LASI, both the Meaning Orientation and the Strategic Orientation, along with their respective subscales, were generally positively related to both measures of academic performance, with the exception of the Strategic Approach subscale. The Reproducing Orientation and its subscales, with the exception of the Fear of Failure score, tended to correlate negatively with both the GPA and the NBME scores. Interestingly, the Non-Academic Orientation correlated negatively with the NBME scores ($r = -.15$) but not the GPA. The Comprehension Learning subscale was also positively related to both

measures of academic performance. Multiple regression analyses using the four major factors of the LASI failed to predict significantly either the GPA ($F = 1.08$; df = 4,74; p, not significant) or the NBME scores ($F = 1.73$; df = 4,42; p, not significant).

Two scales of the ILP, Synthesis Analysis and Elaborative Processing, were positively (though not significantly) related to both the GPA and the NBME scores. Neither Study Methods nor Fact Retention correlated substantially with either measure. Again, multiple regression analyses using ILP scores failed to predict significantly either the GPA ($F = 1.14$; df = 4,74; p, not significant) or the NBME scores ($F = 2.13$; df = 4,42; p, not significant).

Discussion

Reliability estimates for learning-style measures ranged from a poor .4055 to an acceptable .7539 for the ILP, with a similar range of .3701 to .7359 for the LASI. In each inventory, one factor (Fact Retention — ILP; Strategic Orientation — LASI) was found to have relatively low reliability estimates. Thus it appears that while the reliabilities of the two learning-style measures are adequate, the reliabilities of two specific factors are open to question. It is interesting, however, to note the similarity of mean values for the ILP factors between this study and those reported by Vu and Galofre.[9] Over time and institutions, the mean values for each factor were surprisingly similar, thus lending additional stability to the findings reported in this study.

The pattern of interrelationships between the two learning-style inventories generally provided good support for the theoretical distinctions between deep and surface approaches to learning. Hypotheses regarding the relationships between the scores on the LASI and ILP inventories were generally well-substantiated. In particular, the Meaning Orientation, or "Deep Learning Factor," of the LASI correlated significantly with three of the four ILP factors (Synthesis-Analysis, Study Methods, and Elaborative Processing). Only Fact Retention failed to correlate significantly. Interestingly, the ILP Fact Retention factor appeared virtually unrelated to any of the LASI subscales.

In contrast to the nature of deep learning as measured by LASI's Meaning Orientation factor, the Reproducing Orientation factor (LASI) describes surface learning, or superficial approaches, to the acquisition of information. As predicted, the Reproducing Orientation factor correlated negatively with all ILP factors except fact retention.

The students employing a Non-Academic approach (LASI factor) were characterized by the lack of an organized study plan and the tendency to go off on tangents while studying. Consistent with predictions, negative correlations were found between scores on the Non-Academic factor and all four of the ILP factors, but the correlations with only two of these were significant: Synthesis/Analysis and Study Methods.

Strategic learning represents selective approaches to learning depending upon the circumstances. Thus, a student with little or no time to learn may adopt a surface approach to rapidly acquire the facts necessary to do well on an exam, whereas that student may use a deep approach (hence learning the material better) if given more time and different circumstances. Predictions regarding the strategic approach in general were not supported. None of the correlations was significant; all were extremely low in value, leading the authors to conclude that the strategic approach is not at all strongly related to the ILP.

The *patterns* of correlations between learning style measures and indicators of academic performance were generally confirmed. Both the GPA and the NBME total Part I scores correlated positively with the Meaning Orientation and Strategic Orientation scores of the LASI and the Synthesis Analysis and Elaborative Processing scores of the ILP. The NBME scores were also negatively related to the Reproducing Orienta-

tion and Non-Academic Orientation scores of the LASI. However, the magnitudes of these relationships were quite small; no correlation reached statistical significance. Thus, it appears that while there are predictable relationships between these measures of learning styles and indicators of academic performance, the relationships are surprisingly weak.

In speculating why these two learning-style measures do not adequately predict academic performance, several issues should be considered. First, it may be that the reliability of the learning-style measures was insufficient. However, as discussed previously, reliability estimates for all but two factors of the LASI and ILP — namely the Strategic Orientation (LASI) and Fact Retention (ILP) factors — seemed to be large enough to detect significant relationships between learning styles and academic performance, should they have existed. Second, sample size was similarly considered. While a small sample might have accounted for the nonsignificant correlations with the NBME scores ($n = 47$), the sample size for GPA ($n = 79$) should have been large enough to have found a significant correlation, had one existed. Third, the GPA and NBME Part I scores may not be adequate measures of academic performance. That is, students' knowledge often may be broader than their test scores indicate. However, the two measures of academic performance used in this study are widely accepted and without comparable alternatives.

Similarly, it may be argued that the LASI and ILP are not valid measures of learning styles. However, the intercorrelations between the two scales and their underlying factors provide support for the construct validity of at least the deep and surface approaches to learning. Finally, it may be that learning styles, while related to academic performance, are not a major factor in explaining academic performance. Previous research has shown that a variety of factors are predictive of academic performance: MCAT scores, preclinical GPA,[11] and other measures of learning style.[12] It

is clear, however, at least so far as the results of this study are concerned, that these two measures of learning style are not predictive of academic performance.

In conclusion, this study has shown that the two learning-style inventories, the LASI and the ILP, even though developed at different times with different purposes, are related. Both inventories may represent an information-processing category of learning-style inventories. While the original authors of the LASI theoretically differentiated their measure from many American learning-style inventories — namely those with personality and information-processing characteristics — it appears that this position may not be valid.

An important initial interest of the authors in these inventories was to ascertain the inventories' diagnostic usefulness in predicting students' academic performances. It had been hoped that individual student profiles on these learning-style measures might make it possible to show students where their strengths and weaknesses lie. It appears that neither measure is much help in this regard, nor do they seem to be useful from a strictly descriptive sense. Mean scores of either measure were extremely difficult to interpret diagnostically. Without either better instructions from the inventories' authors on how the mean scores can be usefully translated into student feedback, or published standardized norms, these two measures appear to have utility primarily from a research perspective.

References

1. Curry L. *Learning Style in Continuing Medical Education.* Ottawa, Ontario, Canada: Canadian Medical Association, 1983.
2. Witzke, D. B., and Rubeck, R. F. Individual Learning Style: The Development of a Reliable Instrument. In *Research in Medical Education: 1984. Proceedings of the Twenty-Third Annual Conference,* Stephanie Kirby, compiler, pp. 97–107. Washington, D.C.: Association of American Medical Colleges, 1984.
3. Schmeck, R. R., Ribich, F., and Ramaniah, N. Development of a Self-Report Inven-

tory for Assessing Individual Differences in Learning Processes. *Appl. Psychol. Meas.* **1**(1977):413–431.

4. Newble, D. I., and Entwistle, N. J. Learning Styles and Approaches: Implications for Medical Education. *Med. Educ.* **20**(1986):162–175.

5. Rezler, A. G., and Rezmovic, V. The Learning Preference Inventory. *J. Allied Health* **10**(1981):28–34.

6. Ramsden, P. *The Lancaster Approaches to Studying and Course Perceptions Questionnaire.* Oxford, England: Educational Methods Unit, 1983.

7. Entwistle, N. J., and Ramsden, P. *Understanding Student Learning.* London, England: Croom Helm, 1983.

8. Myers, L. B. *The Myers-Briggs Type Indicator Manual.* Princeton, New Jersey: Educational Testing Service, 1962.

9. Vu, N. V., and Galofre, A. How Medical Students Learn. *J. Med. Educ.* **58**(1983):601–610.

10. Curry, L. *Learning Style in Continuing Medical Education.* Ottawa, Ontario, Canada: Canadian Medical Association, 1983, p. 423.

11. Leonardson, G. R., and Peterson, L. P. Relationship between Subject Examination Scores in Clerkships and Academic and Demographic Factors. *J. Med. Educ.* **60**(1985):719–721.

12. Markert, R. J. Learning Style and Medical Students' Performance on Objective Examinations. *Percept. Motor Skills* **62** (1986):781–782.

Differences in Residency Performances and Specialty Choices between Graduates of Three- and Four-year Curricula

L. K. GUNZBURGER, Ph.D., THOMAS LOESCH, M.Ed., R. LEISCHNER, M.D., and EILEEN HALL

Abstract—This study identified differences in the specialty choices and residency program directors' performance ratings of residents graduated from two different curricula of the same medical school. One curriculum was three years long, and compressed two years of the basic sciences into one year of study. The other was a four-year program devoting two years each to the basic and clinical science, but with elements unifying the two areas. Using an 18-item form, the program directors rated the performance of 42–96% of the residents who had graduated in the classes of 1982, 1984, 1985, and 1986. (1982 was the only class of the three-year curriculum that was studied.) Graduates of the three-year program showed less strength in background medical knowledge and in their experience of using research data; their greatest strengths seemed to be in the sorts of skills that normally would be acquired during the course of residency experiences. Graduates of the four-year curriculum seemed more able to integrate background medical knowledge and effective care of patients. Their weaknesses appeared to be in those skills that would be developed during the course of the residency experience. The only marked differences between the two groups in terms of residency specialty choice were in surgery and medicine. *Acad. Med.* 66(1991):47–48.

This study was made to identify differences in specialty choices and performance ratings between residents who were graduated from two different curricula. In the early 1970s, the Loyola University of Chicago Stritch School of Medicine, in Maywood, Illinois, moved from a traditional, four-year curriculum consisting of two years of basic sciences followed by two years of clinical sciences to a three-year curriculum that covered essentially the same material but included only one year of basic sciences. Two previously reported studies[1,2] compared differences among graduates of these curricula who had completed their medical training and who were practicing physicians. Problems with the compressed, three-year curriculum necessitated a return to a four-year curriculum in 1980, but elements of an experimental track unifying the basic and clinical sciences were incorporated in the new program. The present study compared differences in performances between the graduates of the last class of the three-year curriculum (the 1982 class) and the first three classes of the revised four-year curriculum (the 1984, 1985, and 1986 classes).

Method

A rating form was developed to evaluate the residents' performances in their first year of residency. Each year the form was sent to the directors of residency programs entered by Loyola graduates approximately seven months into the residencies. The form contained 18 items concerning various medical care situations; each item consisted of a statement describing the resident's performance in a specific task or competency. Program directors were asked to rate each statement according to a five-part scale ranging from "strongly agree" to "disagree." Their ratings were based on one or more of the following sources: personal observation, patients' reports, verbal reports of faculty, and evaluation reports. Data concerning the residents' specialty choices also were obtained.

Results and Discussion

Ratings were received for 63 graduates (42%) of the 1982 class, 133 (96%) of the 1984 class, 97 (80%) of the 1985 class, and 108 (87%) of the 1986 class. (There was no 1983 class.) The following results were based on the obvious differences between the classes' responses to each item using the mean score or percentage for each class.

There was no substantial difference among the four classes in terms of a number of supplemental questions concerning the bases upon which the ratings were assigned. Since the 1986 class had much better ratings, the lower ratings for the first two classes (1984 and 1985) of the revised, four-year curriculum compared with those received by the three-year curriculum group (1982 class) most likely can be attributed to the normal effects of a major curriculum transition, and thus the data for those two classes have been omitted from the discussion.

The following comparisons are based (in most cases) on the last class of the three-year curriculum group (1982 class) and the third class of the revised, four-year curriculum group

Dr. Gunzburger is professor and associate dean of curriculum and educational research and development, the University of Health Sciences/The Chicago Medical school, and formerly at Loyola University of Chicago Stritch School of Medicine (LUCSSM), Maywood, Illinois; Dr. Leischner is acting dean and pathology course director, and Ms. Hall coordinator of educational research and development, both at LUCSSM; and Mr. Loesch is a fellow, College of Education, University of Illinois at Chicago.

Correspondence and requests for reprints should be addressed to Dr. Gunzburger, Associate Dean, Curriculum and Educational Research and Development, University of Health Sciences/The Chicago Medical School, 3333 Green Bay Road, North Chicago, IL 60064.

Other articles about specialty choices appear on pages 41, 44, and 49.

(1986 class). On five items, the residents in the four-year group received the same mean ratings as did those in the three-year group. These items concerned interviewing skills, patient relationships, handling anxiety, evaluating research data, and using opportunities for continuous learning.

On eight items, the four-year group received slightly better mean ratings than did the three-year group. These items concerned using laboratory and test procedures, having a fund of medical knowledge, understanding pathogenesis, identifying issues and setting priorities, selecting appropriate therapies, writing good medical records, acting effectively in emergencies, and working well with others.

On five items, the four-year group received much higher mean ratings than did the three-year group. These items concerned pursuing symptomatology during history taking, performing a physical examination, maintaining up-to-date medical records, applying learning in patient care, and asking challenging, thoughtful questions.

The frequencies of the residency directors' agreements or disagreements with individual rating form items also were inspected to identify graduates' areas of strength and weakness in training. Raters of the 1982 and 1984 classes indicated that their graduates' strengths lay in day-to-day floor experiences, the kind of skills they would gain with time on the floors. Their weaknesses lay in background medical knowledge to support their practical skills, as well as in experience using the kinds of data found in journals and through independent investigation of topics. Ratings of the 1985 class indicated that these graduates began to show benefits from the four-year curriculum, developing medical insight rather than only being strong in practical skills. This overall trend in ratings of individual items continued for the 1986 class, suggesting that areas of graduates' skill needing to be strengthened are those that improve with time and floor experience, skills that are not absolutely essential qualities to have as a new intern.

The specialty choices for all four classes were examined. The most notable trend was the selection of medicine over surgery specialties. Of the 1982 class, 42.9% chose internal medicine or a medicine subspecialty residency program, while only 15.9% reentered a surgery residency program, fewer than the number who entered a pediatrics specialty (17.5%). In contrast, the 1984 class had an increase (to 25.6%) in graduates choosing a surgery residency, and a substantial decrease (to 27.1%) in those entering internal medicine or its subspecialties. The percentage of graduates entering surgery residencies then declined from 1984 (25.6%) to 1986 (19.3%), while that of graduates entering medicine residencies increased from 27.1% in 1984 to 34.2% in 1986.

There also was a substantial increase in the number of residencies taken in family practice for the 1984 to 1986 classes (13.5%, 13.4%, and 14.8%, respectively), compared with the 1982 class (6.3%). Graduates electing pediatrics residencies rose from 12% in 1984 to 18.6% in 1986. Except for surgery, medicine, and pediatrics, these trends mirror national data.[3] Loyola residents entered pediatrics at higher rates in 1982 and 1986, entered surgery residencies more frequently in 1984 to 1986, and chose medicine at lower rates in 1984 to 1986.

These findings suggest that many of the recommendations of the Project Panel on the General Professional Education of the Physician and College Preparation for Medicine (GPEP)[4] can be instituted and appear to have some impact on graduates' attitudes and practices.

References

1. Gunzburger, L., Yang, L., and Tobin, J. Effect of Three-Year and Four-Year Curricula on Physicians' Attitudes and Medical Practice. *J. Med. Educ.* **59**(1984):373–379.

2. Barbato, A., et al. Comparison of Graduates of Regular Curriculum and Unified Basic-Science–Clinical Curriculum. *J. Med. Educ.* **63**(1988):505–514.

3. Data from the National Residency Matching Program, published in the *J. Med. Educ.* **57**(1982):420–422; **59**(1984):442; **60**(1985):499; and **61**(1986):618.

4. Muller, S. (Chairman). Physicians for the Twenty-First Century: Report of the Project Panel on the General Professional Education of the Physician and College Preparation for Medicine. *J. Med. Educ.* **59**, Part 2 (November 1984).

Teaching and Clinical Education

Attitudes of Faculty and Clinical Physical Therapists Toward Teaching as a Career

Carolyn K Rozier, PhD, PT
Basil L Hamilton, PhD

ABSTRACT: *The purpose of this study was to identify aspects of a teaching position that could be used to recruit clinicians and to help alleviate the faculty shortage. Inventories were developed to determine attitudes toward and satisfaction with a clinical position as opposed to a faculty position and to determine attitudes toward teaching in a faculty position. These inventories were sent to all physical therapists teaching in education programs and to 1,000 clinicians. The clinicians who felt they would be most satisfied in a teaching position believed that teachers had more influence on the profession, served as role models, and had more prestige and respect. Faculty believed more strongly than clinicians that academic salaries are inadequate and that too much time is spent in non-teaching activities. Clinicians believed more strongly that there is not enough patient contact in a faculty position and that assigning grades is stressful. Clinicians who had taught during their undergraduate or graduate program or in a continuing education program indicated that they would be more satisfied in a teaching position. The findings of this study are discussed in terms of faculty recruitment implications.*

INTRODUCTION

Difficulty in recruiting physical therapists for positions in physical therapist and physical therapist assistant education programs is a problem facing our education programs and the profession.[1,2] Clinicians facing a shortage of therapists want more graduates from education programs. These programs lack a sufficient number of faculty to increase the number of students.[3] Effective ways to recruit faculty must be identified to alleviate the current shortage of faculty in education programs.

Dr Rozier is Professor and Dean, School of Physical Therapy, Texas Woman's University, Box 22487, TWU Station, Denton, TX 76204. Dr Hamilton is Professor, Department of Psychology and Philosophy, Texas Woman's University.

Survey research can be used to determine the degree of agreement or disagreement with certain statements about attitudes toward teaching or toward clinical work that are most attractive to faculty and clinicians.[4] These attitude statements can be grouped into inventories to identify congruent attitudes that determine satisfaction with teaching or clinical practice in physical therapy.[5–7] Measurement of attitudes also can reveal a person's underlying beliefs and ultimately indicate intentions and behavior.[8]

Measurement of certain attitudes held by clinicians toward a teaching position might identify clinicians who are interested in teaching. If one can identify positive attitudes held by clinicians toward teaching, these can be used in a marketing plan to recruit faculty from among interested clinicians. Because people tend to work in environments where others hold similar attitudes or in environments that meet their needs,[9–12] one can determine which attitudes toward a teaching position and toward the clinic are common to faculty and to certain clinicians. Faculty and clinicians can be expected to have some differing attitudes toward teaching and the clinic, because research has shown that teachers of a profession hold differing attitudes from practitioners in the profession.[13,14]

To determine effective ways to recruit clinicians as faculty, it would be useful to know how satisfied current faculty are and what attitudes they hold toward teaching or the clinic. The level of job satisfaction perceived by clinicians, together with how satisfied they believe they would be in a faculty position and what attitudes they have toward a faculty position, also are factors to be identified. These responses then can be compared between faculty and clinicians to correlate attitudes and background information to determine which aspects of a faculty position should be emphasized in a recruitment plan.

METHOD

Subjects

The subjects of this study were 1000 physical therapists working in clinical positions

and 876 physical therapists teaching full-time in education programs for physical therapists or physical therapist assistants. All education program directors of accredited programs were sent questionnaires to distribute to full-time faculty who were physical therapists. Clinicians were randomly selected from the latest active membership lists of the American Physical Therapy Association (APTA), excluding members of the Section for Education because many faculty were members of that section. Because of the high response rate, follow-up mailings were unnecessary.

Questionnaire Development

The questionnaire was developed after a review of the literature on attitude related to job satisfaction.[6,15–22] The questionnaire was exempt from human subjects review board approval. Suggestions for a draft questionnaire were generated via interviews of three physical therapy faculty members and an open-ended questionnaire mailed to 15 physical therapy faculty members. A draft questionnaire consisting of 40 Likert Scale items was developed. The draft questionnaire was mailed to 24 physical therapist faculty members at a physical therapy education program, and responses were subjected to multiple regression analyses. Questions that did not contribute to predicting the overall sum of the scores on each inventory were deleted or reworded.

Final Questionnaire

The final survey contained two 21-item attitude inventories (Appendices A,B). Questions on both inventories were phrased according to guidelines for attitude inventory construction.[23–25] A 5-interval Likert Scale was used. The first inventory asked for agreement or disagreement with statements about why a faculty member chose to teach rather than to remain in the clinic and about why a clinician might choose to teach. The statements in this inventory were phrased differ-

Reprinted with permission from the *Journal of Physical Therapy Education*, Vol 6, No 2, pp 47-51, 1992.

ently for clinicians because clinicians were indicating why they might teach and faculty were indicating why they decided to teach. Additionally, the statements were phrased to imply differences between a clinic position and a faculty position, and answers were higher on the Likert Scale if respondents believed they would like teaching more than working in the clinic.

The second inventory asked for agreement or disagreement with statements related to what a person likes or might like about a faculty position. The final internal reliabilities were .70 and .77 for faculty and clinicians for the first inventory, and .77 and .73 for faculty and clinicians for the second inventory. In addition to the inventories, demographic information was collected and clinicians were asked about plans for graduate education. One question on job satisfaction in the clinic and one question on projected or actual job satisfaction in teaching were included. These questions were intended to indicate a person's global satisfaction with the job as a whole.[20]

Data Analysis

The SPSS Statistical Package* was used for data analyses. Ranges, means, standard deviations, and percentages were calculated for the demographic items for both faculty and clinicians. Demographic differences between faculty and clinicians for continuous variables were analyzed with two-tailed independent t tests and for categorical variables were analyzed with chi-square analyses.

The Likert Scale responses were coded so that a score of 5 indicated a positive attitude. For positively worded items, this scoring procedure meant that a response of "strongly agree" received a score of 5. For negatively worded items, this scoring procedure meant that a response of "strongly disagree" received a score of 5. Derived measures of job satisfaction were generated by summing all items on each of the two inventories. Differences between faculty and clinicians on each item on each of the two inventories, on the summed inventory scores for the two inventories, and on the two global satisfaction items were analyzed with two-tailed independent t tests. Because many statistical tests were performed, a .01 level of significance was used for each test to control somewhat for the inflation of the Type I error rate, or false rejections of null hypotheses.

The associations between the satisfaction items and the summed inventory scores and the associations between the satisfaction items and individual items on each of the two inventories were analyzed with Pearson product-moment correlation coefficients for both faculty and clinicians. The resulting correlations were tested for significance with two-tailed t tests.

RESULTS

Subject Characteristics

Questionnaires were returned from 613 faculty and 566 clinicians for a return rate of 69% and 57%, respectively. Demographic information is presented in tables 1 and 2. The faculty tended to be older than the clinicians, but both groups had received their entry-level education at similar ages. Both faculty and clinicians had backgrounds with some experience in teaching (Tab. 2). A higher percentage of faculty reported involvement in teaching activities while a graduate student than did the clinicians. This was expected, because a higher percentage of faculty had graduate degrees. A higher percentage of clinicians had received a baccalaureate degree as entry into the profession; however, faculty did not have the correspondingly higher percentage of entry-level master's degrees. Faculty did have a higher percentage of certificates as entry level. Only 28 clinicians were enrolled in graduate education, while 49% of clinicians reported that they would not want to go to graduate school, 31% of clinicians responded that they would like to go to graduate school, and 20% of clinicians were uncertain.

Group Comparison of Inventories

Table 3 lists the items on Inventory One where faculty and clinician responses differed significantly. The groups did not differ on statements that teachers had more opportunities to serve as role models and had more flexible hours, and both groups had tried teaching and liked it. Both groups were neutral on whether a clinician or a faculty member received more respect, exerted more control over his or her job situation, or had more opportunity for continuing education. Faculty and clinician responses differed significantly on 11 of the 21 items on Inventory Two (Tab. 4). Faculty were more positive than clinicians in response to statements such as teaching offers a challenge, more flexible hours, more status, more opportunity for advancement, and a pleasant environment.

*SPSS Inc, 444 N Michigan Ave, Chicago, IL 60611.

Table 1

Characteristics of Subjects (N=1179)

Item	Group	Range	$\overline{X}$	SD	t	P
Age (yr)	clinicians	22–65	34.59	8.14	11.66	.001
	faculty	24–67	40.32	8.69		
Age highest degree received	clinicians	18–54	24.61	4.33	20.26	.001
	faculty	17–53	31.17	6.63		
Age entry-level degree received	clinicians	17–47	23.58	3.58	1.25	.210
	faculty	17–53	23.32	3.54		
Years in clinical practice	clinicians	0–40	10.02	7.30	39.27	.001
	faculty	0–32	7.54	3.55		
Years in administration	clinicians	1–29	5.39	4.92	3.17	.002
	faculty	1–34	4.54	4.21		

Table 2

Educational Background and Experience of Respondents (N=1179)

Education/Experience	Clinicians (%)	Faculty (%)	X^2	P
Highest degree				
Certificate	2			
Baccalaureate	77	12		
Master's	21	62	505.93	.001
Doctorate		26		
Entry-level degree				
Certificate	11	23		
Baccalaureate	82	68		
Master's	7	9	34.51	.001
Teaching background				
Taught while in entry-level program	37	27		
Taught while in graduate program	15	54		
Taught as clinical instructor	51	65	195.81	.001

Faculty tended to be more negative in their responses to whether salary was adequate or whether too much time was spent on non-teaching activities.

There was a significant difference between faculty and clinician responses on the question of general clinical satisfaction. Clinicians reported significantly higher satisfaction than faculty (Tab. 5). Faculty indicated significantly more satisfaction with a teaching position than clinicians. Faculty and clinician responses differed significantly ($P=.001$) on the sum for Inventory Two but not on the sum for Inventory One. For clinicians, the sum for Inventory One had a significant ($P=.001$) inverse relationship of $-.18$ with satisfaction in the clinic. The negative relationship theoretically occurred because the inventory contained statements related to whether a person thought a faculty position would be more advantageous than clinical work. For clinicians, the sum of Inventory One did correlate significantly ($r=.47; P=.001$) with the question of general satisfaction with a teaching position. The same significant correlation was not true for faculty. There were significant correlations of the sums for Inventory Two with the question on satisfaction with a teaching position for both faculty ($r=.43; P=.001$) and clinicians ($r=.46; P=.001$).

Correlations to Teaching Satisfaction

Thirty-one percent of clinicians indicated that they would not enjoy teaching; 28% indicated that they felt neutral toward teaching, and 41% felt positively toward teaching. Sixteen of the 21 questionnaire items from Inventory One correlated significantly with the question on teaching satisfaction for clinicians and 7 items for faculty. Most of the correlations were low (below .45) and may be of little practical importance, but some correlations were of interest. Clinicians who felt that they would be satisfied as teachers believed that teachers had more influence on the profession ($r=.36; P=.001$), served as role models ($r=.31; P=.001$) and had more prestige and respect ($r=.25; P=.001$) than clinical counterparts. Clinicians who believed that they would be satisfied teaching also indicated that they had always wanted to teach ($r=.25; P=.001$) and that they had tried teaching ($r=.44; P=.001$). Although many of these items on Inventory One also were significantly correlated for faculty to teaching satisfaction, the correlations were of lesser magnitude ($r < .15$).

There were 15 individual items on Inventory Two for clinicians and 17 items for faculty that correlated significantly ($P=.01; r <.45$) with the question on general satisfac-

tion with teaching (Tab. 6). Some characteristics of faculty and clinicians also correlated with teaching satisfaction. Clinicians would not be as likely to be satisfied with a faculty position if they did not anticipate enrolling ($r=-.36; P=.001$), or wish to enroll ($r=-.42; P=.001$) in a graduate degree program; or the longer they had been in practice ($r=-.14; P=.001$); or the older they were ($r=-.14; P=.001$). There was a positive correlation to perception of satisfaction with a teaching position of the clinicians ($r=.44; P=.001$) and faculty ($r=.14; P=.001$) who had tried teaching.

Faculty who had the opportunity to teach in some type of program prior to becoming a faculty member indicated that they would expect more satisfaction with teaching ($r=.20; P=.001$). Clinicians who said that they had always wanted to teach had a significant correlation ($P=.001$) with their perception of

satisfaction with teaching ($r=.64$), as was also true for faculty ($r=.12$).

DISCUSSION

Attitudes Toward Clinical Physical Therapy

Various reasons are given by clinicians as to why they are satisfied with clinical physical therapy, and patient contact is one.[26] It was hypothesized along with Pearl[27] that lack of patient contact for clinicians would be a negative aspect of teaching. In this study, clinicians believed that there was not enough patient contact in teaching ($\overline{X}=2.16$; SD=.77; note that Likert Scale is reversed). Faculty also agreed with the perception of less patient contact, but this item did not significantly correlate with their teaching satisfaction. One explanation might be that 67.7% of faculty members are reported by the APTA[3] to participate in clinical practice.

Table 3

Results of t Test for Faculty/Clinicians on Inventory One[a] (N=1179)

Statement	Faculty ($\overline{X}$)	SD	Clinicians ($\overline{X}$)	SD	t	P
Influence others more in teaching	3.84	.91	3.69	.77	−3.03	.001
More prestige in teaching	2.95	.96	2.50	.78	−8.92	.001
Learning enjoyable	4.57	.54	4.11	.67	−12.84	.001
Like to publish	3.05	1.13	3.33	.88	4.73	.001
Research	3.18	1.13	3.51	.91	5.69	.001
Influenced to try teaching	3.24	1.17	2.85	.90	−6.70	.001
Inspired by teacher	3.09	1.17	2.88	.95	−3.30	.001
External event required flexible hours	2.56	1.04	2.89	.91	5.53	.001
Teaching less physical	2.88	1.19	3.21	1.03	4.99	.001
Summers off appealing	2.81	1.35	4.02	.87	18.22	.001
Less stress in teaching	2.06	1.01	2.42	.89	6.60	.001
Clinic not stimulating	2.51	1.18	2.13	.83	−6.53	.001
Work not pleasant	2.02	1.00	1.76	.75	−5.08	.001
Family obligations made teaching more convenient	2.51	1.23	2.71	.88	3.28	.001

[a]Likert Scale: 1=strongly disagree; 2=disagree; 3=neutral; 4=agree; 5=strongly agree.

Table 4

Results of t Test for Faculty/Clinicians on Inventory Two[a] (N=1179)

Statement	Faculty ($\overline{X}$)	SD	Clinicians ($\overline{X}$)	SD	t	P
Teacher salary not adequate[a]	1.96	1.02	2.22	.88	4.70	.001
Too much time non-teaching[a]	2.56	1.12	2.90	.73	6.16	.001
No opportunity for advancement in teaching[a]	3.47	1.00	3.14	.87	−6.04	.001
Not enough patient contact[a]	2.57	1.02	2.16	.77	−7.69	.001
Assigning grades is stressful	2.98	1.09	2.71	.89	−4.59	.001
Challenge	4.30	.63	3.50	.83	−18.27	.001
Pleasant environment	3.85	.87	3.41	.75	−9.19	.001
Flexible hours	4.12	.81	3.56	.68	−12.92	.001
Status	3.49	.85	3.28	.74	4.33	.001
Too many demands[a]	2.03	.96	2.45	.77	13.28	.001
Constraints interfere[a]	2.36	1.03	2.45	.76	1.69	.001

[a]Likert Scale reversed on these statements: 1=strongly agree; 2=agree; 3=neutral; 4=disagree; 5=strongly disagree.

Attitudes Toward Teaching

Some clinicians responded that they would be satisfied in teaching and that they also were satisfied with the clinic. It could be that these people most likely would report satisfaction wherever they were employed.[4] These people believed that teaching would let them expand their own knowledge, influence students, and design learning experiences in a pleasant, challenging environment, but still were satisfied with their clinic position. This study also found that clinicians who indicated the least perceived satisfaction with teaching had certain demographic items that were negatively correlated with teaching satisfaction, such as not wanting to enroll in graduate school the longer they had been in practice or the older they were. Occupational changes may indeed occur in specific phases of a person's life, and older individuals are less likely to change.[9]

Opportunities to use one's abilities are important in job satisfaction.[4,9] Clinicians who had tried teaching or who had always wanted to teach had a positive correlation with perceived satisfaction with a faculty position. This agreed with the results of a survey of physical therapy clinicians who revealed strong positive attitudes toward teaching in the clinical setting.[28]

In a study of engineers,[13] researchers found that the issue of salary amount was more important to practitioners than to faculty. In previous studies of physical therapy clinicians, salary was found to be the primary reason for choosing a particular position.[29,30] In the present study, both clinicians and faculty agreed that faculty salaries were inadequate, but this item did not correlate significantly with teaching satisfaction. Clinicians also believed less strongly than faculty that teaching salaries were inadequate. There-

fore, we might still be able to recruit faculty from the clinical environment if other work activities in teaching were stressed that were pleasing to clinicians: being a role model, influencing the profession, and gaining respect.

Recruitment Implications

The results of this study can be used in marketing plans to recruit more clinicians into teaching in physical therapy education programs. To market teaching as a product, we should recruit those who already have favorable attitudes and stress the positive aspects of teaching and the needs of the individual that teaching would fill.[4,8] For clinicians who currently do not feel positively toward teaching, a marketing plan could stress the positive attitudes that faculty hold toward teaching, including more autonomy with one's time, prestige, and opportunities for advancement.

Research has shown that a person dissatisfied with a job is likely to want to change.[10,11,31] In this study, only 2.5% of clinicians indicated that they were very dissatisfied with their clinic work. A major recruitment plan should not be based on individuals dissatisfied with clinic work in general.[12,31] For clinicians who are not satisfied or who are not stimulated by their clinic position, an emphasis could be placed on the various positive aspects of a teaching position. According to a survey by the APTA, therapists do change clinic jobs in search of better working conditions.[3] Persons wanting a change could be the target of a marketing plan stressing the flexibility and autonomy of education.

CONCLUSION

Faculty and clinician attitudes toward teaching indicate the types of statements to high-

light in a marketing plan to recruit clinicians for faculty positions. Both groups believed that they could influence the profession more as teachers and that academia offered a pleasant work environment with flexible hours. Clinicians who had taught in an undergraduate or graduate program had a significant positive correlation with perceived teaching satisfaction; therefore, one might want to recruit clinicians who have had some teaching experience.

One potential methodology worth investigating is for physical therapy education programs to provide opportunities for clinicians or entry-level students to teach to stimulate interest in teaching as a career for the physical therapist.

REFERENCES

1. *The Plan to Address the Faculty Shortage in Physical Therapy Education: Final Report of the Task Force.* Alexandria, VA: American Physical Therapy Association; 1985.

Table 6

Pearson Correlation: Individual Items on Inventory Two with Question on Teaching Satisfaction (N=1179)

Group/Item	n	r	P
Clinicians:			
Not enough patient contact[a]	553	.17	.001
Students not motivated[a]	552	.11	.005
Assigning grades is stressful[a]	552	.17	.001
No satisfaction in teaching[a]	552	.43	.001
Clinic more rewarding[a]	552	.46	.001
Designing learning	552	.36	.001
Autonomy	552	.22	.001
Challenge	556	.33	.001
Pleasant environment	556	.38	.001
Students grow	557	.29	.001
Influence students	557	.17	.001
Flexible hours	557	.22	.001
Status	557	.27	.001
Research exciting	557	.37	.001
Expand own knowledge	555	.32	.001
Faculty:			
Too much time non-teaching[a]	572	.16	.001
No advancement in teaching[a]	575	.23	.001
Students not motivated[a]	576	.14	.001
Immediate feedback lacking[a]	575	.18	.001
No satisfaction in teaching[a]	574	.41	.001
Clinic more rewarding[a]	574	.32	.001
Design learning	576	.14	.001
Expand own knowledge	576	.12	.003
Autonomy	574	.15	.001
Challenge	576	.20	.001
Pleasant environment	574	.46	.001
Students grow	575	.25	.001
Influence students	575	.14	.001
Flexible hours	575	.21	.001
Status	574	.13	.001
Too many demands[a]	574	.22	.001
Constraints[a]	576	.23	.001

[a]Negative statement and Likert Scale reversed on these items.

Table 5

Responses to Satisfaction Ratings (N=1179)

Question	$\bar{X}$	SD	t	P
Rate your actual/predicted satisfaction with a teaching position.				
Faculty	4.11	.88		
Clinicians	3.11	1.13	5.54	.001
Rate your satisfaction with your previous/current clinical work.				
Faculty	4.50	.68		
Clinicians	4.32	.72	−16.82	.001
Sum of Inventory One				
Faculty	65.66	8.59		
Clinicians	64.27	8.09	5.56	NS
Sum of Inventory Two				
Faculty	74.47	7.68		
Clinicians	68.16	7.06	−14.60	.001

2. *Action Plan to Address the Faculty Shortage.* Alexandria, VA: American Physical Therapy Association Board of Directors; 1988.

3. *Faculty Activity Survey.* Alexandria, VA: Department of Education, American Physical Therapy Association; 1989.

4. Vroom VH. *Work and Motivation.* New York, NY: John Wiley & Sons, Inc; 1964:79,88,102,154,173.

5. Aiken LR. Attitude measurement and research. In Payne DA (ed): *Recent Developments in Affective Measurement.* San Francisco, CA: Jossey-Bass, Inc.; 1980:1–20.

6. House RJ, Wigdor LA. Herzberg's dual factor theory of job satisfaction and motivation. *Personnel Psychology.* 1967; 20(4):369–389.

7. Gothard WP. *Vocational Guidance.* New Hampshire: Croom Helm; 1985:28.

8. Ajzen I, Fishbein M. *Understanding Attitudes and Predicting Social Behavior.* Englewood Cliffs, NJ: Prentice-Hall, Inc; 1988:154.

9. Osipow SH. *Theories of Career Development.* Englewood Cliffs, NJ: Prentice-Hall, Inc; 1983:11,218,313–314.

10. Hilton TL. Career decision making. *J Counsel Psychol.* 1962; 954:291–298.

11. Holland JL. *The Psychology of Vocational Choice.* Waltham, MA: Blaisdell Publishing Co; 1966:6.

12. Holland JL. *Making Vocational Choices: A Theory of Careers.* Englewood Cliffs, NJ: Prentice-Hall, Inc; 1973:4–9.

13. Erez M, Shneorson Z. Personality types and motivational characteristics of academics versus professionals in industry in the same occupational discipline. *Journal of Vocational Behavior.* 1980;17:95–105.

14. Goodwin L. The academic world and the business world: a comparison of occupational goals. *Sociology of Education.* 1969;42(2):170–175.

15. Marsh JF, Stafford FP. The effects of values on pecuniary behavior: the case of academicians. *American Sociological Review.* 1967;32:740–754.

16. Culbertson HM. Potential female and minority communication education: an exploratory study of their views on teaching as a profession. Presented at the Annual Meeting of the Association for Education in Journalism and Mass Communication; 1984; Gainesville, FL.

17. Hale C. Measuring job satisfaction. *Nursing Times.* 1986;82(5):43–46.

18. Body KL. Dental hygiene job and career satisfaction. *Dental Hygiene.* April 1988; 170–175.

19. French RM, Rezler AG. Personality and job satisfaction of medical technologists. *Am J Med Tech.* 1985;39(6):392–396.

20. Florian V, Sheffer M, Sachs D. Time allocation patterns of occupational therapists in Israel: implications for job satisfaction. *AJOT.* 1985;36(6):392–396.

21. Brollier C. A multivariate predictive study of staff OTR job satisfaction: some results of importance to psychosocial occupational therapy. *Occupational Therapy in Mental Health.* 1985;5(6):13–27.

22. Davis GL, Bordieri JE. Perceived autonomy and job satisfaction in occupational therapists. *AJOT.* 1988;42(9): 591–595.

23. Edwards AL. *Techniques of Attitude Scale Construction.* New York, NY: Appleton-Century-Crofts Inc; 1957:2–15.

24. Guilford JP. *Psychometric Methods.* New York, NY: McGraw-Hill; 1954:263–280.

25. Converse JM, Presser S. *Survey Questions.* Beverly Hills, CA: Sage Publications; 1986:39–79.

26. Atwood CA, Woolf DA. Job satisfaction of physical therapists: *HCM Review.* Winter 1982; 81–86.

27. Pearl MJ. *A Marketing Approach to the Physical Therapy Faculty Shortage in Higher Education.* Atlanta, GA: Georgia State University; 1987. Dissertation.

28. Sotosky JR. Physical therapists' attitudes toward teaching physical therapy. *Phys Ther.* 1984;64:347–349.

29. Simonton TE. Survey finds better pay, working conditions key to keeping physical therapists on job. *Progress Report.* 1989;18(6):3.

30. Harkson DG, Unterreiner AS, Shepard KF. Factors related to job turnover in physical therapy. *Phys Ther.* 1982;62:1465–1470.

31. Heddesheimer J. Modal motivation for mid-career changes. *Personnel and Guidance Journal.* 1976;55:109–111.

Appendix A

Inventory One

Responses:

Strongly Agree (SA)	Agree (A)	Uncertain/ Neutral (N)	Disagree (D)	Strongly Disagree (SD)

Reasons why I chose to teach:

Teaching would allow me to have more influence on the profession as a whole.

A teacher can serve as a role model for students.

There is more prestige in teaching than in clinical work.

There would be more respect for one's expertise in teaching.

There would be more control of the situation available in the classroom than in the clinical setting.

Studying and learning are enjoyable.

There are more opportunities for continuing education in teaching than in clinical work.

There is more time to publish while teaching.

There is more time to do research while teaching.

There was influence by others to try teaching.

I have always wanted to teach.

An excellent teacher in school had been an inspiration to go into teaching.

An external event in life required a more flexible work schedule.

A try at teaching had resulted in a feeling that a good job had been done.

Teaching is less physically demanding than clinical work.

The opportunity to take summers off is appealing.

Working hours would be more flexible in an academic setting than in a clinical setting.

There would be less stress in an academic setting than in a clinical setting.

The clinic is not stimulating, and trying something different would be attractive.

Working so closely with patients all day long is not pleasurable.

Family obligations made teaching more convenient than clinical work.

Appendix B

Inventory Two

Responses:

Strongly Agree (SA)	Agree (A)	Uncertain/ Neutral (N)	Disagree (D)	Strongly Disagree (SD)

As a teacher, I believe that:

The salary of a teacher is not adequate.[a]

Too much time is spent on non-teaching activities.[a]

There is no opportunity for advancement in teaching.[a]

There is not enough patient contact in teaching.[a]

Students are often not motivated.[a]

Immediate feedback from students is lacking.[a]

Assigning grades to students is often stressful.[a]

There is not much satisfaction with teaching.[a]

Doing clinical work is more rewarding than teaching.[a]

Designing learning experiences is rewarding.

Teaching offers autonomy.

Teaching is a challenge as opposed to a routine.

Academia offers a pleasant work environment.

Seeing students grow intellectually is rewarding.

Teachers can have an influence on students.

The flexible working hours for teachers are satisfactory.

The status of a teacher in the community is attractive.

Performing research projects is exciting.

Teachers have too many demands on their time.[a]

Constraints of the higher education institution often interfere with teaching.[a]

Teaching offers the opportunity to expand the teacher's own knowledge.

[a]Likert Scale for these questions is as follows:
SA=1; A=2; N=3; D=4; SD=5. For all other questions, SA=5, etc.

Group Work and Reflective Practicums in Physical Therapy Education: Models for Professional Behavior Development

Jody Gandy, MS, PT
Gail Jensen, PhD, PT

ABSTRACT: As the professional role of the physical therapist continues to evolve, physi- cal therapy educators are faced with the task of preparing professionals who can solve problems and make decisions in an often ambiguous, complex health care setting. They also, however, are faced with curriculums that are already content rich and that leave little room for new additions. The authors suggest alternative teaching methods that focus on active learning strategies applied in small group process and reflective activities. Small group process can facilitate development of profes- sional behaviors through the use of collabo- ration, collegiality, goal setting, decision mak- ing, divergent thinking, peer evaluation and self-evaluation, and creative problem solving. Reflective activities can be used to help bridge theory with practice. Reflection allows time for analyzing, synthesizing, and integrating complex information and examining alterna- tive strategies and their consequences. Exam- ples of specific classroom activities of these two teaching methods include group expert techniques, game activities, provocative is- sues, student-designed evaluations, and reflec- tive practicums.

INTRODUCTION

How do we as physical therapy educators prepare students to meet the demands of practice? Greatly expanded services and op- portunities for physical therapists, the con- tinuing movement toward direct access, and the changing context of health care require that graduates have the knowledge, attitudes, and values that represent professionals.

Ms Gandy is Associate Director, Department of Educa- tion, American Physical Therapy Association, Alexan- dria, VA. This work was done while she was a faculty member, Department of Physical Therapy, Temple Uni- versity, Philadelphia, PA. Dr Jensen is Associate Profes- sor, University of Alabama at Birmingham, Birmingham, AL. This work was done while she was a faculty member, Department of Physical Therapy, Temple University.

The competent physical therapist has been described by experts as one who can solve problems and analyze patients' needs, dem- onstrate accountability and responsibility, seek consultation, handle ambiguity, communicate effectively, and work in collegial and interde- pendent relationships.[1,2] While recognizing that these behaviors are essential for clinical practice, educators also face the dilemma of presenting an expanding body of knowledge. This places extraordinary demands on the student and the educator in an already satu- rated curriculum. In general, knowledge dou- bles in less than three years.[3] If that is true in physical therapy, it may be difficult to avert the pressure to succumb to the "banking concept of education"[4]; that is, the deposi- tion of more information as quickly as pos- sible into students' minds.

This article discusses the use of alternative teaching methods in physical therapy educa- tion. These methods employ active learning strategies that may help counteract the bank- ing concept of education and, in turn, foster the development of professional behaviors necessary to meet the demands of practice.

As educators we often attend to our con- cerns for course content first, before thinking about the teaching methods we employ. Sev- eral investigators have reported that when undergraduate college students are asked to describe what they understand the term *learn- ing* to mean, the majority—more than two thirds—view learning as knowing more, mem- orizing for later production, or acquiring and using facts. This is in contrast to the one third who believe learning involves insights into subject matter, new ways of thinking about reality, and personal growth.[5-7] Bloom, in referring to the cognitive taxonomy of edu- cational objectives, stated that much aca- demic learning still focuses on the memori- zation of facts.[8] He lamented that—even after a quarter of a century and the sale of over one million copies of his book on the cognitive taxonomy—our instructional ma- terial, our classroom teaching methods, and

our testing methods rarely rise above the lowest category of the taxonomy—knowl- edge.

The learning model frequently used in professional education also stresses knowl- edge acquisition through sequential learning by first providing scientific knowledge, then applied skills, and finally some type of practi- cum.[9] This model focuses on primarily the individual's needs in the classroom or clinical setting. The students' role in this model often is passive listening to lectures, practicing techniques in a laboratory setting by imitat- ing and repeating the technique, and demon- strating academic and clinical competence by satisfactorily completing short-answer writ- ten and practical examinations using simu- lated patient problems. Finally, students progress to clinical experiences where they apply and integrate classroom knowledge in the real world with real patients. One has to ask what can be done within the professional education learning model to adequately pre- pare students to meet the professional de- mands of practice.

Physical therapy is not the only profession struggling with balancing an expanding knowl- edge base with the need for skill develop- ment and appropriate professional behav- iors. Teacher education is a useful example because the field has had ongoing research focused on the area of teaching and learning as it relates to the development of profes- sional behaviors. The mid-1970s were the height of competency-based teacher educa- tion when several large-scale studies investi- gated the link between teacher behavior and student learning.[10-12] The research in this area was highly behavioral and positivistic, trying to link teacher behaviors to student learning as indicated by gains in test achieve- ment.[13] A positivistic research approach usu- ally employs quantifiable research methods to relate facts, establish direct relationships, and determine cause and effect. Eventually the competency approach was highly criti- cized for its proliferation of competencies;

the growing inability to validate the competencies; and its narrow, instrumental view of what teachers do.[14,15]

Critics of the competency-based system, and the positivistic research that went along with it, argued that teaching, like other professions, is driven by decisions and judgments made in uncertain, complex environments.[15,16] They argued that teacher education programs must be about the business of preparing the teacher as thinker and decision maker.[13]

In his investigations of professionals at work (eg, architects, managers, clinical psychologists, and town planners), Schon made a powerful argument against overemphasis on technical rationality or on the technical knowledge base for professions.[17] He argued that overreliance on technical skills may not solve the problem of preparing students to meet the demands of their profession and often overlooks the broader context of the problem. We all can think of situations when our physical therapy techniques were applied without any effect and perhaps without considering all possible factors contributing to the problem. Schon called these problem areas the *indeterminate zones of practice*. The problems often are fraught with uncertainty, uniqueness, and value conflict, and therefore escape the applications of strict "technical knowledge." It is these indeterminate zones of practice that many observers of professions see as central to professional practice.[5]

Physical therapy, like teaching, now has increased concern for preparing therapists who are not only technically competent but able to make decisions in a rapidly changing clinical environment.[18,19] What teaching methods could be used in our classrooms and laboratories to facilitate the development of professional behaviors necessary for today's practice? In this article we suggest two alternative teaching methods for physical therapy educators—the use of small group process and reflective activities to develop professional behaviors in the student. These teaching methods have been used successfully by the authors in their educational settings.

Small group process can facilitate the development of professional behaviors through the use of collaboration, collegiality, goal setting, decision making, divergent thinking, peer evaluation and self-evaluation, communication, and creative problem solving.[20-23] Group work can be an effective technique for achieving intellectual, technical, and professional social goals.[20,24-26] This approach emphasizes active, participatory learning through group interaction and cooperation where individuals learn from each other as well as on their own. Students learn how

to balance the needs of the group with their personal needs.

The second method uses reflective practicums, which can bridge the two worlds of theory and practice. Specific examples given are the use of inquiry field work, clinical education journals, and patient case seminars. Students' responses to the use of these alternative strategies have been very positive but not without some level of initial skepticism and anxiety because the activities were new to them and required a change in their thought processes and behavior patterns.

GROUP WORK

Bion noted that the use of small groups allows the individual to develop and experiment with professional behaviors within a "safe" group environment.[22] Group work is an excellent technique for increasing conceptual learning, creative problem solving, individual accountability, leadership skills, the ability to take risks, and oral communication skills.[23,26,27] Our society recognizes individual achievement, but creative problem solving often is performed better by groups than by individuals working alone.[23,26,27] An example of creative problem solving among small groups is collaborative research, a frequently used model in many research endeavors.

For group work to be successful, physical therapy educators must be comfortable in relinquishing some control, thus allowing groups to become more independent in their creative thinking and group processing. Group work alters the teacher's role dramatically, changing it from a position of power and authority to one of facilitator and colleague. The educator must be comfortable delegating some authority to students.[23] Students have difficulty changing from their familiar

role of dependency or counterdependency to an active group role that functions independently using the educator as a consultant. In addition, time must be available for students to struggle with their group's development to function more effectively.

Group Expert Technique

One way to facilitate group process within a class is to begin with an activity that builds confidence and collegiality among group members. The group expert technique allows for coverage of different topics as well as total involvement of each student.[26] Figure 1 illustrates the implementation of this technique. In the first division of groups, each group discusses a different problem and arrives at a consensus. The teacher's role is to circulate among the groups to make sure each group is on the right track and that individuals in the group are not providing each other with erroneous information.

A second division of groups occurs so that there is one expert from the five groups in each of the new groups. A combined numeral and letter system can be used when handing out the original assignments. In the first division, all group members should have the same numeral but a different letter (A through E). On the second group division, groups are arranged by the same letter so that all the A's are together and their group contains members with numerals I through V. The task for the second group division is to discuss each of the five different cases with a resident expert available to facilitate the discussion and respond to questions.

This technique gives the class a wide variety of patient problems to discuss in a short time and gives each student a leadership role and the opportunity to experience collegial exchange in a creative problem-solving environment.[23]

Figure 1

Example of classroom implementation of group expert technique.

STEP I:	Assume 25 students in the class.
STEP II:	Divide into equal groups.
	<p align="center">**GROUPS**</p><p align="center">I II III IV V</p>
STEP III:	Assign each group a task (eg, Each group must analyze a different patient problem such as, I: s/p right ACL repair; II: spinal cord injury; III: left below-knee amputee; IV: left CVA; V: pediatric idiopathic scoliosis).
STEP IV:	Teacher circulates among the groups to make sure each group is "on track" and moving to appropriate conclusions.
STEP V:	Divide groups a second time so that each group in this second division has a member from Groups I–V.
	<p align="center">**GROUPS**</p><p align="center">A B C D E</p>
STEP VI:	The groups (A-E) now discuss each of the five patient problems. They will have a resident expert (a member from Groups I-V) for each patient problem who can facilitate the discussion.

Group Game Activities

When we succumb to the banking concept of education, we find the task overwhelming and no longer fun. Game activities allow students to experience the fun of learning while reinforcing and integrating information obtained from courses during the semester or throughout the year. This group activity also teaches students about learning in situations where cooperation and competition coexist.[28] The game activity used by one author was the television show "Jeopardy" with some modifications.

"Jeopardy" is a game that uses a visual board with categories across the top of the board (Fig. 2). Under each category are five monetary values ranging from $100 to $500 in the first round. The player selects a category and dollar amount, and the announcer reads the answer under that selection. The participant must "buzz in" first to respond to the question in that category in the form of a question. In round two, the dollar value doubles ($200 to $1,000), and the game is played the same way as in the first round. Finally, the players are given a final Jeopardy category and must secretly select their final wager according to their earnings thus far. The players respond to the final Jeopardy question in writing so the other players are unaware of their answer as well as their wager. The winner of the game has the correct final Jeopardy answer and the largest earnings remaining (Tab. 2).

At Temple University, the class was divided into two large groups by laboratory section. The two groups self-selected two different teams, each with five student members to play single and double Jeopardy. The categories were generated from the semester's courses, with faculty providing questions for the game board at various degrees of difficulty. The categories used were anatomy, physiology, neuroanatomy, physical agents, psychosocial aspects of rehabilitation, and potpourri. The game board was fabricated from a large piece of cardboard. The category headings, dollar values, and questions were attached to the board using thumbtacks so that all parts were removable. The class instructor acted as the game show host and even tape recorded the music from the "Jeopardy" program to make it more authentic. (If the technology is available, each of the categories and questions can be programmed into the computer. The computer monitor can then be projected onto a large screen so both teams can easily read the question at the same time the instructor reads the question.)

Each team used a cowbell to be recognized to respond to the question. If the student did not answer the question correctly, the other team had the opportunity to confer and respond to the question. Each team selected a scorekeeper for the game. Each team accrued money with every correct response, while an incorrect response detracted money from the total. After the first Jeopardy board was completed, the two groups changed their players to play double Jeopardy using new categories. After the second game board was finished, each large group decided how much it was willing to wager without revealing the amount to the other team.

The final Jeopardy question was a patient problem that required students to integrate their knowledge from all the categories. Each team discussed the final Jeopardy answer and collectively determined its response to the question. The team that finished with the most money won the game. This game activity encourages individual students to take a risk by responding to questions, while the group's role is to foster support, cohesion, and group cooperation while making learning enjoyable.

Provocative Issues

Another small group technique is focused around current provocative issues in physical therapy and health care. The class is divided into two groups that research a specific controversial topic, such as physician-owned physical therapy services, autoimmune deficiency syndrome, practice without referral, and the use of diagnostic-related groups in physical therapy and their impact on the quality of health care. Each group collects information from a variety of resources, including the library, personal interviews, organizational materials, and case presentations. Each group presents the specific issue and its pros and cons using a "fishbowl" technique. In the fishbowl technique, the class forms two concentric circles. The students in the inner circle present the positive issues advocating for change while the students in the outer circle listen. Students exchange seats and present the opposing arguments while the other group listens. Following the presentation of all information, the entire group interacts and discusses the topic based on the information provided.

This technique assists students in learning how to analyze and discuss multidimensional issues using divergent thinking, how to deal with ambiguity and value conflict, and to recognize that not all issues are readily solvable. This activity helps to address those areas identified as part of the indeterminate zones of practice.

Student-designed Evaluations

The last small group activity assists students in enhancing their skill in self-appraisal, self-examinations, and peer evaluations. Students complete course evaluations that not only evaluate the educator but also evaluate their own performance during the course. A technique that enhances student self-examination consists of students writing their own test questions on a specific topic and critiquing each other's questions in terms of clarity, ability to test for appropriate knowledge, taxonomy levels, and written communication skills. To develop skill in peer evaluation, students design an evaluation tool as a group to be used to critique each other's classroom presentations. This instrument can assess the individual's ability to convey information based on content, clarity, organization, creativity, and applicability. Students learn to both give and receive feedback through the evaluation process.

This technique enhances the student's ability to design and perform peer evaluation and self-evaluation. This process requires the student to develop skill in receiving as well as in giving feedback. These professional behaviors are necessary for the student to perform effectively in the clinic.

Figure 2
Illustration of game board used to play Jeopardy, a game activity.

Jeopardy Game Board					
Anatomy	Neuroanatomy	Physiology	Physical Agents	Psych Rehab	Potpourri
$100	$100	$100	$100	$100	$100
$200	$200	$200	$200	$200	$200
$300	$300	$300	$300	$300	$300
$400	$400	$400	$400	$400	$400
$500	$500	$500	$500	$500	$500

Double Jeopardy: The game board doubles in value in increments of $200 from $200 to $1,000.

Final Jeopardy: Each team can wager a portion or all of its earnings. The group must answer the complex patient problem as a team effort. The team left with the greatest residual sum of money after responding to the final Jeopardy question wins.

REFLECTIVE PRACTICUM EXPERIENCES

The second teaching method suggested is the development of reflective practicums that bridge the two worlds of the professional—theory and practice. The typical clinical experience emphasizes the development of students' technical expertise rather than reflective ability. In clinical practice we want a reflective practitioner, one who can deal with the uncertainties of practice by not relying only on their technical efficiency but also by reflecting on the nature of the clinical problem.[29] The practitioner must be able to deal with problem setting as well as problem solving. *Problem setting* involves identifying the appropriate problem to solve. This is a conceptual process rather than a technical process. Once a description and explanation of the problem is formulated, then the plan for action can be laid. The problem-solving process involves technical procedures that are not necessarily applied in a precise, regimented fashion. The reflective therapist fluctuates between the results of the treatment and the original description of the problem. Schon called this conceptualization of the problem and appraisal of the treatment effects "reflective conversation of the situation." Experienced competent clinicians often perform this type of problem solving rapidly and almost unconsciously.[30] What kind of learning experience could be integrated into physical therapy education programs to facilitate development of a reflective practitioner? Three ideas may enhance the student's ability to become a reflective practitioner: inquiry field work, use of a journal, and case seminars.

Inquiry Field Work

Inquiry field work may help students enhance their understanding of the complexity of the practice environment and appreciate that elements of behavioral science are essential to their future work as physical therapists. The goal of this learning experience would be to have a health care situation serve as a social laboratory, not just a practice environment. Students could be involved in small group field work where data collection methods such as observations and interviews are used to complete a small qualitative study. The purpose of this project would be for students to look beyond the technical aspects of physical therapy toward the social and political issues that affect the delivery of physical therapy in the context of health care. The students would observe and interview to try to understand what occurs in the organization, identify potential problems, and

discuss solutions. The written project could be shared in seminar groups, given the benefits discussed earlier regarding the use of small groups.

Reflective Journal

A second learning experience focusing on developing reflective orientation in students could be integrating a meaningful journal experience. Students keep a journal according to a set of guidelines throughout their clinical experiences. Students' insights during their clinical experiences provide clinical educators with information about the ways students think about physical therapy practice, their development as practitioners and problem solvers, and information about their practice environment.[31]

Case Seminars

A third idea is to use seminars to discuss patient cases going through the problem-setting and problem-solving phases. Selected faculty and clinicians could be used as consultants and role models in their combined analysis of the patient cases. For example, discussion of the case would include all aspects of the patient's disposition, including physical (all related aspects of medical care), emotional, socioeconomic, cultural, and ethical issues. The patient's case would be examined from the onset of the problem through the transition of the patient to work and/or home. Faculty and clinicians would serve as experts for students to use as a resource as well as role modeling reflective thinking in action. These experts assist students in learning the process of being a reflective practitioner in the clinical setting.

The goal of implementing learning experiences that focus on developing a reflective orientation in students is increased emphasis on experiences that represent the complex, ambiguous nature of clinical practice, and giving permission to students to move beyond mastery techniques and to critically examine what was done and why.[32]

CONCLUSION

In physical therapy education, the objective of the learning process is to see that graduates have the knowledge, attitudes, and values that represent professionals in their fields. Professional behaviors necessary for physical therapy clinical practice have been described as problem-setting and problem-solving abilities and the ability to handle ambiguity, communicate effectively, and work in collegial relationships while still being accountable for one's actions.[20-23]

We have presented two alternative teaching methods and several learning activities that we believe have been helpful in facilitating professional behaviors. Incorporation of these approaches at Temple University has enhanced students' understanding of these required behaviors and has provided them with the opportunity to be comfortable with and develop skill in using these professional behaviors. The use of small groups and reflective learning as teaching alternatives has been substantiated in the literature.[26,28,32]

Qualitative research methodologies currently are being used to understand more fully the nature of the teaching-learning process as it unfolds in the classroom.[13] Similar investigations should be undertaken in physical therapy education. As professional practice continues to evolve, physical therapy educators must examine their teaching strategies in relation to outcome performance measures. This examination will help to determine whether the efficacy of what we provide students to practice effectively within the context of health care is the best that we can offer.

REFERENCES

1. *Physical Therapy Education and Societal Needs: Guidelines for Physical Therapy Education.* Alexandria, Va: American Physical Therapy Association; 1984:19–27.
2. Houle C. *Continuing Learning in the Professions.* San Francisco, Calif: Jossey Bass; 1984:34–75.
3. Chaffee E. *Remarks on the Current Efforts to Implement a Postbaccalaureate Entry Requirement for Physical Therapy.* Position paper. Alexandria, Va: American Physical Therapy Association; October 1987.
4. Friere P. *Pedagogy of the Oppressed.* New York, NY: Heider and Heider; 1970.
5. Marton F. Describing and improving learning. In: Schmeck R, ed. *Learning Strategies and Learning Styles.* New York, NY: Plenum; 1988:53–82.
6. van Rossum E, Schenk S. The relationship between learning conception, study strategy, and learning outcome. *British Journal of Educational Psychology.* 1984;54:73–83.
7. Iran-Nejad A. Active and dynamic self-regulation of learning processes. *Review of Educational Research.* 1990;60(4):573–602.
8. Bloom B. The 2 sigma problem: the search for methods of group instruction as effective as one-to-one tutoring. *Educational Researcher.* 1984;13(4):4–16.
9. Dinham S, Stritter F. Research on professional education. In: Wittrock M, ed. *Handbook of Research on Teaching,* ed. 3. New York, NY: MacMillan Publishing Co; 1986:952–970.
10. Haberman M, Stinnett T. *Teacher Education and the New Profession of Teaching.* Berkeley, Calif: McCutchan Publishers; 1973.
11. Shalock H. Closing the knowledge gap. In: Houston W, ed. *Competency Assessment, Research, and Evaluation.* Syracuse, NY: National Dissemination Center for Performance-Based Education; 1974.
12. Houston W. Competency-based teacher education. In: Dunkin M, ed. *The International Encyclopedia of Teaching and Teacher Education.* New York, NY: Permagon Press; 1987:3–19.
13. Richardson V. The evolution of reflective teaching in teacher education. In: Clift R, Houston W, Pugach

M, eds. *Encouraging Reflective Practice in Education: An Analysis of Issues and Programs.* New York, NY: Teachers College Press; 1990:3–19.

14. Short E. The concept of competence: its use and misuse in education. *Journal of Teacher Education.* 1985;36(2):2–6.

15. Sykes G. Teacher education and the predicament of reform. In: Finn C, Ravitch D, Fancher R, eds. *Against Mediocrity: The Humanities in America's High Schools.* New York, NY: Holmes and Meier Publishers; 1984.

16. Shulman L. Paradigms and research programs in the study of teaching: a contemporary perspective. In: Wittrock M, ed. *Handbook of Research on Teaching,* ed 3. New York, NY: MacMillan Publishing Co; 1986:3–36.

17. Schon D. *Educating the Reflective Practitioner.* San Francisco, Calif: Jossey-Bass; 1987:3–21.

18. Myers RS, Rose S. Introduction: clinical decision making in physical therapy practice, education and research. *Phys Ther.* 1989;69:523.

19. Magistro C. Clinical decision making in physical therapy: a practitioner's perspective. *Phys Ther.* 1989;69:525–534.

20. Bennis WB, Shepard HS. A theory of group development. *Human Relations.* 1956;9:415–457.

21. Lippitt GL. How to get results from a group. In: Bradford LP, ed. *Group Development.* Washington, DC: National Training Laboratories, National Education Association; 1961.

22. Bion WR. *Experiences in Groups.* New York, NY: Basic Books; 1961.

23. Rice AK. *Learning for Leadership in Selections in Group Relations Reader 1.* Coleman AD, Bextopn, eds. Washington, DC: AK Rice Institute; 1975:71–73.

24. Cartwright D, Zander A. *Group Dynamics: Research and Theory,* ed 2. New York, NY: Harper and Row; 1960.

25. Tuckman BW. Developmental sequence in small groups. *Psychological Bulletin.* 1965;63:384–399.

26. Cohen E. *Designing Groupwork: Strategies for the Heterogeneous Classroom.* New York, NY: Teacher's College Press; 1986:1–20, 87–90.

27. Mosey AC. *Occupational Therapy: Configuration of a Profession.* New York, NY: Raven Press; 1981.

28. Deutsch M. The effects of cooperation and competition upon group process. In: Cartwright D, Zander A, eds. *Group Dynamics: Research and Theory,* ed 2. New York, NY: Harper and Row; 1960.

29. Claxton CS, Murrell PH. Learning styles: implications for improving educational practices. In Fife JD, ed: ASHE Eric Higher Education Report 4. Washington, DC: George Washington University Press; 1987.

30. Schon D. *The Reflective Practitioner: How Professionals Think in Action.* New York, NY: Basic Books Inc; 1983:3–69.

31. Jensen G, Denton B. Teaching physical therapy students to reflect: a suggestion for clinical education. *Journal of Physical Therapy Education.* Spring 1991;33–38.

32. Zeichner KM, Liston DP. Teaching student teachers to reflect. *Harvard Educational Review.* 1987;57(1):23–48.

The Clinical Learning Spiral: a model to develop reflective practitioners

Lynette Stockhausen

Reflective practice in clinical nursing is an exciting concept. Much of the literature on reflection has been derived from education. Recently the Australasian Nurse Registering Authority Committee (ANRAC) endorsed reflective practice as a registering prerequisite competency for beginning nurse practitioners. This paper examines the concept and development of an action research clinical learning spiral to foster reflective practice of both undergraduate students and their clinical teacher in the practice setting. The innovation of a mutual group, that is, teacher and students interacting through reflection to create a co-operative learning environment is explored. In designing the spiral a number of models were consulted and incorporated.

The action research clinical learning spiral adds structure and focus to the process of reflection-on-action and provides an avenue for students and the clinical teacher to set mutual goals of action to trial for future experiences. This process of reflection allows the clinical facilitator to be an integral component of success to the students learning in the clinical context.

REFLECTIVE PRACTICE

Reflective practice in nursing is an exciting concept. Although practised by nurses for many years, only recently has available literature regarding reflective practice in nursing emerged (Garrett 1991, Jarvis 1992). However, the concept of reflection is not new. Philosophers, educationalists and practitioners have been developing views of reflection since Aristotle first introduced practical judgement and moral action (McKeon

1974). Since then much has been written and researched regarding reflection. Some of the significant contributors to this school of thought include Dewey (1933), Kolb and Fry (1975), Kemmis (1985), Boud, Keogh and Walker (1985), Zeichner (1983), Schon (1983) and Benner (1984).

The process of reflection is an integral factor in the organisation of our daily activities. From the first time we look in the mirror, to when we retire at night, we replay on our minds the days events, often analysing them and re-examining what has occurred in our lives. Boud et al (1985) note that 'reflection comprises of those intellectual and affective activities in which individuals engage to explore their experiences in order to lead to new understandings and appreciation'. Their definition implies that reflection is goal orientated and

Lynette Stockhausen RN DipTeach-Nsg BEd-Nsg MEdSt, Senior Lecturer, School of Nursing, Griffith University–Nathan Campus, Kessels Road, Nathan, Brisbane, Australia 4111

(Requests for offprints to LS)

Manuscript accepted 9 February 1994

that feelings and cognitive abilities are interwoven. The underlying assumptions being that individuals are in control of the activity, that reflection can take place in isolation or in association with others, such as peers or the clinical teacher, and finally that reflection is not an end in itself, but, preparation for new experiences.

Learning through practice and reflective processes have been expounded by Kolb (1984) within the terms of his experiential learning theory. The theory suggests that learning, change and growth are facilitated by cyclic processes. Such experiences involve direct experiences, reflection on the experience, and abstract concept formation from which behaviour may be modified to aid new experiences. Similarly, reflection has been viewed as the link between theory and practice (Schon 1987).

Reflection as perceived in this context suggests that learning is facilitated by early active engagement in practice. Without reflection, experiences would remain unexamined, with the full potential for learning by the participants not fully realised. Within the education literature on reflective practice there is a dimension of an 'elusiveness' to learning that is personal, developmental and embedded in the experience of the learner (Boud 1988). In order to actualise these learning episodes the role of the clinical teacher becomes an integral part of the reflective process. As such, the clinical teacher, rather than being external to the process of learning, is an essential and strategic component to that learning. The clinical teacher has the opportunity to become captured in the developmental and cyclic nature of the total experience, facilitating, not controlling, the clinical experience.

A FRAMEWORK FOR REFLECTIVE PRACTICE

Reflection has been identified as a prerequisite competency for beginning nurse practitioners in Australia (ANRAC 1990). In order to facilitate students' achievement of this competency, a framework to encourage reflection within nursing curricula was required. As such, the Clinical Learning Spiral (Stockhausen 1991) was developed for the purpose of incorporating and developing reflective processes in undergraduate nursing clinical practice. The spiral has been trialed successfully with a cohort of second year students and their clinical teachers in a Bachelor of Nursing programme.

The framework of the spiral incorporates the theoretical elements of clinical education and structures the management of the clinical experience. Inherent within this framework are those elements necessary to successfully prepare, induct, implement and evaluate reflective clinical practice experiences.

The Clinical Learning Spiral was developed utilising other models of experiential learning with particular reference to the Action Research Cycle (Carr & Kemmis 1986), the Reflective Process Model (Boud 1985) and the Critical Experiential Learning Model (Chuaprapaisilp 1989). Each of these models when integrated provides a framework that incorporates all aspects of undergraduate clinical experiences. It was felt that no one model alone consolidated features of clinical experiences that captures the balance, transference and significance of theory and practice and is uniquely nursing orientated.

An overview of the development of the Clinical Learning Spiral with reference to the previous models are contained in the following discussion.

The Action Research Model (Carr & Kemmis 1986) has four cyclic phases of planning, acting, observing and reflecting. These four phases are linked into a cycle that recreates itself into a self reflective spiral (Figs 1 & 2). In this sense no component of the model can be conducted independently of the other. The Carr and Kemmis model premises that a group and its members, collectively and collaboratively undertake the four phases of the cycle. Practice is viewed within a political, economic, historical and social context. From this perspective, examination and reflection of practice leads to a new social consciousness and change. Bartlett (1990) suggests 'that actions are intentional and are to be understood in the social context of their occurrence'. As such, deliberation and analysis of ideas about 'nursing' as a form of action, based on our changed understanding, is highlighted.

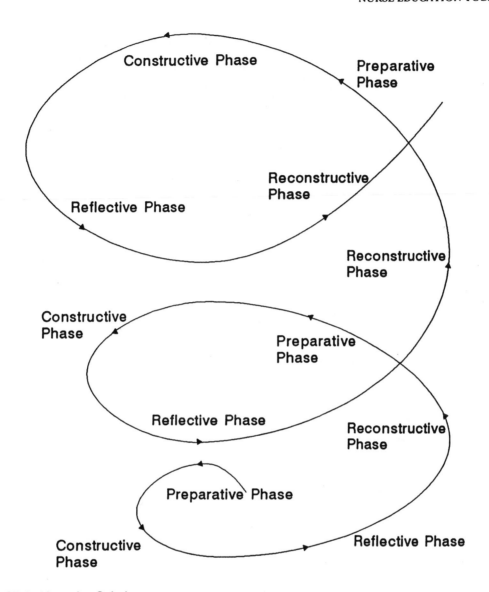

Fig. 1 The Clinical Learning Spiral

The process of reflective learning as postulated by Boud et al (1985) involves three stages that are inter-related and cyclic in nature. Following an initial experience the first stage of the reflective process is 'returning to the experience'. Here students recollect the events that have occurred and re-examine their reactions to those events. The chronological sequence of events is recalled in a descriptive rather than judgemental manner. The second stage is 'attending to feelings', which allows for emotions to be identified, examined and challenged. The focus on feelings heightens the learner's self awareness and enables them to enhance and retain positive emotions and discard negative feelings. The final phase is that of 'processing', where the events that occurred during the experiential phase are re-constructed by the learner in order to make sense of them. This phase requires indepth reflection and introspection.

As the learner processes their experiences, Boud et al (1985) suggest that a re-evaluation occurs. During this activity students link new data to what is already known (association), seek relationships amongst this data (integration), determine the authenticity of ideas and feelings (validation) and create a personal understanding or knowledge about the event (appropriation).

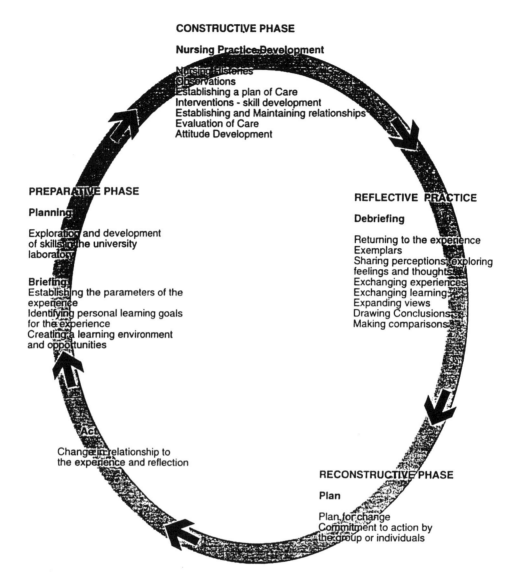

Fig. 2 The Clinical Learning Cycle

Through the use of the Reflective Process Model students are able to actively construct and arrange their knowledge of the world thus developing their own interpretational schema.

The Critical Experiential Learning Model (Chuaprapaisilp 1989) uses elements of the Carr and Kemmis model. It was developed specifically as a framework for learning from clinical experiences in nursing. Chuaprapaisilp's model has three phases: preparation for practice, managing the experiential learning process and reflecting on the experience.

During the first phase, students undertake several preparatory activities. This may include ori-

entation to the clinical environment and the delineation of structures and procedures (development of personal learning objectives and undertaking client assessments) at the commencement of the experience.

The second phase involves the facilitation of the learning experience. There are five strategies in this phase which provide a plan to the total process. These are: structuring, organising, controlling, facilitating and emancipating. In the structuring phase of the clinical experience, the clinical teacher assesses the clinical environment and then facilitates activities within a set time frame. The second strategy of organising involves prioritising activities in order that students receive adequate supervision in meeting their objectives. The clinical teacher and students also decide at this stage the format of debriefing sessions.

During the subsequent facilitating stage the clinical teacher provides on-going individual consultation and explores avenues to provide successful clinical experiences for the student. The facilitation of student learning requires clinical teachers to control their own teaching within a set time frame. In this sense the clinical teacher does not provide all the answers for the students. Instead teaching strategies which foster self-directed learning and critical analysis of issues is encouraged, such as student learning contracts. The final strategy is emancipation which encourages students to challenge approaches to nursing care and make decisions for change.

The final phase of reflection, as outlined by Chuaprapaisilp, is similar to the Boud et al (1985) model but with the inclusion and introduction of a critical theory approach to experiential learning. In this phase the clinical teacher attempts to create a democratic atmosphere where, together, students and clinical teacher, clarify objectives, structures, processes, roles and assumptions during debriefing sessions.

THE CLINICAL LEARNING SPIRAL

The Clinical Learning Spiral (Fig. 1), developed by the author (1991), draws on the previously discussed models and personal reflective experience as a clinical teacher. The model was developed to emphasis the importance of reflective practice to the professional growth of a beginning nurse practitioner. The integration of Carr and Kemmis, Chuaprapaisilp and Boud et al's key concepts provides a model that is clinically and goal orientated. This acknowledges practice by the self and others as a central tenet of professional education for nurses.

The Clinical Learning Spiral detail (Fig. 2) is represented by the preparative, constructive, reflective and reconstructive phases.

The Preparative Phase begins as the individual considers the demands of the experience ahead, the resources required, the environment (sight, sounds, smells), the people (roles, relations, reactions and conflicts), the climate (social, political) and their role as learners in the clinical setting (reflector, participant, observer, facilitator) (Emden 1991).

There are two components to the preparative phase. The first is related to on campus classroom teaching and university laboratory sessions. This incorporates the development and exploration of nursing skills within a controlled learning environment. The second component is the briefing session which is conducted before the commencement of a clinical experience or day. This first phase assists the teacher of the clinical experience and the students to establish the parameters of the experience. During the briefing students are given the opportunity to identify personal and professional objectives to achieve during the clinical experience. At this time the clinical teacher fosters a climate for the students to achieve their objectives and may explore possibilities for creating new learning opportunities.

The Preparative Phase allows the students to identify other resources (such as specific client needs or specialist departments) within the clinical environment that would create learning opportunities. The benefits of student initiated personal objectives highlights the students own learning needs and creates motivation to learn. The Preparative Phase can also be conducted on a one-to-one basis between students and the clinical teacher. Students have identified that this process of individual negotiation has been beneficial in providing them with the opportunity to set personal goals for their experience and plan the care for their clients (Stockhausen 1991).

Each phase throughout the spiral is facilitated by journal writing which has been identified as the most widely used expression of reflection (Zeichner 1986). Students and clinical teachers are encouraged to write about events of significance which occur whilst undertaking clinical experiences.

The Constructive Phase allows students to undertake actual nursing skill development. This second phase incorporates the experience or actual practice of nursing which takes place during the practicum. The clinical experience is viewed from a perspective of 'completeness' (beginning, middle and end). Observation of the students during this phase is crucial as reflections between the observer and the observed can heighten the experience and reveal different perspectives of the same experience.

The Constructive Phase is the actual experience the students and the teacher share in the clinical environment. This phase takes into consideration the dimensions of practice such as care planning, psychomotor skills, attitude and interpersonal communication development and evaluation of care. The establishment and maintenance of relationships, especially with the client and staff of the agency, is also highlighted within this phase.

The third phase of the clinical spiral is the Reflective Phase. Time is allocated for purposeful inquiry so students can deliberate on aspects of their development as a nurse. Consideration is given to others involved in the student's practice such as the patient, peers, registered nurses, the clinical teacher and other health care professionals.

The reflective phase is facilitated by a debriefing process. This allows the students the opportunity to 'return to the experiences' of the Constructive Phase and highlight significant exemplars and events from the day. Debriefing may occur at intervals throughout the day, but always at the end of a clinical day or experience.

The reflective phase can be initiated at anytime on a one-to-one basis between a student and clinical teacher, peer or registered nurse. It is particularly important to provide a reflective phase for constructive feedback to students following some aspect of their nursing practice development. This may be, for example, a psychomotor skill, interpersonal interaction or professional enquiry. Later, during the group reflective phase, students have the opportunity to share personal reflections from their previous one-to-one reflection or share extracts from their journals. During the group reflective phase the rest of the group share their experiences. The students sense of excitement, anxiety and relief, or how the patient felt or responded is explored. Horsfall (1990) notes that as students 'share each others' challenges, achievements and experience' it is possible that

vicarious learning takes place. This phase also sets the scene to examine complexities, differences and subtleties not found in text books but learnt, or made explicit, as a direct result of being submerged in the experience.

The learning processes espoused by Boud et al (1985) identify the importance of allocating time during which students can share feelings, thoughts and perceptions of their experiences. In this forum, students have the opportunity to exchange ideas, consider other points of view, draw conclusions and make comparisons from their clinical experiences. As a consequence of this planned reflection students arrive at a deeper and more meaningful understanding of the practice of nursing.

The final stage of the Clinical Learning Spiral involves the reconstruction of the learning experience. The Reconstructive Phase provides the students and the clinical teacher the opportunity to plan for change. The change may be in the form of alternate nursing strategies/interventions in patient care, or changes in behaviour that foster interpersonal relationships or personal and professional development. There is a commitment to action as a result of the constructive and reflective phases. This is akin to the Action Research Cycle (Carr & Kemmis 1986). Re-evaluation of the experience helps expand views and develop strategies for future action (Boud 1988).

The Reconstructive Phase ideally develops into a set of negotiated, mutual goals set by the group as a consequence of reflections on experiences, journal entries and discussions during debriefings. Hedin (1989) notes that at the heart of clinical practice is 'the development of meaning to the learner and the avoidance of imposing an other meaning on the learner'. It is the participants of the clinical experience who decide if reflections develop into action. Not every day will produce a new action as some reflections will not lead to any new consequences. Mutual goals are reconstructed from the constructive and reflective phases of the clinical learning spiral, as a direct result of practice. The intention is to make modifications to, or develop goals that can be acted upon. It is imperative that a commitment to action as a consequence of reflection is realised. For action to occur without reflection leads to uninformed, unintentional behaviour. Reflection prior to and subsequent to action can ensure mutual goals are carried forward to the next situation or spiral.

THE CLINICAL LEARNING SPIRAL IN ACTION

Using the Clinical Learning Spiral has provided structure to promote and develop reflective practitioners, enabling the ANRAC competencies within the reflective practice domain to be achieved. With active participation in all phases of the spiral students have begun to develop the art of reflection. Through self expression using journal writing and involvement in debriefing sessions students have had the opportunity to examine their practice, feelings and beliefs, and the consequences of these for patient care. This has been achieved through active participation in all aspects of the spiral. Students and the clinical teacher reflect on what is important to them and then contribute towards the maintenance of a supportive group as they pursue mutual goals of clinical practice.

The phases of the spiral and the processes involved are highlighted by using an example from previous research, by the author, for which the spiral was developed.

Spiral 1

Preparative phase
During the briefing students identify their anxieties at being accepted by the staff of the organisation. Some students have used their journals to write about their impending experience. Students also explore strategies to overcome their fears. To help establish the parameters of the experience and rapport with the organisation and ward staff, as clinical teacher, I undertook the hospital's orientation programme and introduced myself to the ward staff prior to the students' first day.

Constructive phase
A number of registered nurses are asked either by the charge nurses or myself (the clinical teacher) to assist students with their learning goals.

Students, registered nurses and clinical teacher interact throughout the day.

Reflective phase
Students record in their journals learning incidents related to interactions and establishing interpersonal relationships with the registered nurses. Some of these reflections are shared with the group at debriefing, 'I found the staff extremely friendly'. As the students' clinical teacher I also wrote and shared my experiences with the students as I had received positive feedback from the staff regarding the students' courtesy and attentive patient care. During debriefing the students were aware that their fears regarding the staff had been unfounded.

Reconstructive phase
The students and clinical teacher decide to set a goal to: 'Maintain and foster the collegial relationships established on the first day'.

Spiral 2

Preparative phase
The students discuss the implications of the previous set goal to their nursing practice development. Students write and discuss their expected interactions with registered nurse. Objectives for the day are identified that incorporate these ideas.

Construction phases
Students and registered nurses interact throughout the day providing patient care and fostering student skill development.

Reflective phase
'I found "my RN" willing to help me, show me procedures', 'The Registered Nurse was receptive and open to my questions' and 'The RN took the time to explain the procedure to me'. These were some of the journal or spoken comments of the reflective phase. Students discussed the significant impact the Registered Nurse, as a role model, made to a perceived positive or negative clinical experience.

Reconstructive phase

Students and clinical teacher examine the implications of their debriefing and aim to: 'Respect the Registered Nurses knowledge and input into the clinical experience'. Action from this goal was recorded as: provide feedback to the Registered Nurses for their invaluable input into student learning.

Whilst the process did not finish after the second spiral it is evident from the example provided that the Spiral is a worthwhile framework to be utilised in the clinical education. It provides the students with evidence of the significance of their lived experience. If students had only been informed about the contribution the Registered Nurse can make to clinical practice this may not have meant as much to the students as actually being immersed in the context. Students experienced first hand that the Registered Nurse can make a positive contribution to their learning.

CONCLUSION

In an environment of trust, students and the clinical teacher expose their actions, thoughts and feelings; hold them up for examination, reconstruct them and then transform them. In so doing, students are likely to question and challenge their preconceived assumptions about nursing practice. The clinical practice experience is facilitated by the clinical learning spiral and a supportive clinical teacher. The clinical experience becomes a time to collect and analyse judgements, reactions and impressions about what is actually going on in a particular setting. Greater exploration of the social, political, historical and economic dimensions to practice are encouraged.

Schon (1983) asserts that through reflective practice students develop a critical understanding of 'the repetitive experiences of a specialised practice', and can make new sense of the situations of uncertainty or uniqueness which they experience. These experiences lie within a lived context which is connected to the learners' reality within that context.

The phases contained within the Clinical Learning Spiral provide a framework for the clinical teacher to use students' experiences as the catalyst for their next learning experience. The spiral is dynamic and flexible. It is not meant to be static or followed strictly from one step to the next. There is no limit to the number of spirals that can occur. Reflection and reconstruction may occur between a student and clinical teacher throughout the experience and may only take a matter of minutes.

Developing reflective practitioners becomes an avenue to generate explanations of practice situations and build upon practice knowledge. Aligning and complementing student and clinical teachers' reflections on clinical experiences has the potential to provide more meaningful learning for students and rewarding teaching experiences in the practicum.

References

ANRAC. Nursing Competencies Assessment Project 1990 Report to Australasian Nurse Registering Authorities Conference. Nurses Board of South Australia, Adelaide

Bartlett L 1990 Teacher development through reflective practice. In: Richards J, Nunan D (eds) Second language teacher education. Cambridge University Press, London, p 203

Benner P 1984 From novice to expert: excellence and power in clinical nursing. Addison-Wesley, Menlo Park

Boud D, Keogh R, Walker D 1985 Reflection: turning experience into learning. Kogan Page, London, p 19, p 30

Boud D 1988 How to help students learn from experience. The Medical Teacher, 2nd Ed. Churchill Livingstone, London

Carr W, Kemmis S 1986 Becoming critical: knowing through action research. Deakin University Press, Melbourne

Chuaprapaisilp A 1989 Improving learning from experience through the conduct of pre and post clinical conferences: Action research in nursing education in Thailand. Unpublished PhD thesis. University of NSW, Sydney

Dewey J 1933 How we think. DC Heath, Boston

Emden C 1991 Becoming a reflective practitioner. In: Gray G, Pratt R (eds) Towards a discipline of nursing. Churchill Livingstone, Melbourne

Garrett S 1992 Reflective practice as a learning strategy. In: Gray G, Pratt R (eds) Issues in Australian Nursing 3. Churchill Livingstone, Melbourne

Hedin B 1989 Expert clinical teaching. In: Curriculum revolution: reconceptualising nursing education. National League for Nursing, New York, p 82

Horsfall J 1990 Clinical placement: prebriefing and debriefing as teaching strategies. The Journal of Advanced Nursing 8(1) (Sept–Nov): 5

Jarvis P 1992 Reflective practice and nursing. Nurse Education Today 12: 174–181

Kemmis S 1985 Action research and the politics of reflection. In: Boud D, Keogh R, Walker D (eds)

Reflection: turning experience into learning. Kogan Page, London

Kolb D 1984 Experiential learning: experience in the source of learning and development. Prentice Hall, New Jersey

Kolb D, Fry F 1975 Towards an applied theory of experiential learning. In: Cooper C (ed) Theories of group processes. John Wiley, London

McKeon R 1974 Introduction to Aristotle. Random House, London

Schon D 1983 The reflective practitioner. Temple Smith, London

Schon D 1987 Educating the reflective practitioner. Jossey-Bass, London

Stockhausen L 1991 Reflective practice: the mutual group. Reflection in undergraduate nursing practice. Unpublished masters dissertation. University of Queensland, Brisbane

Zeichner K 1983 Alternate paradigms in teacher education. Journal of Teacher Education 334(3): 3–8

Zeichner K 1986 Preparing reflective teachers: an overview of instructional strategies which have been employed in preservice teacher education. International Journal of Educational Research 11(5): 565–575

Survey of Academic Programs: Exploring Issues Related to Pediatric Clinical Education

Jody Shapiro Gandy, PhD, PT

American Physical Therapy Association, Division of Education, Alexandria, Va

The purposes of this study were to: (1) determine if academic programs are providing adequate opportunities for physical therapist (PT) and physical therapist assistant (PTA) students to obtain clinical education experiences with pediatric populations in a variety of settings; (2) discover where, within the curriculum, the pediatric experiences are offered and/or provided; and (3) generate areas for additional research in clinical education and pediatrics. A survey instrument was developed and mailed to 218 PT and PTA Academic Coordinators of Clinical Education (ACCEs) with 82 valid responses returned. Data were analyzed using SPSS/4.0 PC-Statistical Package for descriptive statistics. Results indicated that although a diversity of clinical sites were used to provide pediatric learning experiences, respondents reported an insufficient number of sites to accommodate students enrolled in PT and PTA entry-level programs in 1991 to 1992. A variety of reasons were cited for these insufficiencies. In addition, students were placed in pediatric learning experiences predominantly during the second or third year of the academic program, thereby creating increased competition for a limited number of clinical sites. Areas for further collaborative research are suggested that address issues, strategies, and outcomes related to pediatric clinical education.

Clinical education is a vital link and integral part of a total physical therapy curriculum. Of greatest importance is that clinical education represents an aspect of curriculum where theory meets reality in the practice environment. During the past 15 to 20 years, the profession has made tremendous strides toward developing a body of literature related to clinical education that addresses clinical faculty, academic and environmental resources, design of clinical education, and evaluation and assessment as evidenced in the publication *Clinical Education: An Anthology.*[1] However, to date, little is known specifically about clinical education and special populations such as geriatrics and pediatrics. Likewise, limited clinical education research studies have been evidenced related to specific practice settings such as ambulatory care centers, hospitals, rehabilitation centers, and private practices. Given the paucity of research in this area, it is important to explore issues related to pediatric clinical education.

To understand contemporary clinical education, it is necessary to first describe four significant trends that impact this aspect of education. These include the increased length of clinical education within the total curriculum, increased

0898-5669/93/0503-0128$3.00/0
PEDIATRIC PHYSICAL THERAPY
Copyright © 1993 by Williams & Wilkins

Address correspondence to: Jody S. Gandy, PhD, PT, Director of Clinical Education, American Physical Therapy Association, Division of Education, 1111 N. Fairfax St., Alexandria, VA 22314.

numbers of physical therapy programs and graduates, dramatic changes in the health care delivery system, and greater specialization within the profession.

From academic year 1984 to 1985 to 1991 to 1992, there was a proportional increase in the time students spent in clinical education as entry-level physical therapist (PT) programs increased in total length from an average of 80 weeks to 88 weeks.[2] The data available on physical therapist assistant (PTA) programs from 1989 to 1990 to 1991 to 1992 demonstrated an overall decrease in average program length from 73 to 69 weeks, respectively, whereas average length of clinical education remained consistent (19–20 weeks).[3,4] This indicates that in PTA programs, clinical education has increased proportionally in relation to the total decrease in average length of the curriculum. From 1984 to 1985 to 1991 to 1992, the clinical education component of PT educational programs increased from 20.1 weeks to 25.7 weeks as total average length of PT academic programs increased from 79.7 weeks to 91.7 weeks, respectively. From 1984 to 1992, PT clinical education increased an average of 5.6 weeks (224 hours) as total curriculum increased an average of 12 weeks.[2,3] Thus, 46.7% of the increase in total length of curriculum can be attributed to clinical education. This may suggest that academic programs and/or practice communities have begun to place greater value or emphasis on clinical education today than perhaps noted in the past.

A second trend is a steady increase in the number of accredited academic institutions offering entry-level PT and PTA programs resulting in increased numbers of graduates entering the profession. In 1980, 95 academic institutions offered accredited entry-level PT programs and 56 academic institutions offered accredited PTA programs. Twelve years later, 136 academic institutions offered PT programs and 124 academic institutions offered PTA programs.[2,4] This reflects a 43% growth in the number of PT programs and 121% increase in the number of PTA programs. This does not, however, account for the 17 PT programs and 24 PTA programs that are currently in various phases of development.[5]

From 1980 to 1985, the number of graduates of entry-level PT programs increased significantly from 2449 to 3499 (43%) and PTA programs increased from 685 to 1137 (66%). From 1985 to 1991, the number of graduates of PT programs increased from 3499 to 4533 (30%) and PTA programs increased from 1137 to 1985 (75%).[2,4] This trend suggests there is still growth in the number of PT graduates per year, with PT programs increasing at a slower rate since the early 1980s, despite the elevated numbers of entry-level programs. In contrast, PTA programs demonstrated significantly more accelerated growth during the 1980s with tremendous expansion in the number of programs and number of graduates.

Given that the number of programs and corresponding numbers of students enrolled in accredited PT and PTA programs has dramatically increased over the past 12 years, and the proportional amount of time spent in student clinical education has increased, it would seem logical that demands on clinical education sites to provide quality student learning experiences would need to demonstrate coinciding patterns of growth. In 1985, PT and PTA academic programs affiliated with 3490 clinical education sites at which 4636 graduates were placed.[6] By comparison, in 1991 6518 PT and PTA graduates were placed at 5572 clinical education sites for student clinical experiences.[7] This represents a 60% growth in the total number of available clinical education sites with a concomitant 41% growth in the total student population during the same 7-year period. More than half (57%) of the clinical education sites available in 1992 were affiliated with one or more academic PT and/or PTA programs.[7] In addition, PT and PTA students completed an average of three to four full-time clinical rotations while enrolled in their program.[8]

On the surface it would seem that the 60% growth rate in the development of clinical education sites has more than kept pace with the 41% growth in the total PT and PTA graduates since 1985. However, this does not account for the three to four clinical rotations that each student is provided during the academic program. Thus, to continue to provide quality learning experiences, demands on clinical sites could increase as much as three- to fourfold. If this is true, academic programs should be experiencing some difficulty adequately placing students in quality learning experiences appropriate to students' needs and interests. This also assumes that supervisory models employed at these clinical sites and the timing of the clinical experiences allow for multiple academic programs to place students concurrently at the same sites.

A third major trend effecting clinical education began in the mid- to late- 1980s. A visible paradigm shift has been evidenced in a currently fluctuating health care delivery system. Buzz words such as cost-containment, resource-based relative value system, quality assurance, controlled or total quality management, and managed care are commonly used in the provision of health care services. Third-party payers have increased demands on practitioners to provide empirical evidence to support the outcome effectiveness of the practice of physical therapy for purposes of reimbursement. Consumers are also more sophisticated and are raising issues related to access, affordability, and delivery of quality services. In addition, recognizing the shortage and/or maldistribution of physical therapists, additional constraints are placed on practitioners to deliver quality care with limited resources and often inadequate time.[9] These demands may often conflict with the clinical site's ability to provide quality student learning experiences.

Finally, a fourth trend recognizes the changes in the practice of physical therapy. The profession has progressively become more specialized and technologically advanced over the past decade as evidenced by the association providing opportunities for its members to belong to 19 areas of special interest (Sections) and to become Board Certified Clinical Specialist in seven different specialty areas.[10] In addition, the profession has become more diversified in its practice providing health care in a myriad of public and private institutions, and profit and nonprofit practice settings that manage clients across the life span. Ideally, the diversity of clinical education sites and experiences should be comparable to contemporary physical therapy practice because those settings represent the environments in which entry-level graduates will be expected to practice.[11]

One of those "specialty life-span populations" in which physical therapy services are essential is pediatrics. Pediatrics will be defined broadly as birth to 21 years of age and includes such practice settings as hospitals, rehabilitation centers, home health care, school systems, early intervention centers, residential centers, developmental disability centers, and extended care facilities. Hence, pediatric physical therapy services also represent a wide diversity of practice settings within a "specialty population." In addition, pediatric physical therapy is the only specialty area of practice governed by federal legislation (PL 94-142, PL 99-457, and PL 102-119) that requires appropriate intervention services, including physical therapy for infants, preschoolers, and school-aged children with disabilities.[12] Consequently, there is a critical demand for qualified physical therapy practitioners who can provide comprehensive care to infants, children, youth, and their families, consult with teachers and other personnel in school systems, participate in interdisciplinary rehabilitation teams, and perform screening assessments and evaluations.

According to APTA's 1990 Active Membership Profile Report, members indicated they typically spend most of their time seeing patients between the ages of 18 and 64 (54.2%). In the pediatric range, however, they typically spend 14.6% of their time seeing infants (less than 1 year); 18.3% preschool (1-4 years); 18.8% school children (5-12 years); and adolescents 10.6% (13-17).[13] Although this population may not comprise the majority of time spent by many practitioners, for some it is the primary focus of their practice. Pediatric physical therapy will continue to be an area of need by society substantiated by federal legislation, advances in scientific technology, and the current demand for services.

In light of the increased proportional time students spend in clinical education, increased numbers of PT and PTA academic programs and entry-level graduates, changes within the health care delivery system, and greater specialization of the practice of physical therapy, the impact on the availability and accessibility of clinical education experiences for students needs to be explored, particularly with special populations.

The purposes of this study were to: (1) determine if academic programs are providing adequate opportunities for PT and PTA students to obtain clinical education experiences with pediatric populations in a variety of settings; (2) discover where, within the curriculum, pediatric experiences are offered and/or provided; and (3) generate areas for further research in clinical education and pediatrics.

METHODS

In October 1991, APTA's Department of Education mailed 218 questionnaires with a return stamped envelope to all Academic Coordinators of Clinical Education (ACCEs) at accredited PT and PTA programs. Of 218 questionnaires mailed to ACCEs, 82 responses were valid. After the deadline, programs were sent only one reminder to complete the questionnaire and return to APTA by January 1, 1992. Because of time constraints to present this information at the 1992 Combined Sections Meeting, the author needed adequate time to analyze the data to ensure that the results would be completed by conference.

A four-page, primarily closed-ended, survey instrument was developed and reviewed by three individuals not participating in the study for content and face validity. Questions were developed that addressed the specific issues posed in this study. The instrument was designed to obtain statistical information about the numbers and proportion of available pediatric clinical sites, distribution of those pediatric sites by setting, where, within the academic curriculum, were students accepted to affiliate at pediatric sites, and if students selecting a pediatric experience were accommodated, and if not, why not.

Data were analyzed using SPSS/4.0 PC-Statistical Package for descriptive statistics.

RESULTS

Of 82 ACCE respondents, 55 (67%) were from physical therapist programs and 27 (33%) were from physical therapist assistant programs. The total response rate to the questionnaire was only 38%. Results will be presented comparing two groups, PT and PTA academic programs. Given the low response rate, the results of this study should not be generalized to all PT and PTA academic programs, however, they may reflect current trends in this area.

The average number of total clinical sites with which a PT program affiliated was 159.2 (range, 52–432; SD, 83.2) of which 20.5% (32.6) were defined as pediatric settings. In this study, the average PT class size was 32 students. The average number of total clinical sites with which a PTA program affiliated were 45.1 (range, 12–95; SD, 23.5) of which 24% (10.8) were considered pediatric settings. In this case, the average PTA class size was 17 students.

Figure 1 compares the average distribution of pediatric clinical sites in both PT and PTA academic programs. Similarly, in both PT and PTA programs acute care hospitals comprised the largest proportion of pediatric sites. In contrast, rehabilitation centers accounted for the next largest proportion of pediatric sites in PT programs whereas school systems were ranked second highest for PTA programs. Neonatal and pediatric home care accounted for the smallest proportion of the pediatric site distribution for both programs with neonatal care not available to students enrolled in PTA programs.

Respondents were asked if pediatrics was a required clinical experience for students to graduate. All PT academic programs indicated that pediatrics was not a required experience and 93% of PTA programs also responded that it was not required of students. Sixty percent of the PT programs felt there were an adequate number of pediatric clinical sites to meet the needs and interests of their students. In contrast, only 33% of the PTA programs felt that pediatric clinical education resources were appropriate to meet the needs of their students. Seven percent of the PT programs and 4% of the PTA programs did not respond to this question.

Examining this issue further, Figure 2 demonstrates that a clear majority (76%–92%) of all pediatric clinical experiences are made available to students as a later affiliation

within the curriculum. "Later" is defined as the second year in a 2-year curriculum or the second or third year in a 3-year program. By comparison, Figure 3 indicates that in all but one setting, the majority (67%-100%) of pediatric clinical experiences are also available to PTA students in their later affiliations (second year). Interestingly, private practice pediatric settings accept PTA students as early affiliates.

Finally, respondents were asked to examine pediatric student placements for the 1991 to 1992 academic year. Figure 4 compares PT and PTA students requesting pediatric affiliations versus those actually placed in pediatric clinical experiences in relation to the total number of students enrolled. For PT programs, 500 (26%) of the 1959 total students enrolled had requested a pediatric affiliation. Of those, 13% were unable to be placed in a pediatric site. Similarly, for PTA programs, 111 (23%) of the 484 total students enrolled had requested a pediatric affiliation with 20% of those students unable to be placed at pediatric clinical sites.

Reasons cited by ACCEs from PT programs for the inability to provide students with pediatric clinical experiences in order of priority were:

1. Limitations because of the variety and number of sites;
2. The timing of the placements;
3. Competition for the same sites and budget demands placed on sites;
4. The level of student able to be accepted by the clinical site;
5. Staff shortages and changes in personnel;
6. The geographical location of the sites, and
7. A high cancellation rate.

In contrast, ACCEs from PTA programs provided some reasons that differed from the PT programs for the inability to place PTAs in pediatric clinical sites. In order of priority these were:

1. Staff shortages and personnel changes;
2. The variety and number of sites;
3. The site did not accept PTA students;
4. An inconsistent patient volume, and
5. The geographical location of the sites.

DISCUSSION

The discussion will specifically address the results in light of: (1) whether there are enough pediatric opportunities in a variety of settings for those students interested in pursuing pediatric experiences; (2) when the experiences are offered by the clinical site and how this may impact the availability of pediatric learning experiences, and (3) future recommended areas of study related to pediatrics and clinical education.

To provide perspective, it is important to first examine the national picture of pediatric clinical education sites. According to the 1992 national APTA clinical education database, there were a total of 5572 nonduplicated clinical education sites affiliated with PT and PTA programs. Of those sites, only 516 (9.3%) sites were categorized as "pediatric." More specifically, 41 were categorized as pediatric residential facilities, 135 school system, and the remaining majority (66%) as all other types of pediatric settings.[7] Between 1984 and 1992, the mean number of full-time clinical sites used for clinical education per PT program increased 103%, specifically from 78 (range, 21–136; SD, 30) to 159 (range, 52–432; SD, 83.2), respectively.[8] Information was not available to compare the average number of pediatric sites used by PTA programs since 1984 to 1985.

The results also revealed that in academic year 1991 to 1992, one fourth (611) of the total respondents requested pediatric clinical experiences of which 14% (87 students)

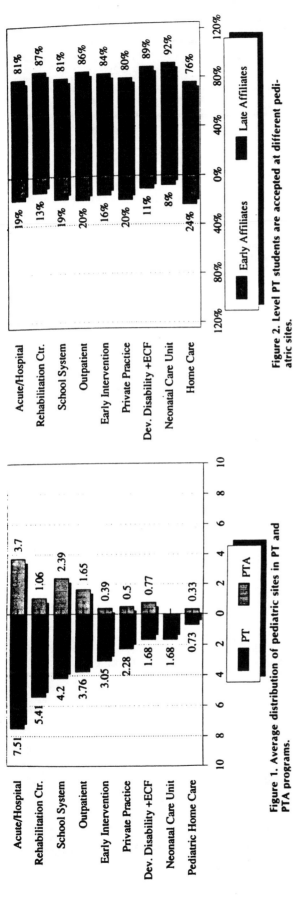

Figure 1. Average distribution of pediatric sites in PT and PTA programs.

Figure 2. Level PT students are accepted at different pediatric sites.

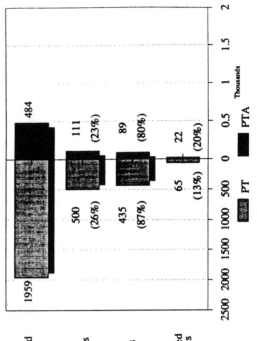

Figure 4. Pediatric placement of 1992 students.

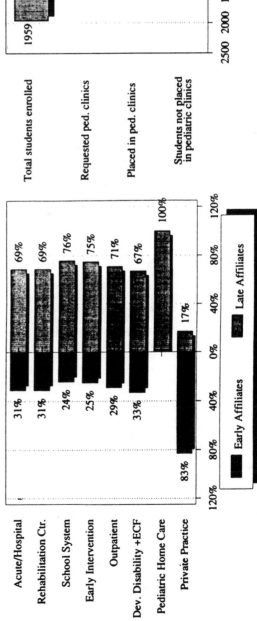

Figure 3. Level PTA students are accepted at different pediatric sites.

were unable to be accommodated. If we were to extrapolate these results to the total number of PT and PTA graduates in 1991 to 1992, the results would indicate that of 6518 graduates, 25% or 1630 might request a pediatric clinical experience. Assuming the same proportions as in the study, if 14% of the students were unable to be accommodated this would mean that 228 students would not be provided with pediatric clinical experiences. On the other hand, if all 1630 students could be accommodated for one full-time rotation, it would necessitate that ideally the 516 available clinical sites would each assume the responsibility for three student affiliates. It would seem that pediatric clinical sites could ideally provide three full-time clinical experiences for 6 to 8 weeks (average length of pediatric experience) and accommodate all students interested in pediatric clinical experiences.[8]

Nevertheless, the results indicate that not all students could, in fact, be accommodated because of a limited numbers of sites, timing of placements, budgetary demands, level of student acceptance, staff attrition/changes, geographical location, inconsistent patient volume, and nonacceptance of PTA students. Many of the reasons cited have been influenced by changes in the health care delivery system, economy, federal legislation governing pediatric physical therapy services, shortage of pediatric physical therapy practitioners, and the level at which students are accepted for pediatric learning experiences. In addition, the level at which students are accepted for pediatric experiences is influenced by the performance expectations for students at entry level and at various levels throughout the curriculum. External factors having an impact on this situation may be more prolonged and difficult to affect as compared with those factors that are managed within the profession. Hence, the profession needs to address the level at which students are provided pediatric experiences, expected outcome performance for pediatric entry-level practice, and the impact the shortage of pediatric physical therapists has on pediatric clinical education. This leads us to the second part of this same issue related to the variety of pediatric sites.

As reported by the ACCEs, the pediatric learning experiences that were available to students reflected the same diversity found in clinical practice ranging from acute care and rehabilitation hospitals to school systems, early intervention centers, and pediatric home care. Students do appear to have ample opportunity to explore pediatric learning experiences in a myriad of clinical settings that adequately represent the current practice of pediatrics. Certainly, it is not surprising to note that pediatric home and neonatal care are the least frequently provided clinical experiences. This is most likely due primarily to the level of risk and liability in managing this patient population and the advanced knowledge and skill required to manage these clients that are often considered beyond entry-level practice.

The second purpose of this study was to examine where within the curriculum students are provided pediatric learning experiences and how timing may impact the availability of pediatric clinical sites. The results indicate that PT and PTA students are provided pediatric full-time clinical experiences predominantly on the later affiliations in the second or third year of study, depending on whether the program is 2 or 3 years in length. It is likely given the limited number of pediatric sites that academic programs use the same clinical facilities to provide student experiences. In addition, academic programs' clinical rotations will frequently overlap because most pediatric clinical experiences were found to be provided later in the curriculum. Thus, there is a strong possibility that increased competition exists for the same clinical sites that are already encountering limited resources.

Assuming there is competition for pediatric clinical sites, exploration of alternative models used to provide clinical education is essential if more students are to be allowed access to pediatric experiences earlier within the curriculum. Examples of some models include early pediatric observation clinical experiences, class field trips to a diversity of pediatric sites, providing different supervisory approaches such as 2 or more students to 1 Clinical Instructor (CI), 2 students (1 PT/1 PTA) to 2 CIs (1 PT/1 PTA), and 2 or more students to 2 or more CIs (eg, split rotations; 2 part-time PTs; 1 experienced CI/1 inexperienced CI [mentor model]). Thus, clinical experiences might be distributed more uniformly throughout the year using the available resources at the clinical site more effectively.

Finally, this study begins to provide future research directions and issues to be explored in pediatrics and clinical education. Below are listed just some of the areas recommended for future initiatives.

- Explore current and alternative models of providing pediatric clinical education and observation. Study the impact these models would have on level of student accepted and overall accessibility.
- Examine and clarify outcome performance measures and expectations for students pursuing entry-level pediatric physical therapy practice.
- Study the impact that a clinical affiliation (early vs late) in pediatrics has on students' career selection in physical therapy.
- Explore reasons why new graduates pursue a career in pediatrics to determine how to influence graduates to become involved in pediatric physical therapy. In a study of Ithaca alumni, 51% sought employment at practices where they had previously affiliated.[14] Perhaps, the likelihood students might pursue employment in pediatric settings would increase if provided a clinical experience in that same environment.
- Explore strategies to develop new pediatric clinical sites to provide quality learning experiences.
- Study the impact of external factors on the provision of pediatric physical therapy. Develop strategies for affecting those factors that directly impact on the provision of quality pediatric physical therapy services to infants, children, youth, and their families.
- Provide longitudinal studies that evaluate the long-term outcome effectiveness of using alternative models of supervision and observation to provide students with pediatric clinical experiences.

CONCLUSIONS

Clinical education and pediatrics was described in this study related to the availability, variety, and accessibility of pediatric clinical learning experiences for physical therapist and physical therapist assistant students in 1991 to 1992. Most significant and most concerning were the number of and reasons cited for students inability to be accommodated with pediatric clinical experiences in the current model. It is critical that issues raised by this study are addressed to enhance opportunities for students to experience pediatric physical therapy and to be capable of making intelligent decisions about future career directions in pediatric physical therapy. Collaborative efforts should pursue additional research investigations and initiatives to clearly identify issues, strategies, and outcomes of any interventions in pediatrics and clinical education.

REFERENCES

1. Department of Education. *Clinical Education: An Anthology.* Alexandria, Va: American Physical Therapy Association; 1992.
2. Department of Education. *Physical Therapy Education Programs Fact*

Sheet. Alexandria, Va: American Physical Therapy Association; September, 1992.

3. Department of Education. *Physical Therapist Assistant Programs Fact Sheet.* Alexandria, Va: American Physical Therapy Association; November, 1990.

4. Department of Education. *Physical Therapist Assistant Programs Fact Sheet.* Alexandria, Va: American Physical Therapy Association; December, 1992.

5. Commission on Accreditation in Physical Therapy Education. *Lists of Accredited and Developing Entry-Level Physical Therapist and Physical Therapist Assistant Programs.* Alexandria, Va: American Physical Therapy Association; November, 1992.

6. Department of Education. *Clinical Education Database.* Alexandria, Va: American Physical Therapy Association; 1985.

7. Department of Education. *Clinical Education Database.* Alexandria, Va: American Physical Therapy Association; 1992.

8. Department of Education. *Report on the Clinical Education Faculty in Physical Therapy Education - 1985.* Alexandria, Va: American Physical Therapy Association; April, 1986.

9. American Hospital Association. *Human Resources Survey: Final Report.* Chicago, Ill: American Hospital Association; 1988.

10. American Board of Physical Therapy Specialties. *Directory of Certified Clinical Specialists in Physical Therapy - 1985–1992.* Alexandria, Va: American Board of Physical Therapy Specialties; 1992.

11. Commission on Accreditation in Physical Therapy Education. *Evaluative Criteria for Accreditation of Education Programs for the Preparation of Physical Therapists.* Alexandria, Va: American Physical Therapy Association, January 1, 1992.

12. Effgen S. IDEA: the individuals with disabilities education act. *Clin Manage.* 1992:12:30.

13. American Physical Therapy Association. *1990 Active Membership Profile Report.* Alexandria, Va: American Physical Therapy Association, 1991.

14. Ciccone C, Wolfner M. Clinical affiliations and postgraduate job selection: a survey. *Clin Manage.* 1988;8:16–17.

INVITED ARTICLES

CHARLES C. LOBECK, M.D., and HOWARD L. STONE, Ph.D.

Class Mentors: A Step toward Implementing the GPEP Report

Abstract—The University of Wisconsin Medical School began a class mentor program in the fall of 1985. Five senior physician faculty members, all in their 60s, have served as mentors thus far, one for each entering class since 1985. Each is asked to spend at least half of his or her time attending courses through four years with the assigned class. The program objectives are to use the experience of senior clinical faculty to help students realize how the information and concepts they learn are important in the practice of medicine, to help with understanding clinical decision making, to provide unique feedback to the faculty and administration on the curriculum and quality of teaching, and to have respected senior faculty serve as advocates for incorporating current education concepts into the medical education program. The mentors have no preset agenda or procedures to accomplish these objectives; each uses his or her own style and interests. Reaction to the program from all parties has been highly favorable: students have been enthusiastic about their encounters with the mentors; the mentors have experienced a new lease on life; and the medical school administration has continued the program as a way of implementing the GPEP recommendation that deans and department chairmen exhibit their commitment to education by their own attitudes and actions. *Acad. Med.* 65(1990):351–354.

Forty years of teaching have taught me this: that it is relatively easy to become a competent specialist, but it is much more difficult to become a good doctor—and it takes much longer.— WILLIAM DOOLIN, *Lancet*, 1958, 2, p.1364

Mentor: a wise and trusted counselor or teacher.— *Webster's Ninth New Collegiate Dictionary*, 1989

The University of Wisconsin Medical School began a class mentor program in the fall of 1985. Its purpose was to make the experience and knowledge of a senior physician teacher available to medical students by providing a mentor to an entire class of students throughout its four years in medical school. The program was not intended primarily as a way for a faculty member to re-experience medical education, as it was in the case of Eichna,[1] although it was assumed

Dr. Lobeck is professor, Department of Pediatrics, and associate dean for academic affairs, and Dr. Stone is professor and director, Department of Medical Education Research and Development, both at the University of Wisconsin Medical School, Madison.

Correspondence and requests for reprints should be addressed to Dr. Lobeck, Associate Dean for Academic Affairs, Medical Sciences Building, 1300 University Avenue, Madison, WI 53706.

that this could occur; nor was the purpose to provide criticism of teaching in the school.

The objectives of the mentor program were:

- to use the many years of experience of senior clinical faculty to help students realize how the information and concepts they learn are important in the practice of medicine and to help them understand the complexity of clinical decision making in modern medical science;
- to provide unique insights on the quality of the teaching and the medical student curriculum to the faculty and administration of the school; and
- to use respected senior faculty as advocates for incorporating current medical education concepts into the school's program of medical education.

It was realized from the beginning that the mentors would become the only faculty knowledgeable about the entire medical curriculum and should be involved in curriculum deliberations, but this purposely was not a stated objective.

Program

Thus far, the program has employed five senior physician faculty members as mentors, one for each class since the entering class of 1985. All of the mentors are in their 60s. Each is asked to spend up to 50% of his or her time attending classes with an incoming class of students through four years of the curriculum. For two of them, this commitment extended past the time of their planned retirements, but in each case they wanted to continue. Another mentor had to retire for health reasons after two years. The school has decided to continue the program for the foreseeable future.

In selecting new mentors, the administration first solicits interest from clinical departments and senior faculty. The associate dean for academic affairs recommends mentors for appointment by the dean. In general, faculty are approached because of the stage they have reached in their professional careers, the distinguished nature of those careers, and their interest in medical education. The selection is not based on faculty members' views of medical education, the clinical disciplines represented, or the closeness of a prospective mentor's relationships with students.

At first, it was not realized that a relatively large number of senior faculty would be interested in being mentors, but experience has proven that the desire to revisit medical student education, particularly basic medical science, is real, and that the example provided by doing it is an exciting prospect. Further, many faculty at or approaching emeritus status find this another way to make a contribution to medical education and their school, a gratifying result of the experiment.

Function

Each mentor attends at least half of the classes during the academic year. They need not take the examinations, and they are asked to be silent during teaching sessions, but they make themselves available to instructors if asked for their criticisms. The actual time spent in classes has varied with individual mentors, but most lectures, small-group sessions, and laboratories are attended by the mentors during the first two years of a more or less traditional curriculum.

All mentors serve as members of the staff of the associate dean for academic affairs and regularly attend staff meetings. They contribute their unique perspective to non-faculty members on the staff and form an important communication link with the administration and as advisers of students.

Although the mentors have no set agenda or requirements to fulfill, except to interact with students and faculty as they see best, each year they must complete a questionnaire before the beginning of the school year. This questionnaire is designed to monitor changes in their perceptions of medical education that have resulted from their experiences as mentors. Before answering the questionnaire, the incoming mentor is asked to read the GPEP Report[2] and respond on a Likert scale as to how he or she perceives the validity of each of the recommendations. The mentors are asked to keep a diary or record of their experiences and to report their

opinions of student and faculty performances to the associate dean for academic affairs.

The mentors are not returning to school to learn the newest medical advances or to learn how students live and think, but to share with the newest students some "barnacles" of wisdom dredged from many years in academic practice. During the first two years, the mentor is visible to the students, but in the clinical third and fourth years, contact is much more attenuated.

Their attendance in classes is readily accepted by students and the faculty, though sometimes this attendance is monitored by departments to assure the accuracy of observations they may make later. Many faculty actively seek advice from the mentors on how to improve their courses or improve specific learning activities for students.

The mentors, depending upon their personal interests, also devise special activities or projects for the students. One has been meeting with students in small ad hoc groups to answer questions about material presented in class or to explain further the relevance of their studies to clinical practice. Another established a weekly get-together that was dubbed "Mentor's Moments." The mentor explains that the sessions were designed to "stimulate the students to think not to keep informing them."

One mentor devised a program for all first-year students to enter their family histories into a computer in the school's computer laboratory, thus creating a "class history." Summaries of the results of these histories became a topic for discussions with the students, allowing them to learn about diseases and discover personal meanings not found in textbooks.

Sometimes a mentor deliberately creates a controversy to get the students to think. One posed the question, "Is alcoholism a medical disorder or an avoidable social ill?" For days heated opinions were aired, experts quoted, and challenges made. Students got the stimulation the mentor sought: "I wanted them to see that there is a world full of contrasting views." At another session a men-

tor showed a slide of pill bottles, enough to fill a small suitcase. They belonged to one very over-prescribed patient. That picture more effectively demonstrated the high cost and possible side effects of drugs than any lecture.

The two mentors who have been through at least one of the clinical years have found different ways to keep contact with the students. One had lunch regularly with his class in the cafeteria of the university hospital; another has regular advising sessions with the students. Both have visited the various locations of third-year teaching distant from the university hospital.

The mentors assume various roles, confidant, counselor, and "pater or mater familias" for class members. There is no requirement that the mentors mix socially with the classes. Some feel it essential to function as a member of the class, attend class functions, and hold social affairs for the students; others have been intellectual advisers and maintained a less intense emotional relationship with members of their classes. It is notable that at third year "skits," both third-year mentors during the past two years have figured prominently as actors in the productions. The one mentor who has "graduated" was a speaker at the special graduation ceremony for medical students and was given a standing ovation by his classmates.

The mentors tend to become spokespersons for the students, though it is rare in this school that the students need urging to speak up. One mentor defended discourteous student behavior at a lecture by agreeing that the speaker had been boring and uninformative, but this is the exception, not the rule.

The mentors have been made ex-officio members of the Educational Policy Council, the curriculum committee of the school. They have been vocal, inserting contrasting views into the deliberations. One, based on his experiences, led an unsuccessful drive in the school to drop the requirement that students pass Parts I and II of the National Board of Medical Examiners examination. Though the views of the mentors can range from dogmatic to very considered, their actions demonstrate the emotional effect the experience has had on them. They defend their positions on issues with vigor and conviction and add an important voice in the deliberations of the council and faculty. Many of their ideas, after modification, are finding their way into the curriculum.

It has become traditional that course directors of the first three years receive a report from the involved mentors on the quality of instruction. Though acceptance of this advice is mixed and the mentors rarely agree completely with each other, their opinions are listened to intently and some instructors ask their help privately.

Evaluation

The impact on the students is impossible to evaluate, since a control group cannot be created without seriously disrupting the educational program. Anecdotal evidence suggests that, in the first semester of the first year, though the mentor has been introduced to the class during orientation, the pressure of learning in the new environment leaves the mentor largely ignored. As the year progresses and when the second year begins, the mentor becomes visible to the students as an ally and aid to their education. By the end of the second year, the mentor is known to all members of the class and his or her value as an adviser in increased. Anecdotes also suggest that students develop great respect for their mentors.

Thus far, evaluation of the program is descriptive. The most easily observable result has been the effect on the mentors, whose comments have ranged from "the enthusiasm of the students really charges my batteries" to "one of the most gratifying aspects of the program is getting to know students well . . . in a non-threatening way." Another mentor commented:

Many of my concepts about medical education at the University of Wisconsin have changed as a result of my experience as a medical student mentor. First, I did not appreciate the enthusiasm, the

energy, or the excitement that the beginning medical student brings as he or she begins medical education. They are excited about becoming a doctor, about learning about medicine. This was a new experience for me, as I sense this in very few of the students that we saw on the wards. We must try very hard to help the students maintain their enthusiasm for learning and their joy at understanding medicine as we help them progress through their education.

Although there have been only five mentors so far, and the results of their experience are too preliminary for firm conclusions, the mentors' questionnaire responses do indicate some interesting trends. From the initial questionnaires completed by the first five mentors, it was clear that they are hardly a homogeneous group of thinkers. This, of course, was not a requirement for selection. (The details of the questionnaire responses are not included here but can be obtained from Howard Stone.)

The most obvious characteristic in the responses is the extremely diverse opinions among the mentors on each of the GPEP recommendations. The mentors thought that the most valid recommendation was that college faculties should make pursuit of scholarly endeavor and the development of effective writing skills integral features of baccalaureate education. They thought the least valid recommendation was that evaluation of student performance should be based in large measure on faculty members' subjective assessments of the students' analytical skills rather than their ability to recall memorized information. Not surprising, these faculty opinions may have changed dramatically during their mentorship.

Further evaluation must wait until more mentors have completed their four-year terms.

Funding

The school provides funds for the second, third, and fourth years of mentorship. Departments provide funding for the first year in its entirety. The dean gives half of the mentor's base salary to the department for the lost services of the mentor during the en-

suing three years. Thus, the additional cost to the school, in a year in which four mentors are employed, is three half-salaries. This amounted to about $120,000 in 1988. The practice supplement, which is guaranteed by the department at this school, is negotiated with the mentor but has not been reduced.

The mentors share an office in the dean's office area.

Conclusions

The mentor program is now in its fifth year. Though some faculty initially expressed concerns that teaching would be reviewed by non-peers, thus potentially impairing academic freedom, the mentors have heeded the warning not to criticize openly, and this concern has subsided.

As of the spring of 1990, only one mentor had completed all four years of the curriculum. The small amount of longitudinal data collected so far indicates that at least one mentor has shown a significant change in attitude toward medical education. He stated:

Before this year I believed most of the GPEP recommendations were foolish, impossible to accomplish, or both. I now believe that our medical school should make implementation of the recommendations a top-priority item, and I would like to see the administration and the faculty develop a commitment to see that such implementation does, in fact, occur.

He goes on to state that Conclusion 5, Recommendation 6 of the GPEP report is by far the most important:

Experience indicates that the commitment to education of deans and departmental chairmen greatly influences the behavior of faculty members in their institutions and their departments. By their own attitudes and actions, deans and departmental chairmen should elevate the status of the general professional education of medical students to assure faculty members that their contributions to this endeavor will receive appropriate recognition.

Obviously, the support of the mentor program by the medical school administration does signify to both students and faculty that a significant commitment is being made to medical student education.

The mentors have suggested that recruiting younger mentors in mid-career would result in their having a greater impact on the school and curriculum. Implementating this proposal would test a number of simmering academic issues. How committed are the faculty to medical student education? Will a faculty career be enhanced or destroyed by time spent this way? The mentors, though aging, have had considerable influence on the educational affairs of the school and tend to underestimate their value.

Steven Muller, chairman of the GPEP panel, stated that one of the purposes of the GPEP Report was to stimulate broad discussion among medical school faculties of the philosophies and approaches to medical education. The mentor program is a way to begin this kind of discussion and has done so at the University of Wisconsin Medical School. A few faculty members have become thoroughly familiar with the medical student curriculum and process of medical education, and they have developed a broader understanding of the eclectic nature of preparing for a medical career and come to espouse many of the GPEP recommendations. Benefits are accruing to students, the school

and faculty, and the mentors themselves. The program's success has done much to elevate the importance of medical student education in the professional lives of our faculty.

The Mentors

The school's five class mentors so far are:

- Entering class of 1985. *William E. Segar*, M.D., is Alfred Dorrance Daniels Professor of Pediatrics and served as chairman of the Department of Pediatrics for 11 years. When retiring as chair, he suggested that he return to medical school as a class mentor.
- Entering class of 1986. *Robert F. Schilling*, M.D., is Washburn Professor of Medicine and an internationally renowned hematologist. A 1943 graduate of the University of Wisconsin Medical School, he served as chairman of the Department of Medicine.
- Entering class of 1987. *Frank C. Larson*, M.D., is professor of medicine and pathology and was director of clinical laboratories of the University Hospital for 30 years. He served as acting dean of the School of Allied Health Professions at its inception, acting chairman of the Department of Pathology for four years, and di-

rector of the School of Medical Technology.
- Entering class of 1988. *Betty J. Bamforth*, M.D., is professor of anesthesiology and has been on the medical school faculty since 1954. She has had a long-time interest in medical students, serving as assistant dean of student affairs from 1973 to 1983.
- Entering class of 1989. *George G. Rowe*, M.D., is emeritus professor of medicine, a research cardiologist, and is well-known by Wisconsin students as a teacher of clinical cardiology. He has decided to return to the employ of the university to be a mentor for this class.

References

1. Eichna, L. W. Medical-School Education, 1975–1979: A Student's Perspective. *N. Engl. J. Med.* 303(1980):727–734.
2. Muller, Steven (chairman). Physicians for the Twenty-First Century. Report of the Project Panel on the General Professional Education of the Physician and College Preparation for Medicine. *J. Med. Educ.* 59, Part 2 (November 1984).

Addendum: Beginning in 1989–90, the class mentor will be appointed to the Admissions Committee during the year in which his or her class is selected. The purpose will be to increase familiarity with the class and provide ongoing review of the admission process.

Legal
Issues/ADA in
Clinical
Education

Introduction to Legal Risks Associated With Clinical Education

Harold G Smith, MEd, EdD, PT

ABSTRACT: *Clinical practice is performed by nonlicensed physical therapy students in health care facilities responsible for providing quality patient care. Individuals participating in the clinical education process must recognize the potential legal liability they may encounter as a result of their role in clinical education. This article introduces common terms and scenarios encountered during clinical education experiences. Every individual involved in clinical education—academic faculty, clinical faculty, supervisor, and student— has some legal risk while participating in clinical education. In addition to providing basic information about potential risks, the article suggests a process to minimize the potential for legal redress if an alleged incident arises while physical therapy students are involved in clincial education.*

INTRODUCTION

In these days of shortages of physical therapy personnel, academic programs are expanding student cohorts, and new education programs are being developed every year. The December 1993 issue of *Physical Therapy* listed 131 physical therapy schools, 135 physical therapist assistant schools, and 49 schools offering a postprofessional degree in physical therapy.[1] All of these programs include a component of clinical education, and they are pressuring clinical facilities to take students for the first time or to take additional numbers of students. The latest debate in physical therapy clinical education involves asking clinical instructors to supervise more than one student at a time during clinical education.

While the physical therapy profession attempts to increase the number of graduates per year, there is a continuing shortage of both academic and clinical faculty. This has resulted in less qualified clinical faculty providing clinical education experiences. In addition, more experienced clinical faculty are

Dr Smith is Associate Professor, Department of Physical Therapy, Medical College of Georgia, Augusta, GA 30912.

being forced to work with more students per year. In the clinical education experience, nonacademic practitioners supervise nonlicensed students who provide treatment. "Defendant," "tort," "plaintiff," and "civil law" are becoming part of the clinical educator's vocabulary. The legal milieu involving health care in the United States has changed.[2] Although physical therapists have not been affected as much as physicians and dentists, Scott pointed out that there has been an increase in the number of claims and court cases involving physical therapists.[3]

It is difficult to secure meaningful statistics about the number of claims filed against physical therapists. Discussion with a representative of a major insurer of physical therapists in February 1991 indicated that the company had processed approximately 200 claims against physical therapists since it began providing physical therapists with malpractice insurance. Scott stated that as of 1990 he was aware of only 20 docketed court cases involving physical therapy practitioners.[3]

This article was written to provide individuals involved in clinical education of physical therapy students with a background of basic legal terms, possible scenarios where legal redress could occur, and a process that should decrease the potential for legal action against those involved in clinical education. The article includes definitions of terms associated with the legal system, including malpractice, negligence, assault, battery, tort, and statutes. Anyone who becomes involved in a court case must understand these terms.

APPLICABLE LAWS
Types of Laws

Bernzweig defined *law* as man-made rules that regulate human social conduct in a formally prescribed and legally binding way.[4] In the United States legal system, laws are derived from two main sources: legislative bodies and court decisions. Laws derived form legislative bodies (usually state governing bodies or the United States Congress) are known as *statutes*, or statutory law. Laws

enacted by a legislative body of one jurisdiction (state) are not binding outside the boundaries of that jurisdiction. Laws governing the practice of physical therapy in one state thus do not apply to the practice of physical therapy in another state. Laws enacted by the United States Congress, however, have precedent over laws enacted by a local or state governing body.

Over time it was impossible for legislative bodies to enact laws to cover all possible social interactions. A second source of laws developed, known as *common* or *case law.* These laws were generated by legal decisions of judges ruling specific cases. After a decision (precedent) was established, it was used to determine the outcome of subsequent similar cases. Both statutory and common law have equal credence, except when a statute is enacted specifically to overrule a common law.

The United States legal system is divided into two major categories, civil and criminal law. *Civil law* involves conflicts between individuals, whereas criminal law regulates behaviors between individuals and governmental jurisdictions. *Criminal law* regulates social actions that impinge on the welfare of society. Examples of criminal misconduct are sexual assault, robbery, murder, rape, and other forms of aggressive behavior that tend to undermine the stability of society. Examples of civil law are contract disputes, boundary disputes between neighbors, and medical malpractice suits.

Civil Law

Both major categories of law have subdivisions that deal with specific areas or behaviors. Bernzweig defined the portion of civil law that includes medical malpractice as the law of torts.[4] A *tort* is a legal wrong committed by an individual against the person or property of another. The usual remedy (result) in a successful tort action is for the court to assess a monetary settlement against the defendant.

Torts

There are three categories of torts: intentional, unintentional (negligence), and strict

Reprinted with permission from the *Journal of Physical Therapy Education*, Vol 8, No 2, pp 67-70, 1994.

liability (liability assessed irrespective of fault).[5-8] Examples of intentional torts are assault, battery, and invasion of privacy. There are two major differences between intentional and unintentional torts. The first is intent. In order to be considered "intentional," the harm must be purposeful, or the wrongdoer must realize with substantial certainty that harm would result from the action. The second difference is that an intentional tort always involves a deliberate act against another, whereas an unintentional tort (negligence) may involve the failure to act when other prudent individuals would have acted in similar circumstances. Most lawsuits arising from the delivery of physical therapy or the provision of clinical education are tort cases that involve unintentional torts (negligence). An example would be letting a patient fall while providing gait training.

Negligence

Pozgar defined *negligence* as the omission or commission of an act that a reasonably prudent person would or would not do under similar circumstances.[6] Bernzweig defined *malpractice* as the negligent acts of persons engaged in professions or occupations in which highly technical or professional skills are employed.[4] The majority of legal actions arising from clinical education involve malpractice on the part of students, clinical instructors, or academic faculty.

Malpractice

To be successful in a malpractice suit, the person initiating the suit (plaintiff) must establish four elements:

1. A duty to act: there can be no negligence without a duty to act.[4] A physical therapist does not have a duty to provide treatment to all persons, only to those individuals with whom he or she establishes a patient-therapist relationship. It is not necessary for there to be a "fee for service" to establish a patient-therapist relationship, merely the exchange of professional services or consultation. In the clinical education setting, if a student is assigned a patient and the patient is a legitimate client of the facility, there is a duty to act.

2. A breach of duty: the failure to provide a duty owed to a patient.[4] The student is expected to treat the patient in a manner that demonstrates competence and conforms to standards of care established for the physical therapy profession. Any breach of this expectation establishes this component of malpractice.

3. Causation: action or lack of action that caused injury to the plaintiff.[4] The student's action or lack of action must have contributed to the harm suffered by the plaintiff. An example would be a fractured hip caused by a fall during gait training.

4. Damages or injury: the plaintiff suffered harm for which the court can assess a monetary value.[4] The action of the student must cause or contribute to the harm suffered by the client, and the court can assess monetary value to the harm. An example would be the patient with the fractured hip suffered during gait training who now is unable to work and loses salary money while the fracture heals.

If any of these elements cannot be established by a preponderance of evidence, the jury or judge should rule against the plaintiff and for the defendant.[8] The plaintiff must prove beyond any question that the defendant was guilty of all four aspects of malpractice.

Although the literature is scant concerning liability actually incurred by physical therapy faculty or students, there are an increasing number of articles regarding the liability of schools, health care facilities, and students involved in other types of clinical education. The majority of legal precedents and rulings have dealt with medical and nursing students. Current writers state that there is no reason to think that various precedents will not be applied to all health care providers.[9-11]

POTENTIAL LIABILITY OF SCHOOLS

Oliver stated that a medical school may be held vicariously liable for negligent patient care performed by its students.[11] Anderson et al noted that one of the problems in determining legal liability in student malpractice suits is determination of who held primary responsibility for supervision of the student at the time of the alleged negligent action.[10]

Felt indicated that there are few cases discussing responsibility of schools for the conduct of students during clinical experiences.[12] According to Felt, a school, under the theory of respondeat superior ("let the master respond"), is not automatically responsible for student conduct in the same way it is for the actions of employees, because students are not employees.[6,12] Unless it can be proven that the student was an agent of the school when the action that resulted in a lawsuit occurred, the school should not be held legally liable.

The school, however, could be held responsible to a plaintiff as a result of its own

negligence. If the school assigned a student to a clinical site knowing that the student was unqualified for activities that the student would be expected to perform at the clinical site, the school may be found negligent for medical and possibly educational malpractice (although most courts have consistently rejected the theory of educational malpractice).

Many facilities accepting students for clinical experiences insist that the affiliation agreement contain a clause specifying the school's responsibility to assign only students who are academically and technically prepared to participate in the clinical experience.[13]

Oliver emphasized the need for the school to be diligent in its evaluation and documentation of student performance.[11] If care is not taken to select students, evaluate student performance, monitor whether the facility is providing adequate supervision in the clinical setting, and select clinical faculty with current knowledge of the program's curriculum, the school may be held liable for negligence.

No court cases specifically implicate physical therapy faculty in any of the above scenarios, but several authors point out that there is a definite possibility that the courts may begin to apply these precedents to schools of physical therapy and to clinical education sites.[10-12]

POTENTIAL LIABILITY OF CLINICAL FACULTY

Clinical faculty are closer in space and time to an alleged negligent incident during a clinical affiliation; hence they are more likely than academic faculty to be named as a co-defendant with a student in a malpractice suit.

Medical students, interns, and residents cannot diagnose or treat a patient without the supervision and control of a licensed clinical faculty member[9]; physical therapy students are under similar restrictions. The Georgia State Practice Act for physical therapy states that students in approved education programs can only perform physical therapy if they are supervised by a licensed physical therapist.[14] The supervisory responsibility defined in the practice act may subject clinical faculty to a potential risk of liability.

Clinical faculty may be found directly liable for their own erroneous acts. If a clinical instructor tells a student to perform an improper or dangerous activity, the clinician could be held responsible for any adverse outcome that may result from the procedure. For example, if a clinical instructor gives a student the wrong weight-bearing status for a patient with a fractured femur, the student could injure the patient based on wrong information, and the clinical instructor could be held liable.

Clinical instructors also may be found liable if they fail to heed information that a student passes on to them after the student's evaluation or treatment of a patient. If a patient proves that he or she had told the student about a problem and the student relayed this to the clinical instructor, who ignored the information, resulting in an injury to the patient, the clinical instructor could be found directly liable.

A potential problem may arise when clinical instructors assign a student to perform an activity in which the student is not competent. Students should tell the clinical instructor when they are not prepared for a specific activity, but if they fail to do so, it is possible that the supervisor will be held responsible for knowing the skill level of students they supervise.[15,16]

Three elements are necessary for the creation of a relationship that could result in vicarious liability for the clinical instructor: (1) the parties must voluntarily consent to an arrangement whereby the student will act for the benefit and under the direction of the clinical instructor, (2) the student must be performing only tasks that are within the scope of direction of the clinical instructor, and (3) the clinical instructor must possess the right to direct the activities of the student.[9] All three conditions exist in clinical education experiences, and thus the clinical instructor may be vicariously liable for the activities of the student. Kapp noted that whether the clinical instructor treats the patient through the student or only offers occasional comments regarding the treatment is of no consequence.[9] The supervisor's direct involvement in case management makes no significant difference from a legal standpoint. Vicarious liability usually arises in employment situations, and in some instances courts have not allowed this doctrine to apply in the teacher-student situation.

POTENTIAL LIABILITY OF CLINICAL FACILITY

Most jurisdictions require that hospitals ensure that health care workers treating patients within the hospital, including students and their instructors, meet applicable standards of professional practice. Scott defined the physical therapy clinician as a "fiduciary," that is, a professional having the legal and ethical duty to act primarily in the patient's best interest.[17] No contract can or should relieve a facility of the responsibility to see that no harm comes to patients.[12]

Authors writing about this topic often refer to *Darling v Charleston Community Memorial Hospital*, a landmark case that established the principle that a health care facility was responsible for negligent acts of a nonemployed physician.[18] The court reasoned that patients could expect a hospital to offer the best health care possible, including monitoring all staff that provided care.

POTENTIAL LIABILITY OF STUDENTS

The author knows of no cases of a physical therapy student being named in a malpractice suit, but there are numerous examples of nursing and medical students being involved in malpractice suits.

Courts have held that students are responsible for their own actions. Every wrongdoer may be liable for harm suffered by another as a result of the wrongdoer's negligence. The training status of a physical therapy student does not allow the student to deliver substandard care.[11] Standards of care for students vary from jurisdiction to jurisdiction, but the common standard states that students must possess the same skill and use the same care and diligence in treatment of patients as a licensed practitioner in similar circumstances. The majority of jurisdictions would hold physical therapy students to the same standard of care as a licensed physical therapist.

Authors point out that every jurisdiction requires that patients be informed when students are involved in their care.[9,11,19,20] Failure to inform patients may subject the student and his or her supervisor to claims of fraud, deceit, misrepresentation, invasion of privacy, breach of confidentiality, and lack of informed consent. Kapp and Oliver acknowledged that they knew of no instances where a student had been sued for failure to disclose student status; however, they argued that failure to disclose the presence of student health care providers could give rise to a finding of liability.[9,11] All individuals involved in clinical education must understand the implication of the patient knowing that he or she is being treated by a student. Students should wear a name tag that identifies them as students, and they should tell the client that they are students before treatment is initiated.

A student should not attempt to provide health care services that he or she is not qualified to perform. The clinical instructor could be found negligent for assigning students to perform inappropriate functions, but the student would not necessarily be absolved of liability by the court trying the case.

RECOMMENDATIONS

Kapp[9] made the following recommendations for limiting the potential liability of individuals involved in clinical education:

1. Clinical facilities should adopt and enforce written guidelines concerning supervisory responsibilities of clinical faculty members.

2. Faculty members, academic programs, and affiliated institutions should require all students and residents to wear name tags clearly identifying them as students and indicating their school. Students should introduce themselves to patients and families as students.

3. Faculty members, academic institutions, and affiliating institutions should devote attention to the activities of their agents. In particular, the academic institution should exercise its power concerning admission, grading, promotion, and discipline of students as conscientiously as possible.

4. Clinical faculty members should provide appropriate supervision of students.

5. All clinical faculty members should use good judgment in assigning students to perform patient care activities. The student should be regarded as a trainee who is an extension of the clinical instructor and not a substitute for the clinical instructor.

6. Medical records should accurately record the role of the clinical instructor in treatment of a patient assigned to a student.

7. Affiliation agreements should accurately reflect the actual functions of the school, affiliating student, and clinical faculty.[9]

Each of Kapp's suggestions is directly applicable to academic faculty, clinical faculty, and students involved in the process of clinical education in physical therapy. Everyone involved in providing clinical education to physical therapy students should remember that if the information has not been documented, in the eyes of the court system it did not happen. It is important that the school, the clinical facility, and the student develop and distribute policies and procedures for all aspects of the clinical experience. The clinical facility also must ensure that the policies are enforced and that any deviation from written procedures is documented.

CONCLUSIONS

Physical therapists have enjoyed relative freedom from malpractice suits, but many authors caution that this condition could change rapidly. The prevailing outlook in the United States with respect to the health care field is for increasing numbers of malpractice lawsuits. As physical therapy attempts to meet the manpower shortages in the profession, increasing numbers of students will be placed in clinical sites.

One area of practice that places physical therapists at risk for liability is the clinical experience of students. Students, by virtue of their educational status, are not as skilled as practitioners, and they are nonlicensed. Clinical faculty must provide ongoing and careful supervision of students' patient care activities.

Every individual involved in physical therapy clinical education must recognize the potential legal pitfalls and take steps to avoid them whenever possible. The seven steps suggested by Kapp are applicable to the physical therapy profession and should become part of the clinical education manual of everyone involved in providing clinical education to physical therapy students.

ACKNOWLEDGMENTS

Special thanks to Carol M Huston, JD, and Clayton D Steadman, JD, for their assistance in preparing this manuscript.

REFERENCES

1. Educational programs. *Phys Ther.* 1993;73:925–942.
2. Horting M. Understanding professional liability. *Clinical Management.* 1989;6:40–46.
3. Scott RW. *Health Care Malpractice: A Primer on Legal Issues for Professionals.* Thorofare, NJ: Slack Inc; 1990.
4. Bernzweig EP. *Nurses' Liability for Malpractice.* New York, NY: McGraw-Hill Book Co; 1969.
5. Ivey FD. Liability issues for occupational health nurses: an overview. *AAOHN J.* 1993;41:16–23.
6. Pozgar GD. *Legal Aspects of Health Care Administration.* 3rd ed. Rockville, Md: Aspen Publishers; 1987:11–28.
7. Peterson RG. Malpractice liability of allied health professionals: developments in an area of critical concern. *J Allied Health.* November 1985:363–372.
8. Jacobson PD. Medical malpractice and the tort system. *JAMA.* 1989; 262:3320–3327.
9. Kapp MB. Legal implications of clinical supervision of medical students and residents. *J Med Educ.* 1983;58:293–299.
10. Anderson JW, Leavell JF, Voss DJ. Tort liability considerations for allied health training institutions. *J Allied Health.* August 1979:133–143.
11. Oliver R. Legal liability of students and residents in the health care setting. *J Med Educ.* 1986;61:560–568.
12. Felt JK. Legal considerations in clinical affiliation agreements. In: Ford CW, ed. *Clinical Education For the Allied Health Professions.* St Louis, Mo: CV Mosby Co; 1978:28–43.
13. Moore M. Legal status of students of health sciences in clincial education. *Phys Ther.* 1969;49:573–581.
14. Official Code of Georgia: Title 43, Chapter 33. Section 43–33–11(2):1992.
15. Fiesta J. Legal update for nurses: part III. *Nurse Management.* 1993;24(3):16–17.
16. Fiesta J. Legal update for nurses: part II. *Nurse Management.* 1993;24(2):14–16.
17. Scott RW. Sexual misconduct. *PT—Magazine of Physical Therapy.* 1993;1(10):78–79.
18. *Darling v Charleston Community Memorial Hospital,* 33 Ill. 2d 326, 211 NE 2d 253 (1965).
19. Banja JD, Wolf SL. Malpractice litigation for uninformed consent: implications for physical therapists. *Phys Ther.* 1987;67:1226–1229.
20. Scott RW. Informed consent. *Clinical Management.* 1991;11:12–14.

Essential Functions Required of Physical Therapist Assistant and Physical Therapy Students

Debbie Ingram, MEd, PT

ABSTRACT: This study was completed to determine whether physical therapist assistant and physical therapy education programs have developed lists of essential functions that students must be capable of performing, with or without reasonable accommodation, while enrolled. A survey was mailed to program directors of all accredited entry-level physical therapy and physical therapist assistant programs (N=253). One hundred ninety responses (75%) were received and analyzed. The results showed that most programs have not developed lists and currently do not request information during the admissions process related to applicants' ability to complete the essential functions of the program, with or without reasonable accommodation. Various tasks are included on the existing lists of essential functions, and consensus has not been reached on the technical skills necessary for program participation. Representatives of 50 programs responded that they plan to begin asking applicants whether they can complete essential functions.

INTRODUCTION

People with disabilities have long been targets of discrimination. They have been denied employment opportunities and access to public facilities. The 1989 US Bureau of the Census report revealed that persons with disabilities had not attained the same work status as persons without disabilities. In 1988, the unemployment rates of men and women with disabilities were both 14.2%. The unemployment rate of persons without disabilities was 6.2% for men and 5.2% for women. In 1987, mean earnings were significantly less for persons with disabilities than for persons without disabilities. The average annual salary for men with disabilities was $15,497, compared with $24,095 for men without disabilities. The average annual salary for all

Ms Ingram is Assistant Professor and Academic Coordinator of Clinical Education, University of Tennessee at Chattanooga, Chattanooga, TN 37403.

employed women with disabilities was $8,075, compared with $13,000 for employed women without disabilities.[1]

The Americans with Disabilities Act (ADA) of 1990 (Public Law 101–336) was established to empower qualified persons with disabilities to seek employment opportunities, transportation, and access to programs and services without fear of discrimination. Institutions of higher education, the preparatory stage for many professions, are affected by the law in various ways. Title I of the ADA prohibits employment discrimination of qualified individuals with disabilities. Title II prohibits discrimination of qualified persons with disabilities for programs and services provided by public entities. Title III requires privately-owned entities to be accessible to persons with disabilities. Title IV ensures that telecommunications relay systems are available to persons with hearing and speech impairments.[2]

To assist universities with implementing the ADA, Rothstein provided legal advice concerning policy development related to students and staff with disabilities. One recommended policy was to develop "technical standards required for admission or participation" in services.[3]

In 1979, the US Supreme Court decided in *Southeastern Community College v Frances B. Davis* (442 US 397) that education programs could develop eligibility requirements and technical standards that all students must be capable of completing during the program. The case concerned an applicant with hearing loss who was denied admission to a nursing program because she was unable to complete all of the program requirements.[4]

A primary responsibility of physical therapy (PT) and physical therapist assistant (PTA) education programs is to graduate qualified persons who can perform the necessary skills safely and competently. During the program admissions process, faculty determine the qualification status of each applicant. Bowman and Marzouk[5] and Mirone[6] suggested that education programs develop lists of essential skills that students must be able to complete, similar to lists of essential

functions in employment settings. Mirone suggested that the lists should be available to all PT applicants, thus allowing each applicant to make the initial determination of his or her qualification.[6]

A review of literature did not reveal any studies related to the essential functions required of PT students with or without reasonable accommodation.

The purpose of this study was to determine whether PTA and PT programs have developed lists of essential functions that students must be capable of performing. The secondary purpose was to determine whether PTA and PT programs ask, during the admissions process, whether students can complete the essential functions of the program with or without reasonable accommodation.

Definitions

Essential functions are defined by the US Equal Employment Opportunity Commission (EEOC) and the US Department of Justice (DOJ) as "fundamental job duties ...and do not include the marginal functions of a position."[7] The EEOC and DOJ define a *qualified individual with a disability* as "one who meets the essential eligibility requirements for the program or activity offered by a public entity. The essential eligibility requirements will depend on the type of service or activity involved."[7]

METHOD

Subjects

The study population consisted of all program directors of PTA and entry-level PT programs accredited by the Commission on Accreditation of Physical Therapy Education (CAPTE). A list of 127 PTA programs and 126 PT programs was supplied by the American Physical Therapy Association (APTA).

Procedure

The data collection instrument was a survey questionnaire developed by the author. The questionnaire was reviewed by two members of the ADA Task Force of the APTA

Reprinted with permission from the *Journal of Physical Therapy Education*, Vol 8, No 2, pp 57-59, 1994.

and was revised based on their feedback. The study received Human Subjects Review Committee approval.

The survey sought the following information:

1. Demographic information (degree awarded by program, class size, and type of institution).
2. Lists of essential functions that students must be capable of performing and requirements during the admissions phase related to capabilities to complete the essential program functions.
3. Plans to change the admissions process as a result of the ADA.

The survey was conducted by mail during March 1993. A cover letter introduced the survey intent and assured respondents of anonymity. To enhance participation, a postage-paid return envelope was included.

Data Analysis

Descriptive statistics, frequency distributions, and percentages were generated from the data. For narrative data, responses were reviewed for summary purposes.

RESULTS

One hundred ninety (75%) of the 253 questionnaires were returned and analyzed. Ninety of the 127 (71%) PTA and 100 of the 126 (79%) PT program directors completed the survey. Of the 100 PT programs represented, 47 awarded entry-level master's degrees and 46 awarded bachelor's degrees. Seven did not respond to the degree-awarded question. The majority of total respondents (74%) represented public institutions. The class size for respondents varied from 12 to 120. The median class size was 32.

A minority of the programs (15%) asked applicants during the admissions process whether they could complete the essential functions of the program with or without reasonable accommodation (Tab. 1). Sixteen PTA programs (18%) and 12 PT programs (12%) asked applicants this question. The majority of programs requesting the information during admission (89%) were public institutions. Eight programs adapted their admissions process to include this question as a result of the ADA. Fifty additional programs (26 PTA and 24 PT) indicated that they planned to begin requesting this information during the admissions process.

Twenty-two respondents (12%) reported that their programs have developed lists of the essential functions that students must be capable of performing while enrolled. The majority of these programs (73%) were af-

filiated with public institutions. Fourteen respondents with lists of essential functions (64%) were PTA programs, and 8 were PT programs (5 entry-level master's and 3 entry-level bachelor's degree).

Programs with lists of essential functions were requested to attach a copy of these lists to the survey. Ten PTA and 3 PT programs submitted lists. Seven programs responded that lists were being developed and could not be released at the time of the study. Twenty programs (13 PTA and 7 PT) requested a copy of the results of this study with the lists of required essential functions.

Various essential functions were noted on the 10 lists for PTA programs (Tab. 2). The tasks of transferring patients and performing physical agents were common to 8 program lists. Six programs addressed effective written and oral communication with patients, families, and coworkers.

One PTA program designed a 13-item essential-functions list after reviewing PTA job descriptions from clinical sites. The list was written in a job-description format, without reference to actual physical requirements to perform the task (eg, "demonstrate ability to set up treatment sessions using laboratory or clinic equipment"). The task was defined

without qualifying the physical means to achieve the task.

Eight PTA programs addressed the lists of essential functions by categorizing the functions with the physical requirement to perform the skill. Examples included adequate vision and hearing to observe and assess patients 10 feet away, vision to accurately read a stopwatch or to set dials on electrotherapy equipment, and digital dexterity to grasp and manipulate objects required to perform job functions.

Four PTA program directors remarked that their interpretation of the *CAPTE Accreditation Handbook* was that all PTA students must be capable of performing all skills listed in the document. It was inferred that these programs had not developed separate lists of essential functions required for their students.

All three PT programs that submitted lists of essential functions award entry-level master's degrees. One program director commented that the submitted list was in draft form and most likely would require changes. This particular list was designed with cognitive, mobility, sensory, and affective abilities defined. Each category listed four to six skills (eg, one skill listed under mobility was, "Must

---

Table 1

Number of Programs With Essential Functions Lists and Relevant Admissions Questions (n=190)

Procedure	Number of Programs		
	PTA[a]	PT[b]	Total (%)
Asks during admissions process whether student can complete essential functions with or without reasonable accommodations	16	12	28 (15)
Has lists of essential functions	14	8	22 (12)

[a]Physical therapist assistant.
[b]Physical therapy.

Table 2

Essential Functions Required by Physical Therapist Assistant Programs (n=10)

Essential Function	Frequency of Response
Transfer patients	8
Perform physical agents	8
Communicate effectively	6
Guard and assist with ambulation	5
Handle the stresses of the work	5
Perform resistance during exercise	4
Assess a patient 10 ft away	3
Respond to a timer	2
Respond to emergencies	2
Perform full-body range of motion	2
Clean whirlpools	1
Perform debridement	1
Perform cardiopulmonary resuscitation	1
Apply universal precautions	1
Monitor vital signs	1

have the agility to move fast enough to ensure patient safety").

Technical standards were defined by one PT program to include six areas: (1) observation; (2) communication; (3) sensorimotor; (4) intellectual, conceptual, integrative, quantitative, and problem solving; (5) judgment; and (6) behavioral and social attributes. Each category defined the requirements. The category of sensorimotor included the statement, "A candidate should be able to execute motor movements required to provide therapeutic intervention (patient transfers, exercise, and application of electrotherapy) and emergency treatment to patients."

The third PT program listed 7 to 10 content areas contained in each semester of the curriculum. The list resembled the standards noted in Section 4.1 of the *CAPTE Accreditation Handbook*.[8] For example, the list for one semester included vital signs, transfers, positioning, range of motion, evaluation tools, and progress notes. In another semester, the list included goniometry, manual muscle testing, massage, and thermal agents.

The only item common to all three PT program lists was the ability to safely transfer a patient from one surface to another. The following essential functions were noted on two lists: effective written and oral communication, ability to respond to emergency or crisis situations, and ability to perform palpations.

Rather than developing lists of essential functions, three programs used the student health form to determine or verify that the student was a qualified applicant. The health forms required physician approval to participate in the programs.

In the comments section of the questionnaire, one PT program responded that extra points were awarded on the admissions evaluation scale to students with disabilities. The length of the program may be extended if necessary from 2 to 3 years for students with disabilities.

DISCUSSION

A primary role of PTA and PT programs is to graduate qualified persons who can safely and competently perform the necessary skills as practitioners. During the program admissions process, it is appropriate for faculty to determine applicants' qualification status. To proceed with this process, lists of essential functions required for the program must be distributed to all applicants. This distribution allows applicants to make the initial determination of their qualifications.

Problems exist for programs without lists of essential functions required of students. The admissions team could make decisions based on misperceptions, rather than allowing applicants with disabilities the opportunity to prove their abilities to perform the tasks. Secondly, qualified applicants with disabilities mistakenly could assume that they could not be accepted into the program because of their disabilities.

The results indicate that few programs have completed the process of developing lists of essential functions. Most programs that do have lists are PTA programs. This could be related to the technical nature of the position. Consensus has not been reached on the items to be included on the lists for PTA and PT programs. Various tasks have been listed by the programs.

Programs may not legally ask an applicant questions related to a personal disability. Various authors have recommended asking all applicants whether they can perform the essential functions of the position with or without reasonable accommodation.[5,6] The results of this study indicate that few PT and PTA programs have added this step during the application and admissions process.

Based on program directors' survey comments, many programs appear interested in developing lists of essential functions and in changing the admissions procedure to include questions related to applicants' ability to complete essential functions.

CONCLUSIONS

Because of the recent passage of the ADA, persons with disabilities can pursue admission to programs of higher education without fear of discrimination. The results of this study indicate that the majority of PTA and PT programs have not developed lists of essential functions and do not request information during the admissions process related to applicants' ability to complete essential functions with or without reasonable accommodation. Additional research must be conducted to reach consensus on the items to be included on lists of essential functions for PTA and PT programs.

ACKNOWLEDGMENTS

The author thanks the directors of the PTA and PT programs for their participation in the study, the members of the ADA Task Force of the APTA, and Dr Richard Metzger for his assistance.

REFERENCES

1. *Labor Force Status and Other Characteristics of Persons with a Work Disability: 1981 to 1988.* US Department of Commerce Bureau of the Census, Series P-23, No. 160; 1989.

2. Americans with Disabilities Act of 1990, PL No. 101-336, 42 USC §12101.

3. Rothstein L. Students, staff and faculty with disabilities. *Journal of College and University Law.* 1991;17(4):471–482.

4. *Southeastern Community College v Davis*, 442 US 397, 408; 1979.

5. Bowman OJ, Marzouk DK. Implementing the Americans with Disabilities Act of 1990 in higher education. *American Journal of Occupational Therapy.* 1992;46(6):521–533.

6. Mirone J. Tricky issues: what educators need to know about the ADA. *Research, Analysis, & Development and Education Divisions Newsletter.* Spring 1993:19–21.

7. *Americans with Disabilities Act Handbook.* Washington, DC: Equal Employment Opportunity Commission and US Department of Justice; 1992.

8. *Accreditation Handbook.* Alexandria, Va: American Physical Therapy Association; 1990.

I N   P R A C T I C E

by   R o n   S c o t t ,   J D ,   L L M ,   P T ,   O C S

CIs and Liability

*Who's responsible for student conduct—student,
CI, site, school? What CIs need to know.*

A number of factors are converging to change clinical education, such as the explosion in the number of professional education programs at different degree levels, governmental health care reform efforts, and managed care. With the use of innovative clinical education models such as the 2:1 collaborative model discussed by Zavadak et al (pages 46-55), in which students supervised by one clinical instructor (CI) may be working as a team to treat patients, now is the time for CIs to strengthen their understanding of liability issues.

What are the basics of malpractice law as it relates to physical therapy?

Any physical therapist who has the legal duty to care for a patient is *primarily* liable (responsible) for physical or mental injury incurred by the patient as a result of 1) professional negligence (substandard delivery of care), 2) intentional (mis)conduct, 3) breach of a contractual promise made to the patient, or 4) use of a dangerously defective modality or piece of equipment. (Sources such as Prosser[1] and Scott[2] elaborate on these basics.)

The clinician who supervises the activities of physical therapist assistants, physical therapy aides, students, and others (eg, athletic trainers) may be *vicariously* (indirectly) liable for patient injury resulting from the liability-generating conduct of these persons when it occurs within the scope of their employment or affiliation.[3,4]

When is the school liable, and when is the site liable?

The party vicariously liable for student conduct usually is the party who has accepted such responsibility under a clinical affiliation agreement, or contract. This contract should clearly delineate the scope of vicarious liability for both site and school and should be undertaken only in consultation with both parties' attorneys. As an additional protective measure for both site and school, the contract also can include language that "memorializes" the mutual understanding that the school will send only those students who are prepared to participate in clinical experiences.

In addition to vicarious liability, sites and schools may incur primary liability for their own negligence in supervising or preparing students who injure patients. A school, for example, may incur primary liability for the negligent instruction or preparation of a student or for the negligent or intentional misrepresentation of a student's competency or status.

In the absence of clear language spelling out who (or whose insurer) is liable for student conduct, a court may rely on the common-law "borrowed servant rule" to assign responsibility, based on whose interests (site or school) the student primarily was serving at the time of an adverse patient incident.

What is the CI's supervisory responsibility?

A CI (or site) may incur primary liability for the negligent failure to review a referral order, a patient's treatment records, or a student's evaluation note before allowing the student to treat a patient. CIs (or sites) also may be primarily liable for the negligent failure to provide on-site and, when appropriate, direct supervision of a student during patient intake, evaluation, and treatment. As Smith[5] noted, the supervisory responsibility defined in certain state practice acts "may subject clinical faculty to a potential role of liability." He cited the Georgia State Physical Therapy Practice Act, which states that physical therapist students "in approved education programs can only perform physical therapy if they are supervised by a licensed physical therapist." Whether the supervision should be "direct" also differs from state to state.

Failure-to-supervise liability often is couched in legal terms, such as "patient or student abandonment." A CI who allows a student to evaluate and treat patients without supervision may face criminal legal action for aiding and abetting physical therapy practice by an unlicensed practitioner in addition to adverse licensure and professional association action for practice and ethical violations.

Malpractice exposure also may occur if a CI gives negligent instruction or guidance to a student that results in patient injury or if there is "negligent failure" to include students in systematic quality monitoring and evaluation processes carried out in the clinic.[6]

Center coordinators of clinical education (CCCEs) and managers need to ensure that CIs understand the rules of appropriate supervision of students and that CIs exercise sound professional judgment when assigning patients to students, based on factors such as student competence and special considerations associated with particular patients.

It is essential that CIs review all student evaluations and countersign their notes before students carry out initial treatment of patients. This precaution helps protect all participants in the treatment process: patient, student, CI, and site. Because students are not licensed health care providers, the "student note" is not legally binding. The CI adopts, or is deemed legally to have adopted, all of the student's patient evaluation and treatment notes as the CI's own. If a malpractice monetary settlement is paid or a court judgement is awarded to a patient, it would be the CI's name, and not that of the student, that would be reported to the National Practitioner Data Bank (a data bank that stores malpractice information on health care practitioners[7]).

CIs have not only an ethical responsibility but a legal duty to honestly and accurately evaluate and report a student's clinical performance to academic coordinators of clinical education (ACCEs). Any critical, candid comments should be accurate, fair, and well-documented in prior written counseling statements given to the student, in which the student was afforded clear notice of deficient performance, an opportunity to respond in writing to the allegation(s), and an opportunity (reasonable time) to remedy any deficiencies. A CI who misrepresents a student's level of competence may be held legally accountable for patient injury that results from that student's conduct.

Remember: Both statutory (legislative) law and common (judge-made) law require that clinical site personnel and academicians handle information about students as confidential.[2,8] Everyone who has official knowledge about students and their performance should understand the gravity of this responsibility.

What role does informed consent play?

As is supported by APTA's *Code of Ethics* and *Guide for Professional Conduct*, the basic rule of law is that all health professionals have the ethical and legal duty to gain a patient's informed consent before treatment.[9] Informed consent is based on the patient's inherent right to self-determination or autonomy. The disclosure elements (ie, the information that must be disclosed to the patient) required for legally sufficient patient informed consent to evaluation and treatment when students are involved include:

1. Type of treatment recommended or ordered.
2. Any material (decisional) risks associated with the proposed treatment.
3. The expected benefit(s) of treatment (ie, treatment-related goals).
4. Information about any reasonable alternatives to the proposed treatment.
5. *The role of a student or students in evaluation and treatment.*

CIs should remember that it is their personal legal responsibility—not the student's—to obtain patient informed consent to physical therapy treatment. (Similarly, this responsibility cannot legally be delegated to a PTA.)

What *is* the student's responsibility?

A student may be *singularly* responsible for patient injury when that student was negligent and failed to follow a CI's instructions or when the student's injurious conduct was malicious.

As may licensed PTs, students may engage in intentional liability-generating conduct. A student, for example, may commit or be accused of *battery* (inappropriate or offensive touching of a patient); *defamation* (false assertions about a patient that damage the patient's good reputation); *invasion of (patient) privacy* and, in particular, public dissemination of confidential patient information; or *sexual harassment*.[1,10]

What about liability in clinical education and the ADA?

The Americans with Disabilities Act may require that facilities make reasonable accommodation for students with disabilities. The burden typically is on the student to apprise the school or site of the disability and request accommodation.[11] Although facilities must show flexibility in providing necessary assistance and accommodation so that qualified students can reasonably meet clinical education requirements for graduation, the ADA does not say that quality and safety standards can be lowered to the point of risking injury to patients.

What risk management strategies can sites use?

- Require students to wear name badges, and instruct and compel them to use identifying initials such as "SPT" after their signatures on patient treatment record entries.
- Assign only seasoned clinicians as CCCEs and CIs.
- On their arrival in the clinic, orient all students to the physical facility and its written policies, protocols, treatment guidelines, and other standardized operating procedures before they begin to evaluate and treat patients.
- Orient students to the equipment they will be using in the treatment of patients.
- Have students sign in an appropriate place that they have read all applicable policies and guidelines.

As Smith[5] wrote in his overview of liability and clinical education, there are "no cases of a physical therapy student being named in a malpractice suit....[and] physical therapists have enjoyed relative freedom from malpractice suits." But CIs (and clinical sites and schools) still should take risk management seriously, both to protect the health interests of the patient and to protect their own professional and legal interests. *PT*

Ron Scott, JD, LLM, PT, OCS, is Assistant Professor, Physical Therapy Department, University of Texas Health Science Center, San Antonio, Tex. He is a member of APTA's Judicial Committee and of APTA's Risk Management—Liability Awareness Program Faculty.

The information in this article should not be interpreted as specific advice for any particular practitioner. Personal advice can be given only by personal legal counsel, based on applicable state and federal law.

References

1. Prosser W. *Prosser on Torts, 4th ed.* St Paul, Minn: West Publishing Co; 1971.
2. Scott R. *Health Care Malpractice.* Thorofare, NJ: SLACK Inc; 1990.
3. Scott R. *Legal Aspects of Documenting Patient Care.* Gaithersburg, Md: Aspen Publishing Co Inc; 1994.
4. Scott R. Vicarious liability. *Clinical Management.* 1991;11(5):14-15.
5. Smith HG. Introduction to legal risks associated with clinical education. *Journal of Physical Therapy Education.* 1994;8(2):67-70.
6. Kearney KA, McCord EL. Hospital management faces new liabilities. *The Health Lawyer.* 1992;6(3):1,3-6.
7. Fraiche D. Peer review and the data bank. *Clinical Management.* 1992;12(3):14-17.
8. Family Educational Rights and Privacy Act of 1974, 20 USC §1232f(a)(b).
9. Rozovsky FA. *Consent to Treatment, 2nd ed.* Boston, Mass: Little Brown & Co; 1990.
10. Finley C. What is sexual harassment? *PT—Magazine of Physical Therapy.* 1994;2(12):17-18.
11. Mirone JA. Cases in higher education. ADA Case Law. *PT—Magazine of Physical Therapy.* 1994;2(6):33.

SPECIAL ARTICLES

LELIA B. HELMS, J.D., Ph.D., and CHARLES M. HELMS, M.D., Ph.D.

Forty Years of Litigation Involving Medical Students and Their Education: I. General Educational Issues

Abstract—An analysis of reported state and federal adjudication from 1950 through 1989 was undertaken to identify trends in litigation involving medical students and undergraduate medical education. Of the 110 decisions cited, 51 (46%) involved disputes over general educational issues. A majority of the decisions affecting general education involved admissions and dismissal processes. Recently courts have begun scrutinizing readmission, course repetition, and cheating. Medical schools have accommodated to judicial scrutiny of general educational issues and have prevailed more often than claimants in litigation during this period, but litigation has not decreased as precedent and procedure have become clearer. Instead, litigation has continued unabated in alternative areas and at different levels of the educational process. *Acad. Med.* 66(1991):1–7.

What has been the general impact of litigation on undergraduate medical education? Have medical schools adapted to judicial intervention? What issues remain to be addressed?

The role of the courts in overseeing, correcting, and setting standards that affect undergraduate medical education has been debated over the past two decades. Careful assessments of how judicial decisions have affected undergraduate medical education are fewer, however. In part, this lack of assessment results from the difficulty of determining the impact of judicial intervention upon policy and of developing methodologies adequate to the task. Traditional legal methodology focuses on a detailed analysis of individual cases and therefore does not provide administrators and faculty with any perspective as to how representative a case is or how frequently the problem occurs. A preoccupation with Supreme Court decisions compounds these limitations. Because traditional legal methodology is predominant in the literature, medical educators often lack perspective about the progress that has been made. Further, they may not develop a framework for understanding the policy implications of litigation or for identifying future problems.

In this review, we applied outcomes analysis to a systematic survey of reported litigation involving medical students and issues of undergraduate medical education over the past 40 years. Outcomes analysis — the examination of specified information contained in all court decisions in one policy sector — allowed us to identify broad litigation patterns and trends. We sought answers to the following questions: How often does litigation occur? What problems of medical education give rise to litigation involving medical students? Which party to the dispute prevails? What implications or conclusions may be drawn from the aggregate case law that can provide guidance in developing policies and procedures for administering medical education?

Method

Reported state and federal cases in which medical students or medical education had been involved were identified for 1950 through 1989. The Westlaw and Lexis computerized legal research services were used to obtain access to all decisions recorded in the state and federal reporting systems through a key word identification system. The key words used were medical student, student of medicine, medical education, undergraduate medical education, medical school, college of medicine, and medical college.

This study included only reported court decisions, which are the sole body of law serving as precedent to guide judicial decisions. In contrast to reported cases, the actual number of suits related to medical students or undergraduate medical education cannot be determined, since present judicial information systems do not collect such information comprehensively. Consequently, an accurate de-

Dr. Lelia Helms is assistant to the dean, College of Education, and Dr. Charles Helms is associate dean for student affairs and curriculum, College of Medicine, both at The University of Iowa, Iowa City.

Correspondence and requests for reprints should be addressed to Dr. Charles Helms, Associate Dean for Student Affairs and Curriculum, University of Iowa College of Medicine, 240 Eckstein Medical Research Building, Iowa City, IA 52242.

Another article about litigation appears on page 39.

Table 1
Cases Involving Medical Students and Issues of Undergraduate Medical Education

Years	Federal Court		State Court		Total	
	General	Finance	General	Finance	All	Finance
1950–1954	—	—	—	1	1	1
1955–1959	—	—	2	—	2	—
1960–1964	—	—	1	—	1	—
1965–1969	1	—	1	—	2	—
1970–1974	1	—	2	—	3	—
1975–1979	7	1	9	5	22	6
1980–1984	6	9	4	—	19	9
1985–1989	9	40	8	3	60	43
Total	24	50	27	9	110	59

termination of the number of cases filed, dismissed, settled out of court, or decided but yet unreported remains beyond the scope of systematic study.

The differences in case reporting of federal and state litigation also limit the study. Although federal district court decisions are generally reported, state district court decisions generally are not. State court reporter systems usually include only appellate-level decisions. These limitations mean that a relatively smaller number of state cases were identified by this search and that there was a bias toward appellate-level decisions. The case law identified in this survey represents, therefore, only the tip of the litigation iceberg.

Results and Analysis

The results of the search can be broken down into three general categories: the volume of litigation, the issues that gave rise to litigation, and the prevailing party.

Volume of Litigation

A general, chronological summary of reported litigation involving medical students and issues of undergraduate medical education from 1950 through 1989 is presented in Table 1. Overall, 110 cases were reported for the 40-year period; of these, 74 were litigated in federal courts and 36 in state courts. Among federal cases, three were decided by the U.S. Supreme Court, 16 by appellate courts, and the

remaining 55 by district, claims, or bankruptcy courts. Reported litigation has become more frequent over these 40 years, with most of this growth involving litigation related to finance (59 cases). Because of the growing importance of financial aid issues in medical education, litigation related to finance is discussed in a separate article.[1]

The part of the study reported here focuses on the 51 cases involving general educational issues unrelated to finance. These cases are shown in the columns entitled "General" in Table 1. The number of these cases reported increased substantially between 1975 and 1979 but appears to have stabilized since 1980. Analysis of medical school enrollment data provides insight into one potential factor accounting for this increase—the expansion of medical education. From 1968 to 1988 medical schools doubled the size of their yearly graduating classes, and the number of accredited schools increased from 86 to 127.[2]

The number of cases involving general medical education thus rose dramatically in a period of medical educational expansion. Interestingly, medical school expansion was part of a general growth trend in postsecondary education that saw a tripling of enrollment between 1960 and 1988 and a 50% increase in the number of institutions.[3] Reported litigation tripled from 1970 through 1979 when higher education was expanding.[4]

Litigation related to general undergraduate medical educational issues

may also have been stimulated in the 1970s by the courts' expanding procedural protections under the 14th Amendment to cover educational institutions.[5] The basic decisions governing how a school could dismiss students and how it could address affirmative action in admissions were enunciated by the Supreme Court during this period in the *Horowitz* and *Bakke* cases, and both involved medical education.[6,7] Economics is the final factor that might account for the increase in litigation related to general educational issues. Medical students have strong economic incentives to sue because they have a great deal to gain financially (both in terms of income and in terms of paying off their debts) in successfully pursuing their medical education.[1]

Issues Giving Rise to Litigation

Analysis of the cited cases provides information about the specific issues in general medical education most subject to litigation by medical students (Table 2). The number of cited cases related to admission to medical school has decreased since 1980: six of the nine admission cases were decided before 1980. This apparent decline in litigation related to admission roughly parallels the 37% decline in the number of medical school applicants from 1974 to 1988, when the ratio of applicants to accepted students fell from a peak of 2.8:1 in 1974 to 1.6:1 in 1988.[2]

Discrimination was at issue in five

Table 2

General Educational Issues Giving Rise to Litigation

| | 1950–1969 | | 1970–1979 | | 1980–1989 | | |
	Federal	State	Federal	State	Federal	State	Total
Admission	—	—	2	4	2	1	9
Dismissal	1	2	5	6	7	4	25
Readmission	—	—	1	—	1	2	4
Retaking work	—	—	—	—	2	1	3
Cheating	—	1*	—	1	2	1	5
Other	—	1*	—	—	1	3	5
Total	1	4	8	11	15	12	51

*Case litigated in 1950–1959 period.

of the admissions cases.[8] One addressed sex discrimination. Three cases were challenges to affirmative action programs and alleged reverse discrimination; these were decided before 1980. By 1980 courts had also decided challenges to admission decisions based on unpublished criteria, on meetings not open to public scrutiny, and on challenges by U.S. students in foreign medical schools who sought admission as transfer students.[9] A more recent case involved false information on the application form discovered after the student had begun his studies.[10]

Not unexpectedly, dismissal from medical school was the academic issue most frequently giving rise to litigation. Cases related to dismissal for failure to meet standards of academic performance were cited throughout the period and constituted 25 (49%) of the 51 cases. Beginning in 1975, reported litigation over dismissal increased substantially, but since 1980 it has leveled off at one to two cases per year.

Several additional smaller clusters of cases were identified. These have occurred primarily since 1980. First were cases dealing with readmission to medical school. Four of these involved the specific issue of readmission after a leave of absence.[11] Second were three cases dealing specifically with policies about repeating courses or examinations.[12] In only one of these did a dismissal motivate the student to litigate. Third were cases of academic dishonesty.[13] Although

cheating is not a recent problem, concerns have been raised about the process due to students accused of cheating. Three cases since 1970 arose as claims that private institutions either violated contract rights under institutional policies or acted in an arbitrary or capricious manner contrary to the U.S. constitution. Another case concerned rights to due process in a public institution where the student was denied the assistance of counsel at a disciplinary hearing on expulsion. Fourth were five cases deciding issues of negligence,[14] alleged fraud,[15] and false imprisonment.[16] In the earliest of three negligence cases, a student was sued by a patient for malpractice. The remaining two negligence cases litigated the responsibility of medical schools for injuries sustained by students participating in student-sponsored and required college activities. In addition, the American University of the Caribbean was charged with fraudulent misrepresentation and breach of contract by a medical student who quit 11 days after entering the first-year class.[15] Finally, a medical student sought damages for unlawful detention by a university security officer when the student was found apparently living in the storeroom of a university building.[16]

Of interest, 11 of the 51 cases litigated allegations of discrimination. Nine of these cases were litigated in federal and two in state courts. Both state cases involved issues of reverse discrimination in admissions, whereas only two of the federal cases

focused on this issue.[17] Of the seven remaining federal cases,[18] three dealt with discrimination based on race, two on sex, one on handicap, and one on age. Six claims of discrimination were decided in the five-year period 1975–1979, but only five occurred in the ten-year period 1980–1989.

Prevailing Party

How litigation turned out is important information that can guide medical schools in developing policies and procedures. Most cases may be categorized by winning party, either student or school (Table 3). Medical students prevailed in 12 (24%) of the 51 cases overall. The students involved in cases that were decided in state court won twice as frequently (eight of 27 cases) as did those in federal court (four of 24 cases). The students' success rate declined substantially between 1970–1979 and 1980–1989. In the earlier decade, the students prevailed in eight of 19 cases (42%), whereas for the 1980–1989 period that ratio fell to three of 27 cases (11%).

In the 1970–1979 period 11 cases litigating dismissals were reported. The students prevailed in almost half, one in federal court and four in state courts.[19] Since 1980, ten cases regarding dismissals were reported, and no student prevailed. Similarly, from 1970 to 1979, medical schools lost half of the challenges to their admission procedures. Since 1980 medical schools appear to have successfully

Table 3
Prevailing Party in Litigation

Issue	1950–1969			1970–1979		1980–1989		
	Student	School	Other Party	Student	School	Student	School	Unclear
Admission	—	—	—	3	3	—	3	—
Dismissal	1	2	—	5	6	—	10	1†
Readmission	—	—	—	—	1	1	2	—
Retaking work	—	—	—	—	—	—	2	1†
Cheating	—	1	—	—	1	1	2	—
Other	—	—	1*	—	—	1	3	—
Total	1	3	1	8	11	3	22	2†

*Malpractice suit against both student and school, won by patient.
†Remand required for retrial under a corrected interpretation of the law.

weathered all admission litigation. In one case — despite the fact that a student won a preliminary injunction permitting him to continue his medical education and graduate before the court issued its final decision about falsifying information on his application forms — the medical school was sustained and the degree rescinded.[10] In the areas of both dismissal and admission, medical schools in recent years appear to have accommodated to judicial standards for adequately protecting students' rights.

Cases involving readmission form a separate group, with outcomes not unlike those involving dismissal. Of the four cases dealing with readmission, three involved illness, either physical or mental, that necessitated the granting of a formal leave of absence from school; the fourth addressed readmission after dismissal for academic reasons.[11] Litigation arose over the status and due process rights of these students when the schools denied them readmittance. In the one case, where the sole reason for the leave was a physical condition, the student was found to have a property interest in the reinstatement procedures. In the two cases where mental illness was in question, though, neither student succeeded in being readmitted. In the *Doe* case this denial occurred after very extensive evidentiary hearings on the student's condition and consideration of the student's rights as a handicapped individual under federal statutes. In the more recent *North* case, no claim was

made for accommodation to a handicap. Instead, the case was decided primarily in contract law over whether a school in authorizing a one-year leave of absence established an express contract for readmission. In rejecting this argument, the court reasserted its traditional deference to academic decision making. *Williams*, the earliest of these cases, explored the property rights and procedures due to a student seeking readmittance after dismissal for academic reasons.

In recent years the courts have been more willing to become involved in processes and issues of medical education beyond admissions and dismissals. Three cases[12] examined policies and practices permitting or denying students the right to repeat courses or examinations; two of these also involved claims of discrimination. A medical student dismissed for academic reasons alleged racial bias in the administration of a school policy of allowing students to rectify course failures by taking make-up examinations. In *Lewis*, a case with an unclear outcome, the student's Title VI claim of discrimination survived a motion for summary judgment. In *Moire*, a claim of sex discrimination and harassment was disallowed for a third-year student who was required to repeat a clerkship in psychiatry. In *Levy*, a court let stand a decision that requiring a student to retake a neurobiology course during the time set aside for studying for the National Board of Medical Examiners examinations was not unreasonable because

the student had not retaken it during previous opportunities.

The courts have also dealt recently with the ongoing problem of cheating.[13] Decisions rendered have focused on ensuring that appropriate procedures are employed to handle cheating, whether under a due-process analysis in public institutions or under a contract theory in private institutions, and on distinguishing between the nature of dishonesty as an academic rather than a behavioral sanction so as to ensure that appropriate procedures are provided in any resulting decision about the student's status. Institutional actions against students have been sustained in all but one egregious case, in which the school was enjoined from summarily expelling the student without any hearing.[20] The courts allowed classification of cheating as an academic offense and permitted dismissal under the less stringent standard governing academic decision-making procedures rather than disciplinary cases.

When less commonly addressed issues related to medical education (such as negligence) were litigated, the outcomes varied.[14] The courts found institutions not liable for the death of an overweight student in a student-sponsored race or for injuries sustained by a student participating in a one-mile run designed as an experiment for a required physiology course. In only one early case was responsibility for patient care by a medical student litigated. In that case, the patient won a malpractice claim against both the student and the school.[21] A student prevailed in an unusual claim of false imprisonment arising from his access to and use of university space for studying and living.[16]

Among the 11 cases dealing with allegations of discrimination, a student prevailed only once, in *Bakke*.[7] In a racial discrimination case dealing with bias in repeating examinations, the outcome is not clear.[22] Both of these cases were litigated in federal courts. Neither claim of discrimination succeeded in the two cases tried in state courts.

Discussion

Litigation involving issues related to general undergraduate medical education has provoked substantial concern and discussion among medical educators over the past decade.[23-27] Our review identified patterns and trends in litigation and thus expands understanding of the role litigation plays in three ways: first, it substantiates the reasons for the ongoing concern about litigation; second, it identifies an apparent pattern of institutional learning in response to litigation; and third, it points to the development of issue areas for future litigation.

An overview of the data on litigation outlines a sharp growth in volume from 1975 to 1979 that has been sustained and consolidated during the 1980s. The focus of concern in the literature on problems arising from dismissals of medical students seems justified. Suits challenging dismissals have been a consistent source of reported litigation since 1970. In a larger context, the 1970s was a period when enrollments were expanding and when the courts were outlining rights and procedures available to students. The relative success of medical students' litigation from 1975 to 1979 reflects the reframing of basic student rights that occurred in all sectors of education during that period.[4,5] By 1980, however, medical schools appear to have adapted to legal expectations by adopting appropriate procedural standards.[23,25,26]

The case law data sustain the idea that faculty have little reason to fear judicial intervention in upholding academic standards.[27]

Contrary to the general trends, challenges to admission decisions appear to be both declining and less successful. We see two possible reasons for this: first, variations in the rates of application may account for some of this decline; and second, reverse discrimination claims that proliferated in the late 1970s were addressed relatively early and thoroughly by the Supreme Court in *Bakke*.[7] A caveat, however, is in order. Litigation challenging affirmative action programs in medical education may be re-energized by recent Supreme Court decisions narrowly construing the leeway available in designing and administering voluntary affirmative action programs in other areas.[28] Such programs must be carefully tailored to respond to demonstrated prior discrimination with minimal harm to those who do not benefit from affirmative action.

These data thus identify what might be described as a learning curve in terms of institutional success in litigation brought by medical students. After initial liability is established, institutions appear to adapt to judicial standards and changing expectations, as occurred in the areas of admission and dismissal during the 1970s, with successful accommodation established by the 1980s.

It is apparent, however, that litigation does not necessarily decrease as precedent and procedural standards become clearer in one area. Instead, precedent is applied to alternative stages and levels of decision making in the educational process. An indication of this is a disturbing pattern of broadening judicial scrutiny of decisions made before or ancillary to the final stage of dismissal. The courts are being asked to resolve a variety of problems related but antecedent to the final dismissal decision. Over the past decade although 20 cases were litigated by students who were dismissed, nine of these challenged acts or decisions preceding actual dismissal. The courts are thus gradually

extending the scope of their review back into the conditions preceding actual dismissal. This finding should be of greatest concern to educators, for it points to an expanding role for the courts in monitoring and regulating basic practices of medical schools.

As courts develop precedent and institutions develop policy in response, continued litigation can be expected to force courts to probe ever more deeply into medical school programs. As institutions adopt policies, they must balance the "dangers" of flexible policy with the "safety" of specific policy. A recent case[29] provides an excellent illustration of this dynamic. In the only dismissal case with an unclear outcome during the 1985–1989 period, a medical school regulation requiring that course instructors issue written grading criteria on the first day of class was used to force a remand for fact finding when, instead, an instructor issued criteria orally. Despite the court's warning that the student "was engaged in a war that could not be won," the school's failure to follow through and issue written instead of oral criteria was enough to withstand a motion for summary judgment.[29] Medical administrators must be willing to permit sufficient leeway for faculty discretion while protecting students' legitimate interests.

The data identified in this survey point to issues and areas likely to be the subjects of additional concern in the future. In this regard medical schools would be wise to review carefully their policies (1) dealing with leaves of absence and conditions for re-admission, (2) requiring repetition of courses and examinations, and (3) on cheating.

Finally, although negligence has not been frequently alleged by medical students against medical schools and there is only one case alleging negligence by a medical student, this relative paucity of cases was somewhat surprising in an era of litigation. Interestingly, no case has been reported in which a medical student claimed that negligence arose from the failure of a medical program to educate. Such claims have been made by residents against hospital programs, chiropractors against schools of chiropractic medicine, and students against the public schools.[30] Allegations of negligence by medical schools in failing to educate students adequately — in areas such as preventive measures for treating patients with AIDS, for example — would appear to be a cause of action ripe for litigation by a student with resourceful counsel. That students are not commonly included in malpractice claims may be explained in part by rather clear-cut judicial allocation of responsibility for patient care to supervising faculty.

Part II of this report, "Issues of Finance," will appear in the February 1991 issue.

References

1. Helms, L. B., and Helms, C. M. Forty Years of Litigation Involving Medical Students and Their Education: II. Issues of Finance. *Acad. Med.* 66(February 1991): in press.
2. *American Medical Education: Institutions, Programs and Issues.* Washington, D.C.: Association of American Medical Colleges, 1989.
3. Ottinger, C. *Fact Book on Higher Education.* New York: MacMillan, 1985.
4. Zirkel, P. A. Commentary: Higher Education Litigation: An Overview. *West's Ed. Law Rptr.* 56(1989):705–708.
5. Wright, T. H. Faculty and the Law Explosion: Assessing the Impact: A Twenty-five Year Perspective (1960–85) for Colleges and Lawyers. *J. College & University Law.* 12(1985):363–379.
6. Board of Curators of the University of Missouri v. Horowitz, 435 U.S. 78, 98 S. Ct. 948 (1978).
7. Regents of the University of California v. Bakke, 438 U.S. 265, 98 S. Ct. 2733 (1978).
8. Cannon v. University of Chicago, 559 F.2d 1063 (6th Cir. 1976). Alevy v. Downstate Medical Center, 348 N.E.2d 537 (N.Y. 1976). Regents of the University of California v. Bakke, 438 U.S.265 (1978). McDonald v. Hogness, 598 P.2d 707 (Wash. 1979). Baker v. Board of Regents of State of Kansas, 721 F.Supp. 270 (D. Ka. 1989).
9. Steinberg v. Chicago Medical School, 354 N.E.2d 586 (Ill. App. 1976). Carl v. Board of Regents of University of Oklahoma, 577 P.2d 912 (Okla. 1978). Selman v. Harvard Medical School, 494 F.Supp. 603 (D.C. N.Y. 1980).
10. North v. West Virginia Board of Regents, 332 S.E.2d 141 (W.Va. 1985).
11. Doe v. New York University, 666 F.2d 761 (2nd Cir. 1981). Williams v. Howard, 528 F.2d 658 (D.C. Cir. 1976). North v. State, 400 N.W.2d 566 (Ia. 1987). Evans v. West Virginia Board, 271 S.E.2d 778 (W.Va. 1980).
12. Lewis v. Russe, 713 F.Supp. 1227 (N.D. Ill. 1989). Moire v. Temple University School of Medicine, 613 F.Supp. 1360 (D.C. Pa. 1985). Matter v. Levy, 450 N.Y.S.2d 574 (N.Y. 1982).
13. Beilis v. Albany Medical College of Union University, 525 N.Y.S.2d 932 (N.Y. 1988). Corso v. Creighton University, 731 F.2d 529 (8th Cir. 1984). Hall v. Medical College of Ohio at Toledo, 742 F.2d 299 (6th Cir. 1984). Pride v. Howard University, 384 A.2d 31 (D.C. App. 1978). People v. Board of Trustees of University of Illinois, 134 N.E.2d 635 (Ill. App. 1 Dist. 1956).
14. Gehling v. St. George's University School of Medicine, 705 F.Supp. 761 (E.D. N.Y. 1989). Turner v. Rush Medical College, 537 N.E.2d 890 (Ill. App. 1 Dist. 1989). Christensen v. Des Moines Still College of O & S, 82 N.W.2d 741 (Ia. 1957).
15. Reimer v. Tien, 514 A.2d 566 (Pa. Super. 1986).
16. Parker v. Downing, 547 So.2d 1180 (Ala. Civ. App. 1988).
17. Baker v. Board of Regents of State of Kansas, 721 F.Supp. 270 (D. Ka. 1989). McDonald v. Hogness, 598 P.2d 707 (Wash. 1979). Regents of University of California v. Bakke, 98 S. Ct. 2733 (1978). Alevy v. Downstate Medical Center, 348 N.E.2d 537 (N.Y. 1976).
18. Lewis v. Russe, 713 F.Supp. 1227 (N.D. Ill. 1989). Watson v. University of South Alabama College of Medicine, 463 F.Supp. 522 (D.C. Ala. 1979). Williams v. Howard University, 528 F.2d 658 (D.C. Cir. 1976). Moire v. Temple University School of Medicine, 613 F.Supp. 1360 (D.C. Pa. 1985). Cannon v. University of Chicago, 559 F.2d 1063 (6th Cir. 1976). Doe v. New York University, 666 F.2d 761 (2nd Cir. 1981). Petock v. Thomas Jefferson University, 630 F.Supp. 187 (E.D. Pa. 1986).
19. Greenhill v. Bailey, 519 F.2d 5 (8th Cir. 1975). Demarco v. University of Health Sciences/Chicago Medical School, 352 N.E.2d 356 (Ill. App. 1976). Maitland v. Wayne State Medical School, 257 N.W.2d 197 (Mi. App. 1977). North v. West Virginia Board of Regents, 233 S.E.2d 411 (W.Va. 1977). Wong v. Regents of University of California, 93 Cal. Rptr. 502 (Cal. App. 1971).
20. Corso v. Creighton University, 731 F.2d 529 (8th Cir. 1984).
21. Christensen v. Des Moines Still College of O & S, 82 N.W.2d 741 (Ia. 1957).
22. Lewis v. Russe, 713 F.Supp. 1227 (N.D. Ill. 1989).
23. Irby, D.M., Fantel, J.I., Milam, S.D., and Schwarz, M.R. Legal Guidelines for Evaluating and Dismissing Medical Students. *N. Engl. J. Med.* 304(1981):180–184.
24. Arkin, H. R., Academic Dismissals: Due Process: Parts I & II. *JAMA* 254(1985): 2463–2466, 2653–2656.
25. Irby, D. M., Fantel, J. I., Milam, S. D., and Schwarz, M. R. Faculty Rights and Responsibilities in Evaluating and Dismissing Medical Students — A Legal Perspective. *J. College and Univ. Law.* 8(1981): 102–119.
26. Milam, S. D., and Marshall, R. D. Impact of Regents of the University of Michigan v. Ewing on Academic Dismissals from Graduate and Professional Schools. *J. College & University Law.* 13(1987):335–352.
27. Irby, D. M., and Milam, S. D. The Legal Context for Evaluating and Dismissing Medical Students and Residents. *Acad. Med.* 64(1989):639–643.
28. City of Richmond V. Croson, 109 S. Ct. 706 (1989).
29. Bergstrom v. Buettner, 697 F.Supp. 1098 (D. N.D. 1987) at 1102.
30. Morgan, D. Liability for Medical Education. *J. Legal Med.* 8(1987):305–338.

Cases Cited

Alevy v. Downstate Medical Center, 348 NE2d 537 (NY 1976).
Baker v. Bd. of Regents of State of Kansas, 721 FSupp 270 (D Ka 1989).
Beilis v. Albany Medical College of Union University, 525 NYS2d 932 (NY AD3 Dept 1988).
Bergstrom v. Buettner, 697 FSupp 1098 (D ND 1987).
Board of Curators of the University of Missouri v. Horowitz, 98 SCt 948 (1978).
Cannon v. University of Chicago, 559 F2d 1063 (6th Cir 1976).
Carl v. Board of Regents of University of Oklahoma, 577 P2d 912 (Okla 1978).
Chism v. University of Kansas, College of Health Sciences & Hosp., 699 P2d 43 (Ka 1985).
Christensen v. Des Moines Still College of O & S, 82 NW2d 741 (Ia 1957).
Connelly v. University of Vermont & State Agr. College, 244 FSupp 156 (DC Vt 1965).
Corso v. Creighton University, 731 F2d 529 (8th Cir 1984).
Demarco v. University of Health Sciences/Chicago Medical School, 352 NE2d 356 (Ill App 1976).
Depperman v. University of Kentucky, 371 FSupp 73 (DC Ky 1974).
Doe v. New York University, 666 F2d 761 (2nd Cir 1981).
Eiland v. Wolf, 764 SW2d 827 (Tex App 1 Dist 1989).
Evans v. West Virginia Bd. of Regents, 271 SE2d 778 (WVa 1980).
Gehling v. St. George's University School of Medicine, 705 FSupp 761 (ED NY 1989).
Giles v. Howard University, 428 FSupp 603 (DC DC 1977).
Greenhill v. Bailey, 519 F2d 5 (8th Cir 1975).
Hall v. Medical College of Ohio at Toledo, 742 F2d 299 (6th Cir 1984).
Heisler v. New York Medical College, 449 NYS2d 834 (1982).
Hines v. Rinker, 667 F2d 699 (8th Cir 1981).

Lewis v. Russe, 713 FSupp 1227 (ND Ill 1989).

Maitland v. Wayne State Medical School, 257 NW2d 197 (Mi Ap 1977).

Matter v. Levy, 450 NYS2d 574 (NYAD 1982).

McDonald v. Hogness, 598 P2d 707 (Wash 1979).

Militana v. University of Miami, 236 So2d 162 (Fla App 1970).

Moire v. Temple University School of Medicine, 613 FSupp 1360 (DC Pa 1985).

Mustell v. Rose, 211 So2d 489 (Ala 1968).

North v. State, 400 NW2d 566 (Ia 1987).

North v. West Virginia Bd. of Regents, 332 SE2d 141 (WVa 1985).

North v. West Virginia Bd. of Regents, 233 SE2d 411 (WVa 1977).

Parker v. Downing, 547 So.2d 1180 (Ala. Civ. App. 1988).

Patti Ann H. v. New York Medical College, 453 NYS2d 196 (NYAD 1982).

People v. Board of Trustees of University of Illinois, 134 NE2d 635 (Ill App 1 Dist 1956).

Petition of Johnson, 114 NW2d 255 (Mich 1962).

Petock v. Thomas Jefferson University, 630 FSupp 187 (ED Pa 1986).

Pride v. Howard University, 384 A2d 31 (DC App 1978).

Regents of University of California v. Bakke, 98 SCt 2733 (1978).

Regents of the University of Michigan v. Ewing, 106 SCt 507 (1985).

Reimer v. Tien, 514 A2d 566 (Pa Super 1986).

Sanders v. Ajir, 555 FSupp 240 (DC Wisc 1983).

Selman v. Harvard Medical School, 494 FSupp 603 (DC NY 1980).

Sofair v. State University of New York Upstate Medical Center, College of Medicine, 406 NYS2d 276 (NY 1978).

Steinberg v. Chicago Medical School, 354 NE2d 586 (Ill App 1976).

Stevens v. Hunt, 646 F2d 1168 (6th Cir 1981).

Stoller v. College of Medicine, 562 FSupp 403 (MD Pa 1983).

Turner v. Rush Medical College, 537 NE2d 890 (Ill App 1 Dist 1989).

Watson v. University of South Alabama College of Medicine, 463 F.Supp. 522 (DC 1979).

Williams v. Howard University, 528 F2d 658 (DC Circ 1976).

Wong v. Regents of University of California, 93 Cal Rptr 502 (Cal App 1971).

Methods of Student/ Clinical Site Placement

Ways of Thinking

Enhancing Clinical Decision Making Through Student Self-selection of Clinical Education Experiences

Becky Wojcik, MHPE, PT
Jean Rogers, MA, PT

In some physical therapy education programs, students select clinical experiences rather than being assigned to experiences by the academic coordinator of clinical education (ACCE). Many parallels can be drawn between the process students use to select clinical experiences and the decision-making process clinicians use to manage patient problems or administrative situations. This paper will identify the similarities in the processes used to make these decisions, discuss the process of student clinical education site decisions, discuss the process of student clinical education site selection used in one entry-level program, and present a rationale for using selection of clinical education sites by students as a strategy for enhancing clinical decision making.

The process of selecting clinical education sites for a student's curriculum is similar to the process used to manage patient problems or administrative issues in clinical practice. Resources often are limited, information must be gathered from various sources, and decisions must be made within defined parameters. The time available for making decisions and prioritizing goals frequently is limited. Assessment of needs also is a crucial component in the decision-making processes used in clinical education site selection, patient management, and administration.

Students in the entry-level curriculum at Northwestern University Medical School Programs in Physical Therapy select four full-time clinical experiences. After being randomly ordered, students assess their individual resources for meeting basic needs during clinical experiences. Students are informed of university requirements for the type and duration of clinical experiences. They review materials that clinical facilities submit for accreditation purposes and other descriptive information including facility brochures, student manuals, and information about the locale. Recommendations about housing and transportation made by students with experience at the facilities are available. Students consult with the ACCEs, other faculty, peers, and significant others as they consider their decision. During individual meetings with the ACCEs, potential matches between the student's and facilities' resources and expectations are discussed.

Varying degrees of skill are noted in accessing and interpreting information, identifying resources, prioritizing goals, weighing options, and managing multiple decisions simultaneously. Conflictual and cooperative interactions with peers increase as students vie for resources. Students also grapple with procedural time constraints and the reality of limited resources. It is hypothesized that students' commitments to clinical facilities are greater with this selection process than if the student's clinical experiences are assigned by the ACCE.

Because the components of the decision-making process used in selecting clinical education sites are similar to those used in patient management and administrative decision making, student selection of clinical education sites may facilitate clinical and administrative problem solving. Students may practice skills in accessing multiple sources of information and interpreting that information in light of prioritized goals. Self-assessment of resources and consultation with others can be encouraged. Skill in managing complex, interrelated decisions given time and resource constraints may be developed. Student self-selection of clinical education experiences may enhance clinical and administrative decision making.

Reprinted with permission from the *Journal of Physical Therapy Education*, Vol 6, No 2, p 60, 1992.

Review of Computerized Matching Program to Assign Physical Therapy Students to Clinical Placements

Richard Ladyshewsky, MHSc, BMR, PT

ABSTRACT: Managing and administrating a clinical education program is a detailed and complicated task, considering the magnitude of assigning large numbers of students to placements. Some of the variables involved are the learning needs of students, their previous placement histories, their place of residence and proximity to placement agencies, and the number and type of available placements within a specified region. This article describes a specific software program (Computer Assisted Student Placement, Evaluation, and Review [CASPER]) designed to manage this administrative task. The properties of the software's database management system are presented, along with the administrative implications for academic coordinators of clinical education, placement agencies, and students.

INTRODUCTION

Assigning students to clinical placements often is a cumbersome and detailed task of the academic coordinator of clinical education (ACCE) throughout the academic year. This task involves planning, selecting, arranging, and evaluating placements while considering the requirements of students, facilities, universities, and professional associations.[1] The ability of ACCEs to meet these tasks and requirements throughout the course of the clinical program is an ongoing challenge, particularly in light of the current acute shortage of placements.

A review of the literature demonstrated that several allied health care programs now use specific computer applications to administrate clinical education placements.[1-6]

At the time of this study, Mr Ladyshewsky was Senior Tutor and University Coordinator, Clinical Education, Division of Physical Therapy, Department of Rehabilitation Medicine, University of Toronto, 256 McCaul St, Toronto, Ontario, Canada M5T 1W5. Address correspondence to the author at 403 Riverton Ave, Winnipeg, Manitoba, Canada R2L ON6.

Through the use of customized computer software, administration of a clinical program can be streamlined and made more efficient. A placement matching system that can handle large volumes of information, store it in an organized manner and allow rapid access, permit sorting and recombination of information, and provide a mechanism for adding to this information would be ideal.[2]

Other desired attributes of a computerized matching system are that it be "user friendly," provide descriptive information about students and clinical facilities, outline the availability of clinical placements, and use a matching strategy that is fair and equitable. The ACCE also should be able to override assignments if any special considerations exist. Statistical summaries and reports also should be part of the computer program to ensure administrative efficiency. For example, reports on the distribution and mix of placements as well as reports on the availability of unused placements throughout the university's affiliated agencies would be extremely useful to an ACCE.

BACKGROUND

The Department of Physical Therapy at the University of Toronto offers a Bachelor of Science Degree in Physical Therapy. It is a 4-year program enrolling 66 students per year. Throughout the course of the program, each student is expected to complete a total of 31 weeks of full-time clinical practice in several separate placements. The ACCE, therefore, must organize over 460 different placements annually. Every student is required to complete one placement in each of the following areas before graduation: (1) acute care/general medicine, (2) outpatient orthopaedics, (3) neurology, (4) cardiorespirology, (5) community care, (6) long-term care/gerontology, and (7) selective placement chosen by the student. Most students are assigned to a different facility for each of the seven placements.

The Department of Physical Therapy is fortunate to have 85 different facilities affiliated with its program. These facilities are located across metropolitan Toronto, in adjacent cities and suburbs, and in more isolated communities in central and northern Ontario. These facilities or agencies are varied enough to allow students to complete their requirements.

COMPUTER-ASSISTED PLACEMENT, EVALUATION, AND REVIEW

The information system used to administer the Department's clinical program is the Computer Assisted Student Placement, Evaluation, and Review (CASPER) program. CASPER originally was developed by the Canadian Association of Occupational Therapists with FAST Microconsulting Limited* in 1986 to administer the association's national placement program that assigns occupational therapy students to placements across Canada. CASPER subsequently was modified and tested in 1988–1989 by the University of Toronto Department of Physical Therapy and FAST Microconsulting Limited to meet specific requirements for Ontario physical therapy programs. The CASPER system now is used in 7 of the 13 physical therapy programs in Canada and in 3 of the 12 occupational therapy programs.

System Methodology

CASPER is a menu-driven system, which makes it user friendly. It functions with a system of codes established by the user. The codes are used to categorize variables such as placement specialty, student's home university, regions within a catchment area, and accreditation status of the teaching facility. The codes are not fixed and can be preset by the ACCE to reflect the unique nature of each academic program.

*FAST Microconsulting Limited, 274 Prince Edward Dr, Toronto, Ontario, Canada M8Y 3X9.

Figure 1
Codes used to describe placement type and area of therapy. These can be altered according to program requirements.

CONSTANTS MASTER FILE (MAINTENANCE)

TYPE OF THERAPY CODES

A	ADULT ACUTE	O	
B	PEDIATRIC ACUTE	P	ADULT MIX - PSYCH
C	PEDIATRIC REHABILITATION	R	ADULT REHABILITATION
D	PEDS. LONG TERM CARE(LTC)	S	ADULT REHAB/LTC
E	PEDIATRICS ACUTE AND REHAB	T	
F	PEDS. REHAB AND LTC	U	
G	PEDS. ACUTE AND LTC	V	
H	PEDS. ACUTE REHAB - LTC	W	
I		X	ADULT ACUTE/LTC
J	PEDS. AND ADULT REHAB.	Y	
K		Z	ADULT ACUTE/REHAB LTC
L	ADULT LONG TERM CARE		
M	ADULT ACUTE AND REHAB.		
N			

AREA OF THERAPY CODES

A	AMPUTEES	O	OUTPATIENT ORTHOPAEDICS
B	BURNS	P	VARIETY OF CONDITIONS
C	CARDIORESPIROLOGY	R	RHEUMATOLOGY
D	DAY HOSPITAL NEUROLOGY	S	SPORTS INJURIES
E	NEUROSURGERY	T	TRAUMA
F	PLASTICS	U	CARDIORESPIROLOGY ICU
G	GERIATRICS	V	DAY HOSPITAL
H	HOME CARE	W	NEUROLOGY/NEUROSURGERY
I	INPATIENT ORTHOPAEDICS	X	GENERAL MEDICINE
J	STEPDOWN UNIT/CARDIORESP.	Y	ONCOLOGY/PALLIATIVE CARE
K	CARDIAC REHABILITATION	Z	UNKNOWN
L	NEUROSURGICAL ICU		
M	PULMONARY REHABILITATION		
N	NEUROLOGY		

Depending on the size of an academic program and the number of affiliations it has, CASPER setup involves entering information about each affiliated facility and the codes that will run the system. This setup time only occurs once, but it involves some preplanning to determine which codes to use. Creating an address file for the facility, along with one or two paragraphs of descriptive text, and entering the placements offered by the facility are the only other data entry required.

Hardware/Software Specifications

The CASPER program requires an IBM™ compatible computer[†] running DOS and a

[†]IBM Corporation, Boca Raton, FL 33432.
[‡]Wordperfect Corp. 288 W. Center St, Orem, Utah 84057.

dot-matrix printer. Required software is the CASPER program and Wordperfect™ (WP) 5.1.[‡] The database functions of CASPER are written in COBOL, a programming language, which manages the bulk of the matching process and stores all codes and files to run the system. The CASPER program operates with the WP 5.1 component, the latter storing the descriptive text information about each agency and the student placement history. This integrative function between CASPER and WP 5.1 allows the ACCE, for example, to retrieve student files stored in WP text while working within the CASPER database. The ACCE can review previous student placement assignments on-line while deciding where to place the student.

The student history file is stored in a WP 5.1 file. This file records all previous placements each student has had during his or her

studies. Because this file is stored in WP 5.1, the ACCE also can enter text about the student's performance in a specific placement. Information on previous placements is entered automatically into the student's file at the end of each academic year by running a year-end backup. This year-end backup clears all existing placement assignments from the CASPER system, allowing the ACCE to reuse them for the next academic year.

Software Menus

Facility record A. The facility record A is the main file of information about each specific agency. The agency's address, names of contact people, descriptive information about the agency, and codes indicating accreditation status are stored in this record. When this record is created, the facility is assigned a five-digit code by the ACCE according to the regional layout of the academic program's placement distribution area. The first digit of the code is an alphabetic or numeric reference and reflects region. Thirty-six regional distributions can be accommodated. The next two digits (numeric) represent cities or towns within that region. Up to 99 communities can be assigned per region. The last two digits (numeric) are specific to the agencies within that region and community. Up to 99 agencies can be assigned a code per community within a specific region. This coding format allows CASPER to store a considerable number of facilities within its system ($36 \times 99 \times 99 = 352,836$).

Facility record B. Facility record B is a separate file from record A. Record B is used solely to enter the placement information specific to each agency. When this record is created for an agency, it is given the same five-digit code as in facility record A, so that the contact name and address information is the same on each record. For example, the file for hospital 11111 that was created originally in record A would be the same number used in creating record B.

The area and type of therapy of the actual placement is entered by the ACCE using a system of codes that reflects the needs of the specific program. An example of a coding system used by the Department of Physical Therapy at the University of Toronto is shown in Figure 1. These codes are entered directly onto facility record B, as illustrated in Figure 2. The remaining codes used in setting up record B specify the dates for each placement session, the level of the student, the language requirement for the placement, and the number of placements available. A message section also is available to further describe details of the placement.

Figure 2

File used to maintain the registry of placements for a specific agency. Type code=type of therapy (Fig. 1); area code =area of therapy; sess code=session (eg, 1=January 1–31); lang code=preferred language; pos code=number of placements available in that particular session.

Service 11111   General Hospital

Jane Smith
Manager, Physiotherapy Service
General Hospital
100 Main Street
Toronto, Ontario   Last Updated 12/12/91 at 15:13

	Type	Session	Language		Message
	Area		Level	Positions	
1.	R	I	1	4	E	1	Inpatient Ortho. eg. THR
2.	R	O	2	4	E	2	Outpatient Ortho.
3.	A	N	2	4	E	1	Neurology eg. CVA, Head Injury
4.	A	G	3	3	E	1	Gerontology - Activation Unit

Figure 3

Agency summary sheet illustrating demographic data, descriptive information about programs and services, and listing of placements and student assignments. This report was developed using information from facility records A and B.

University of Toronto
Department of Physical Therapy

FACILITY 11111 General Hospital   Printed on 10/11/92

General Hospital   Jane Smith
100 Main Street   Manager, Physiotherapy Service
Toronto, Ontario
M5Y 1X5   CONTACT
Attn: Physiotherapy Dept.   John Doe
                             Centre Coord. Clinical Ed
                             PHONE (416) 555-5555, ext. 123
                             FAX (416) 555-4444

Catchment Area = University of Toronto

General Hospital is a 200-bed general treatment center catering to the needs of a multi-cultural area in the heart of Toronto. Programs within the hospital include: general surgery (25) beds, general medicine (50) beds, orthopedics (20), obstetrics and gynecology (30), pediatrics (15), chronic care (30), and rehabilitation (30).

Special physical therapy programs: prenatal program, fracture clinic, hydrotherapy, back wellness program, and sports clinic.
Staffing: 1 manager, 2 senior therapists, 6 full-time therapists, 2 physical therapist assistants.

Type		Session		Language		Message
	Area		Level		Positions	
R	I	1	4	E	1	Inpatient orthopaedics (eg, THR) (TO-4) Frank Peters
R	O	2	4	E	2	Outpatient orthopaedics (TO-4) Sharon Brown (TO-4) John Green
A	N	2	4	E	1	Neurology (eg, CVA, HI) (TO-4) Tina Washington

After data entry, most of the information from facility records A and B are merged to produce a placement database sheet (Figure 3). This sheet is shared between facilities and students in planning placement assignments.

Student record. The student record includes information specific to the student such as name, university affiliation, student identification number, and level within the program. The student's placement requests are entered in this file. Students make their requests from a directory listing all of the placements offered for a specific session. The directory is generated by CASPER and is developed using the placements offered by the various agencies for that particular session.

Each student may make up to five requests per session. This information is entered into his or her file with any important information that may affect the placement assignment. When the student record is created for a particular session, a number from 1 to 9999 is assigned randomly to the student's file by the computer. This number is the student's lottery number and is the basis on which CASPER matches a student to a particular placement. An example of the student's placement request file is shown in Figure 4.

Matching Process

In preparation for running the matching program, all students complete a form indicating their top five placement choices for a particular session. Students obtain placement information from a catalog printed out by CASPER that lists all placement options in various agencies. Students then submit their choices to the ACCE, and a separate file for each student is created in the CASPER system.

After all students requests are entered into the system, the ACCE runs the matching program. CASPER assigns placements during the matching process on a student-by-student basis. As described earlier, each student automatically is assigned a random number when his or her placement requests are initially entered into a file. The student with the lowest random number for that particular session has his or her placement requests processed first. The student with the second lowest number then would have his or her placement requests processed, and so on until the last student. If two or more students request the same placement, the student with the lowest number receives the placement.

The matching process attempts to place students within one of their five selected placements. The system continues down the student's list of choices until a match is made. During the process, the student's choice for "type of therapy" and "area of therapy" are considered. If no match is found for the student during this first run, CASPER then looks at different options using the information stored in the student's file (eg, a similar type of placement in a different facility within the student's preferred city). If this review does not result in a match, CASPER searches for a placement in any city in the region specified by the student. If a student does not receive a placement assignment, the system indicates that there is no match for this student, and the ACCE assigns the student at that time.

This process ensures a fair and equitable process for students and allows the ACCE to remain at "arm's length" from the matching process. The ACCE, however, can override the matching process for a specific student by placing the student in a specific agency before the matching process is initiated or by altering assignments after the matching process has been completed.

Reporting Functions

When the matching process has been completed, the ACCE can generate a report from the computer listing all students and their placements for the various sessions. The ACCE then can post this list for students to record their placement assignments. A copy of each agency's student assignment list also is generated by the computer and mailed to the agency by the ACCE. This report matches the information sheet reviewed by students as part of the placement directory except that the names of students assigned to each placement appear as part of the agency's summary sheet (Fig. 3).

One of the most useful reports generated by CASPER is a list of unused placements. This provides the ACCE with a current summary of available placements should a student's placement be canceled later. The other report that CASPER generates is a list of all placements by area, type, and session. This report is very useful in planning the administration of the selection process. For example, if students must complete a neurology placement and this report lists 44 neurology placements spread over two sessions (22 in each session), you can stratify your student population of 40 into two groups. One group (n=20) must select its neurology placement in the first session, and the other group (n=20) must select its neurology placement in the second session. This ensures that your match runs smoothly by allowing you to spread your distribution of placements across the student population.

Figure 4
Student placement request file illustrating the student's name and number (890473881), random number assignment (9952), five placement requests, and the actual placement assignment after the matching process was completed.

Identification TO Smith D 2 University of Toronto # 890473881

Student Given Name   Debbie
            Surname   Smith
            University   Toronto

Level   4   Language   E

Assigned Number   9952

Last Updated   21/06/93
Auto Placed   21/06/93
Manually Placed   / /

	Region	City	Facility	Type	Area	Session	
1.	1	00	16	R	N	2	Downtown Hospital
2.	1	00	26	R	N	2	Queen Elizabeth Centre
3.	1	00	38	A	W	2	General Hospital
4.	1	00	34	A	E	2	Main Street Hospital
5.	2	00	15	R	G	2	North Toronto Hospital

PLACED
1	00	26	R	N	2		Queen Elizabeth Centre

Stroke Unit Rehabilitation

RESULTS

The CASPER system has been used by the ACCE of the Department of Physical Therapy at the University of Toronto for 3 years. The time requirements to enter the data, run the match, and review the assignments were audited by the ACCE for fourth-year placements for the 1992–1993 academic year. Every fourth-year student must complete three placements in the final year of the program. Of a total of 183 placements, 85% of the students received one of their five choices for all three sessions. Thirteen percent of the students received one of their five choices for two of three sessions. Two percent of the students received one of their five choices for only one session.

The overall assignment rate was considered acceptable, given that all students had to complete one musculoskeletal, one cardiorespirology, and one neurology placement. These latter two placement specialties traditionally are in short supply in the catchment area. CASPER was, for the most part, able to efficiently accommodate most student requests according to their five choices. An adequate number and distribution of placements stored within the CASPER database, of course, is necessary to ensure that all students receive an assignment.

CASPER allocates students only to placements listed in the system. It can, however, manage the administrative aspects of the matching process far more efficiently and accurately than an ACCE. For example, prior to the implementation of CASPER, organization of the placement inventory and manual assignment of the fourth-year students to placements often required 150 to 200 hours of ACCE time. The actual nature of the task has not changed over the years. With the implementation of CASPER, however, the total amount of time spent by the ACCE to organize senior placements during the 1992–1993 academic year (n=183) was only 16.5 hours. This included meeting students as a group to explain the coding and selection process, revising the previous year's placements, entering student's requests, running the matching process, and reviewing/editing the matches. This encompassed approximately 5.4 minutes of administrative time per placement. The total time spent by the ACCE to complete data entry and to run the match was 4 hours, or 1.5 minutes per placement.

DISCUSSION

CASPER allows the ACCE to maximize all placement options in a fairly extensive region while ensuring that students have some input in their clinical program. The CASPER system allows the ACCE to objectively assign placements to students. The lottery method ensures that the process is fair and equitable. Most importantly, the system frees time for the ACCE to engage in other academic initiatives, such as program evaluation and teaching.

The information maintained within the system has been useful in preparing reports measuring the contribution of each facility to the program. For example, the CASPER system stores the total number of placements provided by facilities as well as each facility's staff complement. Using this information, the ACCE produced a report outlining each facility's contribution compared with other affiliated agencies. The measure used across all facilities is the number of offered placements to the number of clinical staff. A facility offering 10 placements a year with five staff would have a 2:1 student-to-staff ratio. Another facility may offer 15 placements annually with a staff complement of 10. They would have a 1.5:1 student-to-staff ratio.

The process of updating placements each academic year is expedited, because each facility reviews its commitment from the previous year and returns any changes to the ACCE. Descriptions of programs and services within each agency also are revised at this time by making changes within the CASPER system. These updates require very little time and typically involve minor adjustments to the number/type of placement offered, altering a message description, or adding a new placement. The facility's descriptive text may require updates as programs or services change. Updating the data ensures that students receive current information about each facility.

CONCLUSION

Use of a computerized matching system for physical therapy student clinical education placements ensures a high rate of successful matching and administrative efficiency. Most students in this operational review of CASPER received one of their five choices for each of their three placement sessions. This was accomplished, in part, by having enough placements in the system to match the students, but the real advantage was the short amount of time it took CASPER to manage this process.

ACKNOWLEDGMENT

The author thanks the Ministry of Health of Ontario, Canada, for its support of this project.

REFERENCES

1. Polatajko H, Ernest M, MacKinnon J. Computerized fieldwork data base: applications and implications. *Canadian Journal of Occupational Therapy.* 1987;54:263–267.

2. Van Swearingen JM. Systematic clinical placement of physical therapy students. *Phys Ther.* 1987;67:394–398.

3. Carey JC, Ellingham C, Chen Y. Computer-based solution to a clinical education problem in a physical therapy course. *Phys Ther.* 1986;66:1725–1729.

4. Duffield C, Donoghue J. Using the computer for clinical placements. *The Australian Nurses Journal.* 1986;15:44–45,57.

5. Hawkins JM, Hawkins B. Clinical placements by computer program. *Am J Occup Ther.* 1978;32:390–394.

6. Dennis JK, May BJ. Computer-assisted student clinical placements. *Journal of Physical Therapy Education.* 1990;4:87–92.

RESEARCH REPORTS

ARTICLES

Investigating the Fairness of the National Resident Matching Program

YUFEI YUAN, Ph.D., and AMIRAM GAFNI, D.Sc.

Abstract—The National Resident Matching Program (NRMP) was established in the early 1950s to bring order and fairness to a previously chaotic application process for internship and residency positions. Over the years many reservations were raised about the fairness of the process, specifically, that hospital programs are doing better than students are (i.e., programs obtain preferred residents more often than students receive preferred programs). This paper presents an analysis of the results of the 1986 Match. The findings do not support the claim that the results of the Match are biased in a way that favors programs. Overall, the students' success was greater (i.e., receiving on average higher-ranked choices) than was the hospital programs' success. In fact, in 20 of 22 specialty programs, the students' degree of success was greater than or equal to the success of the programs. This finding raises the question of fairness toward programs rather than students. The authors analyze factors that affected both the hospitals' and the students' degrees of success in the 1986 Match and suggest strategies for improving the Match results. *Acad. Med.* 65(1990):247–253.

The National Resident Matching Program (NRMP) was established in the early 1950s to bring order and fairness to a previously chaotic application process for internship and residency positions.[1,2] In brief, from the turn of the century until 1945, the competition by hospitals for interns and residents manifested itself in a race to sign employment contracts earlier and earlier in medical students' careers. In some cases students were subjected to direct pressure from programs and were forced to decide prematurely. The adoption of a centralized matching mechanism seemed to resolve most of these problems.

The NRMP requires each of the participants (students and hospital program directors) to supply a rank-order list of preferences. Based on these rank-order lists, a computerized algorithm is used to assign the students to hospital positions. The assignment algorithm used is described in general terms in the NRMP directory[3] and is equivalent to the one described by Gale and Shapley.[4] The use of the algorithm provides a "stable solution," namely, the outcome of the matching process is such that after the Match, there exists no student and hospital program (who are not assigned to each other) who would *both* prefer each other to their assigned partners.

In spite of this theoretically stable solution, many reservations were raised during the years about the fairness of the NRMP process. For example, some said that residency program directors understand the Match system better (stemming from past experience resulting from participating in many Matches) and thus are able to receive better students because they know which ones to rank higher[5]; that due to lack of satisfaction with the "official" program (NRMP), "unofficial" arrangements have appeared[6]; that there is dishonesty in some recruitment interviews from program directors[7]; and that the current computer algorithm treats students and programs unequally in a way that favors programs.[8]

Nevertheless, the NRMP has been praised as an equitable system of residency matching. Some proponents insist that it is a far fairer system than the routine admission-rejection system used by colleges, medical schools, or other schools.[9] Since most complaints indicate a bias in favor of hospital programs, it is important to examine whether the criticism is supported by evidence. In this paper we present an analysis of the results of the 1986 NRMP.

Method

The data about the hospital programs and students who participated in the 1986 Match were provided to us by the NRMP with special permission. Unless otherwise stated, "student" is being used as a general term for all the types of applicants: U.S. senior students, U.S. citizens who are graduates of foreign medical schools, and others. In order to keep the data confidential, the students' and hospitals' names were omitted. In addition, the students' and programs' identifications were reformulated so they could

Dr. Yuan is assistant professor, Area of Management Science and Information Systems, Faculty of Business, and Dr. Gafni is associate professor, Centre for Health Economics and Policy Analysis, Department of Clinical Epidemiology and Biostatistics, Faculty of Health Sciences; both at McMaster University, Hamilton, Ontario, Canada.

Correspondence and requests for reprints should be sent to Dr. Gafni, Department of Clinical Epidemiology and Biostatistics, Room 2C12A, McMaster University, Health Sciences Centre, 1200 Main Street West, Hamilton, Ontario, Canada L8N 3Z5.

not be recognized.

The data were organized in three files: the students' ranking file, the hospital programs' ranking file, and the Match result file. The students' ranking file provided ranking information about all the students who participated in the Match. Each record consisted of the student's identification, programs listed by the student, the rank assigned to the student, whether the student was a U.S. senior, whether he or she was part of a couple for matching, and whether the student was active in the Match (that is, did not withdraw from the Match process). Similar information for the hospital programs is found on the hospital programs' ranking file. Each record consisted of the hospital program's identifications, the type of program (specialty), the students listed by the program, the ranks assigned to them, the number of positions offered, and the number of positions filled. The Match result file provided information about all the Match pairs (the programs and the assigned students), the unmatched students, and the unfilled positions.

The analysis consisted of three tasks: (1) To compare the students' and the hospitals' Match successes; (2) to identify factors that affected the hospitals' Match success; and (3) to identify factors that affected the students' Match success.

To compare the students' success with the hospitals' success we calculated the mean value and standard deviation of the program's rank for the matched student and the student's rank for the matched position. Hospital programs have different quotas. Thus, for a student to be ranked as the third candidate by a hospital program that offers only one position is not the same as being ranked third candidate by a hospital program that offers ten positions. Therefore, to make meaningful comparisons, we standardized the rank order by using the following strategy: the rankings submitted by a hospital program were divided into subgroups. The size of each subgroup was equal to the number of positions (quota) offered by that program. Thus, the first

subgroup consisted of a number of students — equal to the quota of that hospital program — who were ranked highest on its list. This subgroup was considered the "standardized first choice." Similarly, the students in the second-highest ranking subgroup were considered the "standardized second choice," and so on. For example, if a program's quota were five, the first- to the fifth-ranked students listed by the program would be considered the "standardized first choice" students for its five positions. The sixth- to the tenth-ranked students would be considered the "standardized second choice" students, and so on. Notice that by using this method, we assumed that (1) all positions offered by a hospital program were identical, and (2) all candidates in each subgroup were equally favorable for all the positions of the hospital program. In other words, if the hospital filled some positions with candidates from the first-choice subgroup, this would be the same as filling one of these positions with a first-choice candidate, and so on.

We calculated the difference between the student's rank and the hospital program's rank (standardized) for each matched pair for the system as a whole (all specialties together) and for each specialty. We employed the t-test to find out whether the mean of the rank difference was zero for all specialties as a whole and for each specialty. Finally, we tried to ascertain whether the mean rank differences were affected by the size of the market and/or demand-supply relations for each program specialty. This was done by calculating the corresponding correlation coefficients.

The Match results are different for individual specialties. To identify the factors that affected individual programs' Match successes, we had to analyze the Match results within each specialty. To keep our study manageable, three program specialties were chosen: internal medicine, surgery, and obstetrics-gynecology. These specialties were selected because a large number of positions were offered to students in each of them. Also, as shown later, they represented three

different cases: one where the students' success in general was better than the hospital programs' success (internal medicine), one where there was no statistical difference between the students' and the programs' successes (obstetrics-gynecology), and one where programs' success in general was better than students' success (surgery).

In our analysis we used the filling rate and mean of each program's ranking to measure each program's success. The filling rate was defined as the ratio of the number of positions filled to the number of positions offered by a program. The mean of each program's ranking was the average of all the standardized program rank orders assigned to the students who were matched to that program. We concentrated mainly on those factors that were easy to measure and thus could be used most easily in practice to improve future success. We selected three factors as independent variables (possible factors affecting success): (1) the number of candidates listed per position, (2) the number of positions offered, and (3) the mean rank order assigned to the program by students who applied for the program. Pearson correlation coefficients between each program's success measures and the independent variables were calculated and a general linear model and F-distribution tests were used to test how these factors affected each program's success.

To identify the variables that affected the students' success, we considered only those students who were U.S. seniors, who applied for only one type of program (specialty), and were not a member of a couple participating in the Match. This subgroup was relatively homogenous and contained the majority of the students (about 70% of all applicants and 85% of all matched applicants). For the reasons previously mentioned, the analysis was carried out only for internal medicine, surgery, and obstetrics-gynecology (about 55% of all positions offered by all specialty programs).

To indicate a student's success or failure to obtain a position, we used a dichotomous variable, where 1 indi-

Table 1

Measurements of Students' and Programs' Successes in the 1986 Match*

Program Specialty†	Positions Filled	A/P Ratio	MPR Mean	MPR SD	MSR Mean	MSR SD	DIFF Mean	DIFF SD	p-value from t-Test
Specialties for which students' or programs' success is demonstrated									
Internal medicine	5,985	8.8	3.25	2.74	2.28	2.60	1.24	3.47	.0001
Anesthesiology	280	5.7	2.56	2.21	1.68	3.17	0.88	3.66	.0001
Pediatrics	1,723	9.0	2.95	2.33	2.22	2.05	0.74	2.72	.0001
Family practice	1,960	6.9	2.62	1.80	1.92	1.86	0.70	2.32	.0001
Radiology—diagnostic	390	8.4	2.79	2.08	2.31	1.94	0.47	2.49	.0002
Psychiatry	782	6.1	1.63	1.09	1.43	1.18	0.19	1.40	.0001
Orthopedic surgery	355	15.4	2.01	1.39	2.58	2.76	−0.57	2.76	.0001
Surgery	1,994	9.2	2.23	1.57	3.39	4.12	−1.15	4.06	.0001
Specialties for which students' or programs' success is not demonstrated									
Obstetrics-gynecology	974	11.2	2.76	2.02	2.95	3.71	−0.19	3.82	.1193
Transitional	1,022	7.0	2.44	0.25	2.34	0.16	0.10	0.26	.6577
Emergency medicine	280	11.2	2.18	1.18	2.23	2.05	−0.05	2.08	.6883
Pathology	276	5.7	1.82	1.23	1.78	2.49	0.04	2.58	.8154
Urology	77	1.7	1.04	1.82	1.03	2.67	0.01	2.90	.2854
Physical medicine and rehabilitation	74	8.2	2.00	1.48	2.39	2.87	−0.39	2.99	.2629
Otolaryngology	40	1.4	1.00	—	1.00	—	—	—	—
Neurology	29	1.6	1.10	0.31	1.07	0.37	0.03	0.33	.5728
Neurologic surgery	29	1.5	1.00	—	1.00	—	—	—	—
Ophthalmology	18	2.6	1.22	0.43	1.11	0.47	0.11	0.47	.3313
Radiology—therapeutic	14	4.4	1.29	0.61	1.21	0.58	0.07	0.27	.3356
Plastic surgery	6	16.8	1.17	0.41	1.50	0.84	−0.33	0.82	.3632
Preventive med/public health	5	8.6	1.60	0.89	2.20	1.30	−0.60	1.82	.5012
Dermatology	5	7.9	1.00	—	1.00	—	—	—	—
Overall	16,318	8.5	2.83	2.28	2.34	2.76	0.49	3.28	.0001

*The authors analyzed data provided to them by the National Resident Matching Program to determine whether the students or the hospitals' specialty programs had greater success in the 1986 Match and to identify the factors contributing to the success of each group. The means of the rankings presented in the table (in the MPR and MSR columns) indicate that for six of the eight specialty programs for which a group's success could be shown, the students had greater success than did the programs. (Note: higher ranks—meaning greater success—are shown by smaller numbers.)

†Data about the specialty programs from the 1986 Match are presented here in two groups: the top group comprises those specialty programs for which the mean difference between the program's rank and the student's rank for the matched pairs was found to be significantly different from zero; the bottom group comprises the specialty programs where this difference was not significantly different from zero. In the bottom group, there is no way to ascertain, from the available data, whether one group was more successful than the other for a given specialty program.

‡The column headings are defined as follows: positions filled = number of positions filled in each specialty program; A/P ratio = number of applications per number of positions available; MPR = the mean rank order assigned to matched students by the programs; MSR = the mean rank order assigned to programs by the students; DIFF = the mean difference between the program's rank and the student's rank for the matched pair.

cated a student who was matched to a position and 0 indicated one who was unmatched. The independent variables considered were the number of programs listed by the student and the highest standardized program rank assigned to the student by all programs that listed him or her. Pearson correlation coefficients between the three variables were calculated for the three specialties considered in this study. A general linear model and F-distribution tests were used to test the impact of those variables.

Results

In Table 1 we present and compare the measurements of the students' and the programs' successes in the 1986 Match for all the specialty programs considered in the Match process that year. The students' mean rank for the position to which he or she was assigned was 2.34 (SD = 2.76). The programs' mean rank for a student assigned to an available position was 2.83 (SD = 2.28). A t-test performed for pair comparison shows that the mean of the rank difference

is not zero ($p \leq .0001$). Notice that higher ranks are represented by smaller numbers; thus a smaller mean rank indicates better performance.

For Table 1 the different specialty programs were divided into two groups. The first group includes all programs where the mean difference between the program's rank and the student's rank for the matched pairs was found to be significantly different from zero. The second group includes the specialty programs where this difference was not found to be significantly different from zero. Notice

Table 2

Pearson Correlation Coefficients between Hospitals' Success Variables and Hospitals' Choice Variables, 1986 Match*

Choice Variable†	Success Variables,† by Specialty Program					
	Internal Medicine		Surgery		Obstetrics-Gynecology	
	FIL	MPR	FIL	MPR	FIL	MPR
CPR	.36770	.59637	.40585	.26764	.37676	.33335
Significance level‡	(.0001)	(.0001)	(.0001)	(.0001)	(.0001)	(.0001)
MSR	.06070	.18739	.02960	.21945	.02050	.10479
Significance level‡	(.1024)	(.0001)	(.5302)	(.0001)	(.7421)	(.1011)
QUOTA	.14821	−.00357	.10016	−.13264	.26564	−.22379
Significance level‡	(.0001)	(.9250)	(.0321)	(.00600)	(.0001)	(.0004)

*The authors analyzed data provided to them by the National Resident Matching Program to determine whether the students or the hospitals' specialty programs had greater success in the 1986 Match and to identify the factors contributing to the success of each group. The correlations of the data above show that in all three specialty programs, the filling rate (FIL) was affected most by the number of candidates listed per residency (CPR). Program size (QUOTA) seems to have been much less important. The students' evaluation of the program (MSR) does not seem to have affected the filling rate. (See the text for additional interpretations of these data and an evaluation of the explanatory power of the three variables.)

† The variables are defined as follows: FIL = filling rate; MPR = the mean rank order assigned to matched students by the programs; CPR = the number of candidates listed per position; MSR = the mean rank order assigned to programs by the students; QUOTA = the number of positions offered by a program.

‡ The numbers in parentheses show the significance level for testing (F-test) such that the coefficient = 0.

that in the first group, the students' success was greater than the programs' in six of the eight specialties. In two specialties (orthopedic surgery and surgery) the programs' success was greater.

Table 1 also contains information about the numbers of positions filled; these numbers can serve as indicators of the size of the market in 1986. We also present data on the ratio of the number of applications to the number of positions available in each program specialty. Notice that since every student could apply to more than one position, the number of applications was greater than the number of applicants (overall, the ratio of active applicants to positions in the 1986 Match was 1.1). We tried to explore whether differences in market size and/or the ability of programs to attract candidates (represented by the ratio of the number of applications to positions) could explain the differences in the mean ranking. No statistically significant relations were found between those variables and mean difference in ranking between matched programs and students.

Table 2 presents the results of our analysis of the three different variables (CPR, QUOTA, and MSR— defined below) that affected the hospital programs' success. An important finding is that in all three specialty programs, the filling rate was affected most by the number of candidates listed per residency position (CPR). This might indicate either the "aspiration level" of accepting a resident or the demand for the program, or both. Program size (QUOTA) seems to have been much less important. The applying students' evaluation of the program, measured by the students' average ranking (MSR), does not seem to have affected the filling rate. It is important to mention, however, that, based on a factor analysis using a general linear model, the explanatory power of these three variables together is about 40% in each of the three specialty programs ($R^2 = 0.383, 0.399, 0.392$ for internal medicine, surgery, and obstetrics-gynecology, respectively).

The effect of the three variables just mentioned on the hospital programs' satisfaction from the students they received (measured by the average ranks of the students matched— the MPR variable) is also presented in Table 2. Again, the number of students listed per position seems to have been an important variable, but with negative impact. However, it was much more important in the case of internal medicine, less so in the case of obstetrics-gynecology, and even less in the case of surgery. The students' evaluation of the program seems to have affected the programs' satisfaction with the students they received, while the size of the program (QUOTA) does not seem to have had any effect. This is different from the effects of these two variables on the filling rate. Using the same type of analysis, we found that, compared with the former analysis, the three variables presented in Table 2 represent only a smaller portion of the explained variance ($R^2 = 0.237, 0.167, 0.251$ for internal medicine, surgery, and obstetrics-gynecology, respectively).

The number of programs listed by the student was found to have been an important factor in determining his or her chance to find a position. It is interesting to note that this factor was more important for internal medicine ($R^2 = 0.371$) and obstetrics-gynecology ($R^2 = 0.350$) than for surgery ($R^2 = 0.183$). The evaluation of students by programs was also found to be an important factor, but less so than the variable just discussed in determining the chances of a student to find a position. This factor, like the one previously discussed, was more important for obstetrics-gynecology ($R^2 = −0.214$) and internal medicine ($R^2 = −0.194$) than for surgery ($R^2 = −0.135$). The significance level for rejecting (F = test) such that the coefficient equals zero was 0.0001 in all cases.

Table 3 further illustrates how the number of candidates per position af-

Table 3

Impact of the Number of Candidates Listed per Position (Offered by Internal Medicine Programs) on the Programs' Success in Having All Available Positions Filled by the 1986 Match*

Programs' Filling Rate†	Number of Candidates Listed per Position					Total and % All Programs§
	0–29 No., %'s of Programs‡	3–5.9 No., %'s of Programs‡	6–8.9 No., %'s of Programs‡	9–11.9 No., %'s of Programs‡	12 or More No., %'s of Programs‡	
0%	20 62.5% 22.7%	9 28.1% 4.1%	2 6.3% 1.1%	1 3.1% 1.0%	0 0.0% 0.0%	32 4.4%
10%	3 42.9% 3.4%	3 42.9% 1.4%	1 14.3% 0.6%	0 0.0% 0.0%	0 0.0% 0.0%	7 1.0%
20%	3 50.0% 3.4%	3 50.0% 1.4%	0 0.0% 0.0%	0 0.0% 0.0%	0 0.0% 0.0%	6 0.8%
30%	15 42.9% 17.1%	16 45.7% 7.3%	1 2.9% 0.6%	3 8.6% 3.1%	0 0.0% 0.0%	35 4.8%
40%	10 52.6% 11.4%	7 36.8% 3.2%	2 10.5% 1.1%	0 0.0% 0.0%	0 0.0% 0.0%	19 2.6%
50%	4 14.3% 4.6%	16 57.1% 7.3%	7 25.0% 3.9%	0 0.0% 0.0%	1 3.6% 0.7%	28 3.8%
60%	2 8.3% 2.3%	15 62.5% 6.3%	6 25.0% 3.4%	0 0.0% 0.0%	1 4.2% 0.7%	24 3.3%
70%	7 28.0% 8.0%	11 44.0% 5.0%	4 16.0% 2.2%	3 12.0% 3.1%	0 0.0% 0.0%	25 3.4%
80%	4 10.3% 4.6%	16 41.0% 7.3%	10 25.6% 5.6%	6 15.4% 6.1%	3 7.7% 2.1%	39 5.3%
90%	5 15.1% 5.7%	12 36.4% 5.5%	11 33.3% 6.2%	5 15.0% 5.1%	0 0.0% 0.0%	33 4.5%
100%	15 3.1% 17.1%	112 23.2% 50.9%	135 28.0% 75.4%	80 16.6% 81.6%	140 29.1% 96.6%	482 66.0%
Total and % all programs‖	88 12.1%	220 30.1%	179 24.5%	98 13.4%	145 19.8%	730 100.0%

* The authors analyzed data provided to them by the National Resident Matching Program to determine whether the students or the hospitals' specialty programs had greater success in the 1986 Match and to identify factors contributing to the success of each group. This table makes clear the observed trend that the more candidates a hospital listed for a specialty program position, the more likely was the position to be filled.

† The filling rate is the ratio between the number of positions filled and the number of positions offered by a program. In this table the programs are grouped by their filling rates, after these rates were rounded to the nearest 10%.

‡ The top value in each group of three values = the number of programs; the middle value = the percentage that this number of programs is of all the programs with the designated filling rate; and the bottom value = the percentage that this number of programs is of all the programs with the designated number of candidates listed per position. For example, in the top left group, there were 20 programs; this was 62.5% of the 32 programs with the filling rate of 0% and was 22.7% of the 88 programs that listed 0–2.9 candidates per position.

§ This is the total number of programs for the row (i.e., added horizontally), accompanied by the percentage that this number is of all the internal medicine programs studied.

‖ This is the total number of programs for the column (i.e., added vertically), accompanied by the percentage that this number is of all the internal medicine programs studied.

Table 4

Impact of the Number of Choices of Internal Medicine Programs That Students Made on the Students' Success in Being Matched to a Program by the 1986 Match*

Level of Students' Choice Matched	Number of Choices Listed by Students					Total and
	1–3	4–6	7–9	10–12	13 or More	
	No., %'s of Students†	No., %'s of Students†	No., %'s of Students†	No., %'s of Students†	No., %'s of Students†	No., %'s % All Students‡
1st	264 12.1% 52.9%	414 19.0% 66.8%	529 24.3% 57.3%	364 16.7% 50.8%	606 27.8% 47.4%	2,177 53.9%
2nd	27 3.8% 5.4%	87 12.4% 14.0%	188 26.7% 20.4%	167 23.7% 23.3%	235 33.4% 18.4%	704 17.4%
3rd	3 0.7% 0.6%	46 10.9% 7.4%	105 24.9% 11.4%	84 19.9% 11.7%	183 43.5% 14.3%	421 10.4%
4th	0 0.0% 0.0%	18 8.2% 2.9%	43 19.6% 4.7	44 20.1% 6.2%	114 52.1% 8.9%	219 5.4%
≥5th	0 0.0% 0.0%	7 3.0% 1.1%	44 19.0% 4.8%	50 21.6% 7.0%	131 56.5% 10.2%	232 5.8%
Unmatched	205 72.2% 41.1%	48 16.9% 7.7%	15 5.3% 1.6%	7 2.5% 1.0%	9 3.2% 0.7%	284 7.0%
Total and % all students§	499 12.4%	620 15.4%	924 22.9%	716 17.7%	1,278 31.7%	4,037 100.0%

*The authors analyzed data provided to them by the National Resident Matching Program to determine whether the students or the hospitals' specialty programs had greater success in the 1986 Match and to identify factors contributing to the success of each group. This table makes clear the observed trend that the more programs a student chose, the more likely was the student to be matched to a program.

†The top value in each group of three values = the number of students; the middle value = the percentage that this number of students is of all the students whose designated choice was matched; and the bottom value = the percentage that this number of students is of all the students who listed the designated number of program choices. For example, in the top left group, there were 264 students; this was 12.1% of the 2,177 students whose first choice was matched and was 52.9% of the 499 students who listed only one to three program choices.

‡This is the total number of students for the row (i.e., added horizontally), accompanied by the percentage that this number is of all the students who applied for internal medicine residency programs.

§This is the total number of students for the column (i.e., added vertically), accompanied by the percentage that this number is of all the students who applied for internal medicine residency programs.

fects the program's filing rate; here, we present more detailed data for one specialty, internal medicine. It is easy to see that those programs that did not fill any position—20 out of total of 32 (62.5%)—listed fewer than three candidates per position. The percentage of the programs that filled all positions in each group significantly increased when the number of candidates listed per position increased (from 17.1% for the first group, with fewer than three candidates per position, to 96.6% for the fifth group, with 12 or more candidates per position).

Table 4 further illustrates the impact of the number of choices on the student's match; here we present more detailed data for the case of the U.S. senior students who applied for internal medicine programs only. The table shows that for those students who listed three of fewer choices, 205 out of 499 (41.1%) were unmatched. However, for those students who listed ten choices or more, fewer than 1% were unmatched. It is clear that listing too few choices does involve a high risk of being unmatched, both from the program's side and from the student's side.

Discussion

Our analysis strongly suggests that the actual results of the 1986 Match do not favor programs, a finding that is contrary to the perception of many investigators[5-7] and to the theoretical argument that the algorithm used for the matching process is biased in favor of programs.[4,8] Overall, in our study, the students performed better than did the programs. Furthermore, the analysis of each specialty program shows that in the majority of cases (20 out of 22 cases) the students' performance was better than or at least as good as that of the programs. The analysis was performed only for the outcome of the 1986 Match; however, we have no reason to believe that 1986 was different from previous or subsequent years. In order to test our conclusion, the same type of data and analysis could be used for the results of the Match in other years.

The NRMP has been praised as an equitable system of residency matching. The two goals of adopting a centralized matching mechanism were to bring order and fairness to a chaotic application process for internship and residency positions. There is general agreement that the first goal was achieved. With respect to the second goal—fairness—the evidence indicates that improvement is still called for. An ideal situation would be that the students success would be equal to the programs' success and that no "sector" could, through superior analysis of publicly available information, through access to non-publicly-available information, or through any other mechanism, bring about superior performance. This issue is dealt with by the authors in more depth elsewhere.[10]

How else can we improve fairness in the system? Our findings in the present study do not supply the answer. We feel that a promising and practical way to reach this goal is to try to improve the assignment algorithm that is currently used. An example for such an effort to improve the algorithm by using the utility approach is described elsewhere by Mehrez and the present authors.[11]

Finally, we should notice that the matching algorithm, although being optimal in terms of stability,[2] does not guarantee to maximize the number expected to assign a student to a ber of matches, since no algorithm can position that is not mutually agreeable, as shown on the rank-order lists of both parties.[12] Every year we find that while some graduates fail to receive their internship positions, there are still vacancies in some hospitals. After the 1986 Match, for example, there were still 2,634 positions (14%) unfilled, and 5,221 graduates (24.4%) did not receive any position. Our analysis of the Match results suggests that for both the programs and students, listing more choices will increase their chances of finding a Match. Those who choose fewer programs could find themselves without a position in spite of their impression (which they might find to be wrong) of being highly ranked by a hospital where they had been interviewed.[7] The impact of the number of choices on the Match rate was also studied elsewhere by using computer simulation.[13] The results were similar to those presented in this paper.

Financial support for this study was provided by the National Resident Matching Program of the United States and the Natural Science and Engineering Research Council of Canada. The authors thank Dr. John S. Graettinger (who at the time of this study was executive vice president, NRMP) for his encouragement and valuable suggestions; Mr. E. Peranson and Mr. G. Spira (National Matching Service, Inc.), for providing NRMP data; and Dr. G. Norman for helpful suggestions. They also acknowledge the constructive comments made by three anonymous referees, which improved the quality of this paper.

References

1. Graettinger, J. S., and Peranson, E. The Matching Program. *N. Engl. J. Med.* **304**(1981):1163–1165.
2. Roth, A. E. The Evaluation of Labour Market for Medical Interns and Residents: A Case Study in Game Theory. *J. Political Economy* **92**(1984):991–1016.
3. *NRMP Directory.* Evanston, Illinois: National Resident Matching Program, 1980: 18–42.
4. Gale, D., and Shapley, S. L. College Admissions and the Stability of Marriage. *Am. Mathematical Monthly* **62**(1962): 9–15.
5. Martz, B. W. Residency Matching. *J. Med. Educ.* **58**(1983):498–499.
6. Polk, H. R. A Time for Reconsideration of Sequential Surgical Matching Programs. *Am. J. Surg.* **151**(1986):195–196.
7. Herman, T. A. Playing Fair in the NIRMP. *N. Engl. J. Med.* **302**(1979):1425.
8. Williams, K. J., Worth, V. P., and Wolff, J. A. An Analysis of the Resident Match. *N. Engl. J. Med.* **304**(1981):1165–1166.
9. Jordan, W. J. Success of Minority Applicants in the National Residency Matching Program. *J. Nat. Med. Assoc.* **78**(1986): 737–739.
10. Gafni, A., and Yuan, Y. Students' Performance vs Hospitals' Performance in the Labor Market for Medical Interns and Residents: Is the Market "Informationally Efficient"? *J. Health Econ.* **8**(1989): 353–360.
11. Mehres, A., Yuan, Y., and Gafni, A. Stable Solutions vs Multiplicative Utility Solutions for the Assignment Problem. *Operations Res. Lett.* **7**(1988):131–139.
12. Roth, A. E. On the Allocation of Residents to Rural Hospitals: A General Property of Two-Sided Matching Market. *Econometrica* **54**(1986):425–427.
13. Yuan, Y., and Kochen, M. Simulation of Matching under Incomplete Information. In *Proceedings of International ASME [Advancement of Modelling and Simulation Techniques in Enterprises] Conference*, pp 61–72. Williamsburg, Virginia: 1 (1986).

STUDENT
ISSUES IN
CLINICAL
EDUCATION

Recruitment/
Retention of
Physical
Therapy
Students

Minority Student Recruitment and Retention Strategies in Physical Therapy Education

Awilda R Haskins, EdD, PT
Colleen Rose-St Prix, MHSA, PT

ABSTRACT: The purpose of this study was to identify recruitment and retention strategies used by physical therapy education programs and to determine which interventions have increased the proportion of minority applicants, students, and graduates. The sample consisted of 22 physical therapy education programs. Data were collected with a questionnaire and a telephone interview. Results were analyzed using descriptive analysis and non-parametric tests of significance. Interventions found to be related to increasing the proportion of minority applicants or students were (1) talking to parent groups, (2) keeping in touch with minority students, and (3) assisting students in completing admissions applications. External funding appears to be related positively to minority student recruitment. Physical therapy programs in medical schools seem more successful in graduating minorities than do programs in schools of allied health.

INTRODUCTION

Minorities (African Americans, Hispanics, Asians, and Native Americans) are underrepresented in physical therapy as they are in other health professions, education, and the total work force.[1-7] Poverty, inadequate education, and racism have been cited as critical factors responsible for the underrepresentation of minorities throughout our society.[8-18]

Court decisions and legislative efforts have mandated that institutions of higher education correct the underrepresentation of minorities.[19-21] Institutions of higher education have attempted to do so through techniques

ranging from simple methods to comprehensive approaches[22-24] and by studying the institutional characteristics linked to minority student achievement.[25-27]

Efforts to correct the underrepresentation of minorities in the health professions include affirmative action programs and early-outreach programs.[28-32] The most successful early-outreach programs have been comprehensive, "shotgun" approaches that are expensive and require external funding. Recently, however, federal funding for minority programs has declined,[9,11,33] and programs receiving federal funds have been aimed disproportionately at medical schools and only rarely at other health professions like physical therapy.[1,34]

In the absence of federal or other external funding, we believe that physical therapy education programs tend to have few (if any) focused interventions for the recruitment, retention, and graduation of minority students. Successful, cost-effective strategies to recruit, retain, and graduate minorities in the health professions must be identified.

Purpose

The literature is replete with examples of regional, statewide, institutional, and programmatic models of minority student recruitment and retention programs, but there is concern regarding the evaluation of these programs.[22,35-36] The lack of validation of these programs is compounded by the diversity of program components found from college to college and from program to program.[37-38]

Few research studies exist to indicate which components of a comprehensive recruitment and retention program are the most effective, particularly when considering cost, time, and effort. For example, while it is commonplace for recruitment efforts to focus on visiting high schools with a high proportion of minority students, the authors found no research indicating that this strategy is any more effective than summer seminars that introduce students to the health professions or than activities such as pre-athletic health screenings of high school athletes as a means

of providing students with contact with health professionals and exposure to health care fields.

The purpose of this study was to identify the techniques used by physical therapy education programs to recruit, enroll, and graduate more minorities and to determine which interventions were most effective. A comprehensive approach to minority student recruitment and retention is the ideal, but many education programs do not have the resources to mount this type of approach. Even institutions that have and employ the resources to retain and graduate minority students, depend on their professional faculty to recruit these students.

Often the same few committed faculty are called on to expend considerable time and effort in what at times may seem like fruitless recruitment endeavors. The common recruitment tactic of high school visits requires extensive time and effort, often on the part of tenure-track minority faculty who will not necessarily benefit in tenure decisions by their participation in these efforts, and who may in fact be penalized by having less time to perform scholarly and research-related activities.

These same faculty members often are called on to provide minority representation on a host of other institutional and community committees. Service activities such as these, while expected and commended verbally, rarely compensate for a weak scholarly or research activity record—the bottom line in most tenure and promotion decisions. It is imperative that cost- and time-effective recruitment and retention activities be identified.

LIMITATIONS

A limitation of this study is the small population from which the sample was drawn. To measure the success of programs in recruiting, enrolling, and graduating minority students, this study considered only programs that kept data regarding the number of minorities who were in the applicant pool, who were enrolled in the first year of professional study, and who graduated from the

Dr Haskins is Associate Professor and Chairperson, Department of Physical Therapy, College of Health, Florida International University, Miami, FL 33199. Ms Rose-St Prix is Assistant Professor and Director of Recruitment and Retention, Department of Physical Therapy, College of Health, Florida International University. This article was adapted from a platform presentation at the Sixty-Seventh Annual Conference of the American Physical Therapy Association, Denver, CO, June 14-18, 1992.

program. Data obtained from the Department of Education of the American Physical Therapy Association (APTA) indicated that only 52 of 125 physical therapy entry-level programs kept all of these data.

Of the 52 programs that did keep data, the University of Puerto Rico (UPR) was eliminated from the study because all of its students are Hispanic. Because Hispanics constitute a majority of the population in Puerto Rico, Hispanics at UPR do not constitute a minority group. Florida International University, the authors' institution, also was eliminated to avoid a conflict (both authors have served as the minority student program coordinator). Thus only 50 of 125 programs were considered in this study.

Because of the small population studied, it is possible that the sample was selected from a population of programs different in some way from programs that did not keep data on minority students. It may be possible that just the act of keeping data on the numbers of minorities indicates an awareness of cultural diversity issues, which subconsciously affects the proportion of minority applicants, students, or graduates. Conversely, programs not keeping data on minorities may be so unconcerned regarding cultural diversity that their proportion of minority applicants, students, or graduates may differ significantly from the programs in the population studied.

A second limitation of this study is that the focus was on the underrepresentation of physical therapists only. No attempt was made to investigate the status of technical-level workers such as physical therapy aides or assistants. A review of the literature showed that minorities are underrepresented in fields requiring more education and overrepresented in fields requiring less education.

Respondents were asked to identify recruitment and retention strategies that affected students who graduated in 1990. Thus, a third limitation is the ability of respondents to recall what recruitment and retention strategies were used several years prior to 1990.

METHOD
Subjects

A preliminary survey of all 50 remaining programs was conducted by telephone to determine which programs made "special efforts" to recruit, admit, or retain minority students. Twelve programs indicated that they made no special efforts, while 35 programs reported that they made special efforts to recruit, admit, or retain minority students. The researchers were unable to contact representatives at three programs.

Special efforts were defined as meeting one of two criteria:

1. The physical therapy program faculty engaged in specific recruitment or retention activities at the program level to increase minority student participation.

2. The physical therapy program faculty actively participated in an institutional minority student program.

Thus, special efforts consisted of active participation by the physical therapy program faculty in minority student recruitment or retention. Some programs did benefit from institutional efforts, such as minority student scholarships, but admitted to not making any special efforts to recruit or retain minorities. These programs were included in the No-effort Group.

Procedure

A questionnaire was sent to all 12 physical therapy entry-level programs in the No-effort Group. Of the 12 questionnaires sent, 8 were returned by the given deadline. Fifteen of the 35 programs in the Effort Group were selected at random to participate in a telephone survey administered by the researcher. Fourteen of the 15 programs from the Effort Group were surveyed, with a lack of response from one program.

All respondents were asked to identify the degree offered; the length of the program; the type of institution (public or private); the administrative structure of the program (where housed; eg, school of medicine or allied health); the average annual cost of tuition; the number of full-time faculty; the number of minority faculty; and whether external funding was received and, if so, the amount of external funding and the level at which external funding was granted (eg, program, college, or institution).

Respondents also were asked to identify for the class of 1990 (1) the total number of applicants and minority applicants for the year of admission (eg, 1987 or 1988); (2) the total number of students and minority students enrolled in the first year of professional study (eg, 1988); and (3) the total number of graduates and minority graduates.

Equity scores were calculated and used to measure the success of programs in recruiting, enrolling, and graduating minority students. The equity scores were modified from formulas derived by Richardson and Skinner to measure institutional success in enrolling and graduating minority students.[39]

The mean equity scores for application (MESA or application scores) and enrollment (MESE or enrollment scores) were calculated using the proportion of minority group members between the ages of 20 and 24 in the state's population to weight the

scores. Mean equity scores for graduation (MESG or graduation scores) were weighted with the proportion of minorities in the first year of professional study for that class (eg, the number of minority students enrolled in 1988 was used to weight the graduation scores for a 2-year program when that class graduated in 1990).

The closer the equity scores were to 100, the greater the program's success in recruiting or retaining minorities. An application score of 100 indicates an equal proportion of minorities in the applicant pool as in the state's population. An enrollment score of 100 indicates an equal proportion of minority students as in the state's population. A graduation score of 100 indicates an equal proportion of minority graduates as enrolled in the first year of professional study for that class. Equity scores exceeding 100 indicate a higher proportion.

Programs making special efforts to recruit, admit, or retain minority students were surveyed on 37 recruitment activities and 31 retention activities identified in the literature[2,4,5,12,19,21–22,28–35,38] as being successful strategies for minority student recruitment and retention in higher education. A panel of experts reviewed the selected recruitment and retention activities to establish content validity. The programs surveyed also were asked to identify any additional methods used that were not included in the survey.

A pilot study was conducted before conducting the telephone surveys. Two physical therapy programs not selected at random to be included in the study sample were chosen to test the face validity of the questionnaire and telephone survey. The pilot study established the length of time required to administer each survey and ensured that the survey instrument was understandable, logical, and complete. Minor changes were made to the survey instrument to clarify the scope and meaning of certain terminology.

Data Analysis

Data were processed using the Statistical Package for the Social Sciences (SPSS).* Nonparametric tests of significance were used because of the sample size, the presence of extreme outliers, and indications that the distribution of the equity scores in the population may not have an underlying normal distribution. The *P* level was set at .05.

Analysis included frequency counts for degree offered, type of institution, administrative structure, whether a special effort is made to recruit or retain minorities, whether

*SPSS Inc. 444 N Michigan Ave. Chicago, IL 60611.

there is external funding, the level of external funding (ie. program. division. school, college, or institution), and the number of programs using each recruitment and retention strategy.

Analysis also included the medians. means, standard deviation, and range for the mean equity scores, the length of the program, annual tuition, total number of faculty positions currently filled, amount of external funding, total number of applicants, total number of minorities in the applicant pool, total number of students enrolled. total number of minority students enrolled. total number of students graduated. and total number of minorities graduated. Because there were only two minority faculty in the study sample, no analyses were conducted on this variable.

Spearman correlation coefficients were used to determine the relationship ($P<.05$) of the mean equity scores to each of the independent variables: degree offered (bachelor's or master's), length of program, type of institution (public or private), administrative structure (medical school or school of allied health), cost of tuition, number of faculty, presence or absence of special efforts to recruit or retain minorities, presence or absence of external funding, level of external funding, amount of external funding. percentage of recruitment and retention activities implemented at the program level, percentage of all recruitment and retention activities implemented, and each specific recruitment and retention activity. Only three programs could report the amount of external funding for institutional or college efforts.

The Wilcoxon Rank Sum Test was used to determine whether the mean ranks for the mean equity scores differed significantly ($P<.05$) for the presence or absence of special effort. degree (bachelor's or master's), type of institution (public or private), administrative structure (medical school or school of allied health), presence or absence of external funding, level of external funding, and presence or absence of each specific recruitment and retention strategy.

The Chi-square test and Fisher's Exact Test were used to determine whether any relationships ($P<.05$) existed among the nominally valued variables of effort, type, degree, administrative structure, presence or absence of external funding, and level of external funding.

RESULTS
Study Sample

Table 1 identifies the study sample characteristics. Table 2 provides medians for length

of program, annual tuition costs, and number of faculty. Of the 168 faculty members in the study, only two were minorities.

Table 3 compares the number of applicants, the number of students enrolled in the first year of professional study, and the number of students graduated from the program in 1990 with the number of minority applicants, students, and graduates.

Table 4 summarizes the MESA, MESE, and MESG. The graduation scores are higher than the application scores and the enrollment scores because, while the application scores and the enrollment scores are weighted with the proportion of the 20- to 24-year-old population of the state, the graduation score

is weighted with the proportion of minorities enrolled in the program during the first year of professional study.

Programs claiming to make an effort to recruit, admit, or retain minority students were examined to determine the frequencies with which specific recruitment strategies were used. Twenty one (56.8%) of the 37 recruitment activities surveyed were reported as implemented by these programs. Table 5 lists the most frequently used recruitment strategies for the Effort Group.

All programs in the Effort Group used faculty and students in recruitment efforts and used brochures, fliers, and pamphlets to provide information about the program. One

Table 1

Study Sample Characteristics (N=22)

Variable	n (Cases)
Effort	
Yes	14
No	8
Degree	
Bachelor's	18
Master's	4
Type of institution	
Public	17
Private	5
Administrative structure	
Allied health	13
Medicine	6
Arts and sciences	2
Graduate school	1
Level of external funding (if any)	
Program	5
College or institution	10

Table 2

Median Length of Program, Tuition Cost, and Number of Faculty (N=22)

Variable	Median
Length (mo)	24
Tuition (dollars)	2450
Faculty (number)	7

Table 3

Number of Program Applicants, Students in First Year of Professional Study, and Graduates (N=22)

Variable	n (Cases)	X̄	SD	Range	Median
Applicants					
Total	22	257.8	119.2	65-450	267.5
Minority	20	19.3	15.2	3-56	13.0
Students					
Total	22	41.5	16.2	20-82	39.0
Minority	22	3.2	2.2	0-7	2.5
Graduates					
Total	22	39.6	16.3	18-81	37.5
Minority	22	2.7	2.2	0–7	2.0

Table 4

Mean Equity Scores for Application, Enrollment, and Graduation (N=22)

Factor	n (Cases)	X̄	SD	Range	Median
MESA[a]	20	46.3	26.6	16-121	41.0
MESE[b]	22	58.2	82.1	0-408	37.0
MESG[c]	22	77.0	39.3	0-106	100.0

[a]Mean equity scores for application.
[b]Mean equity scores for enrollment.
[c]Mean equity scores for graduation.

Table 5

Top Recruitment Strategies Used by Physical Therapy Programs in the Effort Group (n=14)

Strategy	Number of Programs (%)
Use brochures, fliers	100.0
Use faculty	100.0
Use students	100.0
Hold career fairs	92.9
Sponsor open houses	92.9
Participate in health fairs	85.7
Use nontraditional admissions criteria	85.7
Have cultural diversity as a goal	78.6
Make visits to high schools	78.6
Use alumni	78.6
Give financial aid information	78.6
Use special or flexible admissions policies	71.4
Keep in touch with potential minority applicants	71.4

Table 6

Top Retention Strategies Used by Physical Therapy Programs in the Effort Group (n=14)

Strategy	Number of Programs (%)
Provide academic counseling	100.0
Discuss cultural differences in the curriculum	100.0
Monitor student grade-point average	100.0
Encourage minority student participation in cultural events	100.0
Provide orientation activities	92.9
Provide tutoring	92.9
Provide personal counseling	92.9
Provide career counseling	85.7
Sponsor minority guest speakers	78.6
Teach to different cognitive styles	78.6
Use learning groups	71.4
Teach test-taking skills	71.4
Teach study skills	71.4
Use flexible retention strategies	71.4

Table 7

Results of Wilcoxon Rank Sum Tests for Mean Equity Scores for Application by Recruitment Strategy for Programs Using or Not Using the Strategy (n=14)

Strategy	Uses Mean (n) Rank	Does Not Use Mean (n) Rank	T	1-tailed P Value
Keep in touch with potential students	8.1 (7)	3.3 (5)	13.0	.027
Talk to parent groups	8.6 (5)	5.0 (7)	43.0	.044

third of the programs that reported conducting open houses or sponsoring field trips, offering introductory courses to physical therapy or allied health, or mentoring minority applicants relied on the college to implement the strategy. More than one third of the programs that reported visiting high schools, giving financial aid information, or visiting middle schools relied on either the college or the institution to do so. Two thirds of the programs that reported visiting minority institutions or community colleges relied on the college or institution to implement the strategy.

All of the programs in the Effort Group were examined to determine which retention strategies were used to retain minority students. Twenty (65%) of the 31 retention strategies surveyed were reported as implemented by at least one of the programs in the Effort Group. Table 6 lists the most frequently used retention strategies for the Effort Group.

Approximately 80% of the programs in the Effort Group that reported providing test-taking skills intervention, study skills intervention, and remediation of basic skills relied on the college or the institution to implement the strategy. Almost 60% of the programs in the Effort Group that reported providing college work-study opportunities for minority students relied on the college or the institution to do so. Seventy-one percent of the programs in the Effort Group that reported providing scholarships for minority students relied on the institution to do so.

Strategies Used by Successful Programs

Programs with higher equity scores were compared with programs with lower equity scores to determine which recruitment or retention activities were associated with success in minority student recruitment and retention. Among programs that made special efforts, programs with high application scores reported giving talks to parent groups, keeping in touch with potential minority applicants, using special or flexible admissions policies, providing pre-professional enrichment courses, setting quantitative goals for minority student enrollment, and disseminating financial aid information to prospective minority students.

A statistically significant difference existed in the mean rank of the application score for only two of the above recruitment strategies—talking to parent groups and keeping in touch with potential minority students—when tested with the Wilcoxon Rank Sum Test. For both strategies, the mean rank of the application scores for the programs that

Table 8

Results of Wilcoxon Rank Sum Tests for Mean Equity Scores for Enrollment by Level of External Funding for Programs Where External Funding Was Present or Not Present (n=14)

Funding Level	Present Mean (n) Rank	Not Present Mean (n) Rank	T	1-tailed P Value
Program	17.4 (5)	9.7 (17)	87.0	.010
Institutional or college level	15.0 (10)	8.6 (12)	150.0	.011

used this strategy was higher than the mean rank of the application scores for programs that did not use the strategy. Table 7 lists the mean ranks, the T statistic, and the one-tailed P value corrected for ties for the significant tests.

More programs with high enrollment scores reported assisting students in completing admissions applications. For this strategy, the mean rank of the enrollment score was greater for programs that did assist students to complete admissions applications (n=6; mean rank=9.7) than for programs that did not (n=8; mean rank=5.9; T=58.0; 1-tailed P<.047). No other recruitment strategies showed a statistical difference in the mean ranks of the enrollment score.

No retention strategies were identified that were used more by programs whose graduation score ranked in the top half of the Effort Group than by programs whose graduation score ranked in the lower half of the Effort Group. There also was no difference in the mean ranks of the graduation score for programs that used any given strategy than for programs that did not when tested with the Wilcoxon Rank Sum Test (P>.05).

There was a statistically significant difference in the mean ranks of the application score of programs that did or did not participate in a larger effort that was externally funded (T=120.5; 1-tailed P<.024) when tested with the Wilcoxon Rank Sum Test. The mean rank of the application score was greater for programs that participated in a larger effort that was externally funded (n=9; mean rank=13.4) than the mean rank of the application score for programs that were not part of a larger effort (n=11; mean rank=8.1). The Spearman Correlation Coefficient indicated a statistically significant relationship between the application score and the amount of funding of a larger effort (n=3; r=1.00; 1-tailed P<.001).

There was a statistical difference in the mean ranks of the enrollment score between programs that did have external funding and programs that did not have external funding when tested with the Wilcoxon Rank Sum Test (Tab. 8). The mean rank of the enroll-

ment score was higher for programs with external funding than was the mean rank of the enrollment score for programs without external funding.

There was a significant difference in the mean ranks of the graduation score for programs with different administrative structures when the Wilcoxon Rank Sum Test was applied (T=81.0; 1-tailed P<.031). The mean rank for medical schools or colleges (n=6; mean rank=13.5) was higher than the mean rank for schools of allied health (n=13; mean rank=8.4).

Other Findings

Fisher's Exact Test was used to examine relationships among dichotomous independent variables. There was a statistically significant difference (n=22; P<.031) between programs that did or did not make special efforts to recruit, admit, or retain minority students in the presence or absence of external funding. Sixty-four percent of programs in the Effort Group participated in a larger effort that was externally funded, but only 13% of programs in the No-effort Group did so.

Spearman Correlation Coefficients showed a significant relationship between the graduation score and the total percentage of retention activities implemented; the application score and the enrollment score; and the total percentage of retention activities and recruitment activities implemented. Spearman Correlation Coefficients for these relationships are shown in Table 9.

When tested with the Wilcoxon Rank Sum Test, programs in medical schools have a higher mean rank for the percentage of retention activities implemented at the program level than do programs not in medical schools, but a lower mean rank for the total percentage of retention activities implemented as compared with programs not in medical schools. Table 10 shows the mean rank, the T statistic, and the P value corrected for ties.

In contrast, programs in schools of allied health have a lower mean rank for the percentage of retention activities implemented at the program level (ie, less strategies are implemented at the program level than at the institutional or college levels) and a higher mean rank for the total percentage of retention activities implemented (ie, use more strategies) than do programs not in schools of allied health when the Wilcoxon Rank Sum Test is applied. Table 11 gives the mean ranks, the T statistic, and the P value corrected for ties. In addition, programs in schools of allied health have a significantly (T=18.5; P<.011) higher mean rank (n=9; mean rank=9.6) for the total percentage of recruitment activities implemented than do programs not in schools of allied health (n=5; mean rank=3.7).

DISCUSSION

When programs with higher equity scores were compared with programs with lower equity scores, certain patterns emerged. Those with higher application and enrollment scores reported giving talks to parent groups, keeping in touch with minority applicants, using special or flexible admissions policies, providing preprofessional enrichment courses, setting quantitative goals for minority student enrollment, disseminating financial aid information to students, and assisting applicants in completing admissions applications.

One could question the validity of the statistical results, given the large number of tests performed to examine the relationship between the equity scores and the recruitment and retention activities.

Table 9

Spearman Correlation Coefficients for MESA,[a] MESE,[b] MESG,[c] Percentage of Recruitment Activities Implemented, and Percentage of Retention Activities Implemented (N=22)

Variable		n	r	P Value
MESG	Percentage of retention activities	14	−.722	.004
MESA	MESE	20	.596	.006
Percentage of recruitment activities	Percentage of retention activities	14	.654	.011

[a]Mean equity scores for application.
[b]Mean equity scores for enrollment.
[c]Mean equity scores for graduation.

Table 10

Results of Wilcoxon Rank Sum Tests for Percentage of Retention Activities Implemented at the Program Level and Overall for Medical Schools and Non-medical Schools (N=22)

Level	Medical Schools Mean (n) Rank	Non-medical Schools Mean (n) Rank	T	P Value
Program	11.6 (4)	5.85 (10)	46.5	.009
Overall	2.9 (4)	9.35 (10)	11.5	.004

The paucity of significant results is consistent with the findings of Bender and Blanco, who reported that no one strategy or method was responsible for success in minority student recruitment and retention.[35] The descriptive findings, however, indicate a trend for the strategies associated with higher application and enrollment scores to be the ones implemented by less than 50% of the programs studied.

When strategies used by programs with higher equity scores were compared with the most frequently used strategies, only three strategies (using special or flexible admissions policies, disseminating financial aid information, and keeping in touch with prospective minority applicants) were implemented at any level by more than 50% of the programs in the Effort Group. Less than 50% of programs in the Effort Group implemented four of the strategies (giving talks to parent groups, providing preprofessional enrichment courses, setting quantitative enrollment goals, and assisting students to complete admissions applications) that are effective in increasing either minority applicants or students.

None of the retention strategies examined were positively associated with the equity score for graduation. However, 65% of the retention strategies surveyed were implemented by more than 50% of the programs in the Effort Group, indicating that physical therapy programs put considerable effort into retention.

The mean for the graduation score of programs in the Effort Group was 72.4,

indicating that most of the programs in the Effort Group (whether in the top half or the lower half) successfully retain most of the students they enroll in the first year of professional study. A further indication of this success is that the cutoff point for comparing the top-ranking programs with the lower ranking programs was a graduation score of 96, a score that by itself indicates a good retention rate.

Two recruitment strategies (keeping in touch with potential minority applicants and giving talks to parent groups) were statistically related to a high application score. One recruitment strategy (assisting students in completing admissions applications) was significantly related to a high enrollment score.

A positive relationship was established between the application score and the presence of external funding at the institutional or college level. A positive relationship also existed between the enrollment score and the presence of external funding, both at the program level and at the institutional or college level. These findings may represent a commitment to minority student participation, or external funding may enable programs to engage in activities that may not have been measured and that increase minority student representation. The presence of external funding may indicate a commitment to cultural diversity, or it may facilitate activities that enhance minority student participation.

External funding at the institutional or college level also was positively associated with programs making a special effort to

recruit, admit, or retain minority students. A positive correlation existed between the application score and the amount of funding at the institutional or college level, but only three programs could report the amount of external funding of the larger effort, so this result was discounted.

It is not clear why the graduation score was higher for programs in schools or colleges of medicine than for programs in schools of allied health.

Programs in medical schools had a higher percentage of retention activities implemented at the program level than did programs not in medical schools. This may be a reason for the association of graduation score and medical schools. It is unlikely that external funding is a factor, as only two programs in medical schools participated in an institutional or college minority student program, and none were funded at the program level.

As shown in Table 9, a negative relationship existed between the graduation score and the total percentage of retention activities measured. Programs having the most difficulty graduating minority students may try many strategies to improve retention.

The application score was positively related to the enrollment score. This may indicate that minority enrollments depend on a large pool of minority applicants or that minority students are more likely to apply to a program if there already are minority students in the program. The latter conclusion is supported by the fact that all of the programs making special efforts to recruit minorities reported using current students for recruitment efforts (Tab. 5).

The total percentage of recruitment activities implemented was positively related to the total percentage of retention activities used. Physical therapy programs seem to act consistently with the theory that recruitment activities alone will not resolve the underrepresentation of minorities in the field.

CONCLUSIONS

The results indicate that some recruitment strategies surveyed are related to success in recruiting minority applicants and/or students. Successful strategies include assisting students in completing admissions applications, giving talks to parent groups, keeping in touch with potential minority students, using special or flexible admissions policies, providing preprofessional enrichment courses, setting quantitative goals for minority student enrollment, and disseminating financial aid information to minority students.

There also is some evidence to suggest that external funding is related to success in recruiting minority applicants and students. Programs in medical schools seem to be more successful at graduating minorities than are programs in schools of allied health,

Table 11

Results of Wilcoxon Rank Sum Tests for Percentage of Retention Activities Implemented at the Program Level and Overall for Schools of Allied Health and Other Schools (N=22)

Level	Allied Health Mean (n) Rank	Not Allied Health Mean (n) Rank	T	P Value
Program	5.6 (9)	10.9 (5)	54.5	.023
Overall	9.2 (9)	4.4 (5)	22.0	.037

possibly because they implement more retention activities at the program level.

RECOMMENDATIONS

Physical therapy programs should more vigorously pursue minority students and faculty. This study found that less than 50% of the programs surveyed keep data on minorities; programs average less than three minority graduates per year; the number of programs that set quantitative goals for the enrollment of minority students is small; and there are very few minority faculty members in physical therapy education. These findings may indicate a lack of commitment of physical therapy programs towards minority efforts or a lack of knowledge regarding the most effective means to achieve cultural diversity.

Physical therapy programs must be more involved in larger efforts that are externally funded, set quantitative goals for minority student enrollment, and ensure active participation by their programs in institutional efforts. Physical therapy educators should evaluate their recruitment and retention activities.

Few programs were involved in activities that put them into close proximity with minorities, such as talking to church groups or parent groups, sponsoring family days for recruitment, or participating in Health Occupations Students of America club activities. Few programs participated in scoliosis or athletic screenings or in teaching at the elementary, middle, high school, or community college levels. These activities would potentially expose the profession to a wide variety of students, provide minority students with role models, and increase college awareness among minorities.

Physical therapy programs should develop a network allowing them to share information about minority applicants. Because most physical therapy programs are limited-access, capped programs, this would ensure that more minorities get considered for admission at a wider range of programs.

Few programs provide preprofessional enrichment programs and assistance in completing financial aid and admissions forms. Preprofessional enrichment programs can compensate for inadequate preparatory education, a factor that will continue to exclude minorities from physical therapy education until educators become more aggressive in their attempts to compensate for it.

This study could be improved by enlarging the study sample, possibly to include all programs accredited by the APTA. It may be advantageous for the APTA Department of Accreditation to require all accredited programs to implement uniform procedures for monitoring the number of minorities applying to the program, enrolled in the program, and graduated from the program. Currently many physical therapy programs do not have a data base available on the number of minorities applying to the program, nor are they consistent in defining what constitutes a minority group.

Future research in this area should concentrate on a longer time span encompassing several years of graduates. A few programs indicated that the class of 1990 was not representative of their past success in minority student recruitment and retention. This problem could be overcome by averaging minority participation over several years.

Future studies could be more selective in the types of recruitment and retention activities surveyed, eliminating those identified in this study as being implemented by all programs. Activities implemented by all programs surveyed included the use of printed materials, such as brochures; and the use of current faculty and students for recruitment, providing academic counseling, and monitoring grade-point averages. Future studies could examine the few variables that the results of this study indicated appeared related to high application and enrollment scores.

The APTA has indicated a commitment to increasing minority representation in the profession. In the absence of more definitive findings, physical therapy educators must continue all efforts to ensure that they are actively pursuing this professional goal.

REFERENCES

1. Committee to Study the Role of Allied Health Personnel. Institute of Medicine. *Allied Health Services: Avoiding Crises.* Washington, DC: National Academy Press; 1989.
2. Lecca PJ, Watts TD. *Pathways for Minorities into the Health Professions.* Lanham, Md: University Press of America; 1989.
3. Hodgkinson HL. *All One System: Demographics of Education, Kindergarten Through Graduate School.* Washington, DC: Institute for Educational Leadership; 1985.
4. United States Task Force on Women, Minorities, and the Handicapped in Science and Technology. *Changing America: The New Face of Science and Engineering: Final Report.* Washington, DC: US Government Printing Office; 1989. GPO item no. 1089.
5. Ward WE, Cross MM, eds. *Key Issues in Minority Education: Research Directions and Practical Implications.* Norman, Okla: University of Oklahoma, Center for Research for Minority Education; 1989.
6. Commission on Minority Participation in Education and American Life. *One-third of a Nation.* Washington, DC: American Council on Education; 1988.
7. Thomas GE. Participation and degree attainment of African-American and Latino students in graduate education relative to other racial and ethnic groups: an update from Office of Civil Rights data. *Harvard Educational Review.* 1992;62:45–65.
8. College Entrance Examination Board. *Equality and Excellence: The Educational Status of Black Americans.* New York, NY: College Entrance Examination Board; 1985.
9. Kolbert E. Minority faculty: bleak future. *New York Times.* September 9, 1985 (Section 12: Education Summer Survey):12.
10. National Commission on Excellence in Education. *A Nation at Risk: The Imperative for Educational Reform.* Washington, DC: US Department of Education; 1983.
11. Orfield G, Paul F. Declines in minority access: a tale of five cities. *Educational Record.* 1987/1988;68(4), 69(1):57–62.
12. Margolis RL, Rungta SA. Training counselors for work with special populations: a second look. *Journal of Counseling and Development.* 1986;64:642–644.
13. Howard J, Hammond R. Rumors of inferiority: the hidden obstacles to black success. *The New Republic.* 1985;193(11):17–21.
14. Rosenfeld G. *"Shut Those Thick Lips!" A Study of Slum School Failure.* Prospect Heights, Ill: Waveland Press; 1971.
15. Washington V. Racial differences in teacher perceptions of first and fourth grade pupils on selected characteristics. *Journal of Negro Education.* 1982;51:60–72.
16. Altbach PG, Lomotey K. *The Racial Crisis in American Higher Education.* Albany, NY: State University of New York Press; 1991.
17. Koretz D. *Trends in the Postsecondary Enrollment of Minorities.* Santa Monica, Ca: The RAND Corp; 1990.
18. Pelavin SH, Kane M. *Changing the Odds: Factors Increasing Access to College.* New York, NY: College Board Publications; 1990.
19. Vera RT. The legal obligation to secure access for minority students in higher education. In Ward ME, Cross MM, eds. *Key Issues in Minority Education: Research Directions and Practical Implications.* Norman, Okla: University of Oklahoma, Center for Research on Minority Education; 1989:13–38.
20. Upton JN, Pruitt AS. *Financial Assistance to Black Doctoral Students in Two Adams States: A Policy Analysis.* Atlanta, Ga: Southern Education Foundation; 1985.
21. Boone, Young & Associates, Inc. *Minority Enrollment in Graduate and Professional Schools* (Contract No. 300-82-0253). Washington, DC: Office of Civil Rights, US Department of Education; 1984.
22. Richardson RC, Bender LW. *Fostering Minority Access and Achievement in Higher Education: The Role of Urban Community Colleges and Universities.* San Francisco, Ca: Jossey-Bass; 1987.
23. Pahnos ML, Butt KL. Ethnocentrism—a universal pride in one's ethnic background: its impact on teaching and learning. *Education.* 1993;113:118–120.
24. Sleeter CE. Multicultural education: five views. *The Education Digest.* March 1993:53–57.
25. Kennedy E. A multilevel study of elementary male black students and white students. *Journal of Educational Research.* 1992;86:105–110.
26. Richardson RC, Skinner EF. *Achieving Quality and Diversity: Universities in a Multicultural Society.* New York, NY: American Council on Education and Macmillan Publishing Co; 1991.
27. Lang M, Ford CA. *Strategies for Retaining Minority Students in Higher Education.* Springfield, Ill: Charles C. Thomas; 1992.
28. Haskins AR. Recruitment of minorities into the health professions. *Journal of Physical Therapy Education.* 1989;3(2):14–17.
29. Tysinger JW, Whiteside MF. A review of recruitment and retention programs for minority and disadvantaged students in health professions education. *Journal of Allied Health.* 1987;16:209–217.
30. Baker J, Baker C. Innovative programs to develop a minority and disadvantaged student applicant pool. *Journal of Physical Therapy Education.* 1989;3(2):9–13.
31. Cohn K. The minority recruitment program at the

Pennsylvania College of Optometry. *Journal of Optometric Education.* 1987;12(3):72–74.

32. Ugbolue A, Whitley PN, Stevens PJ. Evaluation of a preentrance enrichment program for minority students admitted to medical school. *Journal of Medical Education.* 1987;62:8–16.

33. Maguire J. Reversing the recent decline in minority participation in higher education. In *Minorities in Public Higher Education: At a Turning Point.* Washington, DC: American Association of State Colleges and Universities; 1988:21–41.

34. United States Health Resources and Services Administration Division of Disadvantaged Assistance, The Circle, Inc. *Revitalizing Pharmacy and Allied Health Professions Education for Minorities and the Disadvantaged: A Pharmacy and Allied Health Deans' Forum on Issues and Strategies* (Contract No. 240-86-0018). Washington, DC: US Department of Health & Human Services, Public Health Service; 1987 (NTIS).

35. Bender LW, Blanco CD. *Programs to Enhance Participation, Retention, and Success of Minority Students at Florida Community Colleges and Universities.* Tallahassee, Fla: Florida State University, State and Regional Higher Education Center; 1987 (ERIC Document Reproduction Series No. ED 288 582).

36. Edmonds MM, McCurdy DP. Variables affecting black students' decision to attend college: a literature review. *Journal of Physical Therapy Education.* 1989;3(2):4–8.

37. Astin HS, Astin AW, Bisconti AS, Frankel HH. *Higher Education and the Disadvantaged Student.* Washington, DC: Human Service Press; 1972.

38. Christoffel P. Minority student access and retention: a review. *Research and Development Update.* New York, NY: College Entrance Examination Board; 1986 (ERIC Document Reproduction Service No. ED 279 217).

39. Richardson RC, Skinner EF. Adapting to diversity: organizational influences on student achievement. *Journal of Higher Education.* 1990;61:485–511.

Recruitment in Geriatrics

An aging population, a shortage of physical therapists, a wide variety of practice options: These realities complicate the recruitment and retention of physical therapists in the geriatrics setting. The solution to this dilemma may rest in the classroom.

By Ann C. Noonan, EdD, PT

By the year 2030, older Americans will comprise about 21 percent of the U.S. population. (*PT Bulletin* 1990) This increase in the geriatric population undoubtedly will result in an increased demand for physical therapists to work with elderly persons. Hospitals, rehabilitation centers, private practices, home health care agencies, and privately owned practice groups already are competing for a limited supply of physical therapists. Because of the changing demographics, the shortage of workers, and the wide variety of available practice opportunities, recruiting and retaining qualified physical therapy personnel in geriatrics settings present a unique challenge.

"In Theory": A Review of Basic Recruitment and Retention Strategies

To flourish, an organization must recruit, manage, and develop its human resources effectively. Research findings show that job satisfaction and personal esteem lead to increased commitment to an organization and to improved organizational effectiveness (Schein 1978, Hall and Lawler 1970). It is important that managers understand what motivates physical therapy professionals so that appro-

priate reward systems can be created to attract and retain qualified personnel. Numerous researchers have developed theories about the kinds of factors that are essential to job satisfaction among workers in any profession, including physical therapy.

Different levels of needs. Maslow (1943) concluded that all workers have five needs that exist in a hierarchy of importance. At the lower level, these needs include physiological, safety, and social needs. At the higher level, these needs include the need for self-esteem and self-actualization. Maslow first assumed that when a need is satisfied, it no longer is a motivator and that each higher-level need becomes activated only after each lower level need has been satisfied; however, a review of the literature indicated that satisfying a need at one level does not necessarily decrease the importance of that need or lead to an increase in importance of a need at the next level (Maslow 1943).

Job satisfaction vs. job dissatisfaction. Herzberg (1968) developed the "Two-Factor Theory of Job Satisfaction," which held that job satisfaction and job dissatisfaction really are separate entities. Herzberg identified "hygiene" or maintenance factors

Reprinted from *Clinical Management.* Noonan AC. Recruitment in geriatrics. 1992;12(1):48-58.
With the permission of APTA.

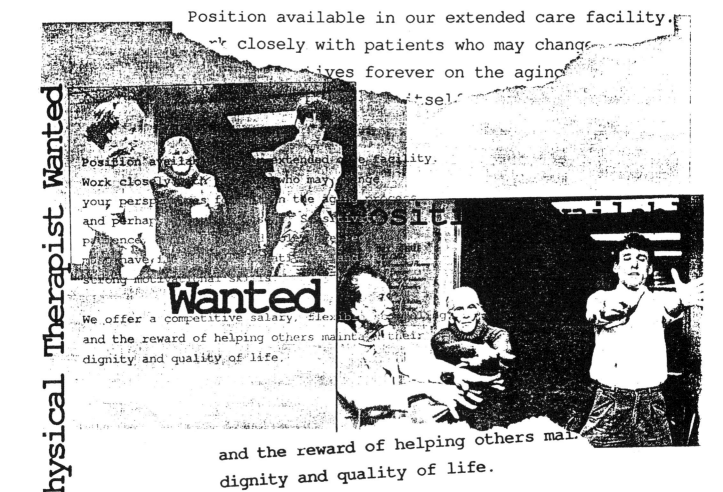

Position available in our extended care facility. Work closely with patients who may change... lives forever on the aging... ...self...

and the reward of helping others mai... dignity and quality of life.

that relate to job dissatisfaction, including job content items, such as salary, working conditions, interpersonal relationships, and organizational policies. He stated that if these needs are not met in the workplace, employees will be dissatisfied and nonproductive. He further stated that, although improving these conditions reduce job *dissatisfaction*, they will not necessarily lead to increased job *satisfaction*. Herzberg believed that to improve job satisfaction among workers, managers must provide "job satisfiers" or moti-

vators. He defined job satisfiers as job-context items, such as recognition for a job well done, a chance for advancement, job growth, and a sense of personal achievement. Herzberg concluded that when job dissatisfiers are low and job satisfaction is high, employees will be motivated to improve individual job performance (Herzberg 1968).

Three basic needs. David McClelland (1961) developed the "Theory of Needs." He concluded that all individuals have three basic needs: a need for achievement, a

need for affiliation, and a need for power. These needs are acquired over time as a result of personal experience, and the individual's level of need determines the type of position with which he or she is most satisfied. Individuals with a strong need for achievement, for example, typically prefer a position that offers the opportunity for individual responsibility. They set high goals for themselves, prefer to work alone, and expect recognition for their personal achievements. This type of individual may prefer working in a home care setting or in a setting in which he or she may work alone and is rewarded on a per-patient or per-visit basis.

Individuals with a strong need for affiliation prefer to work with others. They thrive on interpersonal relationships and are good team members. They enjoy a reward system that recognizes group achievements. These individuals may avoid taking a position of authority because they are uncomfortable unless they are accepted as part of the group.

Individuals with a strong need for power like to have control over situations or people. They prefer an authoritative position in which they can delegate tasks to other individuals. They want to be recognized for developing and improving the effectiveness of the group. These individuals seek leadership roles.

Matching the needs of the individual with the needs of the organization. An individual's needs vary depending on his or her career stage and family situation, on the size of the employer organization, and on geographical location, among other things. Individuals whose needs match the needs-and-rewards system of the organization are attracted to that organization and will remain and grow

with it. Those individuals whose needs and values conflict with those of an organization go elsewhere (Schein 1978). To recruit and retain qualified personnel, the manager must recognize the needs of both the organization and the individuals whom he or she supervises and develop and support a work setting in which individuals have the opportunity to satisfy their own needs while contributing to fulfill the needs of the organization.

When it comes to recruiting and retaining physical therapists in geriatrics settings, matching individual therapists' needs with those of the organization or facility may be especially difficult because of the attitudes and expectations that therapists may have about their professional goals and about working with elderly persons.

Recruitment in Geriatrics Settings: A Matter of Attitudes

Physical therapy graduates traditionally choose to work in large teaching hospitals and rehabilitation settings that offer the opportunity to rotate through various treatment environments and work with different types of patients and different types of health care professionals (Buchanan and Noonan 1988).

These settings may be especially stimulating to new graduates. A review of the literature indicates that after a few years in these traditional settings, many physical therapists leave to work in health maintenance organization, private practice, home health care, or school settings (American Physical Therapy Association 1988). This shift of the workforce, however, does not apply to geriatrics settings, where recruitment and retention remains a challenge. To understand why, we first must understand our attitudes toward aging and elderly persons.

Society's attitudes toward aging. According to Kerlinger (1984), *attitudes* are enduring social beliefs that predispose individuals to think, feel, perceive, and behave selectively. Attitudes are developed and formed as part of our life experiences and influence how we behave in any given situation.

Life experiences in the United States have changed. Years ago, many children grew up with extended families. Grandparents either lived with the family or lived nearby in the neighborhood. Grandchildren had the opportunity to see their grandparents age slowly and gracefully. They interacted with them on a regular basis and developed a respect for

A Review of What Attracts Physical Therapists—In Any Setting

A review of the literature indicates that salary is the number one consideration and location is the number two consideration when physical therapists—both new graduates and experienced professionals—make career choices. Other highly rated items include benefits; job flexibility; opportunity for professional growth, autonomy, and participation in administrative decision making; and a well-equipped and well-staffed department in which peer groups respect and get along well with

one another. Sign-on bonuses surprisingly ranked extremely low as incentives for both new graduates and experienced staff (American Physical Therapy Association 1988, Pearl 1990).

The results of these studies tell us that we *can* do things to encourage recruitment and retention of professional staff.

1. Salary. Facility location cannot be changed. We therefore first must ensure that salary ranges are appro-

their age and their experience. Today many children grow up never knowing their grandparents. Their experience with elderly persons is extremely limited. In addition, society has changed so rapidly that the experiences of the elderly often are unrelated to modern lifestyles, and children no longer respect the experience and knowledge of their seniors.

The physical therapist's attitudes toward aging. In 1990, Wong cited one review of the literature of medical and nursing research that indicated practitioners in general have negatives attitudes toward working with elderly persons. Wong further stated that, although physical therapists have done little research in this area, initial findings indicate that physical therapists have negative attitudes toward working with elderly patients.

It is not surprising that many health care professionals—including physical therapists—choose to work with younger individuals whose goals may be to return to work, to return to athletics, and to return to a healthy, modern lifestyle. In my experience, individuals who work in nursing home settings and extended care facilities often feel the need to apologize for their choice of work because they believe that it is not as highly

skilled or valued as that of their counterparts working in acute care settings. Now director of physical therapy at an extended care facility in Romulus, Michigan, Miller reported that as a graduate student working in that setting, she felt she had to defend her position—even though she enjoyed her work and received great satisfaction from her job (*Geritopics* 1990).

It starts with students. Health care education and practice in our society emphasizes acute care, not chronic care. Goodwin-Johansson (1990) stated that health care workers often assign low priority to patients who will never be "cured" and whose goals simply are to improve function, not to "return home."

Coren et al. (1987) stated that many students believe that elderly patients are unmotivated and unable to make substantial gains. Because goals often focus on maintenance of function, students may believe it is unchallenging and depressing to work in this field for any length of time.

In a study of junior and senior physical therapy students, Wong (1991) found that the majority of students expressed low interest in working in a chronic care setting. Students with prior positive nursing

home work experience did show a much higher interest in working in this type of setting than those who had no prior nursing home experience; however, even among this group, interest was low and barely reached the neutral score of 4 on a 7-point Likert scale. Students who said they had had negative nursing home work experiences indicated that working with elderly persons was frustrating and limited to helping patients ambulate. The students believed that, in the geriatrics setting, they would not be able to use the physical therapy professional skills they were learning in the classroom.

In a study of factors that influence physical therapy students' decisions to work with elderly persons, Coren et al. (1987) found that many students were uncomfortable with the thought of growing old. Working with elderly persons reminded them of their own mortality; the geriatrics setting therefore was something they wanted to avoid.

Retention in Geriatrics Settings: A Matter of Expectations

Voices from the field. In 1990 I was asked to be a guest speaker at the 1991 Conference for Geriatric Allied Health Professionals at the

priate and at least equitable with those of our competition. A study by the American Physical Therapy Association (1988) found that a higher paying salary is the *only* factor that decreases recruitment time in hospital settings.

2. Benefits package. Benefits should include adequate sick leave, vacation time, maternity and family leave, a choice of health care plans, a good retirement plan, and reimbursement for continuing education. Whenever possible, benefits packages should be flexible enough to meet the individual employee's needs. Not all employees desire the same benefits. One employee may depend on the employer for health care insurance; another employee may have insurance through his or her spouse and would rather receive a

higher hourly wage. To some individuals, an increase in vacation time would be preferable to a raise. Employers should develop equitable but variable benefits packages from which employees may choose.

A survey of physical therapy managers in the greater Boston area indicated that most facilities provide an eight-week unpaid maternity leave for their employees. The managers of these facilities unanimously agreed that eight weeks was an inadequate amount of time and advocated at least 12 weeks. They also stated that when an employee resigns, it takes an average of six months to find a replacement (Noonan 1989). Increasing the length of maternity leaves and encouraging return to employment even on a part-time basis may help facili-

University of Connecticut-Storrs. To prepare for my presentation on factors influencing recruitment and retention of health care professionals in geriatrics settings, I scheduled appointments with physical therapy managers who work in geriatrics facilities in the greater Boston area. I asked them why they had accepted positions in geriatrics and why they chose to remain in them. Their answers had a common theme.

The majority of these therapists had entered the field of geriatrics for different personal reasons, but none of them did so because of an interest in that field. Their perspectives changed, however, when they became involved with the geriatric patients. Most of them talked about the adjustments they had made in their expectations for patient progress—adjustments that cannot be taught in the classroom.

"Getting to the bathroom on time." A manager in an extended care facility for eight years, one physical therapist told me that she had accepted a position in geriatrics because the position offered her the opportunity to develop her managerial skills. She admitted that she had had reservations about working with elderly persons and that she had planned to seek a new position when she had

obtained enough management experience. She found, however, that she enjoyed working with elderly patients. She explained that physical therapists who work in geriatrics must be mature and flexible. Because the patients have multiple problems, therapists cannot expect to maintain a rigid schedule. The working environment is not very structured; changes must be made daily to accommodate the daily needs of the patients. "Therapists must be tuned in to the total person, not just to one disease process or problem," she emphasized. "The focus is on functional outcomes, and goals must relate to individual needs. It doesn't matter if a patient develops a perfect gait pattern. What matters to the patient is whether he or she is able to get to the bathroom on time."

In this manager's experience, the value of these functional goals was not taught in the classroom. Students may come to believe that a treatment regimen must be followed perfectly to be acceptable and valuable.

"Eager to please." Two physical therapy managers—who have remained in their positions for an average of 12 years now—indicated that they had accepted a job in geriatrics *only* because they wanted a part-time job with a flexible schedule, which was not available in a teach-

ing or rehabilitation setting at that time. They said that when they began working with geriatric patients their negative feelings about these patients changed.

Many of the therapists I interviewed mentioned that one-to-one, hands-on experience with the geriatric patient was much more rewarding to them than working with modalities and equipment. Some therapists indicated that elderly patients are extremely motivated and try desperately to please. Working with this type of highly motivated patient offers personal satisfaction and has intrinsic rewards.

Accepting limitations. Other therapists I interviewed, however, stated that elderly patients are *not* always motivated and may often be depressed. Because of the multiple medical problems of most geriatric patients, treatment programs must constantly be reevaluated and new methods must be developed to motivate the patient. These therapists emphasized that it is imperative for patients to understand their own limitations and for therapeutic goals to be translated into a language that the patient understands. Expectations must be clear—and agreed upon both by the patient and by the therapist.

ties retain qualified and experienced professionals—and reduce the amount of time that a position is vacant.

On-site day care centers. Schaffer (1986) reported that after the establishment of an on-site day care center for employees, a manufacturing plant documented six dollars in cost containment for every dollar spent on the facility. In addition, she reported that applications for positions increased dramatically. A study of physical therapy managers in the greater Boston area showed that the establishment of day care centers for health care workers resulted in decreased time off for maternity leave and enhanced recruitment outcomes (Noonan 1989).

Day care for elders also is an important benefit. Many working women today take care of not only their children

but their elderly parents. Geriatrics facilities provide an ideal environment for day care for elderly persons.

3. Job flexibility. The American economy and family life style have changed; we therefore must accept and promote flexibility on the job.

In the 1970s, the economic survival of the family began to depend on two incomes (Appelbaum 1981). As early as 1976, Miller indicated that if job scheduling were rearranged to allow couples to serve the family's needs, there would be less conflict between home and work. In 1988, however, the staff of *Business Week* magazine reported that, although it had been anticipated that employers would take major steps to accommodate the needs of working parents, little was being done dif-

Taking the time to listen. Geriatric patients struggle for independence and a sense of control of their own lives, just as any of us do. Listening is a key skill identified by all the therapists I interviewed. When a patient is happy with his or her functional status in a wheelchair, it may be impossible to motivate that patient to use a walker. On the other hand, when patients are in pain, they may not be willing to push themselves to reach 90 degrees of knee flexion. However, when they understand that reaching 90 degrees of knee flexion may allow them to rise from a chair to a standing position independently, they may be more willing to fight through the pain.

Creative problem solving. These therapists all agreed that creativity is essential. One therapist offered this example: An elderly patient who ambulated with a walker constantly fell to the right side. There was no apparent physiological or neurological reason for this. The therapist decided to try raising the right side of the walker to make it higher than the left side. Surprisingly, the patient stopped falling! This kind of problem solving was not something that the therapist learned during ambulation class in PT 101.

The therapists I interviewed believed that many students do not understand the rewards of working with elderly patients. Several physical therapy supervisors stated that although students often complete geriatrics affiliations only because they are required to do so, some students leave the clinic with a new perspective on and appreciation for working with elderly persons.

Recruitment and Retention Strategies in Geriatrics

Redesign the curriculum. It is my belief that physical therapy education programs emphasize acute care rather than long-term care. We teach students that it is the physical therapist's job to diagnose a problem, plan a course of action, and help the patient reach both short-term and long-term goals in a "reasonable" length of time. When a practitioner is unable to accomplish this task, a sense of failure and frustration develops (Perkins 1986). The practitioner may become disinterested in the client and move on to work with other patients. Changes in physical therapist's attitudes toward geriatrics practice therefore must begin in the classroom.

Philips and Smith (1990) proposed that six components should be

To Find Out More

Those interested in developing research projects regarding the need and potential for rehabilitation among the elderly should contact the National Institute on Aging (NIA) in Bethesda, MD. The NIA recognizes the need for more research in geriatrics and provides grant monies for studies in this area.

For those interested in reading more about the problems of the geriatric patient and about research in the field, see the Spring 1990 issue of *Geritopics*, which reviews many of the journals that are devoted to age-related topics.

—*A. C. N.*

included in all allied health professional curricula to improve attitudes toward and care of the elderly person:

1. Students should be given realistic information about health and the aging process. They need to understand that aging is a normal part of life and does not necessarily lead to frailty or dementia.

ferently from the way it had been done before. Despite changes in actual employment patterns,, attitudes about employment policies have lagged far behind.

In 1989, Brazelton called for improved working conditions for working parents. According to Brazelton, when employers identify and meet the needs of working parents, employees display less burnout and show more interest in their jobs, and absenteeism decreases. Employers should begin restructuring organizations to provide equal opportunities to both working mothers and fathers.

Nollen (1982) concluded that new work schedules, carefully designed and executed, are the best investment an employer can make. Improvements in morale,

attendance, and performance levels far outweigh the costs involved.

In 1978 Arkin and Dobrofsky showed that job sharing is one way of helping employees combine work and family life. When two individuals share one position, creativity, resources, and talent are doubled. In addition, problems of sick leave, vacation coverage, and absenteeism are reduced. Although administrative costs are somewhat increased, gains in flexibility, morale, productivity, and efficiency far outweigh the costs.

Lee (1983) indicated that creative work schedules such as job sharing reduce staff turnover rates, and when staff turnover rates are reduced, the costs for advertising and retraining also are reduced. When

Studies have shown that personal experience with elderly individuals and improved knowledge about them results in an increased interest in working with elderly patients.

2. Students must learn how to provide comprehensive assessments of conditions related to aging. These assessments should include not only physical factors but also psychological and social factors that may affect patient response to treatment.
3. Students must begin to understand that improvement and maintenance of function often is the most appropriate goal for many elderly patients. Because elderly clients have multiple conditions, students must learn that treating one symptom may only exacerbate another symptom. In this way, students may begin to understand and treat the whole person, not just a "total hip" or a "total knee."
4. Students must recognize the importance of health education and disease prevention. They must learn to recognize risk factors among various cultural and ethnic communities to provide the best and most appropriate information to their clients.
5. Students must learn to develop effective communication skills both with patients and with patients' families. They must learn to deal with the visual, hearing,
and sensory problems that are related to aging and that may require modification of a treatment plan.
6. Students must become aware of community resources such as social services—Meals on Wheels, elder day care, group walking programs, homemaker services, health education programs—that may be available to their patients. They must learn to use these resources to enhance not only their treatment programs, but also their patient's quality of life.
Enrich classroom experiences. Faculty members should include

employees have more time for family life, stress and fatigue decrease. This results in improved quality and quantity of work.

Job sharing should be implemented at both the staff level and the supervisory level in health care facilities.

Professional growth and autonomy. Individuals' needs vary. Not everyone wants to become a department manager, but everyone wants to be recognized and rewarded for achievement. We must work to develop career ladders and specialty areas that allow individuals to attain levels of increasing responsibility—without forcing them into administrative positions they do not want.

Professional development. Managers should provide stimulating opportunities—both on and off the job—

for interaction with other health care professionals. Inservice education programs and staff meetings should be scheduled on an ongoing basis, with meeting times rotated to allow part-time staff members to participate. If facilities are very small, they may contact similar neighboring facilities to develop joint meetings. Staff members should be encouraged to use their own expertise to develop educational programs for other staff members. In addition, funds should be made available for staff members to attend continuing education programs outside their own facility. If funds are not available through the administration, staff members should consider holding their own fundraising events.

readings and discussions on the normal aging process. Healthy elderly individuals should be invited to attend class and to participate with students in these classroom discussions. Students should be encouraged to discuss their attitudes toward elderly persons and their personal experiences with elderly family members. Special medical problems related to aging should be covered. Students should gain an understanding that the specific goals of elderly individuals vary. What may seem insignificant to a young and healthy student may be a major accomplishment for an elderly individual and make a great deal of difference in that individual's quality of life.

Recently conducted at Northeastern University as part of a required senior course, one classroom program—the "Senior to Senior Project"—matched physical therapy students with appropriate elders (Hamel and Lake 1991). The students and elders met one hour a week over a period of five to six weeks. The purpose of the project was to promote communication and mutual learning. Although students were prohibited from providing hands-on physical therapy care to the elders, they were encouraged to discuss life experiences, including the impor-

tance of physical fitness and exercise in maintaining good health.

At the end of the project, students generally showed an increased awareness of the aging process and an improved understanding of the problems of elderly persons. A number of students expressed a new interest in working with the geriatric client. Although some students indicated that they were still not interested in working in geriatrics settings, they stated that they "no longer feared" working with that particular population (Hamel and Lake 1991).

Classroom discussions also must cover the cultural and ethnic factors that may have an effect on the health needs of elderly persons. Accidents, for example, are the number one cause of death among older American Indians and Native Alaskans, rates of certain types of cancer and diabetes are higher among Mexican Americans, and hypertension is twice as prevalent among older blacks than older whites (Phillips and Smith 1990). Socioeconomic factors, which also may have an effect on the treatment of elderly persons (see "Patient Compliance" in this issue of *CM*), also should be addressed in the classroom.

Increase the number of available clinical education sites. In addition to

increasing and improving students' classroom knowledge of geriatrics, physical therapy education should include at least one clinical education experience in a geriatrics setting.

Studies have shown that personal experience with elderly individuals and improved knowledge about them results in an increased interest in working with elderly patients. Peach and Pathy (1982) found that medical students who completed a geriatrics clinical rotation were more likely to consider a career in gerontology than those who had not done so. Another research study conducted by Coren et al. (1987) showed that a correlation exists among the existence of courses on geriatrics, student experience in working with elderly patients, and student intentions of working with elderly patients. Further results of this study indicated that a large number of students have neutral attitudes toward working with the elderly. With appropriate education and experience, these "neutral" students might be encouraged to pursue careers in geriatrics.

Results of a 1988 American Physical Therapy Association survey as reported by Schunk (1990) indicated that 67 percent of the responding schools reported an inadequate number of geriatrics affiliation sites.

Subsidize staff participation in professional organizations. Staff members should be encouraged to belong to and participate in both local and national professional organizations. Whenever possible, funding should be provided to help with the costs of active participation. Yearly membership fees or registration fees for national conferences may be included as options in benefits packages or as bonuses for a job well-done.

Encourage student education programs. Clinical affiliation students may stimulate staff members and encourage them to look at their routine in a new way. Students may bring new ideas from the classroom. Students may choose to accept positions at the facility before they graduate, which may decrease recruitment and training

costs. A study of 100 Ithaca College physical therapy graduates showed that 51 percent of the respondents had actively sought employment at a former clinical affiliation site (Ciccone and Wolfner 1988).

If staff members enjoy teaching, they should be encouraged to contact local universities. Many colleges welcome clinicians as guest speakers for various programs. In addition, some universities hire clinicians to assist with laboratory courses on an ongoing basis. Allowing clinicians the time to teach not only stimulates their professional development and prevents burnout, but also makes students aware of the facilities in which the clinicians work and may spur a student to apply for a position upon graduation.

Only 11 percent of these schools had as many as 20 percent of their clinical sites in geriatrics settings. Ciccone and Wolfner (1988) found that a strong relationship exists between clinical education and the types of work settings that students choose upon graduation. Increasing the number of clinical education sites in geriatrics settings eventually may help fill vacant positions in those settings.

Increase the visibility of physical therapist who works in the geriatrics setting. Physical therapists who work in geriatrics settings must become more vocal. They should be proud of their clinical expertise and become active in their professional organizations. This activity will help promote the value of geriatrics practice and also help enhance the prestige of working in geriatrics settings. Geriatrics clinicians should consider becoming clinical faculty members in physical therapy programs. Their insight and expertise is needed to help students understand the challenges and rewards that exist in the growing specialty area of geriatrics.

Increase research efforts in geriatrics. Physical therapy students must be encouraged to develop clinical research projects with faculty members and clinicians who have expertise in geriatrics.

In 1988, Wong completed a historical review of articles related to the topic of geriatrics published in *Physical Therapy* from January 1980 through June 1987. She found that although the geriatric population at that time made up 25 percent of the patient population, only five percent of the journal articles were related to that topic. Although she acknowledged that the number of articles related to geriatrics was on the increase, she concluded that, to meet the needs of the aging client, we must examine our attitudes toward elderly persons, restructure our physical therapy curricula, and increase and improve our clinical knowledge base as it relates to the geriatric patient.

As more research findings in geriatrics become available, and as more recognition is given to the specialists in the field, more graduating students and physical therapists may be encouraged to seek employment positions with the elderly patient, rather than simply "ending up" in these settings because the position offered them flexibility to combine their career and family lives.

Teach the Value of the Work

To attract and retain qualified personnel in any type of setting, a manager must create a work environment in which the work that contributes to the organization's needs also is valued by individuals as a path toward expected personal outcomes or rewards.

For geriatrics physical therapy, recruitment and retention strategies must begin in the physical therapy curricula, with classroom and clinical education experiences that help students understand the aging process and develop positive attitudes toward elderly persons. With this type of exposure, physical therapy students may be more likely to choose the geriatrics setting as a career path. And, because they have been taught about the value of physical therapists' work in that setting, they may be more likely to stay there. **CM**

Ann C. Noonan, EdD, PT, is an associate professor in the Department of Cooperative Education, Northeastern University, Boston, MA. She served as director of physical therapy at Milton Hospital, Milton, MA, for 15 years.

REFERENCES
Appelbaum, E. 1981. *Back to work: Determinants of Women's Successful*

Encourage staff participation in department decision making. Studies also have shown that health care professionals seek positions in facilities in which their ideas are respected and sought out. The reasons most often cited for leaving a position were a rigid administration and inflexible departmental decisions (American Physical Therapy Association 1988). Including staff members in discussions regarding problems and potential solutions may result in discovering and or avoiding potential future problems, allows individuals to share their personal experiences and expertise, results in more effective and appropriate solutions, and leads to increased commitment to the organization and its goals. When staff members are involved in decision making, they develop a sense of shared responsibility and increased job motivation.

REFERENCES
Appelbaum, E. 1981. *Back to work: Determinants of Women's Successful Re-entry.* Boston, MA, Auburn House.
Arkin, W., L.R. Dobrofsky. 1978. Job sharing. In R. Rapoport & R. Rapoport (Eds.), *Working couples* pp. 122-158. New York, NY, Harper and Row.
Brazelton, T. B. 1989. Working parents. *Newsweek* February 13: pp. 66-70.
Business Week. 1988 Human capital. The decline of America's work force. September 19:112-114, 118, 120.

Re-entry. Boston, MA, Auburn House.

Arkin, W., L.R. Dobrofsky. 1978. Job sharing. In: R. Rapoport & R. Rapoport, eds. *Working couples* pp. 122-158. New York, NY, Harper and Row.

Brazelton, T. B. 1989, Working parents. *Newsweek* February 13: pp. 66-70.

Brimer, M.A. 1984. To recruit and retain therapists: Consider their needs. *Clinical Management* 4(6): 38-39.

Business Week. 1988. Human capital. The decline of America's work force. September 19:112-114, 118, 120.

Buchanan, E., A.C. Noonan. 1988. *Factors Affecting Job Selection of Physical Therapy Graduates at Northeastern University*. Presentation at the Annual Meeting of Massachusetts Chapter of the APTA, Falmouth, MA.

Ciccone, C.D., M. L. Wolfner, 1988. Clinical affiliations and postgraduate job selection: A survey. *Clinical Management* 8 (3):16-17.

Coren, A., M. Andreassi, H. Blood, B. Kent, 1987. Factors related to physical therapy students' decisions to work with elderly patients. *Phys Ther* 67:60-65.

Fox, M. F., S. Hesse-Biber, 1984. *Women at Work*. Boston, MA, Mayfield Publishing.

Goodwin-Johansson, C. 1990. Therapy in the nursing home—A personal and professional challenge. *Physical Therapy Forum* 9(45) pp. 1-6.

Hall, D. T., E. E. Lawler. 1970. Job characteristics and pressures and the organizational integration of professionals. *Administrative Science Quarterly*, 15:271-281.

Hamel, P. C., D.L. Lake. 1991. *Senior to Senior Project: Intergenerational Awareness Exercise as Communication Facilitator*. Platform presentation. Boston, MA, American Physical Therapy Association Annual Conference, June.

Herzberg, F. 1968. One more time: How do you motivate employees? *Harvard Business Review* 46 (January-February):53-62.

Kerlinger, F. N. 1984. *Liberalism and conservatism. The nature and structure of social attitudes.* Hillsdale, NJ, Lawrence Erlbaum Assoc. Inc.

Lee, P. (1983). *The Complete Guide to Job Sharing*. New York, NY, Walker and Co.

Maslow, A. 1943. A theory of human motivation. *Psychol Rev* 50:370-396.

McClelland, D. 1961. *The Achieving Society*. New York, NY: Van Nostrand Reinhold.

Miller, G. D. 1990. Nursing homes—A viable challenge for the motivated therapist. *Geritopics* Spring:22.

Miller, J. B. 1976. *Toward a New Psychology of Women*. Boston, MA, Beacon Press.

Nollen, S. D. (1982). *New Work Schedules in Practice: Managing Time in a Changing Society.* New York, NY, Van Nostrand Reinhold.

Noonan, A. C. 1989. Physical Therapy Managers' Assumptions Regarding Working Mothers in the Physical Therapy Profession. Dissertation. Boston, MA, Northeastern University.

Peach, H., M.S. Pathy. 1982. Attitudes towards the care of the aged and to a career with elderly patients among students to a geriatric and general firm. *Age Aging* 11 196-202.

Pearl, M. J. 1990. Factors physical therapists use to make career decisions. *Phys Ther* 70:105-107.

Perkins, D. N. 1986. *Knowledge as Design*. Hillsdale, NJ, Lawrence Erlbaum Assoc. Inc.

Ciccone, C.D., M. L. Wolfner, 1988. Clinical affiliations and postgraduate job selection: A survey. *Clinical Management* 8 (3): 16-17.

Lee, P. (1983). *The Complete Guide to Job Sharing.* New York, NY, Walker and Co.

Nollen, S. D. (1982). *New Work Schedules in Practice: Managing Time in a Changing Society.* New York, NY, Van Nostrand Reinhold.

Noonan, A.C. 1989. Physical Therapy Managers' Assumptions Regarding Working Maothers in the Physical Therapy Profession. Dissertation. Boston, MA, Northeastern University.

Pearl, M. J. 1990. Factors physical therapists use to make career decisions. *Phys Ther 70:105-107.*

Recruitment and Retention of Physical Therapists in Hospitals. 1988. Alexandria, VA, American Physical Therapy Association, Inc.

Schaffer, S. 1986. The Response of Small Business to the Employment Generated Needs and Problems of Working Parents. Dissertation. Washington, DC, George Washington University.

Philips, B. U., D.L. Smith. 1990. Issues in aging: The curricular agenda of the 90's in schools of allied health sciences. In: Price, G. D., P. A. Fitz, eds. *Cultural Diversity and the Allied Health Curriculum Issues in Aging*, pp. 34-39. Storrs, CT, University of Connecticut.

PT Bulletin. 1990. August 22:3.

Recruitment and Retention. 1988. Alexandria, VA, American Physical Therapy Association, Inc.

Schaffer, S. 1986. The Response of Small Businesses to the Employment Generated Needs and Problems of Working Parents. Dissertation. Washington, DC, George Washington University.

Schein, E. H. 1978. *Career Dynamics: Matching Individual and Organizational Needs*. Reading, MA, Addison Wesley Publishing Co. Inc.

Schunk, C. 1990. Geriatric curriculum in physical therapy education. Entry level education. Results of APTA Survey. *Geritopics* Fall:13-14.

William, A. K. 1990. Keeping current with aging: A review of selected journals in gerontology and geriatrics. *Geritopics* Spring:15.

Wong, R. A. 1990. Negative attitudes toward chronic care intervention: Overview of a growing challenge. *Geritopics* Spring:11-14.

Wong, R. A. 1991. Impact of previous nursing home experience on students physical therapists' employment interest. *Journal of Physical Therapy Education* Fall:56-59.

Wong, R. A. 1988. Geriatric emphasis in physical therapy. A historical survey. *Phys Ther* 68:360-363.

Factors Related to Career Selection

Factors Influencing Job Selection of New Physical Therapy Graduates

Cindy I Buchanan, MS, PT
Ann C Noonan, EdD, PT
Mary L O'Brien, MPH, PT

ABSTRACT: The purpose of this study was to identify factors that influence new physical therapy graduates in job selection. Senior-year students from 14 randomly selected physical therapy programs were surveyed one month prior to graduation. Respondents were asked to rank order 14 factors that may have influenced their decision to select a particular job. Data were analyzed using the Kruskal-Wallis Test for significant rank order followed by the Mann-Whitney Test to compare specific variable medians. Students ranked salary, location, and type of clientele significantly higher (P<.05) than they ranked benefits and physical facilities. Benefits, however, were rated significantly more important (P<.05) than advancement opportunity, continuing education, and tuition assistance. Sign-on bonuses, previous employment at the facility, and relocation expenses were ranked as the least important factors influencing job selection.

INTRODUCTION

To prosper, an organization must recruit, manage, and develop its human resources effectively. Managers must identify individual needs and develop an organizational work environment that allows individuals to satisfy their needs while contributing to the needs of the organization. Job satisfaction and personal esteem will lead to increased commitment to an organization and improved organizational effectiveness.[1,2] Recruitment problems may be alleviated by developing new programs to satisfy, motivate, and retain existing personnel.[3] When hiring staff, employers must consider individuals who will work well within the organization. Identification of factors influencing job choice may help administrators recruit optimal employees.

In response to the proliferation of alternative work sites and reports that hospitals were experiencing difficulties recruiting and retaining physical therapists, the American Physical Therapy Association identified recruitment and retention of physical therapists in hospital settings as an important topic requiring research attention. As a result, the APTA began a study to determine whether such a problem did indeed exist, and if so to discover what factors contributed to the problem.

In 1988, survey instruments measuring job-satisfaction levels were sent to physical therapists and physical therapist assistants currently working in hospital environments and to therapists and assistants identified as having left the hospital environment within the past year. Results of the survey indicated that the number of vacancies for physical therapists in hospital settings was very low. The survey further showed that it took an average of 8 months or longer to fill a vacant position.[4]

Among the variables investigated, higher salaries was the only factor that decreased recruitment time. Therapists cited rigid working conditions as the reason for leaving the hospital setting. Strong correlations were found among feelings of professional autonomy, high staff morale, and satisfaction with salary. Therapists indicated that in searching for a new position they looked for adequate income and an environment that promoted autonomy, flexibility, and staff interaction and input into decision making.

In 1977, Barnes and Crutchfield[5] compared job-satisfaction levels of physical therapists working in private practices with those of therapists working in hospital settings. Their results indicated that levels of personal achievement, job responsibility, and salary contributed to positive job satisfaction among therapists in both settings. Problems with administrators and peers were dissatisfiers among hospital-based therapists, while working conditions led to dissatisfaction among some private practitioners.[5]

Pearl[6] investigated factors considered by physical therapists in making career decisions. She surveyed a random sample of 500 clinicians who were APTA members. Results of her study indicated that 56% of the responding therapists were employed outside traditional hospital and rehabilitation settings. Salary (51%) and location (38.2%) ranked highest as factors influencing present job selection. The job itself and the level of autonomy also were ranked very highly. Dissatisfiers included paperwork, excessive hours, and lack of benefits.

Respondents indicated that salary (52%) and location (28%) were factors they would most consider in making a career move. Benefits and professional development also rated highly. Less than 1% of respondents indicated that a sign-on bonus would be effective in recruiting them to a new position.[6]

Ciccone and Wolfner[7] conducted an informal survey to determine the relationship of clinical affiliation to job selection after graduation. They completed a telephone survey of 100 graduates chosen at random from the physical therapy program at Ithaca College in New York. Results of their survey indicated that over half of the alumni had applied for a position at a facility in which they had completed a clinical affiliation. They concluded that clinical internship does affect job selection and could be effective as a recruitment tool.[7]

Joseph Benanti, Jr.,[8] indicated that in today's job market, physical therapy managers must be innovative and flexible. He stated that the market for physical therapists will become even more competitive in the future. His suggestion to physical therapy administrators was to be resourceful and proactive in developing aggressive recruitment and retention strategies.[8]

This study was developed to assist managers in developing and implementing effective recruitment strategies by identifying factors

Ms Buchanan is Clinical Specialist, Department of Physical Therapy, 6 Robinson Hall, Northeastern University, 360 Huntington Ave, Boston, MA 02115. Dr Noonan is Associate Professor, Department of Cooperative Education, Northeastern University. Ms O'Brien is Clinical Specialist, Department of Physical Therapy, Northeastern University.

influencing new physical therapy graduates in the job-selection process.

METHOD

In 1989, a pilot study of factors influencing job choices of graduating physical therapy students was conducted by distributing a written survey to 100 senior-year students at Northeastern University in Boston, Mass. Students were asked to rank each of 14 factors, including location, type of clientele, salary, and prior experience at the facility, on a Likert Scale. In analyzing the results of that survey, we found that most students rated all factors as either most important or least important, with few responses in the middle portion of the scale.

Based on the results of the pilot study, the survey instrument was modified so that students were instructed to rank order the 14 factors, ranking the most important factor as 1 and the least important factor as 14 (Tab. 1). In addition, important characteristics of the job selected and demographic information were requested. Demographic information included the student's gender, state of residence, the name of the physical therapy program attended, and the degree they would obtain on graduation. Respondents also were asked how they had learned about their first job, the type of setting in which they would work, and their starting salary.

For this study, the names of 19 physical therapy education programs were randomly drawn from a hat containing the names of all accredited US physical therapy programs. The programs selected were representative of all geographic areas within the United States. A faculty member from each of these

Table 1

Kruskal-Wallis Rank Order of Factors Influencing Employment Decisions of New Graduates (N=216)

Factor	Median Rank[a]
Location	3
Salary	4
Clientele treated	4
Benefits	5
Physical facilities	6
Advancement opportunity	7
Continuing education	7
Tuition assistance	7
Clinical experience	10
Interview process	9
New-graduate training program	9
Sign-on bonus	11
Previous employment	11
Relocation expenses	11

[a]1=most important; 14=least important.

Table 2

Job-Choice Settings of New Graduates (N=216)

Setting	Number of Graduates (%)
Hospital	52.9
Private practice	18.3
Rehabilitation center	11.3
School system	2.8
Travel	2.1
Other	10.5

19 programs was contacted by one of the authors and asked to participate in the study. Fourteen programs had clinical affiliation and graduation schedules that met the time frame of this study, which took place during the spring of 1990.

A faculty member from each program was asked to distribute the survey to graduating seniors on completion of the clinical education component of the curriculum but before graduation. Of 428 surveys mailed to faculty members, 224 were returned, for a response rate of 52%. Eight of the returned surveys were incomplete and could not be used. Data analysis was conducted on the remaining 216 surveys.

Data Analysis

The Kruskal-Wallis Test was used to detect significant differences in the rank order of the 14 factors influencing employment decisions. Specific pairs of influencing factors then were analyzed using the Mann-Whitney Test (Figure). Descriptive statistics were determined for demographic and job-information variables.

RESULTS

Of the 216 respondents, 146 (67.5%) had accepted a job to be assumed on graduation. Of the 146 respondents who already had accepted jobs, 6 did not provide information on gender or salary, and 2 did not provide information on the type of job selected. Ninety eight (70%) of the respondents were female, and 42 (30%) were male. One hundred seven (76.4%) of the respondents would receive a bachelor's degree on graduation, and 33 (23.6%) would receive an entry-level master's degree.

Of the respondents, 52.9% had accepted an employment opportunity in a hospital (Tab. 2); 18.3% would be working in private practice settings; 11.3% would be working in rehabilitation centers; and 2.1% had chosen to work in pediatric settings. The remaining

10 students had accepted employment in sports, geriatric, psychiatric, corporate, or traveling facilities. None of the students chose to work in a home health setting.

One fourth (28.6%) of the students had learned about the job they selected as a result of a previous clinical affiliation at the site (Tab. 3). Fifteen percent had learned of the job through previous employment at the site, and 15% had learned of the job they eventually accepted by "word of mouth" from other students, friends, family, or therapists. Sixteen students (11.4%) became aware of employment opportunities through school-related job fairs, and 15 students were committed to their future job because of scholarship programs. Ten students simply called job sites themselves to apply for a position. The remaining students learned of available physical therapy positions through various forms of advertising. Only one student learned of his or her future job through *Physical Therapy*. Advertisements in *PT Bulletin* accounted for the job choices of six students.

The results of the Kruskal-Wallis Test indicated that students consistently rated some factors as more important than others in influencing job selection (P<.05). Location was the variable rated most important in

Table 3

Method by Which Respondents Learned of Selected Jobs (N=216)

Method	Number of Respondents (%)
Previous clinical affiliation	28.2
Previous employment at the site	14.8
Word of mouth	14.8
Job fair (school related)	11.3
Tuition-assistance program	9.8
Called facility	7.0
Newspaper advertisement	5.6
PT Bulletin advertisement	4.9
Recruiter	1.4
College/university placement office	1.4
Physical Therapy journal	0.7

influencing job selection, followed in importance by salary and type of clientele treated. Availability of a new-graduate training program was rated as the least important variable influencing job choice (Tab. 4).

Further analysis by the Mann-Whitney Test indicated which variables differed significantly in rank (P<.05). Five groups of factors were found to exist with no significant difference in the ranks of the factors within each group. All factors within a specific group, however, differed significantly in rank from factors belonging to another group

Table 4

Differences Between Groups Based on Results of Mann-Whitney Test (P<.05)

Groups	P
Clientele vs Benefits	0.0048
Benefits vs Advancement Opportunity	0.00015
Tuition vs Clinical Experience	0.0075
New-graduate Program vs Bonus	0.0135

Figure

Grouping of factors based on Mann-Whitney Test.

Group 1	Group 4
Location	Clinical experience
Salary	Interview process
Clientele treated	New-graduate training program
Group 2	**Group 5**
Benefits	Sign-on bonus
Physical facilities	Previous employment
	Relocation expenses
Group 3	
Physical facilities	
Advancement opportunity	
Continuing education	
Tuition assistance	

Differences within these groupings were not significant (P<.05).

(Tab. 4). No significant differences were found between students' ratings of salary, location, and type of clientele treated; however, these three factors were significantly more important than all other factors in job selection.

The employee-benefits factor was rated as significantly more important than the remaining 10 factors influencing job selection, with the exception of physical facilities and equipment. Rankings for facilities, opportunity for advancement, continuing education funds, and scholarship money did not differ significantly; however, all were rated as more important than the remaining six factors listed. Clinical experience at the facility, interview impressions, and new-graduate training programs were rated significantly higher than sign-on bonus, previous employment, and relocation expenses, the latter three factors being rated as the least important in the decision to choose a particular job opportunity.

DISCUSSION

Results of this study indicate that salary and location are the most important factors new graduates consider in job selection. This is in agreement with the results reported by Pearl[6] in a study of factors influencing experienced therapists in new-job selection. As a result of her findings, Pearl concluded that therapists who currently are working may be less altruistic than their predecessors. Although we are not discounting her conclusions, we believe that there may be some alternative explanations for our findings regarding new graduates.

Many students are faced with large school loans and few location options. They may be living with family to save money or may have no mode of transportation. Brimer[9] postulated that new graduates anticipate their weekly paycheck to begin recovery from the financial burden of school. The positive influence of a high salary on the job selection of new graduates may reflect the rising cost of education rather than a lack of altruism.

Further comparison of these results with those of Pearl[6] indicate that employee benefits and opportunity for advancement are of secondary importance in job selection for both experienced therapists and new graduates. Both groups listed factors such as relocation expenses and sign-on bonuses as having minimal influence on their decision to accept a particular employment opportunity.

Although previous clinical experience at a facility was not rated as highly important in selecting a job, this is the avenue by which the majority of students learned of the job they had accepted. This finding supports Ciccone and Wolfner's statement that an "important aspect of the clinical education/ job selection relationship . . . is that having a student program provides the institution with an applicant pool from which to fill vacant staff positions."[7] Our results also concur with those of Pearl[6] in that few participants learned of the job they selected through advertisements in professional literature or newspapers.

A discrepancy exists between the low rank (ninth) of clinical experience as a factor in job selection and the high proportion of students who accepted jobs at facilities where they had completed a clinical affiliation. This discrepancy may indicate that students do not behave in ways in which they say they behave when looking for a job. This certainly would make the validity of the survey questionable. On the other hand, students may have formulated ideas about important factors in job selection before selecting clinical affiliation sites. These factors then may have been important not only in selecting their first job, but also in selecting the clinical affiliation site. Where they completed a clinical affiliation thus may have been influenced by preconceived important job-selection factors, rather than the choice of affiliation site influencing job selection.

The majority of new graduates chose to work in hospital settings. This trend is quite different from that of experienced therapists, who most often seek jobs in private practice.[6] Directors of hospital-based physical therapy departments may fill vacancies more readily by designing recruitment strategies aimed at new graduates rather than at experienced therapists.

CONCLUSION

Salary and location are highly important job-selection factors for new graduates of physical therapy programs. The majority of new graduates accept jobs in hospital settings and learn of employment opportunities through previous clinical experience at the site. Hospital-based physical therapy departments may fill staff vacancies more efficiently if they offer clinical affiliation programs, provide competitive salaries, and market their recruitment programs to new graduates.

REFERENCES

1. Schein EH. *Organizational and Cultural Leadership.* San Francisco, Calif: Jossey Bass; 1985.
2. Hall DT, Lawler EE. Job characteristics and pressures and the organizational integration of professionals. *Administrative Science Quarterly.* 1970; 15:271–281.
3. Curtis C. Career development: innovative management solutions to staff attrition. *Rehabilitation Management.* June/July 1989: 65.
4. American Physical Therapy Association. *Recruitment and Retention of Physical Therapists in Hospital Settings.* Washington, DC: American Physical Therapy Association; 1988.
5. Barnes MR, Crutchfield CA. Job satisfaction-dissatisfaction: a comparison of private practitioners and organizational physical therapists. *Phys Ther.* 1977; 57:35–41.
6. Pearl MA. Factors physical therapists use to make career decisions. *Phys Ther.* 1990; 70:105–107.
7. Ciccone CD, Wolfner ML. Clinical affiliations and post-graduate job selection: a survey. *Clinical Management.* 1988; 8(3):16–17.
8. Benanti JA. Turbulent times call for innovative management. *Clinical Management.* 1984; 4(6):14–15.
9. Brimer MA. To recruit and retain therapists: consider their needs. *Clinical Management.* 1984; 4(6):38–39.

Student Attitudes Toward Rural Physical Therapy Practice

Patricia A Hageman, MS, PT
Robert H Fuchs, MA, PT

ABSTRACT: This survey study identified student attitudes toward physical therapy practice in a rural setting. Rural was defined as cities with less than 10,000 population and counties with less than 25,000 population. One hundred eighty-one students, enrolled in one of three state-supported physical therapy programs in Nebraska, South Dakota, and North Dakota, responded to the survey. The results indicated that students from rural areas were more likely to indicate interest in future rural practice than students from urban areas. Early exposure to rural physical therapy practice influenced most students favorably toward future rural practice. Student concerns about rural practice focused on referral issues. Strategies for physical therapy educators to increase interest in rural practice include recruiting students from rural areas, promoting early student exposure to rural practice, and assisting students in managing perceived obstacles toward rural health practice.

INTRODUCTION

Residents of rural areas encounter difficulty obtaining physical therapy services because of the lack of physical therapy providers. Rural residents in general usually are assumed to be at a distinct disadvantage for health care services because fewer providers are available to them and they often are required to travel long distances to obtain services.

The north central states of North Dakota, South Dakota, and Nebraska are geographically large, yet they have total populations of 639,000, 696,000 and 1,578,000, respectively, according to the 1990 US Census. The majority of the population within these states is concentrated within a few cities, and the remaining population is scattered across the

Ms Hageman is Director and Assistant Professor, Division of Physical Therapy Education, University of Nebraska Medical Center, 600 S 42nd St, Omaha, NE 68198-4420. Mr Fuchs is Assistant Professor, Division of Physical Therapy Education, University of Nebraska Medical Center.

state where distances between communities frequently are greater than 40 miles. Shortages of physical therapists exist within these states, especially in rural areas.[1-3]

The distribution of active physical therapists in this area is documented in the 1989 *Nebraska Manpower Report* prepared by the Nebraska Department of Health.[3] That study revealed that 44 of 93 counties did not have any active therapists, and 27 counties had only one active physical therapist. The remaining counties had 2 to 15 therapists, except the two most populated counties in Nebraska, which reported 70 and 154 active physical therapists, respectively.[3]

Physical therapists' decisions for location of practice and factors affecting those decisions are not well documented. Interest in rural health has generated several research studies to determine the most effective strategies for recruiting and retaining health professionals, with the focus of most of these studies on physicians. Some evidence supports the contention that physicians and physician assistants tend to locate in areas where their professional education took place.[4-6]

Madison suggested that physicians select a practice site based on influences from early life.[7] Research has shown a strong correlation between the types of communities that physicians choose for their practices and the types of communities in which they were raised.[8,9] The results of several studies indicate that physicians raised in rural areas who have early contact with rural practices are positively influenced toward rural practice.[10,11] The literature suggests that the greater the number and duration of prior contacts, the more likely it is that a physician would establish a practice at that site.[12] Whether physical therapists consider similar factors when deciding where to practice is unclear.

Because of the need for rural-practicing physical therapists within this region, strategies are being sought to interest physical therapy students in rural health practice. The purpose of this study was to identify student attitudes toward physical therapy practice in a rural setting, where *rural* was operationally defined as cities with less than 10,000 popu-

lation and counties with less than 25,000 population. The study addressed student interest in rural health practice, student perceptions about rural physical therapy practice, and factors influencing future practice decisions.

METHOD

The study population consisted of 196 students enrolled in one of three state-supported physical therapy programs in Nebraska, South Dakota, and North Dakota during the 1990–1991 academic year. These programs were selected for this initial project because of the similarity between the states in geography and population distribution. Each of these states had only one active physical therapy education program at the time the surveys were administered.

Data Collection

A three-page questionnaire with an open- and closed-question format was used to collect students' interests and beliefs about practice in a rural health setting. The study received appropriate Institutional Review Board approval. A cover letter was sent to directors of the physical therapy programs seeking permission to distribute the questionnaires. Each student received a cover letter explaining the survey instrument.

Data Analysis

The frequencies of the responses were calculated. A Spearman rank correlation was used to test for a significant relationship between students' home-town population size and the level of interest in future rural physical therapy practice.

RESULTS

The rate of return for the questionnaire was 92.3%, with 181 of the 196 students responding.

Previous Contact

A total of 118 (65.2%) of the respondents indicated that they had previous contact with physical therapists in rural practices. Among those with previous contact, 73 (61.9%) respondents indicated that the prior contact influenced them positively toward a possible rural practice, 44 (24.3%) respondents indicated that the contact had no effect on their future practice, one individual did not respond, and none of the respondents reported that the contact influenced them negatively toward rural practice.

Rural Health Opportunities

To determine students' awareness of manpower shortages, students were asked whether they believed that opportunities were available for physical therapy practice in the state where they were attending physical therapy school. Only one student responded that opportunities were very limited. The remainder of the respondents replied that there were many opportunities (145 students, 80.1%) or that there were a few opportunities (35 students, 19.3%) for rural physical therapy practice.

The majority of students (124 students, 68.5% of respondents) believed that it would not be difficult to find a position in a rural community, although 44 students (24.3%) thought it might be somewhat difficult and 12 students (6.6%) thought it might be moderately difficult to find a position. One individual felt that it would be extremely difficult to find a position.

Perceptions of Rural Practice

Students were asked to respond to an open-ended question about what aspects of a rural physical therapy practice they considered rewarding or advantageous. The respondents could leave the question blank or could provide one or more remarks. The comments received were categorized into one of seven areas. Sixty-nine comments indicated that the rural setting allowed closer relationships between patients and therapists. Fifty-four comments stated that rural practices permitted treating a variety of patient types. Students reported that rural practice permitted more freedom with better physician interaction (45 responses). Additional rewards or advantages mentioned related to small community lifestyle (40 responses), a less stressful environment (19 responses), and a challenging practice (8 total). Thirteen responses were categorized as other.

When asked about their perceptions of obstacles to finding a position or beginning a practice in a rural area, the responses were focused in several areas. Most citations (85 comments) related to concerns about the referral base. These referral base concerns were as follows: (1) the need for physical therapists was filled, (2) the population was too low to support a physical therapy practice, (3) the demand for physical therapy was low in rural areas because physicians and the community lacked familiarity with the pro-

fession, (4) people go to larger cities because they believe the care is better, and (5) the difficulty in determining where open positions are located.

Students also reported concerns about finding the capital to begin a rural practice (19 comments) and concerns that the pay scale would not be competitive (20 comments). Several responses indicated fears about being isolated without peer support (10 comments), lacking access to quality equipment (8 comments), and difficulty for spouse and family members to find employment (4 comments). Obstacles cited with fewer than 4 comments included frequent travel required, limited supply of suitable housing, the large effort needed to start a practice, and the difficulty of "breaking into" the community. Ten respondents remarked that there would be no obstacles or difficulty in beginning physical therapy practice in a rural area, although one individual added that it would be frightening.

Students identified their perceptions of the primary types of practice opportunities in rural and/or small communities as employment or contracts with community hospitals (129 responses; 71.3%) and nursing homes (20 responses; 11%). The remaining responses related to types of opportunities in rural and/or small communities were distributed among private practices, school systems, and physician offices.

Interest in Rural Practice

Students were asked how interested they were in rural health practice both immediately after graduation and sometime in the future. The results are listed in Table 1. A total of 103 students (56.9% of responses) indicated moderate to strong interest in rural practice immediately after graduation. The number rose to 141 students (78.4% of responses) indicating moderate to strong interest in rural practice sometime in the future but not immediately after graduation.

A Spearman rank correlation was completed between the students' interest level in rural health practice and their hometown population. Analysis of the data revealed that students from smaller hometowns had a stronger interest than students from urban areas in rural health practices for practice after graduation ($r=0.199$, $P<0.01$) and for future practice although not immediately after graduation ($r=0.158$, $P<0.05$). The numbers and percentages of students expressing interest in rural practice are displayed in Tables 2 and 3.

Reasons for Practice Selection

Complete data about reasons for practice selection are included in Table 4. The most

Table 1
Interest in Rural Physical Therapy Practice After Graduation

Interest Level	Percentage of Responses	
	Immediately After Graduation (n=181)	Sometime in Future (n=180)
Strong	9.9	22.8
Moderate	47.0	55.6
Very limited	33.1	17.8
None	9.9	3.3

Table 2
Interest in Rural Physical Therapy Practice Immediately After Graduation by Hometown Population Size

Hometown Population Size	Number of Responses (n=181) with Percentage of Total for Each Population Category			
	Strong Interest	Moderate Interest	Limited Interest	No Interest
<1000	3 (9.7)	16 (51.6)	11 (35.5)	1 (3.2)
1000–5000	7 (11.9)	33 (55.9)	16 (27.1)	3 (5.1)
5000–10,000	3 (15.8)	10 (52.6)	4 (21.1)	2 (10.5)
10,000–50,000	3 (7.5)	17 (42.5)	13 (32.5)	7 (17.5)
50,000–200,000	0 (0.0)	4 (26.7)	7 (46.7)	4 (26.7)
>200,000	2 (11.8)	5 (29.4)	9 (52.9)	1 (5.9)

frequently cited reasons provided by respondents for possible future consideration of a rural/small community health practice were that they enjoyed living in a rural/small community area (29.2% of responses) and that it was a practice setting they would enjoy (25% of responses).

Only 21 respondents (11.6%) indicated that they had no interest in rural physical therapy practice. The primary reasons among that group for not considering a rural physical therapy practice were that it is not a practice setting they would enjoy (61.9% of responses), they had no family or friends in rural areas (19.0% of responses), and the financial incentives are limited (19.0% of responses).

DISCUSSION

The questionnaire response rate of 92.3% was excellent. No follow-up reminder was mailed to the students.

Interest in Rural Practice

Within this study, physical therapy students from rural areas were more likely than those from urban areas to express a strong or moderate interest in a rural practice. This finding is consistent with the research results of physician and physician assistant studies where students from rural areas were more likely than urban students to practice in rural areas.[4,5,8,9]

Prediction of the percentages of those surveyed who actually will enter rural practice is difficult because, although interest in rural health practice was high, projected interest does not guarantee actual settling into a rural health practice. An Illinois study of physicians found that although initial interest in rural health was at 50%, only 8% actually settled into a rural setting.[13] Several researchers suggest that attitudes and interests of both faculty and students may be important in increasing the number of graduates interested in rural health practice.[9,14]

The correlations between students' interest in future practice and students' hometown size were statistically significant, but the specific correlation coefficients (r values) did not reflect a high correlation. We believe that statistical significance was found because of the large subject sample (n=181). Nonetheless, Tables 3 and 4 show slightly more interest in rural practices by students from communities defined as rural according to our operational definition.

Early professional socialization was recommended by several researchers as a method to enhance future practice patterns.[6,11,12] The results of this study support this concept

where prior contact to rural physical therapy was perceived as a positive influence or at worst a neutral influence toward future rural practice.

Rural Health Practice Perceptions

The results indicate that the students in this study were aware of manpower shortages in rural areas. The majority of physical therapy students did not feel that it would be difficult to find a position, but a large percentage (31%) indicated that it would be somewhat or moderately difficult to find a position.

The benefits of a rural practice described by physical therapy students in this study were similar to published reports of factors influencing physicians toward rural practice. Rural lifestyle, adequate income, professional freedom, and proximity to family were factors listed by respondents in this study and in studies of the satisfaction of rural physicians.[4,15]

Whereas physicians listed dissatisfaction with factors such as travel, income, and long working hours in a rural health practice, the majority of physical therapy students listed concerns about establishing a sufficient referral base as obstacles for beginning a rural health practice.[15] The concern raised by students in this study that rural communities and physicians are not familiar with physical therapy has been substantiated by a situation analysis study conducted by the Northern Outreach Program in Ontario, Canada.[16]

Implications

The physical therapy education admissions process should focus on recruiting and selecting students from rural areas. Programs should foster early exposure to rural health practices, and education is needed to assist students in managing their perceived obstacles toward rural health practice. The student responses suggest that physical therapy programs may need a heavier focus on topics such as marketing services to the physician and public, establishing a financially sound practice, and networking strategies. Because so many respondents reported uncertainty about the number of available opportunities for physical therapists in rural communities, marketing efforts by rural communities should be improved.

Care must be taken when applying the results of this study to other programs or regions of the country. Future research should focus on the relationships between student attitudes within the program and actual practice locations after graduation. Future research also should specifically ask students to define their interests to more clearly predict which students will choose rural practice. For example, asking students whether they have made rural contacts and whether they have made actual plans for future practice would be useful. Currently the authors are analyzing data from an expanded version of the questionnaire that was sent to other physical therapy programs.

Table 3

Interest in Rural Physical Therapy Practice Sometime in the Future by Hometown Population Size

Hometown Population Size	Number of Responses (n=179) with Percentage of Total for Each Population Category			
	Strong Interest	Moderate Interest	Limited Interest	No Interest
<1000	5 (16.7)	20 (66.7)	4 (13.3)	1 (3.3)
1000–5000	16 (27.6)	35 (60.3)	7 (12.1)	0 (0.0)
5000–10,000	7 (36.8)	11 (57.9)	1 (5.3)	0 (0.0)
10,000–50,000	9 (22.5)	20 (50.0)	8 (20.0)	3 (7.5)
50,000–200,000	1 (6.7)	9 (60.0)	4 (26.7)	1 (6.7)
>200,000	3 (17.6)	5 (29.4)	8 (47.1)	1 (5.9)

Table 4

Reasons for Considering Future Physical Therapy Practice in a Rural Setting (n=160)

Reason	Percentage of Responses
Enjoy rural/small community areas	29.4
Enjoyable practice setting	25.0
Lifestyle	15.6
Family/friends	10.0
Able to establish own practice	8.1
Need for physical therapists	8.1
Financial incentives	2.5
Other	1.2

CONCLUSION

The results of a questionnaire study completed by 181 of 196 students enrolled in three state-supported physical therapy programs within the north central states of North Dakota, South Dakota, and Nebraska demonstrated the following:

1. A relationship existed between students' hometown population size and their interest in future rural practice. Students from rural areas were more likely to indicate interest in future rural practice than students from urban areas.

2. Prior exposure to rural health physical therapy practice influenced the majority of students favorably toward future rural practice. No responses indicated that prior exposure was a negative influence.

3. Factors considered as advantageous to rural practice by students were the opportunity for closer relationships between therapists and patients, the variety of patient types, and greater professional freedom. Factors considered as obstacles to rural physical therapy practice included concerns about an adequate referral base.

4. The primary reasons that students would consider a rural physical therapy practice were enjoyment for living in a rural area and for the practice setting. The primary reasons students would not consider a rural physical therapy practice were that it was not a practice setting they would enjoy and no family or friends lived in rural areas.

REFERENCES

1. University of Nebraska Medical Center. *Study of Allied Health Professionals in the State of Nebraska.* Omaha, NE: School of Allied Health Professions; 1987.

2. Roberts J. Survey of Nebraska hospital manpower needs. Lincoln, NE: Nebraska Hospital Association; 1990.

3. *Nebraska Health Manpower Report.* Lincoln, NE: Nebraska Department of Health; 1990.

4. Rhodes JF, Day FA. Location decisions of physicians in rural North Carolina. *Journal of Rural Health.* 1989;5:137–153.

5. Stratton TD, Geller JM, Ludtke RL, Fickenscher KM. Effects of an expanded medical curriculum on the number of graduates practicing in a rural state. *Acad Med.* 1991;66:101–105.

6. Fowkes VK, Hafferty FW, Goldberg HI, Garcia RD. Educational decentralization and deployment of physician assistants. *J Med Educ.* 1983;53:194–200.

7. Madison DL. Managing a chronic problem: the rural physician shortage. *Ann Intern Med.* 1980;92:852–854.

8. Leonardson G, Lapierre R, Hollingsworth D. Factors predictive of physician location. *J Med Educ.* 1985;60:37–43.

9. Rabonowitz HK. Evaluation of a selective medical school admissions policy to increase the number of family physicians in rural and underserved areas. *New Engl J Med.* 1988;319:480–486.

10. Breisch WF. Impact of medical school characteristics on location of a physician practice. *J Med Educ.* 1970;45:1068–1070.

11. Chaulk CP, Bass RL, Paulman PM. Physicians' assessment of a rural preceptorship and its influence on career choice and practice site. *J Med Educ.* 1987;62:349–351.

12. Rabinowitz HK. The relationship between medical student career choice and a required third-year family practice clerkship. *Family Med.* 1988;20(2):118–121.

13. Summey JH, Loftin VC, Loftin EV. Illinois medical school graduates: initial practice location choice. *Illinois Med J.* 1986;169:238–241.

14. Hafferty FW, Boulger JG. Medical students view family practice. *Family Medicine.* 1988;20(4):277–281.

15. Movassaghi H, Kindig D. Medical practice and satisfaction of physicians in sparsely populated rural counties of the United States: results of a 1988 survey. *Journal of Rural Health.* 1989;5(2):125–136.

16. Beggs C. The Ontario Northern Outreach Program in physical therapy. *Physiotherapy Can.* 1988;40(2):80–85.

Building Student Interest in Acute Care

The hospital is one of the most necessary and remarkable organizations within our health care system. Regardless of the severity of illness or the type of disease, the hospital provides around-the-clock, seven-days-a-week services. It is the fundamental mechanism through which our society cares for those who are unable to care for themselves.

Within this institution, we as physical therapists work with members of other health care disciplines to provide high-quality, efficient patient care. Within this institution, we constantly are challenged by life-and-death situations, ethical dilemmas, complex medical problems, ongoing new admissions and unexpected discharges, scheduling conflicts, ever-changing technology, and complicated medical record keeping. It should come as no surprise to us, then, that many students who choose health care as a profession—and who have the option within their profession to work in health care settings with a more medically stable, cooperative, or motivated patient—choose those less stressful settings. These alternative settings ironically may offer a

By Daniel Dore, PT, MPA

higher salary and a more controllable work week.

Observations of an Interviewer

During the past several years, I had the opportunity to interview more than 200 newly graduated and licensed therapists for acute care staff positions at a large university medical center. These therapists ranged in age from 21 to 43 years and represented more than 38 physical therapy education programs across the United States. Of the more than 200 applicants, *only 7 expressed that acute care hospital work was a long-term career goal.* The vast majority of the applicants viewed the acute care experience as an opportunity to be exposed—through a rotation system—to patients with a variety of medical and surgical conditions. Their goal: to develop a solid, broad foundation for the time when they "move on" to a position in an outpatient or rehabilitation setting.

When confronted with rotations that included pulmonary care, cancer care, or any patient profile involving multiple disease processes, these applicants typically stated that their curriculum had not focused on the patient who is hospital-based but rather on the ambulatory patient with musculoskeletal

problems or on the patient who is medically stable and has neurological problems. There may be various sociological reasons why this focus may have evolved in some physical therapy education programs. One theme recurs, however, among the new graduates I encounter, regardless of their level of schooling: They feel unprepared and unmotivated to pursue work in acute care.

What Do We Do? One Example

We know we must prepare our entry-level physical therapists for the acute care setting. But how can we foster, within the education program, a sense of fulfillment and purpose in choosing the acute care setting for employment?

Using concepts that also may be applied to clinical education settings, our acute care senior clinical staff developed an acute care elective for second-year, master's degree entry-level physical therapy students. The objective was for the student to appreciate and participate in the unique role that the physical therapist plays as a member of an interdisciplinary health care team managing the care of the patient who is acutely ill.

Because the work of the physical therapist in the hospital-based setting is characterized by a high degree of autonomy and responsibility in clinical decision making, student learning in this setting must result in a sound knowledge of pathology and the disease process and a proficiency in evaluation and treatment planning. This course was designed to allow the student with an interest in acute care to develop additional knowledge and skills in the evaluation and treatment of the patient who is acutely ill and to become comfortable and fulfilled within this setting.

To accomplish the goals of the course, information was applica-

Reprinted from *Clinical Management*. Dore D. Building student interest in acute care. 1992;12(6):12-13. With the permission of APTA.

tion-oriented and presented by experienced therapists whose day-to-day patient care responsibilities centered on the acute care setting. In addition, the class was geared toward open group discussion regarding specific patients and information pertinent to a variety of acute care settings and problems.

Prior to class, each student was expected to review a specific patient's chart assigned by the clinician and to be ready to present that case to the group. This format was very similar to making rounds on a hospital floor and provided the opportunity for others in the class to ask questions or add information. This format also allowed the clinician to have a base of practice information to which more detail or explanation could be added or from which leading questions could be posed. Discussion of each chart included:

1. *Patient profile,* from preadmission status through hospital course, including medications, tests, laboratory values, and physical therapy intervention.

2. *Problem list,* with recognizable links made between cardiovascular, neurological, cardiopulmonary, and musculoskeletal systems.

3. *Short-term and long-term functional goals* and plans to achieve those goals.

4. *Discharge* planning.

These items were discussed with the senior therapist or clinical resource therapist teaching in that particular subject.

Following this discussion, the senior therapist presented the topic of the day in an informal and practical manner. Topics included: critical care units, focusing on the recognition of various lines and leads and equipment functions; precautions; problem solving; com-

mon errors in practice and patient relations; universal precautions and their practical application to day-to-day acute care situations; patients' rights, with attention to verbal and nonverbal communication with patients; the needs of the family; "do not resuscitate" orders; occupational stress; the logic of discharge

---

We know we must prepare our entry-level physical therapists for the acute care setting. But how can we foster, within the education program, a sense of fulfillment and purpose in choosing the acute care setting for employment?

---

planning; and the prioritization of patients. In addition, presentations were made on selected topics in hematology, cardiopulmonary, orthopedics, neurology, pediatrics, wound care, and coronary care.

The last hour of each class focused on the care of specific patients, with each student working with a senior therapist in that therapist's area of clinical expertise. During the course, each student could choose a surgical procedure or diagnostic test to observe and

could present a specific topic relevant to the acute care setting.

Patients as Instructors

One of the most valuable teaching methods may involve the use of "patient panels." Former patients may be invited to the clinic classroom to speak to students about the impact that physical therapy had on them during their hospital stay.

A patient who had undergone bone marrow transplantation and a patient who had been in and out of the intensive care unit as a result of AIDS complications have shared their physical therapy experiences with our students. Now in the end-stage, the patient with AIDS has told students that he finds physical therapy to be the most meaningful part of his home health program. Interactions like this one between student caregivers and patients can only reinforce student understanding of the importance of acute care work.

Stop the Migration!

Health care has undergone drastic changes in the past few decades. The migration of health care personnel from the acute care setting is one of the most disturbing.

Helping people when they are too ill to care for themselves certainly is one of the noblest professional choices a person can make. I would hope our curricula and our prospective physical therapy clinicians never lose sight of this truth. **CM**

Daniel Dore, PT, MPA, is Director of Clinical Services, Department of Physical and Occupational Therapy, Duke University Medical Center, Durham, NC, and Clinical Associate, Graduate Program in Physical Therapy, Duke University.

Physical Therapy Employment Practices Comparing Baccalaureate- and Postbaccalaureate-Degree Entry Levels

Joyce MacKinnon, EdD, PT
Laurie Gould, PT
Lynn Herchenroder, PT
Arlene Morse, PT
Diane Seabury, PT

ABSTRACT: With economics as a focus, the purpose of this study was to gather data on physical therapy employment practices, with entry-level education as the variable of interest. The subjects in this study were 77 physical therapy directors of various types of health care facilities selected randomly from the University of New England Physical Therapy Department's list of clinical affiliation sites. The design of the study was primarily descriptive; a questionnaire was used to gather information. Data from the returned questionnaires were tallied manually and reported numerically as percentages or analyzed using chi square. Results demonstrated no statistically significant differences in employment practices with regard to hiring, work load, professional responsibilities, remuneration, benefits, or career advancement when baccalaureate entry-level degree physical therapy graduates were compared with postbaccalaureate entry-level degree therapists. This information should be considered by current and prospective students and faculty in the discussion surrounding physical therapy entry-level education.

INTRODUCTION

A person's choice of a career and the way in which that person prepares for his or her chosen career are influenced by many factors, one of which is economic. According to

Dr MacKinnon is Professor and Chair. Department of Physical Therapy, University of New England, Hills Beach Rd. Biddeford, ME 04005. Address all correspondence to Dr MacKinnon. Ms Gould, Ms Herchenroder. Ms Morse. and Ms Seabury were students in the undergraduate program. Department of Physical Therapy, University of New England, when this study was completed in partial fulfillment of their degree requirements. This study was approved by the Institutional Review Board of the University of New England.

principles of basic economic theory, a person choosing a career considers the total cost of one career investment compared with others, and then looks at the expected return on the investment.[1] The cost:benefit ratio of one career can be compared with another, or the cost:benefit ratio of various methods of preparing for the same career can be compared.

To determine total career cost, for example, a person deciding between nursing and physical therapy can investigate the cost involved in obtaining the appropriate education, the cost of licensure, and the cost of years of unemployment or underemployment experienced while obtaining the appropriate degree. That person then can estimate the expected economic return for both career choices, which frequently is expressed in terms of salary, and can use this information as one factor in making a career decision.

Once a career choice is made, that person also can look at the cost:benefit ratio involved in the choice of educational routes available. For example, a person interested in nursing can obtain a diploma, an associate degree, or a baccalaureate degree in nursing to be eligible to sit for licensure and enter the practice arena.[2] A person interested in physical therapy can choose between a baccalaureate degree or an entry-level master's degree to be eligible to sit for licensure and enter the practice arena. As of 1993, students also can add an entry-level doctoral degree to these choices.

Cost:benefit ratios for careers and methods of preparing for careers have been demonstrated to affect educational enrollment decisions.[3] As stated, both nursing and physical therapy are careers with multiple educational entry levels. The nursing profession has attempted to look at the various cost:benefit ratios involved in the choice of entry-level education,[2,4-7] but the physical therapy profession has not done similar stud-

ies. Instead, therapists assert opinions such as, "Frankly, as a 3-year department head with 10 years in various clinical settings, I smile every time an entry-level master's new graduate thinks he or she should be paid more than a grad (sic) with a bachelor's degree. There is no difference between the two at 1 month or 5 years out."[8]

The purpose of this study was to gather information on employment practices with entry-level education as the variable of interest, focusing on the economic aspects of choice of entry-level degree. Students interested in becoming physical therapists may attend an accredited baccalaureate-degree entry-level (BEL) program or a postbaccalaureate-degree entry-level (PBEL) program. As more programs open at the PBEL,[9] and as BEL programs make a transition to PBEL,[10] current and prospective physical therapy students and faculty are interested in the practice ramifications of entry-level degrees. If documented differences in employment practices based on entry-level education can be demonstrated to exist, or if it can be demonstrated that no differences exist, this information could markedly affect student choice of programs (as has been seen in other academic majors[3]) and have a profound impact on physical therapy education.

Economic ramifications are only one factor in deciding on a career or on the appropriate way to pursue career preparation. It is beyond the scope of this article to discuss the many other factors involved in the support of the American Physical Therapy Association and its membership to move the profession to postbaccalaureate-degree entry level.[11-14]

The null hypothesis for this study was that no statistically significant differences would exist in employment practices with regard to hiring, work load, professional responsibili-

Reprinted with permission from the *Journal of Physical Therapy Education*, Vol 8, No 1, pp 11-17, 1994.

ties, remuneration, benefits, or career advancement when BEL physical therapy graduates were compared with PBEL graduates, either at the time of first employment or subsequently. The investigators believed that support for the null hypothesis would stem from employers' perception that both BEL and PBEL therapists were educated to competently begin to practice physical therapy.[8] Because both BEL and PBEL programs are accredited using the same standards, this would be a logical assumption.[15] We also thought that the national shortage of physical therapists available for the number of positions open would encourage employers not to differentiate between BEL and PBEL graduates.[16]

Support for the alternate hypothesis, that there would be a statistically significant difference when BEL physical therapy graduates were compared with PBEL graduates, would rest on the assumption of employers that a master's degree would connote a higher level of competence than a baccalaureate degree.[17,18]

The independent variable in this study was entry-level degree program, either BEL or PBEL. There were six dependent variables:

1. *Hiring.* Respondents to a questionnaire were asked to rank physical therapy applicant attributes, with entry-level degree being one of the attribute choices.

2. *Work load,* which was operationally defined as the average number of patients seen daily by a physical therapist at the end of the first year of employment.

3. *Professional responsibilities.* This category was operationally defined as whether a physical therapist would be expected to supervise students, supervise physical therapist aides and assistants, provide in-service education, be involved in clinical research, or chair department or hospital/facility committees by the end of the first year of employment.

4. *Remuneration,* which was operationally defined as the starting salary range for an entry-level therapist at the time of first employment.

5. *Benefits,* which was defined as money allocated for continuing education.

6. *Career advancement,* which included the opportunity to supervise staff, students, the department, or a research project.

METHOD
Subjects

The subjects in this study were 100 physical therapy directors of various types of health care facilities selected randomly from the University of New England (UNE) Phys-

ical Therapy Department's list of 207 clinical affiliation sites. The majority of respondents were directors of physical therapy in general hospitals, with directors of physical therapy in rehabilitation hospitals or clinics comprising the next largest category of respondent. We also had representation from private practice, home health, and nursing homes, and one respondent each from a college health center, a school system, and a developmental center (Tab. 1). Geographically, our respondents were primarily from New England, although other parts of the country also were represented (Tab. 2).

Instrument

We developed a questionnaire to assess physical therapy employment practices, with entry-level degree as the variable of interest. Initially a pilot questionnaire was sent to 152 randomly selected directors of physical therapy departments in New England, with a request to complete the questionnaire and provide feedback concerning the instrument. From this feedback, and with consultation from a sociologist nationally recognized as an expert in survey research design (John Allan, PhD), the questionnaire was modified and used in this study.

The questionnaire first asked the respondent to indicate the type of facility with

which he or she was affiliated, the state in which the facility was located, and which of the two types of entry-level graduates the respondent had supervised. The respondent then was asked to answer five paired questions. The question was asked first with the BEL physical therapist as the subject of interest, and then was asked using the PBEL physical therapist as the subject of interest.

To look at differences in expected work load, the respondent was asked to indicate the average number of patients seen daily by a physical therapist employed at his or her facility by the end of the first year of employment. The respondent then was provided with a list of professional responsibilities and was asked which ones a physical therapist at his or her facility would be expected to perform by the end of the first year of employment. To examine the area of remuneration, the respondent was asked to indicate the starting salary range for a physical therapist at his or her facility at the time of first employment.

Because it is difficult legally for an employer to offer differing health care benefits based on an employee's educational level, *benefits* were defined as money allocated for continuing education. The respondent was asked to indicate the amount of money allocated to a physical therapist at his or her facility for continuing education at the time

Table 1

Type of Facility With Which Respondent Was Affiliated (N=77)

Type of Facility	Number of Respondents
General hospital	35
Rehabilitation hospital or clinic	18
Clinic, private practice	8
Other	7
Home health	3
Nursing home	3
College health center	1
School system	1
Developmental center	1
Residential care facility	0

Table 2

State in Which Facility Was Located (N=77)

State	Number of Respondents
Maine	19
New Hampshire	12
Massachusetts	6
Florida	6
New York	5
Pennsylvania	4
Connecticut, Rhode Island, New Jersey	3 (each state)
Arizona, Louisiana, Vermont, West Virginia	2 (each state)
Alabama, Delaware, Georgia, Kentucky	1 (each state)
Maryland, Michigan, Tennessee, Washington	0

of first employment. The final paired question addressed intradepartmental advances available to physical therapists at the respondent's facility, including supervision of staff, students, the department, or a research project.

Questionnaire respondents considered both BEL and PBEL physical therapists at their facilities when asked whether any salary differences, differences in advancement opportunities, or differences in available benefits existed when the two groups were compared, either at the time of first employment or at any subsequent time. Respondents also were asked what types of students (BEL or PBEL) they had accepted for clinical affiliation.

To explore employer perceptions of entry-level graduates, especially with regard to hiring, we asked respondents to rank employee attributes from most to least important, from a list that included age, clinical experience, entry-level degree, additional degrees, continuing education, references, personal attributes, and the institution from which the applicant received his or her degree. We deliberately chose these attributes to differentiate between the entry-level degree itself and other attributes that might be more characteristic of one type of entry-level degree physical therapist versus the other. For example, because the PBEL therapist may be older than the BEL therapist, we listed age as an attribute choice. We thought that employers might be more inclined to hire PBEL therapists merely because they are older, and we wanted questionnaire respondents to be clear about the attribute choices they were making.

The final question asked the respondent to indicate the type of entry-level physical therapy program from which he or she graduated. Respondents had the choice of three types of entry-level programs: BEL, certificate, or PBEL. In the past, physical therapy students could attend and graduate from a certificate program, as well as BEL and PBEL programs. A certificate program essentially was a PBEL program without a degree. These programs now have been phased out.

Procedure

The surveys were mailed to the physical therapy directors as described, along with a cover letter and a stamped return envelope. Two weeks after the initial mailing, a follow-up notice was mailed to the directors asking them to respond if they had not already done so.

Data Analysis

Percentages were calculated and reported for demographic items of interest, such as type of facility, state in which the facility was

Table 3
Education Level of Physical Therapists Supervised by Respondents (N=77)

Education Level	Number of Respondents Who Supervised at this Level (%)
Both BEL[a] and PBEL[b]	43 (55.7)
Only BEL	34 (44.3)
Only PBEL	0 (0)

[a]Baccalaureate entry level.
[b]Postbaccalaureate entry level.

Table 4
Education Level of Physical Therapy Students Accepted for Clinical Affiliations (N=77)

Education Level	Number of Respondents Who Accepted Students for Affiliation at this Level (%)
Both BEL[a] and PBEL[b]	50 (65)
Only BEL	24 (30.75)
Neither	3 (3.85)[c]
Only PBEL	0 (0)

[a]Baccalaureate entry level.
[b]Postbaccalaureate entry level.
[c]Some sites on the clinical affiliate list were added recently and had not yet accepted students for clinical affiliation. Three of these sites were included in our sample.

Table 5
Type of Physical Therapy Entry-Level Education Program From Which Respondents Graduated (N=77)

Type of Program	Number of Respondents (%)
Baccalaureate entry level	64 (83)
Certificate	10 (13)
Postbaccalaureate entry level	3 (4)

located, type of entry-level graduate supervised, and the entry-level degree of the respondent. Percentages also were reported when questionnaire respondents were asked to compare BEL and PBEL graduates with regard to salary differences, differences in advancement opportunities, or differences in available benefits.

When respondents were asked to rank applicant attributes, the final ranking reported in this article was calculated by taking each attribute, adding the ranking of each individual respondent for that attribute to reach a total score, and then using that total to rank attributes from most to least important. If an attribute had a total score of 88, and that score was the lowest score compared with all other totals, that attribute would be ranked first in importance.

A chi square analysis was performed on questions relating to 1) average number of patients seen daily by a physical therapist by the end of the first year of employment, 2) responsibilities that a physical therapist would be expected to assume by the end of the first

year of employment, 3) the starting salary range for a physical therapist at the time of first employment, 4) money allocated to a physical therapist for continuing education at the time of first employment, and 5) intradepartmental advancements available to a physical therapist at any time in the therapist's career, comparing PBEL and BEL physical therapists.

RESULTS

Seventy seven of the 100 surveys were returned and analyzed. Results are listed in Tables 1–8. The highest number of respondents worked in general hospitals, but all facility choices were represented with the exception of the residential care facility (Tab. 1). Nineteen states were represented in our sample, with Maine having the highest number of respondents (Tab. 2). These distributions accurately reflected the sample population. The majority of directors in our sample were located in general hospitals, and the majority were from the northeastern part of the country, with Maine being the state most highly represented.

The majority of respondents had supervised both BEL and PBEL physical therapists (Tab. 3) and had accepted both BEL and PBEL students for clinical affiliations at their facilities (Tab. 4). The majority of respondents had graduated from a BEL program (Tab. 5).

The ranking of applicant attributes from most to least important based on the educational level of the therapist being supervised (BEL or PBEL) is shown in Table 6. In both ranking schemes, entry-level degree is ranked as below the midpoint of the attribute list in importance. The ranking of applicant attributes from most to least important based on the entry-level education of respondents (BEL, PBEL, and certificate) is found in Table 7. While the respondents who held BEL degrees ranked entry-level degree below the midpoint in order of importance, the respondents who had graduated from a certificate program ranked this attribute at the midpoint, and respondents who held PBEL degrees ranked the attribute second in importance.

All results of our chi square analyses supported the null hypothesis that there would be no statistically significant differences in employment practices related to work load, professional responsibilities, remuneration, benefits, or career advancement when BEL and PBEL physical therapists were compared (Figs. 1–5). When asked to compare BEL and PBEL graduates at their facilities, 100% of the respondents reported no differences in benefits available to the two groups, 92% reported no advancement differences, and 84% reported no salary differences (Tab. 8).

DISCUSSION

The results of our study indicate that physical therapy employment practices are not affected by therapist entry-level education when considering work load, professional responsibilities, remuneration, benefits, or career advancement either at the time of first employment or at any time subsequently (Tabs. 7, 8). Our results are similar to the results obtained in studies that scrutinized employment practices for nurses with various entry-level degrees. In a study by Lowry, she found that the economic benefits of having a baccalaureate degree in nursing, as compared with a diploma or an associate degree in nursing, were not realized until the completion of a lifetime of employment and certainly were not present 1 to 5 years after first employment.[2] Link found that while some facilities offered an increased salary for baccalaureate-degree educated nurses, this practice was not consistent among facilities.[5]

Table 6

Ranking of Applicant Attributes Based on Education Level of Therapist Supervised (N=77)

Attribute	Rank[a]
Ranking for respondents who had only supervised BEL[b] physical therapists (n=34)	
Clinical experience	1
Personal attributes	2
References	3
Continuing education	4
Entry-level degree	5
Additional degrees	6
Institution	7
Age	8
Ranking for respondents who had supervised both BEL and PBEL[c] physical therapists (n=43)	
Clinical experience	1
Personal attributes	2
References	3
Continuing education	4
Additional degrees	5
Entry-level degree	6
Institution	7
Age	8

[a]1=most important; 8=least important.
[b]Baccalaureate entry level.
[c]Postbaccalaureate entry level.

Table 7

Ranking of Applicant Attributes Based on Entry-Level Education of Respondents (N=77)

Attribute	Rank[a]
Ranking for BEL[b] respondents (n=64)	
Clinical experience	1
Personal attributes	2
References	3
Continuing education	4
Entry-level degree	5
Additional degrees	6
Institution	7
Age	8
Ranking for PBEL[c] respondents (n=3)	
Clinical experience	1
Entry-level degree	2
Additional degrees	3
Personal attributes	4
Continuing education	5
References	6
Institution	7
Age	8
Ranking for certificate respondents (n=10)	
Personal attributes	1
Clinical experience	2
References	3
Entry-level degree	4
Continuing education	5
Additional degrees	6
Institution	7
Age	8

[a]1=most important; 8=least important.
[b]Baccalaureate entry level.
[c]Postbaccalaureate entry level.

Figure 1

Chi-square analysis comparing responses to the paired question: Please indicate the average number of patients seen daily by a baccalaureate entry-level and/or postbaccalaureate entry-level physical therapist by the end of the first year of employment.

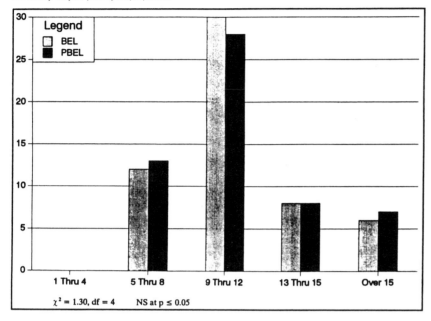

$\chi^2 = 1.30$, df = 4   NS at $p \leq 0.05$

Figure 2

Chi-square analysis comparing responses to the paired question: Which of the following responsibilities would a baccalaureate entry-level and/or a postbaccalaureate entry-level physical therapist be expected to perform by the end of the first year of employment?

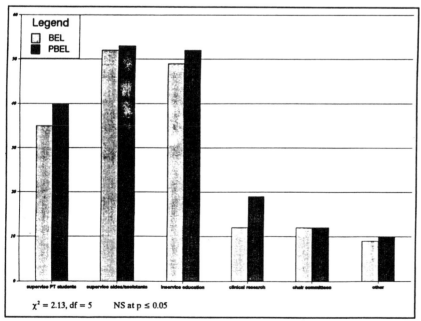

$\chi^2 = 2.13$, df = 5   NS at $p \leq 0.05$

Table 8

Comparison of Baccalaureate Entry-Level and Post-baccalaureate Entry-Level Physical Therapy Graduates at Any Time During Employment (N=56)

| | Respondents (%) | |
Factor	Yes	No
Salary differences	16	84
Advancement differences	8	92
Benefits differences	0	100

When we collated responses to the question concerning the ranking of employee attributes as a function of the entry-level degree of the respondent (Tab. 7), we found great similarity in the rankings provided by BEL and certificate graduates. The list generated by the PBEL graduates, however, put greater weight on the entry-level degree and additional degrees as applicant attributes to be considered when hiring a physical therapist. It would be interesting to explore this ranking scheme further to determine whether PBEL graduates are biased towards hiring other PBEL graduates or therapists with additional degrees. The small number of respondents in our sample who graduated from PBEL programs also might have influenced our results.

In reviewing the data of our study, we considered possible reasons for the results we obtained and implications concerning the lack of differences in physical therapy employment practices when BEL and PBEL graduates were compared. We believe that economics is a factor in employment practices. The national shortage of physical therapists[16] may lead employers to hire a qualified therapist without regard for entry-level degree. Because physical therapy accreditation standards do not differentiate between BEL and PBEL graduates,[15] prospective employers also may not distinguish between the two academic levels in the hiring process.[8] Another factor that may affect employer perceptions is the proliferation of program configurations among both BEL and PBEL physical therapy programs. Baccalaureate programs range in length from 4 to 6 years, while PBEL programs range in length from 4 years 3 months to 7 years, including both preprofessional and professional education.[19] Under these circumstances, it is difficult for employers to understand what the differences would be between the two types of graduates.

The results of our study should be considered within the context of its limitations. One limitation is that we used a sample of convenience. We knew that all of the respondents

Figure 3

Chi-square analysis comparing responses to the paired question: Please indicate the starting salary range for a baccalaureate entry-level and/or a postbaccalaureate entry-level physical therapist at your facility at the time of first employment.

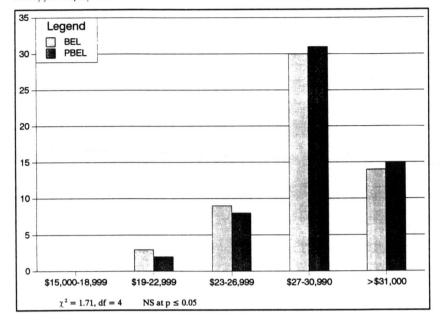

$\chi^2 = 1.71$, df = 4   NS at $p \leq 0.05$

Figure 4

Chi-square analysis comparing responses to the paired question: Please indicate money allocated to a baccalaureate entry-level and/or a postbaccalaureate entry-level physical therapist at your facility for continuing education at the time of first employment.

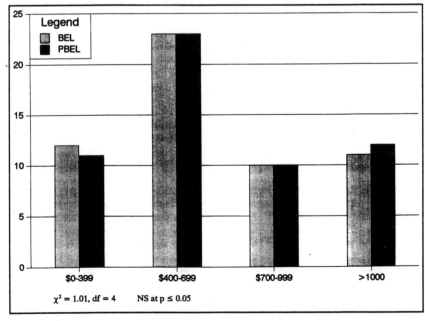

$\chi^2 = 1.01$, df = 4   NS at $p \leq 0.05$

had accepted BEL students because we chose our sample from our university's clinical affiliation sites. A sample where respondents had more exposure to PBEL students might have influenced the outcomes of this study. The majority (83%) of the questionnaire respondents also were BEL graduates. Including more supervisors who were PBEL graduates may have influenced this study's outcomes. The fact that the majority of our respondents were from the northeast may have influenced the results of our study, but the questionnaire responses from directors outside that geographical area did not differ noticeably from those of the directors located in the northeastern states.

Another limitation involves the survey instrument used to collect data. As previously noted, the questionnaire used in this study was self-designed. It was, however, pilot tested with a limited sample, and concerns about the instrument's validity were addressed by a person knowledgeable in survey research design.

Based on the results of this study, physical therapists may want to discuss whether there should be any differences in employer policies or perceptions regarding BEL and PBEL physical therapists. If we as a profession think that differences should exist, then we need to be more articulate about our educational process. We also need to consider the economic realities surrounding the shortage of qualified physical therapists and the monetary incentives for employers to hire a qualified therapist regardless of degree level. Conversely, we may take the position that a graduate of an accredited physical therapy entry-level program is qualified to practice irrespective of the degree granted.

CONCLUSION

The results of this study would indicate that graduates of BEL and PBEL physical therapy programs are treated equally in the employment setting with regard to the variables studied. A future study with a larger representation of PBEL graduates should explore the possible hiring bias of PBEL supervisors with regard to entry-level and advanced degrees.

ACKNOWLEDGMENT

The authors thank John Allen, PhD, for his assistance in questionnaire preparation.

REFERENCES

1. Freeman RB. *The Market for College-Trained Manpower.* Cambridge, Mass: Harvard University Press; 1971.
2. Lowry LW. Is a baccalaureate in nursing worth it? *Nursing Econ.* 1992;10(1):46–52.

Figure 5

Chi-square analysis comparing responses to the paired question: Are the following intradepartmental advances available to a baccalaureate entry-level and/or a postbaccalaureate entry-level physical therapist in your facility at any time in his or her career?

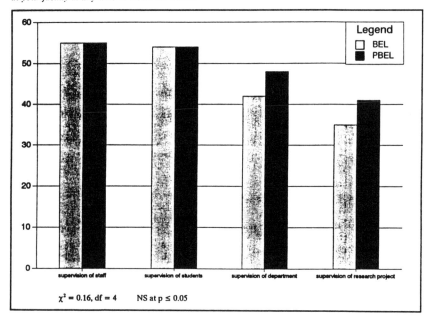

$\chi^2 = 0.16$, df = 4   NS at p $\leq$ 0.05

3. Matilla JP. Determinants of male school enrollments: a time series analysis. *Rev. Econ and Stats.* 1982:64:242–251.

4. American Association of Colleges of Nursing. The economic investment in nursing education: student, institutional and clinical perspectives. Washington, DC: American Association of Colleges of Nursing: 1989.

5. Link CR. What does a BS degree buy? An economist's point of view. *Am J Nurs.* 1987:87(12):1621–1627.

6. DeGroot HA, Forsey L, Cleland VS. The nursing practice personnel data set: implications for professional practice systems. *J Nurs Admin.* 1992:22(3):23–28.

7. Koerner JG, Bunkers LB, Nelson B, et al. Implementing differentiated practice: the Sioux Valley Hospital experience. *J Nurs Admin.* 1989:19(2):13–20.

8. Kuponis P. Free for all: set up three years of PT school for a BS, add three years, clinical exposure for DPT. *PT Bulletin.* 1992: December 2:9.

9. American Physical Therapy Association. *Physical Therapy Education Programs.* Alexandria, Va: Department of Education, American Physical Therapy Association: 1992.

10. American Physical Therapy Association. *Academic Administrator's Survey: Transition to Postbaccalaureate Degree Entry Level.* Alexandria, VA: Department of Education, American Physical Therapy Association: 1991.

11. American Physical Therapy Association. *Position Paper. House of Delegates Handbook.* Washington, DC: American Physical Therapy Association: 1979.

12. American Physical Therapy Association. *Raising Entry Level Education for Physical Therapists.* Washington, DC: Department of Education, American Physical Therapy Association: 1981.

13. American Physical Therapy Association. *A Future in Physical Therapy.* Alexandria, Va: American Physical Therapy Association: 1991.

14. Matthews J. Preparation for the twenty-first century: the educational challenge. *Phys Ther.* 1989:69:981–986.

15. Commission on Accreditation in Physical Therapy Education. *Evaluative Criteria for Accreditation of Educational Programs for the Preparation of Physical Therapists.* Alexandria, Va: American Physical Therapy Association: 1990.

16. American Society of Allied Health Professions. AHA survey of human resources. *Trends.* November 1991:4.

17. MacKinnon J. Review of the post baccalaureate degree for professional entry into physical therapy. *Phys Ther.* 1984:64:938–942.

18. Spurr S. *Academic Degree Structures: Innovative Approaches.* New York, NY: McGraw Hill: 1970.

19. American Physical Therapy Association. *Physical Therapy Education.* Alexandria, VA: Department of Education, American Physical Therapy Association: 1991.

What Consumers Say About Physical Therapy Program Graduates

Mary Ann Dettmann, MS, PT
Diane S Slaughter, MS, PT, SCS, ATC
Richard H Jensen, PhD, PT

ABSTRACT: *Patients' perceptions of physical therapists were studied in southeastern Wisconsin. Five hundred seventy patients were surveyed who were receiving physical therapy services in one of 22 facilities (hospitals, nursing homes, outpatient centers, sports clinics, and rehabilitation services). Over 95% of patients reported having a positive opinion about their physical therapist. No statistical difference existed between patients' opinions about graduates of one program and patients' opinions about all therapists in the geographical area. Opinions about physical therapists did not differ based on therapists' years of experience. Accreditation bodies and promoters of educational accountability are encouraging educational institutions to assess and use patient opinion as a source of feedback on graduates.*

INTRODUCTION

Assessment, educational outcomes, and quality assurance are terms commonly used when discussing measurement of the results of the teaching and learning process.[1,2] The US Department of Education requires information about learning outcomes from the institutions and programs it reviews.[2] From kindergarten through graduate school, institutions, administrators, and teachers measure student performance.

The Commission on Accreditation in Physical Therapy Education (CAPTE) sets standards for assessing and evaluating physical therapy education programs.[3] The CAPTE self-study guide provides specific recommendations for educational institutions to use in evaluating graduate performance. Section 4.0 in the self-study guide states, "Evidence which supports compliance may include surveys of program graduates, surveys of clinical faculty, and information received from employers and patients or clients of program graduates."[3] Graduate performance is described in three categories: patient care, the physical therapy delivery system, and the health care system and society.

Many physical therapy curricula collect data on the opinions of clinical faculty, employers, and program graduates regarding student performance.[4] Because patient feedback is included in the accreditation standards, we decided to explore that feedback. Literature reporting direct patient feedback on program graduates is sparse. Although patient feedback may not be as relevant as assessment by employers or peers, it is an available resource to consider.[5] Patient opinion may be valuable in assessing specific consumer-centered criteria such as "feeling safe" and "receiving quality care."

The purpose of this study was to assess patients' opinions of physical therapist performance in southeastern Wisconsin. Issues addressed included patients' opinions of whether the therapist shared information with the patient about treatment goals; whether the therapist used good interpersonal skills, managed time well, was able to teach, and seemed to enjoy his or her work; and whether the patient felt safe during therapy. A secondary purpose was to compare patients' opinions about the performance of graduates from Marquette University with opinions about the performance of physical therapists in general within the same geographic area.

METHOD

A questionnaire survey was developed based on information provided in the CAPTE Standards and Criteria for Physical Therapy Educational Programs. Section 4.1.1 of the Accreditation Guidelines regarding patient care asks whether program graduates practice in an ethical, legal, safe, caring, and effective manner.[3] Survey questions asked patients whether they believed that their therapist was caring and ethical and whether they felt safe and comfortable during treatment. In addition, based on material in sections 4.2 and 4.3, patients were asked about their therapist's communication, time management, evaluation skills, goal setting, treatment-plan modification, and ability to teach.

A pilot survey was conducted with patients at two local facilities. Forty patients were interviewed using the survey to assess question clarity. Based on this pilot survey, the questions were refined, and a 1-page, 13-question survey was constructed. Patients were asked to indicate in what type of physical therapy facility they were receiving care (eg, outpatient clinic, nursing home) and how many physical therapy treatments they had received. In the first seven questions, respondents rated specific qualities about their therapist. Responses were made on a scale from "strongly agree" to "strongly disagree" (Table 1). The remaining six questions about therapist attitudes and behaviors were of the fixed-answer, yes-or-no format (Table 2). Space was provided at the end for patient comments.

Construct and content validity were considered when developing this survey and the subsequent study. The basic premise in designing the survey was to ascertain patients' opinions about their therapist. To obtain construct validity, we designed a tool that would allow consumers to express their opinions about their therapist. We selected qualities that an effective therapist should demonstrate, such as ability to use good communication skills and to create a safe and comfortable environment. We asked consumers to rate their therapist on these qualities. The qualities we selected closely paralleled those qualities suggested in the accreditation self-study (Tables 1, 2). Survey questions contained terminology similar to that used in the self-study, which supported content validity.

All physical therapy services listed in the telephone company yellow pages in the greater Milwaukee area were asked to participate in the study (N=49). Twenty-two sites (45%)

Ms Dettmann is Associate Professor, Program in Physical Therapy, Marquette University, Milwaukee, WI 53233. Ms Slaughter is Administrative Assistant, Program in Physical Therapy, Marquette University. Dr Jensen is Director, Program in Physical Therapy, Marquette University. Address correspondence to Ms Slaughter.

Reprinted with permission from the *Journal of Physical Therapy Education*, Vol 9, No 1, pp 7-9, 1995.

Table 1

Frequency of Patient Responses to Questionnaire Items (N=570)

Item	Rank[a]					
	1	2	3	4	5	NA
My physical therapist (PT) seems interested in me as a person.	356	160	15	3	1	35
I find it easy to talk with my PT.	386	140	10	3	2	29
My PT is a good listener.	374	146	18	3	1	28
My PT seems to enjoy his or her work.	396	129	15	0	1	29
My PT is able to manage time well.	351	162	19	3	1	34
My PT seems ethical.	356	153	20	1	0	40
My PT is able to teach me and my family about my condition.	328	159	31	2	2	48

[a]1=strongly agree; 2=agree; 3=no opinion; 4=disagree; 5=strongly disagree; NA=don't know or not applicable.

Table 2

Frequency of Patient Responses to Yes/No Questionnaire Items (N=570)

Item	Rank[a]		
	1	2	NA
My therapist evaluated my problem the first time I came in.	476	23	71
My therapist set up treatment goals that I understood.	503	21	46
My therapist explained the goals of therapy to me.	497	27	46
My therapist changed my treatment if needed as my condition changed or stayed the same.	446	21	103
I feel safe and comfortable during treatment.	527	6	37
My therapist communicates well with my physician and with others.	382	11	177

[a]1=yes; 2=no; NA=not applicable.

agreed to participate and were sent copies of the one-page survey, a cover letter, and a return envelope for each patient. During a 1-week period, each patient who was capable of completing the form (with or without assistance) was given the cover letter, survey, and envelope. The person distributing the survey indicated on the survey whether the patient was being treated by a Marquette University graduate and indicated the therapist's number of years of experience. The cover letter explained that the survey was part of a curriculum evaluation, that the information would be confidential, and that responses would not affect patients' treatment or the therapist providing treatment. Patients placed the completed survey in the envelope, sealed it, and returned it to the person who had distributed the survey.

At the end of the week, the physical therapy departments returned the sealed surveys to Marquette University in plain envelopes. Efforts were made to ensure confidentiality to both the site and the patient. Results were tabulated, and statistical analyses were performed.

RESULTS

Five hundred seventy completed surveys were returned. The frequency by location of patients who responded is reported in the Figure. The mean number of years of physical therapists' experience was 9.1 (range=1–36). Marquette University graduates had treated 341 (60%) of the respondents. Sixty-six percent of respondents indicated that their primary diagnosis was an orthopedic or spinal condition; other conditions were neurologic (10%), arthritic (3%), cardiac (3%), pediatric (3%), and unknown or unable to classify (15%). More than 30% of respondents had already experienced 20 or more physical therapy visits, with most experiencing 8 to 12 treatments.

Responses to the 13 questions were overwhelmingly positive (Tables 1, 2). More than 95% of respondents answered "strongly agree" or "agree" to the first seven questions and answered "yes" to the six remaining questions.

Several 2x2 and 2x3 chi-square analyses were completed to compare patients' ratings. No difference existed between patients' opinions of Marquette-educated physical therapists and their opinions of graduates from other curricula. Significant differences existed in sample sites and populations. There were significantly more Marquette graduates practicing in nursing homes than other graduates and fewer Marquette graduates employed in sports clinics ($P<.001$). Graduates with 16 or more years of experience were predominantly from Marquette ($P<.001$).

Many patients did not respond to the item, "My therapist communicates well with my physician and other persons providing care for me." Although the majority of respondents answered "yes" to the question, 177 respondents indicated "don't know or not applicable." Therapists may not always inform patients about interaction with other members of the health care team.

Eighty-five patients wrote comments on the survey, and 82 of these comments were complimentary. Frequently made comments included "I enjoyed therapy" and "my therapist is [very] good." Almost 50% of comments related to therapists' affective characteristics (eg, friendly, caring, warm, and personable). Twenty-one comments (25%) were in the cognitive or psychomotor domain, addressing therapists' skill and knowledge. The remaining comments addressed a combination of the therapist's affective, cognitive, and psychomotor skills.

DISCUSSION

The results indicate that consumers in southeastern Wisconsin are pleased with their physical therapists. Consumers indicated that they were comfortable with their therapists, valued the service provided, and felt safe and comfortable during treatment.

The 22 sites that responded to the survey represent nearly half of the sites where physical therapy is provided in this area. We would have preferred that more facilities and more patients participated in the study. Several individuals responded that the week we selected was too busy (eg, staff shortages). Other facilities refused to participate without comment, perhaps because of concerns about current patient attitudes or staffing problems.

The person distributing the survey at each facility may have influenced the results. That person was asked to determine patients' ability to complete the survey; all patients capable of completing the questionnaire were asked to participate. The person may have become a "gatekeeper" and may have given the survey only to "satisfied" consumers.

Another possible problem with this type of survey is that some dissatisfied persons may have chosen not to participate. The favorable responses from 570 patients, however, allowed us to conclude that patients in southeastern Wisconsin are pleased with their physical therapists.

Consumer feedback may be helpful to educational institutions and is suggested as

Figure

Treatment locations of patients listed by frequency and percentage (N=570).

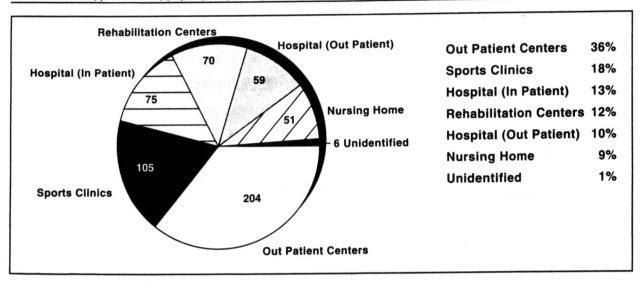

Out Patient Centers	**36%**
Sports Clinics	**18%**
Hospital (In Patient)	**13%**
Rehabilitation Centers	**12%**
Hospital (Out Patient)	**10%**
Nursing Home	**9%**
Unidentified	**1%**

one assessment option by the CAPTE. Patient opinion can be included with other evaluations of graduate performance made by employers, clinical instructors, and the graduates themselves. Institutions should establish a baseline of patient opinion about the physical therapy care provided by program graduates. Assessments of future graduates then can be compared with this norm.

The instrument we designed provides educational institutions with a tool to obtain consumer opinion and adds to the literature available. This type of study can quickly and inexpensively provide information to CAPTE about the value and necessity of consumer feedback. Patient opinion may not be a definitive determinant of quality, but it may be the best available measure of comfort and satisfaction.

Future studies could assess consumer opinion of other therapist qualities. Predictive validity and reliability also could be tested by comparing the results of this study with assessments of consumer opinion of other program graduates using this tool.

Accreditation, educational accountability, and curriculum assessment are three reasons to seek patients' opinions. Brimer[6] reported that the success of any practice is influenced by the physical therapist's ability to keep patients satisfied. As the health care dollar is scrutinized, public opinion about health care providers and their services may determine whether those services are continued.

ACKNOWLEDGMENTS

We thank the patients and staff of all of the facilities that participated for their time and efforts and Dr Guy Simoneau for his help with the statistical analysis.

REFERENCES

1. Langsley D. Medical competence and performance assessment. *JAMA*. 1991:266:977–980.
2. Hutchings P, Marchese T. Watching assessment: questions, studies, prospects. *Change*. September/October 1990:13–38.
3. *Standards and Criteria for PT Educational Programs*. Alexandria, Va: Commission of Accreditation in Physical Therapy Education; American Physical Therapy Association; March 1992.
4. Perry JF, Lee CE. Model for curriculum evaluation. *Journal of Physical Therapy Education*. 1988:2:13–17.
5. Breaden DG. Markers and indicators of physical performance and fitness: an overview. *Federal Bulletin*. 1988:75:67–73.
6. Brimer MA. In the patient's shoes. *Clinical Management*. 1991:8(5):11–13.

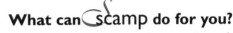

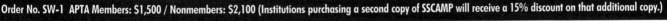